Mosby's Basic Science

FOR

SOFT TISSUE

AND

MOVEMENT THERAPIES

Mosby's Basic Science
FOR
SOFT TISSUE
AND
MOVEMENT THERAPIES

SANDY FRITZ, BS
Founder, Owner, Director, and Head Instructor
Health Enrichment Center
School of Therapeutic Massage and Bodywork
Lapeer, Michigan

KATHLEEN MAISON PAHOLSKY, MS, PhD
Director of Education
Health Enrichment Center
School of Therapeutic Massage and Bodywork
Lapeer, Michigan

M. JAMES GROSENBACH, EdD
Clinical Psychologist
Administrative Director
Health Enrichment Center
School of Therapeutic Massage and Bodywork
Lapeer, Michigan

with 665 illustrations and photos

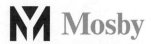

St. Louis   Baltimore   Boston   Carlsbad   Chicago   Minneapolis   New York   Philadelphia   Portland
London   Milan   Sydney   Tokyo   Toronto

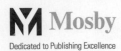
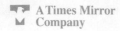

Publisher: John Schrefer
Executive Editor: Martha Sasser
Senior Developmental Editor: Amy Christopher
Project Manager: Linda McKinley
Production Editor: Jennifer Furey
Designer: Renée Duenow
Manufacturing: Debbie LaRocca
Original illustrations by: Graphic World
Cover illustration by: Jim Carroll

Composition by Top Graphics
Printing/binding by World Color Book Group

Mosby, Inc.
11830 Westline Industrial Drive
St. Louis, MO 63146

Library of Congress Cataloging-in-Publication Data

Fritz, Sandy.
    Mosby's basic science for soft tissue and movement therapies /
Sandy Fritz, Kathleen Maison Paholsky, M. James Grosenbach.
      p.   cm.
    Includes bibliographical references and index.
    ISBN 0-323-00284-6
    1. Human physiology.   2. Human anatomy.   3. Pathology.   4. Human locomotion.
5. Movement therapy.   6. Physical therapy.
I. Paholsky, Kathleen Maison.   II. Grosenbach, M. James.
III. Title.
    [DNLM: 1. Musculoskeletal Physiology. 2. Musculoskeletal System—anatomy & histology.
3. Movement. 4. Holistic Health. WE 102 F919m 1998]
QP34.5.F75 1998
612—dc21
DNLM/DLC
for Library of Congress
                                             98-14479
                                              CIP

98 99 01 02 03 / 9 8 7 6 5 4 3 2 1

To all of those who read and read and read.

And to the Health Enrichment Center
School of Therapeutic Massage and Bodywork's graduating class of 1998
—for being guinea pigs.

Foreword

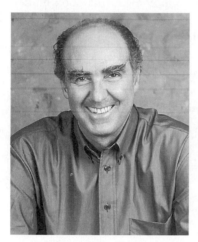

In order to be able to treat pain and dysfunction, utilizing manual methods, it is an essential prerequisite that therapists should have a sound understanding of the territory on, and with which, they are working. There is an absolute requirement for an intimate familiarity with structural patterns, attachments and functions of the muscles, ligaments, tendons, fascia and joints being treated, as well as with the bodily systems they support and which service them.

It is obvious that it is not necessary to understand the intimate workings of an automobile in order to drive one, however there would be little confidence in a auto mechanic who did not fully understand the construction and functioning of the motor he or she was attempting to repair. Where human health and well-being are concerned it is clear that many individuals understand their own body workings as imperfectly as do many drivers their cars. The therapist, however, must have a sufficient degree of knowledge in order to ensure safety and efficacy in what is being offered therapeutically.

What Sandy Fritz, Kathy Paholsky, and Jim Grosenbach have achieved in this landmark text is to set out all the ingredients required for an entry to intermediate level student to experience the wonderful adventure which exploration of the inter-related systems and subsystems of the body represents. They have managed to make this material come alive, to lift it out of the mere presentation of facts, without compromising on the scientific and academic requirements of such a text. They have also done something quite remarkable in producing the information in an easily accessible manner while at the same time encouraging a personal growth experience as the reader is challenged to relate what is being discussed to themselves and their own experience.

It is one thing to present information and quite another to do so and to ask the reader to explore both the topic and its relationship to health and disease as well as to their own belief systems, health status and understanding of how the body works. From such challenges, which are peppered throughout the book, only one result can be anticipated of anyone who diligently works their way through the systematic unfolding of this anatomy and physiology exploration — a sound understanding of how the body works, where the constituent parts are to be found and how they interact in health and disease. With this knowledge and the tools which are available to the skilled modern soft tissue or movement therapist, the future of these emerging professions will become far more assured.

This is a most important time for these professions, as realisation of their value becomes established via research and as national standards are evaluated and improved. As the soft tissue and movement professions encroach on territory which other professions hold to be their own, it is vital for training standards to be enhanced, reinforced and constantly upgraded so that critics and potentially hostile professional organisations are denied the ammunition which weak standards offer.

The existence of this text, following on from the superb *Mosby's Fundamentals of Therapeutic Massage* is precisely the ammunition needed to counter any attempt at denigration of these modalities as such. There remain major tasks in the arena of educational and personal and professional growth; however, this book makes such effort far less arduous. Mosby and the authors are to be congratulated on the effort that has gone into the writing and production of this important text.

Leon Chaitow ND, DO
Senior Lecturer
University of Westminster, London

Preface

Mosby's Basic Science for Soft Tissue and Movement Therapies presents the science basics—anatomy, physiology, and pathology, with clinical application—to a specific population—future soft tissue and movement professionals. This population views the body in a holistic manner. Because philosophy and practices from ancient healing wisdom often form the basis for bodywork modalities, an introduction to the common thread of ancient healing wisdom is carried through the text. This wisdom is related directly to body structure and function and does not represent any particular spiritual discipline.

Two themes are woven through this text:

1. Dynamic balance or homeostasis
2. Analysis and reasoning that honors both the scientific model of cause and effect and the larger picture of intuition, possibilities, and the feelings of the people involved

This textbook presents the objective facts and information base about human beings as they currently exist. Information is not static, but dynamic and like life, every changing. Teachers and students are encouraged to question and explore the information to make it their own. The information was selected to best serve the beginning and intermediate student of soft tissue and movement modalities. Decisions were made as to what to include based on the authors' experiences of many years of training entry- and intermediate-level bodywork students, and several expert reviewers who analyzed the original manuscript content.

This book has been developed to serve two roles. It can be used as follows:

1. As a complete basic science textbook/workbook combination—This book can stand alone without the use of additional support materials for the muscles/skeletal system and other key topics.

or

2. As a companion text to a more general anatomy and physiology book—As a companion, this text will guide the learning and application of the material specifically for the bodywork student.

The format of this text has been designed to address various learning styles. In addition, throughout the text are activities that assist the student in transferring new information from short-term to long-term memory and developing clinical reasoning skills. These activities do not have only one correct answer. Instead they are designed for the student to use what is familiar from past experience as a vehicle to transport the new or unfamiliar information to a level of understanding through a gentle and effective learning process. This enhances the student's ability to utilize creative problem-solving skills. Because there is seldom only one correct way to do anything, developing a process to determine the most effective decision at the time is important. This more gray approach, while more like the body, professional practice, and life, is not the familiar black/white textbook format. This may seem uncomfortable for some at first. An example is often provided to give the student direction.

<u>Understanding is the learning goal of this text.</u> Memorization is not the goal. Instead, the activities identify the fundamental material and ask the student to manipulate it in a personal way to enhance the learning process. The bulk of the text is designed as reference material. The workbook section at the end of each chapter can act as a self-evaluation if desired, or as a reinforcement of the information presented. The answers to these sections are provided at the end of each chapter.

A conversational tone has been used whenever possible, and supported by metaphors and practical applications. Indications and contraindications for clinical practice have also been included. The word *indications* in the context of this book is defined as when treatment is appropriate and beneficial. The word *contraindications* encompasses both avoidance and cautions for the application of treatment. The result is a user-friendly text that relates to daily professional life.

The workbook exercises and activities presented do not represent any specific curriculum design or learning mode other than to address various learning styles. Instead, an attempt has been made to be as generic and as inclusive as possible to allow the instructor and student to individualize the application of the material.

The linear flow of the text begins with a section that includes the fundamentals and a big picture look at the body, health, disease, terminology, and a clinical reasoning model.

The second section presents the mechanisms of physiologic function and control by the nervous system and endocrine system. This is a major deviation from traditional presentations and is presented based on 15 years of teaching experience indicating that if the systems of control are understood first, then it is much easier to understand the rest of the body's anatomy and physiology.

Section Three represents the core portion of the text from a movement science perspective, and the learning includes the musculoskeletal system, kinesiology, and biomechanics. Should this information flow seem out of order, the instructor may decide to simply switch the presentation of Sections Two and Three.

The last section briefly covers the remainder of the body systems, including the integumentary, cardiovascular, lymphatic, and immune systems, as well as the digestive, respiratory, urinary, and reproductive systems. Only the information most applicable to the soft tissue and movement student is presented.

Each chapter in the book contains key terms with definitions and chapter objectives.

A more detailed glossary appears at the end of the book for quick reference. Of course, there is no single correct way to use this book. The sections do not need to be presented in any specific order; however, Chapter One does set the stage for learning. The activities, exercises, and workbook sections can all be used at your discretion.

It is our greatest hope that the material in this book will come alive with the careful guidance of a skilled teacher and with the patient commitment of a dedicated student.

This text is designed for a 500 to 1500 hour curriculum (approximately 15 to 30 credits). A more generalized approach will need to be taken with the shorter curriculums, while additional class time will allow for a more in-depth integration process. Since the text is student-friendly and self-directed, much of the work can be assigned in a self-study format.

This text is written by teachers seeking a more efficient and gentle way to help students understand and use this information. Credit and appreciation is given to the authors of the reference texts consulted in the development of this textbook. Without their efforts, this book never could have been written. Special thanks also goes to those who reviewed the manuscript. Their dedicated attention added to the quality of this text.

Have fun with the book.

Sandy Fritz
Kathleen Maison Paholsky
M. James Grosenbach

Contents

Mosby's Basic Science
FOR
SOFT TISSUE
AND
MOVEMENT THERAPIES

Section One

Fundamentals

CHAPTER 1 THE BODY AS A WHOLE

CHAPTER 2 MECHANISMS OF HEALTH AND DISEASE

CHAPTER 3 MEDICAL TERMINOLOGY

Section One lays the foundation in the study of functional anatomy and physiology that the soft tissue and movement professional must have. The study begins in Chapter 1 with the big picture—a look at the body as a whole. This chapter explores functional balance and the body's ability to maintain a relatively constant internal environment, regardless of external influences. Chapter 2 discusses mechanisms of health and disease. Stress, a primary factor in imbalances in the body, is highlighted, because stress management is a major benefit of soft tissue and movement therapies.

The ability to speak the language of another is essential for effective communication. In Chapter 3, the student will study Western-based scientific language and will be introduced to the language of systems based on ancient healing wisdom.

The first major theme of this text is understanding self-regulating mechanisms, which allow the body to maintain homeostasis, or dynamic balance.

The second major theme is using clinical reasoning, which enables the student to apply the information learned to the therapeutic setting. Without the ability to reason clinically and to problem solve, information becomes little more than a collection of facts.

The journey begins.

ACTIVITY

Identify three personal goals that will motivate you during the study of anatomy and physiology. An example is provided to get you started.

Example: I will learn about my body so that I can age well and remain vital into my elder years.

Your Turn

1. _____

2. _____

3. _____

Chapter 1

The Body As a Whole

CHAPTER OUTLINE

CHAPTER OBJECTIVES

After completing this chapter, the student should be able to perform the following:

- Define the terms *anatomy* and *physiology*.
- Explain the importance of understanding the relationship of the structure and function of the body as a whole.
- Compare the yin/yang theory to anatomy and physiology.
- Define the characteristics of life.
- List and discuss the body's levels of organization.

KEY TERMS

Adenosine triphosphate (ATP) (ah-DEN-o-seen tri-FOS-fate) A compound that stores energy in the muscles. When ATP is broken down during catabolic reactions, it releases energy.

Anabolism (ah-NAB-o-lizm) Chemical processes in the body that join simple compounds to form more complex compounds of carbohydrates, lipids, proteins, and nucleic acids. The processes require energy supplied from adenosine triphosphate (ATP).

Anatomy (an-NAT-o-mee) The study of the body's structures and the relationship of its parts.

Atom The smallest particle of an element that retains and exhibits the properties of that element. Atoms are made up of protons, neutrons, and electrons.

Atrophy (AT-ro-fee) A decrease in the size of a body part or organ caused by a decrease in the size of the cells.

Basement membrane A permeable membrane that attaches epithelial tissues to the underlying connective tissues.

Carbohydrates (kar-bo-HY-drates) Sugars, starches, and cellulose composed of carbon, hydrogen, and oxygen.

Cardiac muscle fibers Smaller, striated, involuntary muscle fibers (cells) in the heart that pump blood.

Catabolism (kah-TAB-o-lizm) Chemical processes in the body that release energy as complex compounds are broken down into simpler ones.

Cell The basic structural unit of a living organism. A cell contains a nucleus and cytoplasm and is surrounded by a membrane.

Collagen (KOL-ah-jen) A protein substance composed of small fibrils that combine to create the connective tissue of fascia, tendons, and ligaments. When combined with water, it forms gelatin. Collagen constitutes approximately one fourth of the protein in the body.

Collagenous fibers Strong fibers with little capacity for stretch. They have a high degree of tensile strength, which allows them to withstand longitudinal stress.

Connective tissue The most abundant type of tissue in the body, connective tissue supports and holds together the body and its parts, protects the body from foreign matter, and is organized to transport substances throughout the body.

Elastic fibers Connective tissue fibers that are extensible and elastic. They are made of a protein called elastin, which returns to its original length after being stretched.

Epithelial (ep-i-THEE-lee-al) *tissues* A specialized group of tissues that cover and protect the surface of the body and its parts, line body cavities, and form glands. Epithelial tissue usually is found in areas that move substances into and out of the body during secretion, absorption, and excretion.

Gross anatomy The study of body structures visible to the naked eye.

Homeostasis (ho-me-o-STA-sis) The relatively constant state of the body's internal environment, which is maintained by adaptive responses.

Hypertrophy (hye-PER-tro-fee) An increase in the size of a cell, which results in an increase in the size of a body part or organ.

Interphase (IN-ter-faze) The period during which a cell grows and carries on its activities.

Lipids (LIP-ids) Fats and oils.

Matrix (MAY-triks) The basic substance between the cells of a tissue. Matrix is composed of amorphous ground substance consisting of molecules that expand when water molecules and electrolytes bind to them. As much as 90% of connective tissue is ground substance. Fibers make up the other component of matrix.

Meiosis (my-O-sis) A type of cell division in which a cell divides its chromosomes in half, forming two reproductive cells.

Membrane A thin, sheetlike layer of tissue that covers a cell, an organ, or some other structure; that lines a tube or a cavity; or that divides or separates one part from another.

Metabolism (me-TAB-o-lizm) Chemical processes in the body that convert food and air into energy to support growth, distribution of nutrients, and elimination of waste.

Mitosis (my-TOE-sis) The period of cell division in which the cell reproduces its DNA and divides into two identical daughter cells.

Molecule (MOL-e-kyool) A combination of two or more atoms. A molecule is the smallest portion of a substance that can exist separately without losing the physical and chemical properties of that substance.

Muscle tissue A specialized form of tissue that contracts and shortens to provide movement, maintain posture, and produce heat.

Nervous tissue A specialized tissue that coordinates and regulates body activity. It can develop more excitability and conductivity than other types of tissue.

Nucleic acids The two types of nucleic acid are deoxyribonucleic acid (DNA) and ribonucleic acid (RNA).

Organelles (or-gan-NELLS) The basic components of a cell that perform specific functions within the cell.

Physiology (fiz-ee-OL-o-jee) The study of the processes and functions of the body involved in supporting life.

Proteins (PRO-teens) Substances formed from amino acids.

Regional anatomy The study of the structures of a particular area of the body.

Reticular fibers Delicate, connective tissue fibers that occur in networks and support small structures such as capillaries, nerve fibers, and the basement membrane. Reticular fibers are made of a specialized type of collagen called reticulin.

Skeletal muscle fibers Large, cross-striated cells that are connected to the skeleton and under voluntary control of the nervous system.

Smooth muscle fibers Muscle fibers that are neither striated nor voluntary. These muscle cells help regulate blood flow through the cardiovascular system, propel food through the gut, and squeeze secretions from glands.

Surface anatomy The study of internal organs and structures as they can be recognized and related to external features.

Systemic anatomy The study of the structure of a particular body system.

Tissue (TISH-yoo) A group of similar cells combined to perform a common function.

The study of the human body in its structure and function is fascinating. For students of soft tissue and movement therapies, the body is the territory of our work. This text provides a map of our territory. A map is a representation of an object, but the map is not the object, any more than this textbook is your body. Our goal is to offer information on which to make decisions as you work with each person you touch. As practitioners, the more familiar we are with the body and its functions, the better able we are to provide the methods used to relax, encourage, and nurture clients with the therapeutic approaches of soft tissue and movement treatments. This first chapter provides information about the body as a whole. Because bodywork professionals deal with the wholeness of each client they serve, this seems to be the best place to begin.

Anatomy and Physiology

Anatomy and physiology are two very distinct yet interrelated biologic studies that combine to present the body's operation as a whole organism. Anatomy is the scientific study of the structures of the body and the relationship of its parts. Physiology is the scientific study of the processes and functions of the body that support life.

The word *anatomy* means "to cut apart." **Anatomy** is a broad field with many subdivisions, each of which is a comprehensive study in itself. The following categories are some of these divisions and subdivisions:

Gross anatomy—The study of body structures large enough to be visible to the naked eye.

Regional anatomy—The study of all the structures of a particular area.

Systemic anatomy—The study of the body divided into its systems.

Surface anatomy—The study of the internal organs and structures as they are recognized from and related to the overlying skin surface.

The term *physiology* is a combination of two Greek words: *physis*, which means "nature," and *logos*, which means "science." **Physiology,** the study of the way the body works, can be divided into two levels:

Organizational (e.g., cellular physiology)
Systemic (e.g., cardiophysiology)

Structure (anatomy) and function (physiology) cannot be separated anymore than a person can be separated into body, mind, or spirit components. Structure and function form a continuum; structure guides function, and function can modify structure.

The concepts of anatomy and physiology are examples of the duality of wholeness, a duality also represented in the yin and yang concept expressed in Eastern terminology. Yin corresponds to structure and yang to function, opposite but complementary qualities.

The idea of wholeness is presented in many cultures and religions as well as in science. Our use of such terminology as yin and yang will be to represent a physiological function, not a spiritual approach (Figure 1-1).

The dual aspects of yin and yang combine to form a whole unit; they are complementary to each other. Yang is said to contain the seed of yin and vice versa. These seeds are represented by the small black and white spots in the yin/yang symbol (see Figure 1-1). Nothing can be totally yin or totally yang (Table 1-1).

The human body and all its functions can be understood through this concept of the relationship of opposites that creates a wholeness. We will use it as one of the main themes throughout this text (Activity 1-1).

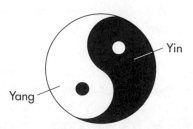

FIGURE 1-1 Yin and yang. (From Fritz S: *Mosby's fundamentals of therapeutic massage,* St Louis, 1995, Mosby.)

✋ PRACTICAL APPLICATION

Students of soft tissue and movement methods must be well versed in gross anatomy. The most effective application of bodywork methods depends on the practitioner's ability to locate, recognize, and understand the structure the hands are manipulating. We must also have a working understanding of both organizational and systemic physiology to understand how and why methods of bodywork are beneficial. Although we touch the anatomy, it is the physiology that produces the benefits of the bodywork. It is not enough to know the location of a muscle; we must also know what the muscle does, the way it functions, and what effects massage or other soft tissue approaches will have on the function of that individual muscle, as well as the effect of the muscle on the whole body. We need to understand how stimulating physiologic changes can influence structure as part of the dynamic process of change that unfolds constantly in our bodies and in our lives as a whole (Activity 1-2).

Characteristics of Life

What constitutes life? No single criterion defines it. Instead, characteristics of life consist of the following:

Maintenance of boundaries—Keeping the internal environment distinct from the external environment

Type—The ability to transport the entire being, as well as internal components

Responsiveness—The ability to sense, monitor, and respond to changes in the external environment

Conductivity—The movement of energy from one point to another

TABLE 1-1 YANG QUALITIES VERSUS YIN QUALITIES

YANG QUALITIES	YIN QUALITIES
Day	Night
Immaterial	Material
Produces energy	Produces form
Hot	Cold
Sun	Moon
Expansion	Contraction
Energy	Matter
Above	Below
Fire	Water
Hollow	Solid
Hard	Soft
Superior	Inferior

ACTIVITY 1-1

Taking no more than 60 seconds, list as many examples as you can of sets of opposites that together reflect wholeness. Two examples are given to get you started.

Example: Black/white
Flexion/extension

Your Turn

ACTIVITY 1-2

Consider this statement:

As the tree is bent, so it grows.
How does the statement reflect the influence of the function on structure?

Your Turn

Growth—A normal increase in size and/or number of cells

Respiration—The absorption, transport, and use or exchange of respiratory gases (oxygen and carbon dioxide)

Digestion—The process by which food products are broken down into simple substances to be used by individual cells

Absorption—The transport and use of nutrients

Secretion—The production and delivery of specialized substances for diverse functions

Excretion—The removal of waste products

Circulation—The movement of fluids, nutrients, secretions, and waste products from one area of the body to another

Reproduction—The formation of a new being; also, the

formation of new cells in the body to permit growth, repair, and replacement

Metabolism—A chemical reaction that occurs in cells to effect transformation, production, or consumption of energy

Each characteristic of life is related to the sum total of all the physical and chemical reactions that occur in the body. It is physiology, or function, that characterizes life.

We can study form (structure) without life, such as in cadaver dissection, but we can study physiology only in terms of living dynamics. This text represents the study of life and the dynamic process of living. Therefore anatomy and physiology are presented together (Activity 1-3).

ACTIVITY 1-3

Reflect on the characteristics of life as a metaphor of your personal life characteristics. Then answer the following:

Your Turn

1. *Maintenance of boundaries.* What are your professional (external) and personal (internal) boundaries?

   _____

   _____

2. *Movement.* How efficient is your movement along life's path?

   _____

   _____

   _____

3. *Responsiveness.* How do you recognize, monitor, and respond to changes in your life?

   _____

   _____

   _____

4. *Conductivity.* What is your explanation for how you make something happen? How do you energize?

   _____

   _____

   _____

5. *Growth.* How would you measure personal and professional growth?

   _____

   _____

6. *Respiration.* How effectively do you breathe?

   _____

   _____

   _____

7. *Digestion.* Describe how you take large, complex concepts and break them into smaller, more understandable pieces.

   _____

   _____

8. *Absorption.* How do you learn? How do you use your learning?

   _____

   _____

   _____

9. *Secretion.* How do you teach? How do you reach a diverse population?

   _____

   _____

   _____

Organization of Body Structure

From the simplest to the most complex, the structures of the body are able to perform their functions in a logical and well-coordinated manner. This organization is one of the vital characteristics of body structure and function.

Patterns of dysfunction also present a logical order of progression in a well-coordinated manner. Disease processes usually begin at the most basic level and, if left uninterrupted, progress to complex, multisystem involvement. On careful assessment, the logic of the progression can be identified. With this information, an intervention process can effectively interrupt the dysfunctional process and move the body toward logical, well-coordinated patterns of health. Our bodies work toward balance, which reflects a logical progression of cause and effect. When we understand the patterns of both effective function and dysfunction, we can create a map to follow for a return to balance and health.

All living and nonliving things are made of the same components. For this reason, a study of anatomy and physiology must begin with an investigation of the basic chemical and physical components.

CHEMICAL LEVEL

Every substance has both chemical and physical properties that give it a unique identity. *Chemical properties* are those that demonstrate the way the substance reacts with other substances or the way it responds to a change in the environment. *Physical properties* are characteristics such as color, taste, texture, and odor.

Atoms and Molecules

An **atom** is a small particle of an element, which is a substance composed of a single kind of atom. Atoms are made up of smaller particles called protons, neutrons, and electrons. Protons, which carry a positive charge (yang), and neutrons, which have a neutral charge, form the nucleus of an atom. They attract electrons, which are negatively charged particles (yin) that travel around the nucleus in specific orbital patterns. The atoms most commonly found in living things are hydrogen, carbon, nitrogen, and oxygen.

Electrons are involved in all chemical reactions that bond atoms to make a **molecule,** a combination of two or more atoms. Molecules can form elements (substances composed of a single type of atom) or compounds (substances made up of different types of atoms). In elements the number of protons in the nucleus of an atom remains the same. This constancy of protons gives the element both its identity and its atomic number. The number of protons and neutrons in the nucleus combine to create the atomic weight. (Because electrons are extremely light, their weight is not a factor.)

The most important structural feature in a chemical reaction is the stability of the outer shell of the atom, where the electrons are located. Shells, or electron shells, are envelopes or layers of electron orbit patterns. An atom can achieve a state of maximal sta-

ACTIVITY 1-3—cont'd

10. *Excretion.* How do you dispose of those aspects of life that no longer serve you?

_____

_____

_____

11. *Circulation.* How do you move physically and mentally in professional relationships?

_____

_____

12. *Reproduction.* How do you maintain, restore, and permit new growth in yourself?

_____

_____

_____

13. *Metabolism.* How do you create your energy and adjust your use of energy in your life?

_____

_____

_____

bility by forming one of three types of bonds (Activity 1-4):

Ionic bond: An atom can gain or lose electrons to fill or empty its outer shell. When this happens, the atom is no longer electrically neutral, because the ratio of protons to electrons is no longer equal. The atom becomes an electrically charged ion with either a negative charge (anion) or a positive charge (cation). Negatively and positively charged ions attract each other to form a stable union.

Covalent bond: When two or more atoms share electrons, a covalent bond is created, the most stable kind of association that atoms can form with one another. This sharing completes the outer shell.

Polar covalent bond: Molecules with polar covalent bonds, called polar molecules, are electrically neutral because they have the same number of protons and electrons. However, the electrons can be arranged in the shells so that one side of the molecule is more negative and the other side more positive. Water is an example of a polar molecule.

ACTIVITY 1-4

Describe a professional, social, or personal relationship that represents the properties of each of the three types of bonds.

Example

Polar covalent bond: A stray cat lives in my barn. The cat feeds with my other barn cats, but I don't think of the cat as part of my family. The weak bond that we have could be broken easily if the cat were drawn to the neighbor's barn and chose to leave.

Your Turn

1. Ionic bond

2. Covalent bond

3. Polar covalent bond

Polar molecules attract each other, with the positive side of one attracting the negative side of a different molecule. These weak polar covalent bonds, sometimes referred to as hydrogen bonds, are abundant in nature. They help create larger molecules such as proteins and DNA.

One or more atoms joined by chemical bonds create a molecule. A molecule is the smallest part of a substance that can exist independently without losing the physical and chemical properties of that substance. If the atoms are of the same type, the result is an element. Atoms of two or more different elements combine to make a compound. The *function* of a molecule is related to its structures. The *structure* of a molecule depends on the patterns of the chemical bonds.

Chemical reactions take place when chemical bonds are broken and new ones are formed. In a chemical reaction, the number of atoms remains the same, but the atoms become linked in a different way, forming a new substance (Figure 1-2).

Metabolism

Metabolism is the word we use to describe all the physiologic processes that take place in our bodies to convert the food we eat and the air we breathe into the energy we need to function. These chemical reactions can be classified into two types:

Catabolism — Chemical reactions that *release* energy as they break down complex compounds

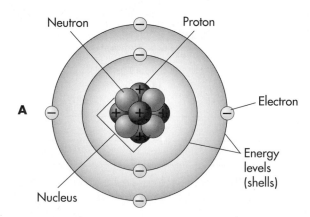

FIGURE 1-2 A, Model of the atom. The nucleus, made up of protons (+) and neutrons, is at the core. Electrons inhabit outer regions called *energy levels.* (**A-C,** From Thibodeau GA, Patton KT: *Structure and function of the body,* ed 10, St Louis, 1997, Mosby. **D,** From Thibodeau GA, Patton KT: *Anatomy and physiology,* ed 3, St Louis, 1996, Mosby.)

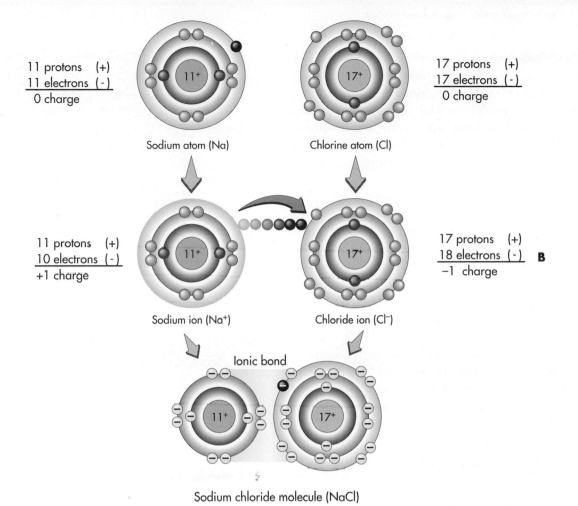

11 protons   (+)
11 electrons (-)
0 charge

Sodium atom (Na)

17 protons   (+)
17 electrons (-)
0 charge

Chlorine atom (Cl)

11 protons   (+)
10 electrons (-)
+1 charge

Sodium ion (Na⁺)

17 protons   (+)
18 electrons (-) **B**
−1 charge

Chloride ion (Cl⁻)

Ionic bond

Sodium chloride molecule (NaCl)

FIGURE 1-2, cont'd B, Ionic bonding. The sodium atom donates the single electron in its outer energy level to a chlorine atom that has seven electrons in its outer level; now each atom has eight electrons in its outer shell. Because the electron-to-proton ratio changes, the sodium atom becomes a positive sodium ion and the chlorine atom becomes a negative chloride ion. The positive-negative attraction between these oppositely charged ions is called an *ionic bond.*

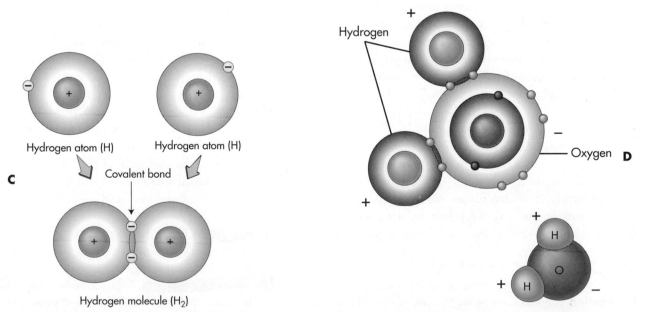

Hydrogen atom (H)   Hydrogen atom (H)

C   Covalent bond

Hydrogen molecule (H₂)

Hydrogen

Oxygen **D**

FIGURE 1-2, cont'd C, Covalent bonding. Two hydrogen atoms move together, resulting in overlapping of their energy levels. Neither atom gains or loses an electron; rather, the two atoms share the electrons, forming a covalent bond.

FIGURE 1-2, cont'd D, Water is a polar molecule. The diagram shows this polar nature. The two hydrogen atoms are nearer one end of the molecule, giving that end a partial positive charge. The opposite end of the molecule has a partial negative charge.

Anabolism—Chemical reactions that *use* energy as they join simple molecules to form more complex molecules of **carbohydrates, lipids, proteins,** and **nucleic acids;** the energy for this process comes from **adenosine triphosphate (ATP).** ATP contains many high-energy bonds that, when broken during catabolism, supply energy for the body's work.

Hydrolysis is a catabolic reaction that uses water to break down larger molecules into smaller ones. Dehydration is an anabolic reaction involving the removal of water while small molecules combine to create larger ones.

🖐 PRACTICAL APPLICATION

In the study of soft tissue and movement therapies, the student must remain mindful of the basic chemical foundations of life and the dynamic processes of change. Change is balanced by the stability of constancy represented in the metaphor of yin and yang, as reflected in the electron and proton relationship. We function in a continual process of old bonds being broken and new ones being formed every millisecond of our lives, whether in cellular functions or social relationships. Each time we apply a massage or other soft tissue method to a client's body, we become part of the stimulus pattern that is the activation process for chemical reactions within the body.

Subtle or "energetic" forms of bodywork may be reflected by the electrical bonding of negatives and positives during chemical reactions that seems to generate the energy of life. The yin/yang concept of a balance of positives and negatives and the duality of wholeness that provides stability during change is also related to the balance of chemical relationships. A more detailed study of the electrical and chemical levels of life, beyond this basic overview, would be valuable not only for an appreciation of the elegance of the simple physical basis of life, but also for an understanding of the metaphor of the way we relate to our clients, our families and friends, and the people of this world.

ORGANELLE LEVEL

Molecules combine in very specific ways to form **organelles,** the basic structure found in cells (Figure 1-3). Each type of organelle performs a specific function within the cell that allows each cell to live. More

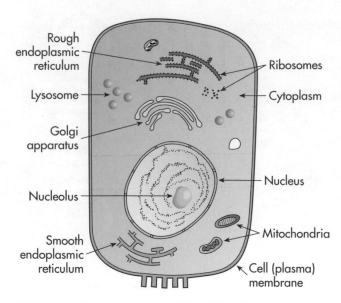

FIGURE 1-3 Generalized cell. (Modified from Williams RW: *Basic healthcare terminology,* St Louis, 1995, Mosby.)

than two dozen organelles have been identified, but the following list includes only the most common ones (Activity 1-5):

- *Cell membrane:* Also known as the plasma membrane, the cell membrane is the outer boundary or skin of the cell. It is composed of phospholipid molecules arranged in such a way that they resemble a sandwich. The function of the cell membrane is to contain the inside of the cell while at the same time allowing transport of certain substances into and out of the cell. Various proteins embedded in the cell membrane allow for this process. Proteins on the surface of the cell act as markers that identify the cell or that work as receptors for chemical signals.
- *Nucleus:* Usually the largest of the organelles, the nucleus contains the chromosomes (threads of DNA). Inside the nucleus is the *nucleolus,* which contains ribonucleic acid (RNA) structures that form ribosomes. The nucleus controls the daily activities of the cell and all cellular reproduction.
- *Ribosomes:* Often the most numerous of the organelles, ribosomes are the sites where amino acids are combined to create various proteins.
- *Endoplasmic reticulum (ER):* Endoplasmic reticulum is a network of interconnected tubes, flattened sacs, and channels distributed throughout the cytoplasm. *Rough ER* is found in cells where

large amounts of proteins are made. *Smooth ER* usually is involved in the metabolism of lipids (fats); it also assists in the detoxification of drugs and the deactivation of steroids. Smooth ER in muscle cells (sarcoplasmic reticulum) uses large amounts of calcium to trigger muscle contractions.

Mitochondria: Mitochondria may be the largest and one of the most numerous types of organelle. They produce ATP, which provides energy for cell activity.

Lysosomes: Lysosomes contain enzymes that function as the cell's digestive system. These enzymes are enclosed in membranes to keep them from breaking down the cell itself.

Golgi's apparatus (or complex): The Golgi bodies process and package protein and some carbo-hydrates for distribution to other parts of the cell or for secretion from the cell.

Cytoplasm: Cytoplasm, which is not classified as an organelle, is the medium that surrounds all the organelles. The fluid portion, *cytosol*, contains many protein enzymes, which function as catalysts in the cell processes. The *cytoskeleton* is an internal scaffolding that anchors the organelles and allows the cells to move and maintain or change their shape.

CELLULAR LEVEL

A **cell** is the basic *structural* unit of an organism. It is also the primary functional unit whose properties reflect the *characteristics of life*. Cells reproduce by cell division. They are surrounded by a dilute saltwater solution. Cells are self-regulating, which allows them

ACTIVITY 1-5

Develop a metaphor for each organelle—think of its function.

Example: The nucleus is the mom of the cell, or the nucleus holds the building plans for a house.

Your Turn

1. Nucleus

2. Ribosomes

3. Endoplasmic reticulum

4. Mitochondria

5. Lysosomes

6. Golgi's apparatus

7. Cytoplasm

8. Cytosol

9. Cytoskeleton

to adjust to constant changes and to interact with their surroundings. The specific activities of any organism depend on both the individual and collective activities of its cells.

Chemically, a cell is composed of carbon, hydrogen, nitrogen, oxygen, and trace amounts of several other elements. Cells are made of approximately 15% protein, 3% lipids, 1% carbohydrates, 1% nucleic acids, and 80% water. Although cells are diverse in both size and shape, they almost all have the same parts and general form. Cells are surrounded by a cell membrane, and all contain cytoplasm and organelles.

Cell metabolism involving catabolism and anabolism can be identified and measured in terms of our recurring theme, the duality of wholeness.

The life cycle of a cell follows a series of changes from the time the cell is formed until it reproduces. The cycle can be divided into two major periods:

1. Growth, or **interphase,** in which the cell carries on most of its activities.
2. Reproduction **(mitosis),** or cell division, in which the cell reproduces itself. **Meiosis** is a form of mitosis that halves the number of *chromosomes* (threads of DNA) in reproductive cells before they combine and multiply.

As mentioned before, disease most likely appears when cellular **homeostasis** (internal balance) has been lost.

Cells change size in response to hormones, nutrient availability, and changes in their function. **Atrophy** is a decrease in the size of a cell; **hypertrophy** is an increase in the size of a cell. Muscle cells in particular can adapt their size to their function. Hypertrophy most often occurs when a person is continually using muscle cells, such as in weight training; atrophy occurs in underused muscle cells, such as when a muscle is immobilized so that a broken bone can heal.

Specialization

No matter what a cell does or where it is located in the body, its basic maintenance functions remain the same. These are nutrition, metabolism, respiration, excretion, organization, and irritability. When a cell needs to adapt to perform specialized duties, the structure of the cell and in turn some of the specialized functions are modified; this form of specialization is referred to as *cell differentiation.* For example, fat cells are modified to store energy, but they have lost the functions of con-

traction and secretion. Muscle cells have very well-developed functions of contractility, but diminished functions of secretion and reproduction. Cells that specialize in certain functions form tissues.

TISSUE LEVEL

A **tissue** is a group of similar cells that are specialized for a specific function. The cells of a tissue are embedded in or surrounded by nonliving material called the *matrix.* The amount and configuration of matrices differ with the type of tissue and the amount of containment or support needed for the tissue.

In most cases, cells directly connect with each other, which allows for better, more stable intercellular communication. Blood plasma, which is a matrix, maintains tissue structure but does not hold it in a solid mass. *Desmosomes* are small contact points of filaments between cells that act like welds. *Gap junctions* are formed when channels of the cells membranes adhere to each other. *Tight junctions* are the type of configuration their name suggests—whole membranes fuse together around the cells to create nonpermeable collars.

The four principal types of tissue—epithelial, connective, muscle, and nerve—can be identified by their structures and functions.

Epithelial Tissue

Epithelial tissues cover and protect the surface of the body and its parts (Figure 1-4). They line cavities, form glands, and specialize in moving substances into and out of the blood during secretion, absorption, and excretion. Because they endure a considerable amount of wear and tear, epithelial cells reproduce very actively. If a person is suffering as a result of stress overload or any homeostatic imbalance, the condition often is first seen in the epithelial tissues because of this fast turnover of cells.

Usually, not much matrix material is found in epithelial tissues. The matrix present tends to form continuous sheets of cells, with the cells held very close together. The surface of most epithelial tissue is

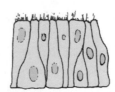

FIGURE 1-4 Epithelial tissue. (From LaFleur Brooks M: *Exploring medical language: a student-directed approach,* ed 3, St Louis 1994, Mosby.)

not in contact with other tissues, but rather is exposed to the external or internal environment. A permeable, thin **basement membrane** attaches epithelial tissues to the underlying connective tissues. Because epithelial tissues contain no blood vessels, they must obtain oxygen and other nutrients from capillaries in the connective tissue.

The epithelial tissues compose three types of membranes, each formed with epithelial tissue on the surface and a specialized connective tissue layer underneath. A **membrane** is a thin, sheetlike layer of tissue that covers a cell, an organ, or a structure; that lines tubes or cavities; or that divides and separates one part from another. The three types of membranes are as follows:

Cutaneous membranes cover the surface of the body, which is exposed to the external environment. The largest cutaneous membrane, more commonly known as our skin, accounts for about 16% of our body weight.

Serous membranes line body cavities not open to the external environment and cover many of the organs. These membranes secrete a thin, watery fluid that lubricates organs to reduce friction as they rub against one another and against the walls of the cavities.

Mucous membranes are found on the surface of tubes that open directly to the exterior, such as those lining the respiratory, digestive, urinary, and reproductive tracts. The film of mucus secreted by these membranes coats and protects the underlying cells.

PRACTICAL APPLICATION

Bodywork therapies focus on the epithelial tissue of the skin as the primary point of touch connections. Of particular importance is the *sensory function of the touch receptors* in the skin. Touch is discussed more extensively in Chapter 11.

Connective Tissue

Connective tissue is the most abundant tissue in the body. Found everywhere, it is the most widely distributed of the four primary types of tissue. Connective tissue is specialized to support and hold together the body and its parts, transport substances through the body, and protect it from foreign substances. All forms of connective tissue are made of matrix, fibers, and cells. The properties of the connective tissue cells and the composition and arrangement of the matrix elements account for the amazing diversity of connective tissues.

Connective tissue cells are often spaced relatively far apart, and the space between cells is filled with large amounts of nonliving **matrix**. Within the matrix of connective tissue is a shapeless ground substance containing molecules that expand when combined with electrolytes and water molecules. The matrix of connective tissue may be 90% ground substance. The remainder is made up mainly of one or more of the following fibers:

Collagenous fibers—Collagenous fibers are tough and strong and have minimal stretch capability. They have a high degree of tensile strength, which allows them to withstand longitudinal stress. These fibers occur in bundles. Because of their color, they are referred to as white fibers. **Collagen** makes up more than one quarter of the body's protein. As we age, the molecular structure of collagen changes, which accounts for the appearance of changes in our tissues.

Reticular fibers—Reticular fibers are delicate fibers found in networks that support small structures such as capillaries, nerve fibers, and the basement membrane. These fibers are made of a form of collagen called *reticulin*.

Elastic fibers—Elastic fibers are extensible and elastic. Found in the stretchy tissues, they are made from a protein called *elastin*, which has the ability to return to its original length, much like a rubber band does after being stretched. Because of their color, these fibers are called yellow fibers.

Each major type of connective tissue has a fundamental cell type that secretes the matrix and fibers (Table 1-2).

TABLE 1-2 CONNECTIVE TISSUE CELL TYPES

CELL TYPE	MATRIX AND FIBERS
Fibroblast	Connective tissue
Chondroblast	Cartilage
Osteoblast	Bone
Hemocytoblast (hematopoietic stem cell)	Blood

Although connective tissue is found in all areas of the body, some areas contain more than others. The brain has very little connective tissue, whereas ligaments, tendons, and skin have high concentrations. The number of blood vessels in connective tissue varies. Cartilage has none, but other types of connective tissue have a large supply.

Three other types of cells also are commonly found in connective tissue:

Macrophages are large, irregularly shaped cells. They develop in the bone marrow and move throughout the body's connective tissue, searching for microorganisms, damaged cells, and foreign particles. When these targets are found, the macrophages dispose of them by ingesting and digesting them, a process known as *phagocytosis.*

Mast cells also develop in bone marrow. Their functions focus on releasing chemicals (heparin and histamine) as part of the inflammatory response, allergic response, and pain.

Adipose cells are large cells stored in white or brown fat in the dermis, or deep layer of the skin, in the gut, and in the colon. When clustered together, they are known as adipose tissue.

Types of connective tissue

Dense regular connective tissue (Figure 1-5)

Structure: The matrix consists mainly of collagen fibers produced by fibroblasts, with fibers oriented in the same direction. The ligaments and tendons formed by this type of tissue have a small number of cells, and blood flow to the area is limited.

Function: Dense regular connective tissue provides strength and resistance while allowing some degree of stretch.

Dense irregular connective tissue (Figure 1-6)

Structure: Collagen and elastin fibers are interwoven and oriented in an irregular pattern to create the matrix. The tissue has little blood flow and is concentrated in the dermis, joint capsules, and surrounding muscles and in some organs.

Function: Dense irregular connective tissues can withstand intense pulling forces and remain impact resistant.

Loose (areolar) tissue (Figure 1-7)

Structure: A loose, irregular configuration of fibroblastic cells, macrophages, and lymphocytes is contained within a fine network of mostly collagen and elastin. Fluid-filled spaces separate the cells and fibers from one another.

Function: Areolar tissue is widely distributed throughout the body and is the substance on which most epithelium rests. It is the packing material between glands, muscles, and nerves, it attaches the skin to the underlying tissues, and it supplies nourishment because of its high vascularity.

Adipose tissue (Figure 1-8)

Structure: Adipose tissue is composed of fat cells with very little matrix between the cells. Support is provided by reticular and collagenous fibers. Adipose tissue is closely associated with the capillaries of both the blood and lymph. Most adipose tissue is found in the buttocks, anterior abdominal wall, breasts, arms, and thighs.

Function: Both the storage and release of fat are regulated by stimulation from hormones and the ner-

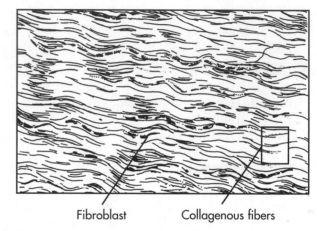

Fibroblast   Collagenous fibers

FIGURE 1-5 Dense regular connective tissue. (From Thibodeau GA, Patton KT: *Anatomy and physiology,* ed 3, St Louis, 1996, Mosby.)

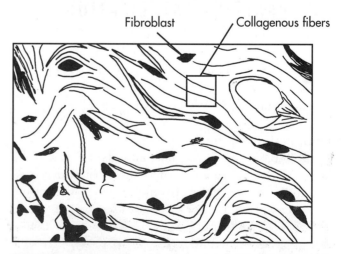

Fibroblast   Collagenous fibers

FIGURE 1-6 Dense irregular connective tissue. (From Thibodeau GA, Patton KT: *Anatomy and physiology,* ed 3, St Louis, 1996, Mosby.)

vous system. Adipose tissue is a source of fuel, it helps to insulate and pad organs and tissues, and it stores fat-soluble vitamins.

Types of cartilage

Cartilage is composed of chondrocytes surrounded by an extensive matrix. Collagen gives cartilage its flexibility, and the strength and water-binding capacity of the ground substance make cartilage rigid yet able to spring back when compressed. Because it has very little blood flow, cartilage heals slowly. The three types of cartilage are hyaline cartilage, fibrocartilage, and elastic cartilage.

Hyaline cartilage (Figure 1-9)

Structure: Hyaline cartilage is semitransparent and has a milky bluish color. It has a very strong and solid matrix. It is flexible and insensitive.

Function: Hyaline cartilage is found at the end of bones in most synovial joints, where it provides additional weight-bearing support or attaches to other bones, such as with costal cartilage. Hyaline cartilage provides the support and flexibility found in the trachea, lungs, and nose.

Fibrocartilage (Figure 1-10)

Structure: Fibrocartilage is composed of large amounts of dense fibrous tissue and small amounts

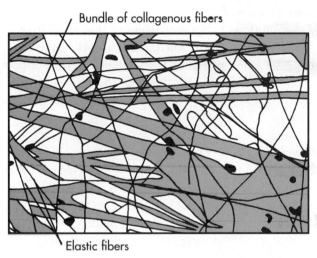

FIGURE 1-7 Loose (areolar) tissue. (From Thibodeau GA, Patton KT: *Anatomy and physiology,* ed 3, St Louis, 1996, Mosby.)

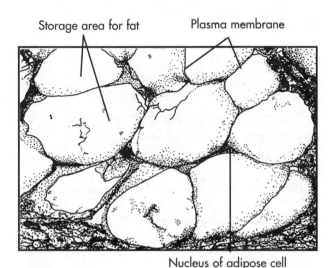

FIGURE 1-8 Adipose tissue. (From Thibodeau GA, Patton KT: *Anatomy and physiology,* ed 3, St Louis, 1996, Mosby.)

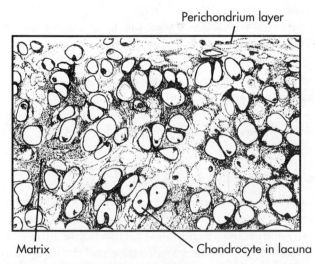

FIGURE 1-9 Hyaline cartilage. (From Thibodeau GA, Patton KT: *Anatomy and physiology,* ed 3, St Louis, 1996, Mosby.)

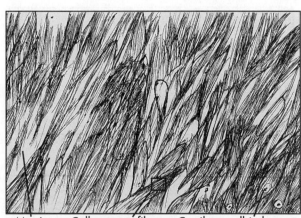

FIGURE 1-10 Fibrocartilage. (From Thibodeau GA, Patton KT: *Anatomy and physiology,* ed 3, St Louis, 1996, Mosby.)

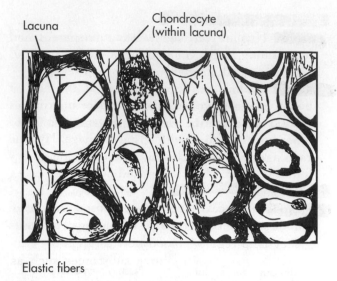

FIGURE 1-11   Elastic cartilage. (From Thibodeau GA, Patton KT: *Anatomy and physiology,* ed 3, St Louis, 1996, Mosby.)

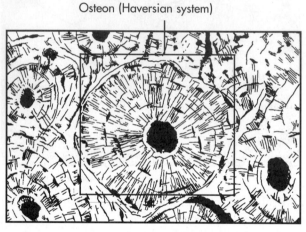

FIGURE 1-12   Bone tissue. (From Thibodeau GA, Patton KT: *Anatomy and physiology,* ed 3, St Louis, 1996, Mosby.)

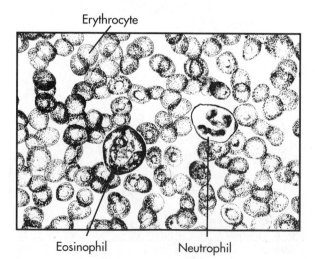

FIGURE 1-13   Blood. (From Thibodeau GA, Patton KT: *Anatomy and physiology,* ed 3, St Louis, 1996, Mosby.)

of matrix, an arrangement that creates a more rigid structure than hyaline cartilage. Fibrocartilage is found mainly in the symphysis pubis, intervertebral disks, and tendon attachments.

Function: Fibrocartilage can withstand compression and impact forces; it diffuses the resultant force so that it is spread over a larger area and is not focused in specific areas of the bone.

Elastic cartilage (Figure 1-11)

Structure: As its name implies, elastic cartilage is a very flexible form of hyaline cartilage with a large concentration of elastic fibers.

Function: Elastic cartilage provides flexibility and support to the external ear and the larynx.

Bone (Figure 1-12)

Structure: Bone is the most rigid of the connective tissues because of its hard, mineralized matrix.

Function: Bone provides the framework for supporting the body; it also protects the internal organs, serves as storage for minerals, and produces blood cells.

Blood (Figure 1-13)

Structure: Blood cells float within an extremely loose matrix, actually a fluid known as plasma, which contains no fibers or ground substances.

Function: Blood helps maintain homeostasis by transporting substances, resisting infection, and maintaining heat.

Connective tissue membranes

Connective tissue membranes are composed exclusively of various types of connective tissue. They are classified as *synovial membranes.*

Synovial membranes line the joint spaces in the mobile synovial joints. This type of membrane is also found in bursae, which are protective sacs found near joints; between layers of muscle and connective tissue; and wherever the body needs extra protection. Synovial fluid is a thick lubricant secreted by these membranes to keep themselves slippery.

✋ PRACTICAL APPLICATION

Many of the benefits of soft tissue and movement therapies derive from these treatments' effects on the connective tissue. Most methods affect the consistency of the ground substance and the directional pattern of the fiber configuration and networks. The gel of the ground substance is considered thixotropic, which means that it liquefies when it is agitated and returns to a gel state as it stands. Manipulating connective tissue seems to soften the ground substance and increase the water-binding capacity, which makes the tissue more pliable (i.e., induces a gel or more liquid state).

When an electrical current is passed through collagen, a slight deforming of the structure results because of the piezoelectric property of the collagen. When collagen itself is compressed, stretched, or twisted, it produces minute electrical currents. Researchers recognize that some forms of electrical stimulation enhance bone growth, but the exact reason why bodywork methods could cause this effect on collagen is under investigation. The body's innate ability to generate electrical current may provide some insight into the body's inherent energy flow, what can be called Qi, or Prana, among other names and may be considered life force, or enlivening energy.

Muscle Tissue

The main characteristic of **muscle tissue** is its ability to provide movement by shortening as a result of contraction. Contraction assists in maintaining posture and produces heat. Contraction occurs as a result of the action of contractile proteins found inside muscle cells. Muscle cells are longer than they are wide, creat-

ing a distinctive pattern that resembles fibers; for this reason the cells are often referred to as muscle fibers.

Muscle tissues (Figure 1-14) may be categorized by their appearance, function, and location as follows:

- **Skeletal muscle fibers** are large, cross-striated cells connected to the skeleton. They are under the control of the nervous system, and their actions are voluntary.
- **Cardiac muscle fibers,** which are found in the heart, are smaller, striated fibers. Their structure is not as organized as that of skeletal muscles.
- **Smooth muscle fibers** are neither striated nor voluntary. Found in the organs and viscera, they help regulate blood flow through the cardiovascular system, move substances such as food and waste through the intestines, and squeeze secretions from glands.

Muscle tissue is discussed in greater detail in Chapter 9.

✋ PRACTICAL APPLICATION

The major element of soft tissue is the muscle and its associated connective tissue. Muscle tissue provides the active aspect of movement. Soft tissue and movement approaches seek to maintain or restore effective movement patterns.

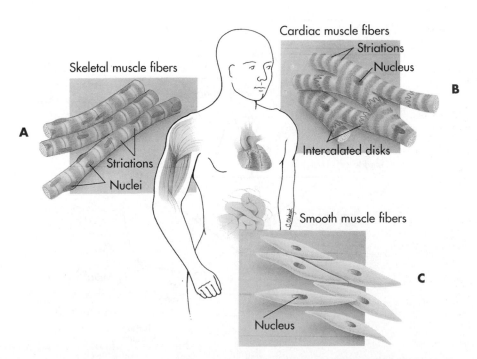

FIGURE 1-14 Muscle tissue. **A,** Skeletal muscle. **B,** Cardiac muscle. **C,** Smooth muscle. (From Thibodeau GA, Patton KT: *Structure and function of the body,* ed 10, St Louis, 1997, Mosby.)

Nervous (Neural) Tissue

The functions of **nervous tissue** (Figure 1-15) are to coordinate and regulate body activity. It can do this well because it has specialized to develop more excitability and conductivity than other types of tissue. Nerve cells are divided into two types: neurons, which are the actual functional units, and neuroglia, which connect and support the neurons. Nervous tissue is discussed in depth in Chapters 4 and 5.

ORGAN LEVEL

Organs are groups of two or more kinds of tissue that combine to perform a special function.

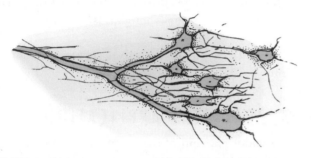

FIGURE 1-15 Nervous tissue. (From LaFleur Brooks M: *Exploring medical language: a student-directed approach,* ed 3, St Louis, 1994, Mosby.)

According to Oriental healing theories, the function of the organs can be associated with energy patterns. Organs that are hollow and work intermittently are thought of as yang organs. Extensions of the yang organs make contact with the exterior of the body. Examples include the stomach, with the mouth opening to the exterior, and the bladder, which empties through the urethra. Organs that are solid and must work all the time to maintain homeostasis are yin organs. Instead of filling and emptying, they store the various essences of life extracted from the food and air. Examples include the heart and lungs. The relationships of the organs are presented in the Five Element meridian theory (depicted in Figure 1-16 as a wheel), which is explained in Chapter 2.

SYSTEM LEVEL

Organs that combine to perform more complex body functions are referred to as *systems.* The number and types of organs found in a system depend on its functions. The 11 systems of the human body are the integumentary, skeletal, muscular, nervous, endocrine, cardiovascular, lymphatic and immune, respiratory, digestive, urinary, and reproductive systems.

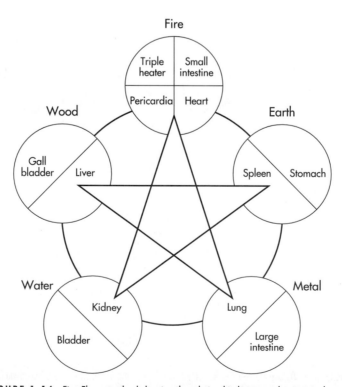

FIGURE 1-16 Five Element wheel showing the relationship between elements and organs.

ORGANISM LEVEL: THE BODY AS A WHOLE

We are more than the sum of our parts. Each part of the body works in combination with the other parts to support the whole. The mutually dependent nature of cells and the organization of complex systems allow us the endless possibilities of diversity that we experience. The cooperation, interdependence, and respect the body displays for itself could be a wise metaphor for the larger organism of the world in which we are the cells—a fundamental unit of life.

After the overview information has been developed in Chapters 1, 2, and 3, this text discusses each of the systems individually. Organizing the book in this manner allows the student to use a more comprehensive anatomy and physiology book that is developed on a systems approach to expand on the knowledge presented in this text.

Summary

This first chapter has laid the foundation for the study of anatomy and physiology. The relationship of structure, function, and homeostasis, in terms of Western and Oriental thought, was presented. The biologic organization of life, from the parts of the atom to the systems of the body, was laid out in a sequential manner, each level made up of the components that build the next level of body organization. On this foundation we will continue to build levels of knowledge as our study of the human body progresses.

WORKBOOK SECTION

1. Explain the importance of understanding the relationship of anatomy (structure) and physiology (function) of the body as a whole.

_____

_____

_____

_____

_____

2. Explain the relationship of yin/yang to anatomy and physiology.

_____

_____

_____

_____

_____

3. List and define the 13 characteristics of life.

_____

_____

_____

_____

_____

_____

_____

_____

_____

_____

_____

_____

_____

4. List and explain the seven levels of organization of the body.

_____

_____

_____

_____

_____

_____

_____

_____

FILL IN THE BLANK

(1) _____ is the scientific study of the (2) _____ of the body and the relationship of its parts. (3) _____ is the scientific study of the processes and (4) _____ of the body that support life.

(5) _____ is the study of body structures large enough to be visible to the naked eye. (6) _____ is the study of all of the structures of a particular area. (7) _____ is the study of the body divided into its systems. (8) _____ is the study of internal body structures as they can be recognized and related to the overlying skin surface.

An (9) _____ is the smallest particle of an element that retains the properties of that element. (10) _____ are the smallest part of a substance that can exist independently without losing its physical and chemical properties.

(11) _____ refers to the chemical reactions in the body. A chemical reaction that releases energy as it breaks down complex compounds into simpler ones is (12) _____.

(13) _____ is a chemical reaction that uses energy as it joins simple molecules together to form more complex molecules. Anabolism requires energy supplied from the molecule adenosine triphosphate, or (14) _____.

(15) _____ are the basic structures of the cells, and they perform specific functions within the cell. A (16) _____ is the basic structural and functional unit of a living organism.

(17) _____ is the period when the cell grows and carries on most of its activities. (18) _____ occurs when the cell divides, the process by which the cell (19) _____ itself.

(20) _____ is a special form of mitosis that halves the number of chromosomes in (21) _____ cells.

(22) _____ is an increase in the size of a cell;

(23) _____ is a decrease in cell size.

A (24) _____ is a group of similar cells that usually have a similar embryologic origin and that are specialized for a particular function.

(25) _____ tissue covers and protects the body's surfaces, lines body cavities, specializes in moving substances into and out of the blood during secretion, excretion, and absorption, and forms many glands. A (26) _____ is a thin, sheetlike layer of tissue that covers a cell, an organ, or a structure, that lines tubes or cavities, or that divides and separates one part from another.

(27) _____ tissue is specialized to support and hold together the body and its parts, to transport substances through the body, and to protect it from foreign substances. Within the (28) _____ of connective tissue is a shapeless or amorphous ground substance containing molecules that expand when bound with electrolytes and water molecules. Of all the hundreds of different protein compounds in the body, (29) _____ is the most abundant, accounting for more than one fourth of the body's protein.

(30) _____ fibers are strong fibers with minimal stretch capacity. They have a high degree of tensile strength, which allows them to withstand longitudinal stress. (31) _____ fibers are delicate connective tissue fibers that occur in networks, which support small structures such as capillaries, nerve fibers, and the basement membrane.

(32) _____ fibers are extensible and elastic. They are made from a protein called elastin, which returns to its original length after being stretched.

(33) _____ tissue provides movement, maintains posture, and produces heat. (34) _____ muscle fibers are made up of large, cross-striated cells connected to the skeleton and under voluntary control of the nervous system. (35) _____ muscle fibers are small, striated, involuntary fibers that enable the heart to pump blood.

(36)_____ muscle fibers are neither striated nor voluntary. They help regulate blood flow through the cardiovascular system, propel food through the gut, and squeeze secretions from glands.

PROBLEM SOLVING

Read the problem presented. There is no correct answer; rather, the exercise is intended to assist the student in developing the analytical and decision-making skills necessary in professional practice.

After reading the problem through, follow the six steps given below:
1. Identify the facts presented in the information.
2. Identify the possibilities presented ("what if" statements), or develop your own possibilities that relate to the facts.
3. Evaluate each possibility in terms of the logical cause and effect and pros and cons.
4. Consider the effect on those involved.
5. Write each answer down in the space provided.
6. Develop your solution by answering the question posed.

PROBLEM

The study of anatomy, physiology, and the mechanisms of health and disease can be both fascinating and frustrating. The student must absorb and understand a tremendous amount of information and remember many details. Textbooks do not always agree, and new research results change the information constantly. Students may find themselves lost in the magnitude of all the information and the implications of what can happen when they delve into this study. If this happens, a student may give up and study merely to pass a test instead of to learn and understand.

Frequently the information does not seem relevant to the career choice or the broader topic the student is studying. As a result, the wonder, fascination, and importance of the information about the body often is replaced with the dread of learning new terms and understanding complex concepts. Unless a direct correlation is established between the acquisition and application of the information they are to learn, students may store data in their minds as interesting but irrelevant facts. When it comes time to actually use the information, it may not be available because it was never integrated as part of a whole process.

QUESTION

What can you do to avoid becoming overwhelmed and to remain excited as you learn about the body?

The first response is provided as a guide to get you started. Fill in at least two more statements.

FACTS
1. The student must learn a tremendous amount of information.

2. _____

3. _____

POSSIBILITIES
1. The student may not know what should be committed to memory.

2. _____

3. _____

LOGICAL CAUSE AND EFFECT
1. The student studies only to pass the test.

2. _____

3. _____

EFFECT

1. The student feels overwhelmed.

2. _____

3. _____

What can you do to avoid becoming overwhelmed and to remain excited as you learn about the body?

_____

_____

_____

_____

_____

_____

_____

_____

FURTHER STUDY

Using a comprehensive anatomy and physiology text (see Works Consulted list at the back of this book), identify the chapters that pertain to the information presented in this chapter. Locate the information presented in this text and then elaborate on it by writing a paragraph of additional information on each of the following:

Atom

_____

_____

_____

_____

_____

Molecules

_____

_____

_____

_____

_____

Chemical bonds

_____

_____

_____

_____

Metabolism

_____

_____

_____

_____

_____

Adenosine triphosphate (ATP)

_____

_____

_____

_____

_____

_____

Organelles

_____

_____

_____

_____

Cell

_____

_____

_____

_____

Tissue types

_____

_____

_____

_____

Membrane types

_____

_____

_____

_____

_____

Answer Key

1. Anatomy and physiology are two very distinct yet Interrelated biologic studies that combine to present the body's operation as a whole organism. Structure (anatomy) and function (physiology) cannot be separated. Structure and function form a continuum; structure guides function, and function can modify structure. The concept of anatomy and physiology is an example of the duality of wholeness.

2. Yin and yang represent opposite but complimentary qualities. Yin corresponds to structure, or anatomy, and yang to function, or physiology. Although they are opposites, yin and yang form a whole unit and are complementary. Yang contains the seed of yin and vice versa. Nothing is totally yin or totally yang; yang transforms into yin and yin into yang. The human body and its functions can be understood by following this concept of the relationship of opposites that creates wholeness.

3. (1) Maintenance of boundaries—Keeping the internal environment distinct from the external environment
   (2) Movement—The ability to transport the entire being, as well as internal components
   (3) Responsiveness-The ability to sense, monitor, and respond to changes in the external environment
   (4) Conductivity—The movement of energy from one point to another
   (5) Growth—A normal increase in the size or number (or both) of cells
   (6) Respiration-The absorption, transport, and use or exchange of respiratory gases (oxygen and carbon dioxide)
   (7) Digestion—The process by which food products are broken down into simple substances to be used by individual cells
   (8) Absorption—The transport and use of nutrients
   (9) Secretion—The production and delivery of specialized substances for diverse functions

   (10) Excretion—The removal of waste products
   (11) Circulation—The movement of fluids, nutrients, secretions, and waste products from one area of the body to another
   (12) Reproduction—The formation of a new being; also, the formation of new cells in the body to permit growth, repair, and replacement
   (13) Metabolism—A chemical reaction that occurs in cells to effect transformation, production, or consumption of energy

4. (1) Chemical level (atoms and molecules): The chemical properties of a substance have to do with the way it reacts with other substances or responds to a change in the environment. Molecules are the smallest part of a substance that can exist independently without losing the physical and chemical properties of the substance. Atoms combine to form molecules. The atoms most commonly found in living things are hydrogen, carbon, nitrogen, and oxygen. An atom can achieve a state of maximal stability by gaining or losing electrons to fill or empty its outer shell. Chemical reactions or chemical change result in the breakdown of substances and the formation of new ones.
   (2) Organelle level: Molecules combine in very specific ways to form organelles, the basic structures found in cells. Organelles perform specific functions within the cell; it is the sum property of these structures that allows each cell to live. More than two dozen organelles have been identified.
   (3) Cellular level: A cell is the basic structural and functional unit of a living organism. Cells are self-regulating, which allows them to adjust to change by attempting to remain constant and maintain homeostasis.
   (4) Tissue level: A tissue is a group of similar cells that usually have a similar embryologic origin and are specialized for a particular function.

Epithelial tissue covers and protects the body's surfaces, lines cavities, specializes in moving substances into and out of the blood during secretion, excretion, and absorption, and forms many glands.

Connective tissue is specialized to support and hold together the body and its parts, to transport substances through the body, and to protect it from foreign substances.

Muscle tissue has the ability to effect movement by shortening as a result of contraction. Muscle tissue enables the body to move, maintain posture, and produce heat.

Nervous tissue is able to regulate and coordinate body activity quickly. Nervous tissue has developed more excitability and conductivity than other types of tissue.

   (5) Organ level: Organs are more complex than tissue. An organ is a group of two or more kinds of tissues arranged so that they can perform a special function.
   (6) System level: Organs that work together to perform more complex bodily functions are called systems. The 11 systems of the human body are the integumentary, skeletal, muscular, nervous, endocrine, cardiovascular, lymphatic and immune, respiratory, digestive, urinary, and reproductive systems.
   (7) Organism level: The body as a whole is an organism. Each part of the body works in combination with the other parts to support the whole. The mutually dependent nature of the cells and the organization of complex systems allow us the endless possibilities of diversity that we experience.

FILL IN THE BLANK

1. Anatomy
2. Structures
3. Physiology
4. functions
5. Gross anatomy
6. Regional anatomy

19. reproduces
20. Meiosis
21. reproductive
22. Hypertrophy
23. atrophy
24. tissue

7. Systemic anatomy
8. Surface anatomy
9. Atom
10. Molecules
11. Metabolism
12. Catabolism
13. Anabolism
14. ATP

25. Epithelial
26. membrane
27. connective
28. matrix
29. Collagen
30. Collagenous
31. Reticular
32. Elastic

Mechanisms of Health and Disease

CHAPTER OBJECTIVES

After completing this chapter the student should be able to perform the following:

1. Define homeostasis, self-regulatory mechanisms, and body rhythms in relationship to bodywork modalities and Oriental and Ayurvedic theories of health.
2. Discuss and contrast the mechanisms of disease and health.
3. Define disease terminology.
4. List disturbances in homeostasis.
5. Discuss risk factors in disease development.
6. List the four primary signs of the inflammatory response.
7. Define pain and list the types of pain.
8. Discuss the pain-spasm-pain cycle in relationship to bodywork methods.
9. Identify viscerally referred pain patterns.
10. Define phantom pain.
11. List the factors influencing health.
12. Identify factors contributing to the stress response.
13. List the stages in the cycle of life.

KEY TERMS

Acute pain   Pain that is usually temporary, of sudden onset, and easily localized. It can be a symptom of a disease process or a temporary aspect of medical treatment. Acting as a warning signal, it activates the sympathetic nervous system.

Afferent (AF-er-ent)   Toward a center or point of reference.

Anaplasia (an-ah-PLAY-zee-a)   Meaning without shape, it describes abnormal or undifferentiated cells that fail to mature into specialized cell types. It is a characteristic of malignant cells.

Benign (be-NINE)   Usually describing a noncancerous tumor that is contained and does not spread.

Biologic rhythms   The internal, periodic timing component of an organism, also known as a biorhythm. Circadian rhythms work on a 24-hour period to coordinate internal functions such as sleep. Ultradian rhythms repeat themselves from every 90 minutes to every few hours, whereas seasonal rhythms function on a yearly basis.

Cancer   Malignant, nonencapsulated cells that invade surrounding tissue. They often break away, or metastasize, from the primary tumor and form secondary cancer masses.

Chronic pain   Pain that continues or recurs over a prolonged time, usually for more than 6 months. The onset may be obscure and the character and quality of the pain change over time. It is usually poorly localized and not as intense as acute pain, although for some it is exhausting and depressing.

Efferent (EF-er-ent)   Away from a center or point of reference.

Entrainment (en-TRAIN-ment)   A coordination or synchronization to a rhythm, especially when a person responds to certain patterns by moving in a coordinated manner to those patterns.

Etiology (e-tee-OL-o-jee)   The study of the factors involved in the development of disease, including the nature of the disease and the susceptibility of the person.

Health   A condition of homeostasis resulting in a state of physical, emotional, social, and spiritual well-being.

Homeostasis (ho-me-o-STA-sis)   The relatively constant state of the internal environment of the body maintained by adaptive responses. Specific control and feedback mechanisms are responsible for adjusting body systems to maintain this state.

Hyperplasia (hye-per-PLAY-zee-ha)   An uncontrolled increase in the number of cells of a body part.

Inflammation (in-flah-MAY-shun)   A protective response of the tissues to irritation or injury that may be chronic or acute. There are four primary signs: redness, heat, swelling, and pain.

Neoplasm (NEE-o-plazm)   The abnormal growth of new tissue. Also called a tumor, it may be benign or malignant.

Pain   An unpleasant sensation. It is a complex, private experience with physiologic, psychologic, and social aspects. Because it is subjective, it is often difficult to explain or describe.

Pathology (pah-THOL-o-jee)   The study of disease as it is observed in the structure and function of the body.

Phantom pain   A form of pain or other sensation experienced in the missing extremity after a limb amputation.

Somatic pain (so-MA-tik)   Pain that arises from the body as opposed to the viscera. Superficial somatic pain comes from the stimulation of receptors in the skin, whereas deep somatic pain arises from stimulation of receptors in skeletal muscles, joints, tendons, and fascia.

Stress   Any external or internal stimulus that requires a change or response to prevent an imbalance in the internal environment of the body, mind, or emotions. It may be any activity that makes demands on mental and emotional resources. Some responses to stress may stimulate neurons of the hypothalamus to release corticotrophin-releasing hormone, or CRH.

Visceral (VIS-er-al) *pain*   Pain that is a result of the stimulation of receptors or an abnormal condition in the viscera (internal organs).

Homeostasis

Our body cells survive and thrive in a healthy condition only when the temperature, pressure, and chemical composition of their fluid environment remains relatively constant. The overall *structure* of our body does not change noticeably from moment to moment. When you go to bed at night, unless there has been major trauma, your body looks pretty much the same as it did when you woke up. This is due to the constant balancing activities of our physiology.

Homeostasis is the relatively constant state maintained by the physiology of the body. Each of us has our own regulatory mechanisms that constantly adjust and adapt to keep the temperature and chemical composition in balance in our fluid environment. When this is interrupted, homeostasis is altered, and the body is more susceptible to a disease process. Homeostasis is the delicate maintenance of the balance of yin and yang we saw in Chapter 1. No matter how complicated, the signs and symptoms in disease can be explained in terms of yin and yang (Box 2-1).

The maintenance of balance between these opposites is homeostasis.

BOX 2-1

CHARACTERISTICS OF YIN AND YANG

Fire is Yang	Hard is Yang
Water is Yin	Soft is Yin
Hot is Yang	Excitement is Yang
Cold is Yin	Inhibition is Yin
Restless is Yang	Rapidity is Yang
Excessive fatigue or	Slowness is Yin
sleepiness is Yin	
Dry is Yang	Transformation/change is Yang
Wet is Yin	Conservation/storage is Yin

Modified from Maciocia G: *The foundations of Chinese medicine,* New York, 1994, Churchill Livingstone.

Most healing arts describe the balanced state of homeostasis in their own terminology. Besides the organ relationship of yin and yang, the Oriental five-element theory is a metaphor of the life elements of fire, earth, metal, water, and wood. They are found in nature and their characteristics are reflected in our bodies.

The ancient healing model of Ayurveda says that an individual is made up of five primary elements. The elements differ from the Oriental model, but the whole picture of balance is similar. The Ayurvedic elements are ether (space), air, fire, water, and earth.

Certain elements can combine to create various physiologic *functions,* called doshas. The *Vata* dosha is formed from ether and air. Vata governs the *principles of movement* and is seen in nerve impulses, circulation, respiration, and elimination.

The *Pitta* dosha is a combination of fire and water. It represents the *process of transformation.* Metabolic transformation begins at a cellular level and moves up through all body functions. One example of Pitta is the transformation of food into usable nutrients.

The *Kapha* dosha blends the water and earth elements. These elements *hold our cells together* and build our muscles, fat, and bones. They also form some of the protective lining and fluids, such as the mucosal stomach lining and cerebrospinal fluid.

Each of us is created of our own unique proportion of Vata, Pitta, and Kapha, which allows for the great diversity of humans. The three doshas and the five elements must be balanced for us to maintain a healthy body. Our character is an expression of the harmonious and smooth interaction between them. The same concept is the foundation of the body/mind

relationship of health and disease that has developed in recent years in Western science.

FEEDBACK LOOP

Every system in our body contributes to maintaining homeostasis, but the nervous and endocrine systems are the most important. For the interaction and communication necessary for the self-regulation to succeed, a well-developed control system is necessary. This system is called a *feedback loop.* Nerve impulses or chemical messengers transmit the information needed to maintain homeostasis through these feedback loops.

One definition of stress states that stress is any stimulus, either internal or external, that creates an imbalance in our internal environment. If we are exposed to such a stress, certain mechanisms attempt to counteract the responses to the stress and bring the conditions back into balance. Thus the body of a person exposed to a stress could respond before any awareness of the stress occurs and bring itself back to a balanced state—homeostasis.

Each feedback loop is made up of the following:

1. A *sensor mechanism* that generates an impulse in response to an afferent electrical or chemical signal
2. An *integration/control center* that analyzes and integrates all signals received and, if needed, initiates a response (efferent)
3. An *effector mechanism* that actualizes the efferent response from the control center

The terms *afferent* and *efferent* are directional terms. They are used to describe movement of a signal from a sensor to an integrating or control center or, in reverse, movement of a signal from the control center to some type of effector mechanism. **Afferent** means that a signal is traveling toward a particular center or point of reference, and **efferent** means that a signal is traveling away from a particular center or point of reference.

Imagine that we put a person in a controlled situation in which we measured the activities that took place during a stress response. When a stress, the stimulus, disturbs homeostasis, receptors immediately send input to an integration center. These signals are interpreted, and corrective responses are sent to effectors.

Negative feedback refers to the feedback that reverses the original stimulus, stabilizes physiologic function, and helps us maintain our constant internal environment. Most systems are of this type. For example, increasing and maintaining the tension in a muscle will help us to later relax the muscle. In soft tissue approaches this is the feedback mechanism used by postisometric relaxation (a muscle energy technique that first contracts a muscle and then lengthens it) to help with lengthening and stretching the tissue.

Positive feedback enhances the original stimulus and thus maintains a disturbed state of homeostasis. In doing so it does not maintain a stable internal environment. The few forms of positive feedback that our bodies use either serve a very specific purpose, such as maintaining contractions during labor and delivery, or continue a cycle that may be harmful. An example of this is when a muscle spasm causes pain, which results in increased spasm. The pain-spasm-pain cycle (pain creates protective spasm, which in turn increases pain) is a positive feedback loop (Figure 2-1).

One premise of Ayurveda is that our body is a projection of our consciousness. Other healing practices have similar underlying principles, including behavioral medicine and mind/body approaches. Self-correcting systems use feedback loops to influence their own expression. Our bodies can use this to coordinate our activities (negative feedback), allowing us to remain in a relatively constant state while immersed in the waves of change (Activity 2-1).

PRACTICAL APPLICATION

Bodywork and other soft tissue approaches can either support or stimulate homeostatic processes. The stimuli from these methods is received by the receptors of the nervous or endocrine systems that send signals through afferent pathways for interpretation in the nervous system control centers of the central nervous system. Messages are returned by way of efferent pathways to the effector targets, where the response is to reestablish balanced function, such as relaxing or tightening a muscle, softening or firming connective tissue, or reducing

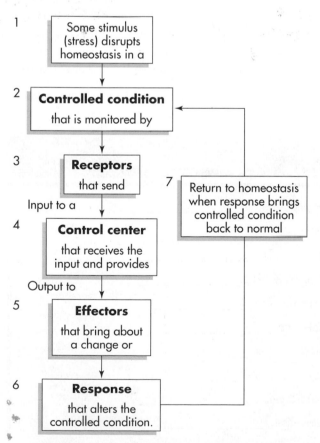

FIGURE 2-1 Components of a negative feedback system (loop).

ACTIVITY 2-1

Many mechanical systems in our homes, autos, and work environment have feedback mechanisms. Identify one and diagram the flow pattern, labeling the sensor mechanism, control center, and effector mechanism. Show afferent and efferent message pathways.

or increasing arousal responses of the autonomic nervous system, whichever restores homeostasis. Bodywork approaches are often nonspecific; the stimuli used usually disrupts the general existing homeostatic pattern, which requires a response through the feedback mechanism. The objective is to reestablish homeostasis the same way we push a reset button on a machine.

Body Rhythms

Biologic rhythms are the internal, periodic timing components of an organism generated within the body. Circadian rhythms work on a 24-hour period to coordinate internal functions such as sleep. Ultradian rhythms repeat themselves every 90 minutes to every few hours, whereas seasonal rhythms function on a yearly basis. Some forms of depressive disorders, as well as many sleep, neurologic, cardiovascular, and endocrine disorders have recently been associated with circadian rhythm dysfunction. Many of the conveniences we use have put us out of sync with the natural rhythms of light, dark, the seasons, and the cycles of the moon (Activity 2-2).

Our biologic rhythms are interconnected. The synchronization of the rhythms of our heart, respiration, and digestion promotes this balance, or homeostasis, to support a healthy body. A balance between sympathetic and parasympathetic portions of the autonomic nervous system influences the sinus nodes of the heart and vascular systems, which in turn modulate heart rate and blood pressure. Our nasal reflexes, stimulated by the movement of air through the nose, rhythmically interact with the heart, lung, and diaphragm (Timmons, 1994).

Our body rhythms are kept balanced through negative feedback loops. When a change occurs in our heart rate, blood pressure, and respiratory rate, efferent nerve receptors called baroreceptors respond to changes in pressure in these systems. The various mental or emotional stressors we encounter daily stimulate the sympathetic system (part of nervous system that responds by fight-or-flight reactions). The central nervous system integrates the information, slows down our brain waves, and decreases the release of cortisol (a steroid hormone of the sympathetic system), thus increasing parasympathetic (relaxation and restoration) activity. Balance is maintained in this manner.

PRACTICAL APPLICATION

When a person experiences positive emotional states, there is a tendency for the biologic rhythms to naturally begin to oscillate together. This process is called **entrainment.** We can also enhance processes with techniques that shift our consciousness

ACTIVITY 2-2

Map your own body rhythms for a 24-hour period.

Write in any other rhythms you recognize.

Waking—Time _____

Elimination (bladder and bowel)—Time _____

Food—Time _____

Alert phase (mental and physical peak)—Time _____

Fatigue phase (mental and physical low) —Time _____

Elimination—Time _____

Food—Time _____

Alert phase—Time _____

Fatigue phase—Time _____

Food—Time _____

Alert phase—Time _____

Fatigue phase—Time _____

Elimination—Time _____

Food—Time _____

Alert phase—Time _____

Fatigue phase—Time _____

Elimination—Time _____

Sleep—Time _____

to our breathing patterns and heart rate. Many disciplines quiet the mind and body during meditation. Other examples include yoga focusing attention on the breath, whereas Qigong focuses on the point below the navel. These systems center attention on body areas that have known biologic oscillators. The location of the chakra system correlates with biologic oscillators (Figure 2-2).

Biologic rhythms can be affected by the rhythm of music. Chaotic or abrupt noise can be a disruptive factor, whereas ocean or other similar nature sounds usually have a calming effect. Studies have shown that the rhythmic physiologic patterns of a dog or cat's breathing or heart rate can benefit elderly persons. The rhythmic patterns of singing, chanting, and

movement in our religious and social rituals interact with biologic patterns, resulting in a calming or exciting organization or disruption of body rhythms.

The rhythmic and ordered approach used in massage and soft tissue methods would seem to have similar effects to those just mentioned, especially when provided by a calm and focused practitioner. The length of application seems to be important as well. A session that lasts between 45 and 90 minutes falls within the ultradian rhythm pattern, thus working within the body's natural balance.

It will take many years before we understand the magnitude of influences that affect our body rhythms. Current research is being done regarding the possibility of disease processes resulting from disruption in body rhythms, as well as the effects of

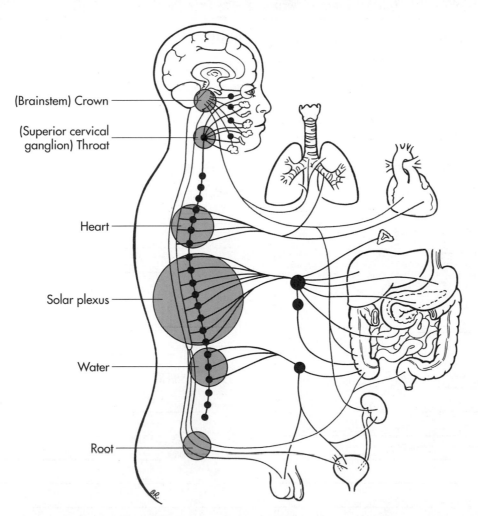

FIGURE 2-2 Comparison of the autonomic nervous system, traditional energy centers, and biologic oscillators. (From Fritz S: *Mosby's fundamentals of therapeutic massage,* St Louis, 1995, Mosby.)

work environments that directly disturb or alter natural body rhythms (Activity 2-3).

Mechanisms of Disease: Pathology

Massage, other forms of soft tissue bodywork, exercise, and movement therapies focus on maintaining health or a balanced state of physical, emotional, social, and spiritual well-being—homeostasis. Health is the result of the organism's effective adaptation to change. Disease occurs when the demand to adapt exceeds the ability of the body and imbalance results. Soft tissue and movement therapies support the body in maintaining or returning it to a "healthy state"—homeostasis. To accomplish both, soft tissue and movement professionals require a knowledge base and understanding of both the normal function of the body and the abnormal body functions of disease states:

- *Disease* can be described as an abnormality in functions of the body, especially when the abnormality threatens well-being.
- *Pathology* is the study of disease.
- *Epidemiology* is the field of science that studies the frequency, transmission, occurrence, and distribution of disease in humans.
- *Pharmacology* deals with the preparation and action of medications and their use to treat or prevent a disease.

ACTIVITY 2-3

The following exercise will demonstrate the entrainment process as part of your understanding of your own body rhythm.

First, take your pulse to measure heart rate.

Next, measure your respiration rate by counting the number of breaths taken in a 60-second period.

Now play some music and listen to it for about 5 minutes. Retake your pulse and recount your respiration rate.

Notice if any change occurs.

Repeat the exercise two more times with different types and tempos of music.

PREASSESSMENT

Pulse rate _____

Respiration rate _____

MUSIC

Type _____

Beats per minute _____

POSTASSESSMENT

Pulse rate _____

Respiration rate _____

Describe the change _____

_____

_____

_____

MUSIC

Type _____

Beats per minute _____

POSTASSESSMENT

Pulse rate _____

Respiration rate _____

Describe the change _____

_____

_____

_____

_____

MUSIC

Type _____

Beats per minute _____

POSTASSESSMENT

Pulse rate _____

Respiration rate _____

Describe the change _____

_____

_____

_____

Signs are objective changes that can be seen or measured by someone other than the client.

Symptoms are the subjective changes noticed or felt only by the client.

A *syndrome* is a group of different signs and symptoms that identify a pathologic condition, especially when they have a common cause.

Acute disease has a specific beginning, signs, and symptoms that develop quickly, last a short time, then disappear.

Chronic disease has a vague onset, develops slowly, and lasts for a long time, sometimes for life.

Communicable diseases can be transmitted from one person to another.

Subacute refers to diseases with characteristics between acute and chronic.

Etiology is the study of all the factors involved in causing a disease.

Diseases with undetermined causes are said to be *idiopathic*.

Pathogenesis follows the development of a disease. For example, flu begins with a latent or nonactive stage, during which the virus becomes established. When a disease is infectious, this stage is called the *incubation* stage. After the disease develops and has run its course, body functions return to normal during the *convalescence* stage.

Remission is a reversal of signs and symptoms that occurs in chronic diseases. This can be a temporary or permanent condition.

Diagnosis occurs when a licensed medical professional categorizes disease by identifying its signs and symptoms.

As stated previously, homeostasis is the relatively constant state of the body's internal environment. If a disease process disturbs homeostasis, a variety of feedback mechanisms usually attempt to return the body to health. A disease condition exists when homeostasis cannot be easily restored. In acute conditions the body recovers its homeostatic balance quickly. In chronic diseases a normal state of balance may never be restored (Thibodeau, 1997).

According to Thibodeau and Patton (1997), disturbances in homeostasis may occur from many different sources:

1. **Genetic mechanisms**—Altered or mutated genes can cause abnormality.

2. **Physical and chemical agents**—Toxic or destructive chemicals, extreme heat or cold, mechanical injury, and radiation can affect the normal homeostasis of the body.

3. **Malnutrition**—Insufficient or imbalanced intake of nutrients can cause a variety of diseases.

4. **Degeneration**—Tissues sometimes break apart or degenerate. The cause is unknown. Degeneration is a normal consequence of aging. Degeneration of tissues can also result from disease.

5. **Hypersensitivity of the immune system**—Some diseases result from the immune system attacking the body (autoimmunity) and from mistakes or overreactions of the immune response. Allergy is the hypersensitivity of the immune system to relatively harmless environmental antigens. Steroid drugs are often used to treat autoimmune disease.

6. **Immune suppression or immune deficiency**—Some diseases are caused by the failure of the immune system's ability to defend against pathogens. The chief characteristic of immune deficiency is the development of unusual or recurring severe infections or cancer.

7. **Pathogenic organisms**—An organism that lives in or on another organism to obtain its nutrients is called a parasite. The presence of microscopic or larger parasites may interfere with normal body functions of the host and cause disease. Pathogenic organisms include the following:

   Viruses—Microscopic, intracellular parasites that consist of a nucleic acid core with a protein coat. Viruses invade a host cell and take over the cell function to produce more viruses.

   Bacteria—Tiny cells without nuclei that secrete toxins, eat body cells, or form colonies of bacteria.

   Fungi—Simple plantlike organisms that lack chlorophyll. Fungi are generally molds or yeast.

   Protozoa—Large one-celled organisms having organized nuclei such as amoebas.

   Pathogenic animals—Large multicellular organisms such as roundworms, flatworms, flukes, mites, and lice.

Medications and herbs used to treat pathogenic organisms are classified by type:

Bacteria—Antibiotics
Virus—Antivirals, vaccines
Fungi—Antifungals
Worms—Anthelmintics
Lice—Pediculicides
Scabies—Scabicides

8. **Tumors and cancer**—Abnormal tissue growths resulting from uncontrolled cell division called **hyperplasia** results in a **neoplasm** or tumor. Tumors can cause a variety of physiologic disruptions.

The **benign** tumor is contained and encapsulated. Benign tumors are relatively harmless, remain localized within the tissue from which they arose, and usually grow slowly. When they do interfere with function, it is because they crowd or block functioning tissue or press on pain-sensitive structures.

A *malignant tumor* (**cancer**) is a nonencapsulated mass that invades surrounding tissue rather than pushing it aside. In addition, malignant cells have the devastating ability to break away from the primary tumor and form secondary cancer masses. This ability of cells to break away is called *metastasis*. Malignant or cancerous tumors tend to spread to other regions of the body. The cells migrate by way of the lymphatic system or blood vessels. Cancer cells that do not metastasize can spread another way by growing rapidly and extending the tumor into nearby tissues. Malignant tumors can replace part of a vital organ with abnormal tissues, a life-threatening situation.

Generally speaking, cells that divide many times display increased mutation rates. Cells in the lymphatic system, epidermis, bone marrow, and gastrointestinal tract are more prone to the development of cancer than cells that do not divide rapidly such as nerve and muscle tissue.

The mechanism of all cancers is a mistake or problem in cell division called anaplasia. **Anaplasia is the reproduction of abnormal and undifferentiated cells that fail to mature into specialized cell types.** Mature specialized cell types display boundary recognition, and therefore they do not invade surrounding tissue. Abnormal undifferentiated cancer cells lack the ability to recognize boundaries and therefore invade and destroy surrounding tissue.

Certainly there is a life metaphor reflected in mature versus undifferentiated cell behavior. Even at the cellular level it is important to grow up and follow our life purpose, living in a way that respects the boundaries of others. When we don't know who we are, we have no purpose in life and act in an immature manner that invades others' boundaries; we function like a cancer in their lives.

At present, the following factors are known to play a role in the development of cancer:

1. **Genetic factors**—More than a dozen forms of cancer are known to be biologically inherited. Cancers with known genetic risk factors include basal cell carcinoma (a type of skin cancer), breast cancer, and neuroblastoma (a cancer of nerve tissue).
2. **Carcinogens**—Carcinogens are chemicals that affect genetic activity in some way, causing abnormal cell reproduction. Many industrial products are carcinogens. A variety of natural vegetable and animal materials are also carcinogenic.
3. **Age**—Certain cancers are found primarily in young people (e.g., leukemia) and others primarily in older adults (e.g., colon cancer). The age factor may result from changes in the genetic activity of cells over time or from accumulated effects of cell damage.
4. **Environment**—Exposure to damaging types of radiation or chronic mechanical injury can cause cancer. For example, sunlight can cause skin cancer, and breathing asbestos fibers can cause lung cancer (Thibodeau, 1997).

Cancer specialists, or *oncologists*, have summarized some major signs of early stages of cancer. Early detection of cancer is important because the stages of development of primary tumors, before metastasis and the development of secondary tumors have begun, are when cancer is most treatable. Several warning signs of cancer are listed in Box 2-2.

Drugs used to treat cancer are called *antineoplastics*. Most of the drugs in this category prevent the growth of rapidly dividing cells. One of the side effects is that they affect epithelial cells, which also rapidly divide, and as a result, antineoplastic drugs interfere with the function of the epithelial tissues and tissue repair.

BOX 2-2

WARNING SIGNS OF CANCER

Sores that do not heal
Unusual bleeding
A change in a wart or mole
A lump or thickening in any tissue
Persistent hoarseness or cough
Chronic indigestion
A change in bowel or bladder function

From Thibodeau GA and Patton KT: *The human body in health and disease*, ed 2, St Louis, 1997, Mosby.

9. Inflammatory response—The body often responds to homeostatic disturbances with the inflammatory response. Inflammation may occur as a response to any tissue injury. The inflammatory response is a normal mechanism that usually speeds recovery from an infection or injury. Disease symptoms can occur when the inflammatory response activates at inappropriate times or is abnormally prolonged or severe, resulting in damage to normal tissues.

The inflammatory response is a combination of processes that attempt to minimize injury to tissues, thus maintaining homeostasis. Inflammation may also accompany specific immune system reactions.

The inflammatory response has four primary signs (Figure 2-3):

Heat and redness—As tissue cells are damaged, they release inflammation mediators such as histamine, prostaglandins, and compounds called kinins. Some inflammation mediators (histamine and bradykinin) cause blood vessels to dilate, increasing blood volume in the tissue. Increased blood volume produces the heat and redness of inflammation. This response is important because it allows immune system cells (white blood cells: neutrophils, monocytes, macrophages) in the blood to travel quickly and easily to the site of injury. These cells attach themselves to the pathogens to be destroyed, especially if tagged with antibodies (proteins that mark pathogens).

Swelling and pain—Some inflammation mediators increase the permeability of blood vessel walls. As water leaks out of the vessel, tissue swelling or edema results. The pressure caused by edema triggers pain receptors. The fluid that accumulates in inflamed tissue is called *inflammatory exudate* and has the beneficial effect of diluting the irritant. Inflammatory exudate is slowly removed by lymphatic vessels. Bacteria and damaged cells are held in the lymph nodes and destroyed by white blood cells. This causes the lymph nodes to enlarge when they process a large amount of infectious material.

TISSUE REPAIR

The processes of inflammation eventually eliminate the irritant, and tissue repair can begin. Tissues have two cell types: parenchyma cells perform the tissue *functions* and stroma cells provide the tissue *structure.* Tissue repair is the replacement of dead cells with living cells. In a type of tissue repair called *regeneration (parenchyma cells)* the new cells are similar to those that they replace. Another type of tissue repair is *replacement (stroma cells).* The new cells are formed from connective tissue. These stroma cells are different from those that they replace, resulting in a scar. Collagen is the chief constituent of scar tissue. Factors that promote collagen formation and health are vitamin C and adequate nutrition, in particular protein. Often, fibrous connective tissue replaces the damaged tissue, resulting in a condition called *fibrosis.* Most tissue repairs are a combination of regeneration and replacement.

Cells regenerate at different degrees and rates. *Labile cells* regenerate easily and quickly. These are cells of the lymphatic system, epidermis, bone marrow, and gastrointestinal tract. *Stable cells,* the most common cell type, regenerate at slower rates. These are the parenchymal or epithelial portion of an organ or gland and the connective tissue or stroma. For example, intestinal cells regenerate in 1 to 2 days, liver cells in 3 to 5 days, and kidney cells in 7 to 14 days.

Total tissue repair can take 4 weeks or longer. Permanent cells, such as nerve and muscle cells, do

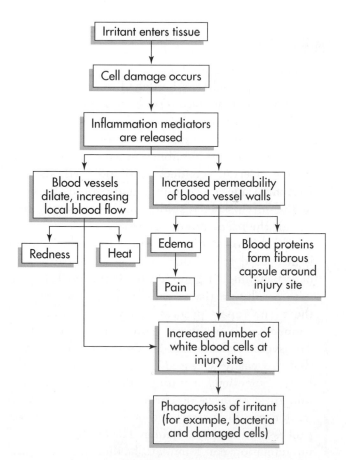

FIGURE 2-3 Inflammatory response.

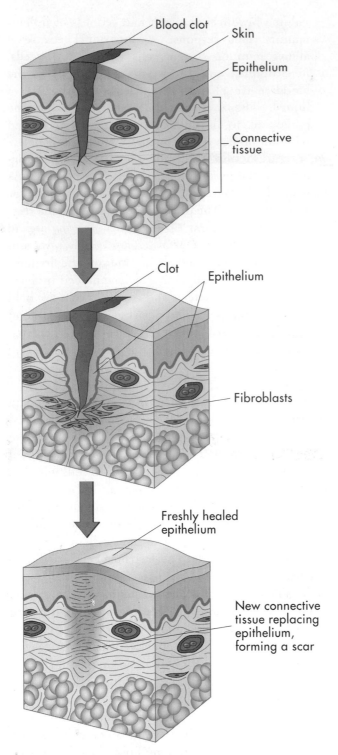

Blood clot

Skin

Epithelium

Connective
tissue

Clot

Epithelium

Fibroblasts

Freshly healed
epithelium

New connective
tissue replacing
epithelium,
forming a scar

FIGURE 2-4 Healing of a minor wound. When a minor injury damages a layer of epithelium and the underlying connective tissue (as in a minor skin cut), the epithelial tissue and the connective tissue can self-repair. (From Thibodeau GA, Patton KT: *Anatomy and physiology,* ed 3, St Louis, 1996, Mosby.)

not regenerate well if at all, and when they do, it is a slow process that takes months. Bodywork practitioners should wait at least 30 to 45 days before working close to an area of tissue repair so as not to disturb the repair formation.

A goal in the healing process is to promote regeneration and keep replacement to a minimum (Figure 2-4).

INFLAMMATORY DISEASE

Local **inflammation** occurs in a small area. If the irritant spreads throughout the body or causes changes in areas other than remaining local, it is called a systemic inflammation. When inflammation becomes chronic and stays active for a longer period than benefits the body or is more intense than seems necessary, it may be called an inflammatory disease. Such systemic inflammations that may become diseases include arthritis, asthma, eczema, and bronchitis.

Treatments

Antiinflammatory and steroid medications are used to treat inflammation. Antihistamines and aspirin can both be used to suppress inflammatory responses.

PRACTICAL APPLICATION

Some soft tissue methods can be used to deliberately create mild and controlled inflammation. Methods such as transverse friction create a localized inflammatory response to stimulate tissue reorganization in areas of adhesion and scarring. Acupuncture and moxibustion cause mild inflammation. Certain connective tissue methods and stretching methods can pull apart microadhesions in the soft tissue, resulting in inflammation that signals the tissue repair process.

The controlled use of therapeutic inflammation is also used to stabilize lax ligaments caused by overstretching, degeneration, or injury. Injection with a solution that creates inflammation signals the tissue repair process to lay down additional connective tissue fibers, reinforcing the ligament. Transverse friction can be used as well in areas that are easily accessed from the surface of the body. Sometimes creating controlled inflammation over an area of chronic soft tissue inflammation can jump start the body into a resolution process and support healing. The controlled use of inflammation can stimulate healing and, coupled with appropriate rehabilitation, is a very effective approach in dealing with these situations.

The key in these methods is to use just enough therapeutic inflammation to encourage the body to restore homeostasis and avoid overstressing the system. These types of methods should not be used on someone with systemic inflammation, such as systemic lupus erythematosus, or when tissue repair mechanisms are compromised, such as in fibromyalgia. Proper training in these methods must include a clear understanding of anatomy to provide specificity, exact application of technique to obtain the desired results, and an understanding of the physiology of the inflammation and healing processes.

RISK FACTORS

Certain predisposing conditions may make a disease more likely to develop. Usually called risk factors, these conditions may put one at risk for a disease but often do not actually cause a disease.

Some major types of risk factors follow (Thibodeau, 1997) (Activity 2-4):

1. Genetic factors—Several types of genetic risk factors exist. An inherited trait can put a person at a greater than normal risk for a specific disease developing. Family history of a disease process and causes of death can usually reveal possible familial genetic traits. Steps can be taken to sup-

ACTIVITY 2-4

Using the aforementioned factors disrupting homeostasis and risk factors, do a personal health assessment.

Example

Genetic mechanisms: My family has a tendency to have strokes, heart attacks, and joint problems.

Physical and chemical agents: I grew up in an environment with heavy secondary cigarette smoke.

Nutrition: I do not eat enough fresh vegetables and I eat on the run all the time.

Degeneration: I have degenerative disk problems.

Immune hypersensitivity: I have some allergy to pollens.

Immune deficiency: I get upper respiratory problems when my immune system is depressed.

Viruses: I am susceptible to flu, colds, and herpes simplex when stressed and tired.

Fungi: I used to get yeast infections in my teens and 20s.

Protozoa: N/A.

Pathogenic animals: N/A.

Tumors and cancer: N/A.

Inflammatory response: I have chronic inflammation in my back.

Environment: I work in a clean environment with natural light. I live in an area I like, but my sleep is sometimes interrupted from highway noise.

Age: I am in my 40s and am experiencing age-related hormone changes and weight gain.

Lifestyle: My lifestyle is extremely busy with demands from many people. I work 60 to 70 hours per week, but I am able to maintain a regular sleep schedule. I exercise moderately, eat too much fat, have never smoked, and do not drink alcohol or use drugs.

Stress: I am a single parent of three. I have many people in my life with many different types of needs. I have many agencies to answer to and feel stressed by the bureaucratic expectations.

Preexisting conditions: I have disk dysfunction, an endocrine problem, and inner ear balance syndrome, hyperventilation tendencies, and dyslexia.

Considering this information, how would you rate your personal health history on a scale of 1 to 10, with 10 being excellent health? To what types of disease processes do you feel you are most susceptible? What could you do to support your personal homeostasis?

Example: In general my health is good, an 8 on the scale. The inner ear problem creates physiologic confusion and nausea that adds to my stress levels. The back and endocrine problems have stabilized but have to be managed. The hyperventilation is under control. I take fairly good care of myself and use some nutritional supplements to balance my diet. If I get enough sleep and exercise, I do better. I feel that I am most susceptible to cardiovascular disease, joint problems, and osteoporosis. Continued attention to diet and exercise, coupled with therapeutic massage to manage my back and stress level, seems to be working.

Your Turn

Genetic mechanisms: _____

_____

Physical and chemical agents: _____

_____

Continued

port the body against the genetic tendency toward a disease process (e.g., changes in diet and lifestyle).

2. Age—Biologic and behavioral factors increase the risk for certain diseases to develop at certain times in life. For example, musculoskeletal problems are common between ages of 30 and 50.

3. Lifestyle—The way we live and work can put us at risk for some diseases. Some researchers believe that the high-fat, low-fiber diet common among people in the "developed" nations increases their risk of certain types of cancer developing. Smoking, excessive use of alcohol, lack of exercise, and poor sleep habits are examples of negative lifestyles.

4. Stress—Stress may be defined as any substantial change in your routine or any activity that causes the body to adapt. This will make demands on mental and emotional resources. Research has shown that as stresses accumulate, an individual becomes increasingly susceptible to physical, mental, and emotional problems and accidental injuries.

5. Environment—Some environmental situations put us at greater risk for getting certain diseases. For example, living in high concentrations of air pollution may increase the risk for respiratory problems.

6. Preexisting conditions—A primary (preexisting) condition can put a person at risk of a secondary condition developing. For example, a viral infection can compromise the immune system and make the person more susceptible to bacterial infection.

ACTIVITY 2-4—cont'd

Nutrition: _____

Degeneration: _____
_____

Immune hypersensitivity: _____

Immune deficiency: _____

Viruses: _____

Fungi: _____

Protozoa: _____

Pathogenic animals: _____

Tumors and cancer: _____

Inflammatory response: _____

Environment: _____
_____

Age: _____
_____

Lifestyle: _____
_____

Stress: _____
_____

Preexisting conditions: _____
_____

Considering this information, how would you rate your personal health history on a scale of 1 to 10, with 10 being excellent health? To what types of disease processes do you feel you are most susceptible? What could you do to support your personal homeostasis?

_____
_____
_____
_____
_____

Pain

Pain is a complex, private, abstract experience, difficult to explain or describe. It is the number one symptom or complaint that causes people to seek health care, and its effective management is a major challenge. Defining pain in descriptive and measurable terms is not easy because pain has a physiologic, psychologic, and social aspect.

PAIN SENSATIONS

We need the sensations we get from pain to live a normal life. These sensations provide us enough information about potential tissue damage to help us protect ourselves from greater damage. It is pain that often initiates the search for medical assistance. The subjective description and indication of the location of the pain helps to pinpoint the underlying cause of disease. The receptors for pain, called *nociceptors*, are simply the branching ends of the dendrites (projections from the nerve cell body) of certain sensory neurons. Pain receptors are found in practically every tissue of the body, and they may respond to any type of stimulus. When stimuli for other sensations, such as touch, pressure, heat, and cold, reach a certain intensity, they stimulate the sensation of pain as well. Injured tissue releases bradykinin, which causes the release of inflammatory chemicals such as histamine and prostaglandins, making peripheral nociceptors more sensitive to the normal pain response. This increased sensitivity to pain is called *hyperalgesia*.

As stated previously, excessive stimulation of a sensory organ causes pain. Additional or excessive stimuli for pain receptors includes distention or dilation of a structure, prolonged muscular contractions, muscle spasms, inadequate blood flow to an organ, or the presence of certain chemical substances. Pain receptors, because of their sensitivity to all stimuli, perform a protective function by identifying changes that may endanger the body. Pain receptors adapt only slightly or not at all. Adaptation is the decrease or disappearance of the perception of a sensation even though the stimulus is still present. An example is getting used to our clothes soon after dressing. If adaptation to pain occurred, the stimuli would cease to be sensed and irreparable damage could result.

Sensory impulses for pain are controlled by the central nervous system along spinal and cranial nerves to the thalamus. From here the impulses may be relayed to the parietal lobe. Recognition of the kind and intensity of most pain is ultimately localized in the cerebral cortex. Some awareness of pain also occurs at subcortical (under the cortex) levels.

Acute pain is either a symptom of a disease condition or a temporary aspect of medical treatment. It acts as a warning signal because it can activate the sympathetic nervous system. It is usually temporary, of sudden onset, and easily localized. The person can frequently describe the pain, which often subsides with or without treatment.

Chronic pain is also a symptom of a disease condition but is identified as a major health problem, with about 25% of the population affected. Chronic pain is a symptom that persists or recurs for indefinite periods, usually for more than 6 months. It frequently has an obscure onset, and the character and quality of the pain change over time. The pain is usually diffused, poorly localized, and often requires the efforts of a multidisciplinary health care team for its effective management.

Intractable pain occurs when chronic pain persists even if treatment is provided or when chronic pain exists without active disease. This represents the greatest challenge to all health care providers. Short temporary symptomatic relief from this type from pain may be provided by soft tissue approaches.

Specific types of pain include the following:

1. Pricking or bright pain—This type of pain exists when the skin is cut or jabbed with a sharp object. It is short lived but intense and easily localized. It is sometimes termed *superficial somatic pain*.
2. Burning pain—This type of pain is slower to develop, lasts longer, and is less accurately localized (e.g., when the skin is burned). This type of pain often stimulates cardiac and respiratory activity.
3. Aching pain—Aching pain occurs when the visceral organs are stimulated. It is constant, not well localized, and is often referred to areas of the body at a distance from where the damage may be occurring. It is important because it may be a sign of a life-threatening disorder of a vital organ.
4. Deep pain—The main difference between superficial and deep pain is the nature of the pain evoked by noxious stimuli. Unlike superficial pain, deep pain is poorly localized, nauseating, and frequently associated with sweating and changes in blood pressure. Deep pain initiates reflex contraction of nearby skeletal muscles. This reflex contraction is similar to the muscle spasm associated with injuries to bones, tendons, and

joints. The steadily contracting muscles become ischemic (lacking in oxygen), and ischemia stimulates the pain receptors in the muscles. The pain, in turn, initiates more spasms, setting up a vicious circle (Figure 2-5).

5. Muscle pain—If a muscle contracts rhythmically in the presence of an adequate blood supply, pain does not usually result. However, if the blood supply to a muscle is occluded (closed off), the same rhythmic contraction soon causes pain. The pain persists even after the contraction until blood flow is reestablished. If a muscle with a normal blood supply is made to contract continuously without periods of relaxation, it also begins to ache because the maintained contraction compresses the blood vessels supplying the muscle and not enough blood is supplied.

Let's look at pain in two other ways: somatic and visceral. **Somatic pain** arises from stimulation of receptors in the skin (*superficial* somatic pain) or from stimulation of receptors in skeletal muscles, joints, tendons, and fascia, (*deep* somatic pain). **Visceral pain** results from stimulation of receptors in the viscera (any of our internal organs).

Superficial somatic pain is transmitted along finely myelinated A delta nerve fibers at a very fast rate. Deep somatic pain and most visceral pain are transmitted slowly by unmyelinated C nerve fibers.

This speed difference in transmission of pain signals is why superficial somatic stimulation transmitted on A delta fibers can block or mask deep somatic or visceral pain. Stimulation of more A-fibers than C-fibers blocks the C-fiber transmission from entering the spinal cord. If the signal does not enter the spinal cord, it cannot be felt as pain. Methods of touch and pressure and most methods of movement are transmitted on A-fibers; any stimuli of this type will increase A-fiber transmission. Treating pain in this way is called counterirritation (Figure 2-6).

REFERRED PAIN

The ability of the cerebral cortex to locate the origin of pain is related to past experience. In most instances of somatic pain and in some instances of visceral pain, the cortex accurately projects the pain back to the stimulated area.

The pain may also be felt in a surface area far from the stimulated organ. This phenomenon is called *referred pain*. In general, the area to which the pain is

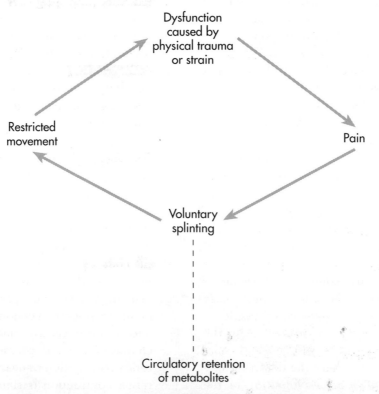

FIGURE 2-5   Pain-spasm-pain cycle. (From Fritz S: *Mosby's fundamentals of therapeutic massage*, St Louis, 1995, Mosby.)

referred and the visceral organ that is stimulated receive their innervation from the same segment of the spinal cord. Because of this, the cortex may misinterpret the source. Consider the following examples. The pain of a heart attack is typically felt in the skin over the heart and along the left arm. The same factor is at work with the referred pain in the shoulder caused by gallstone pain. Figure 2-7 illustrates cutaneous (skin) regions to which visceral pain may be referred. If the client has a recurring pain pattern that resembles patterns on the chart, refer him to the physician for an accurate diagnosis.

As already stated, irritation of the viscera frequently produces pain that is felt not in the viscera but in some somatic structure that may be a considerable distance away from the viscera. Such pain is said to be referred to the somatic structure. Deep somatic pain may also be referred, but superficial pain is not. When visceral pain is both local and referred, it sometimes seems to spread (radiate) from the local to the distant site.

Visceral pain, like deep somatic pain, initiates reflex contraction of nearby skeletal muscle. Because somatic pain is much more common than visceral pain, the brain has "learned" to project the pain to the somatic area and initiate the reflex contraction there.

Obviously, a knowledge of referred pain and the common sites of pain referral from each of the viscera

are very important to bodywork practitioners and other health care professionals. The most common example of referred pain is that of a heart attack, which often appears as chest pain. Another example is pain in the tip of the shoulder, which may be due to irritation in the central portion of the diaphragm. However, it is important to remember that sites of reference are not stereotyped, and unusual reference sites occur with considerable frequency. Heart pain, for instance, may be experienced as purely abdominal, may be referred to the right arm, and may even be referred to the neck.

As previously noted, past experience plays an important role in referred pain. Although pain originating in an inflamed abdominal organ is usually referred to the midline, in clients who have had previous abdominal surgery, the pain of an inflamed abdominal organ is frequently referred to their surgical scars. Pain originating in the maxillary sinus is usually referred to nearby teeth, but in clients with a history of traumatic dental work, such pain is regularly referred to the previously traumatized teeth. This is true even if the teeth are a distance away from the sinus.

When pain is referred, it is usually to a structure that developed from the same embryonic segment or is located in the same dermatome as the structure in which the pain originates. For example, during embryonic development, the diaphragm moves from the neck to its adult location in the abdomen and takes its nerve supply, the phrenic nerve, with it. One third of the fibers in the phrenic nerve are afferent, and they enter the spinal cord at the level of the second to fourth cervical segments, the same location at which afferent nerves from the tip of the shoulder enter. Similarly, the heart and the arm have the same embryonic segmental origin (Fritz, 1995) (Figure 2-8).

PHANTOM PAIN

A kind of pain frequently experienced by people who have had a limb amputated is called **phantom pain.** They experience pain or other sensations in the extremity as if the limb were still there. It is suspected that phantom pain occurs because the remaining proximal portions of the sensory nerves that previously received impulses from the limb are being stimulated by the trauma of the amputation. Stimuli from these nerves are interpreted by the brain as coming from the nonexistent (phantom) limb.

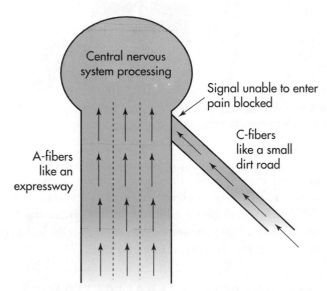

Central nervous system processing

Signal unable to enter pain blocked

C-fibers like a small dirt road

A-fibers like an expressway

Touch, pressure, movement or moderate acute pain purposefully applied = counter irritation which may provide hyperstimulation analgesia.

FIGURE 2-6 Gate control theory of pain (based on Melzack and Wall's gate control theory of pain).

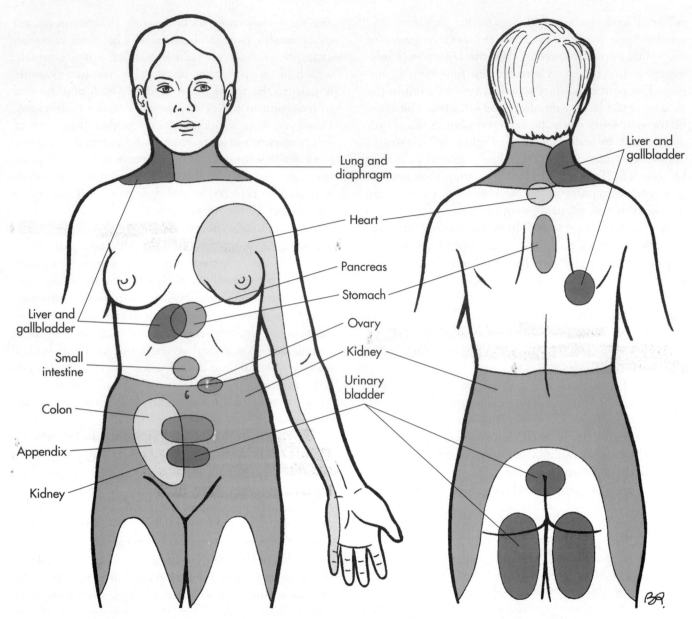

FIGURE 2-7 Referred pain. The diagram indicates cutaneous areas to which visceral pains may be referred. The professional encountering pain in these areas needs to refer the client for diagnosis to rule out visceral dysfunction. (From Fritz S: *Mosby's fundamentals of therapeutic massage,* St Louis, 1995, Mosby.)

PAIN THRESHOLD AND TOLERANCE

Pain may be brought on by mechanical, electrical, thermal, or chemical stimuli. We do not appear to adapt to pain or accommodate to it. We all have about the same threshold for pain. A pain threshold is when stimulation becomes intense enough to initiate the firing of pain receptors. Pain tolerance is how we respond to pain (Activity 2-5). Pain tolerance varies considerably and is heavily influenced by cultural and psychologic factors. Pain tolerance is modified by age and emotional and mental state. Subjective measurements of pain intensity are more reliable than the observable ones. Only the person in pain can determine the amount of

severity experienced. Pain is rarely the same at all times. It is felt (perceived) differently over time and differs with various precipitating and aggravating factors. Pain can range from excruciating to mild and may be difficult for the person to verbalize.

🖐 PRACTICAL APPLICATION

Pain is a complex problem with physical, psychologic, social, and financial components. The vast difference in the experience of pain in humans suggests that natural neural mechanisms must exist to modulate pain transmission and percep-

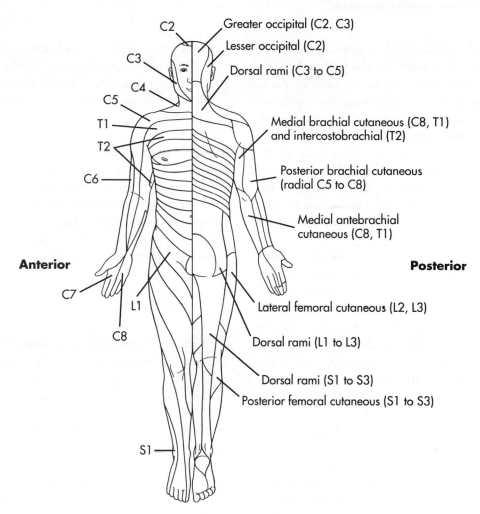

FIGURE 2-8 Dermatomal map (anterior view) and cutaneous nerve distribution (posterior view) of the human body. (From Greenstein GM: *Clinical assessment of neuromusculoskeletal disorders*, St Louis, 1997, Mosby.)

ACTIVITY 2-5

List three personal factors that could change your pain tolerance.

Examples

THINGS THAT COULD INCREASE PAIN TOLERANCE

1. Reading a good book
2. Going for a walk
3. Practicing relaxation techniques

THINGS THAT COULD DECREASE PAIN TOLERANCE

1. Being tired and upset with the kids
2. Driving in heavy traffic
3. Loud music

Your Turn

THINGS THAT COULD INCREASE MY PAIN TOLERANCE

THINGS THAT COULD DECREASE MY PAIN TOLERANCE

tion. Beta-endorphins and enkephalins, both natural opiates, are released in the body when we are in pain and reduce our perception of pain. Stimulus-induced forms of analgesia such as acupuncture, massage, and other forms of bodywork, hydrotherapy, and exercise are all believed to tap into these natural opiate pathways. Counterirritation from touch and movement therapies are viable explanations for why these approaches are effective in pain management because they release endorphins and enkephalins.

Alleviation of pain can be accomplished in many ways. The bodywork professional, as part of a health care team, can contribute valuable manual therapy for various painful conditions with direct tissue manipulation and reflex stimulation of the nervous system and the circulation. Touch and movement, when used as a therapeutic intervention, may help reduce the need for pain medication, thus reducing its resultant side effects. Clients in intense pain must have their therapy monitored by a physician or other appropriate health care professional. Most people experience less extreme pain occasionally throughout life. Bodywork approaches may provide temporary symptomatic relief for moderate pain brought on by daily stress, reducing or eliminating over-the-counter pain medications, but if any pain persists, the client should be referred to a physician.

Medications called analgesics are the most commonly used to treat pain; they may be narcotic or nonnarcotic. Aspirin and other nonsteroidal anti-inflammatory medications inhibit the action of prostaglandins (tissue hormones) and relieve pain. Herbs such as meadowsweet, passion flower, and red pepper may provide some relief.

NOTE: For sufficient information to deal with pain situations presented by clients, a pathology text and a reference text of pharmaceuticals would be helpful. Texts written for nurses often provide the most useful information for both pathology and pharmaceuticals. Suggestions are included in the Works Consulted list at the back of this book.

Mechanisms of Health

A state of health is supported by a balanced lifestyle. Whereas disease reflects states of the "too much" or "not enough" ends of the continuum of imbalance; health is that state of "just right" or homeostasis.

Health is influenced by many factors, including inherited and constitutional conditions. Lifestyle, activity level, rest, loving relationships, exercise, diet, empowering beliefs and attitudes, self-esteem, authentic personality, and freedom from self-hindering patterns all support health.

Each individual will need to understand his own body, mind, and spiritual self as he seeks balance to allow the body to maintain a dynamic state of homeostasis (Activity 2-6).

ACTIVITY 2-6

This affords you an extensive look at your health profile. Complete the following statements by providing three different responses to each statement.

Example

My lifestyle supports health in the following ways:
1. I am involved in work that I love.
2. I am surrounded by information.
3. I am financially stable.
My lifestyle does not support health in the following ways:
1. I work too many hours.
2. I am overwhelmed with too much to know and understand.
3. I have a lot of debt.

Your Turn

My lifestyle supports health in the following ways:

1. _____

2. _____

3. _____

My lifestyle does not support health in the following ways:

1. _____

2. _____

3. _____

ACTIVITY 2-6—cont'd

My activity level supports health in the following ways:

1. _____
2. _____
3. _____

My activity level does not support health in the following ways:

1. _____
2. _____
3. _____

My rest pattern supports health in the following ways:

1. _____
2. _____
3. _____

My rest pattern does not support health in the following ways:

1. _____
2. _____
3. _____

My relationships support health in the following ways:

1. _____
2. _____
3. _____

My relationships do not support health in the following ways:

1. _____
2. _____
3. _____

My aerobic exercise supports health in the following ways:

1. _____
2. _____
3. _____

My aerobic exercise does not support health in the following ways:

1. _____
2. _____
3. _____

My diet supports health in the following ways:

1. _____
2. _____
3. _____

My diet does not support health in the following ways:

1. _____
2. _____
3. _____

My beliefs and attitudes support health in the following ways:

1. _____
2. _____
3. _____

My beliefs and attitudes do not support health in the following ways:

1. _____
2. _____
3. _____

My self-esteem supports health in the following ways:

1. _____
2. _____
3. _____

My self-esteem does not support health in the following ways:

1. _____
2. _____
3. _____

My personality supports health in the following ways:

1. _____
2. _____
3. _____

My personality does not support health in the following ways:

1. _____
2. _____
3. _____

Stress Management

Maintaining and supporting health requires us to effectively manage stress and stressors. A stressor is not always a negative event. A wedding and a funeral may be equally stressful.

Exposures to intense or extreme stressors (too much) and deprivation of necessary stimuli (too little) can cause imbalance and thus many problems. Too much heat, cold, noise, activity, exercise, food, or social demands, or not enough food, touch, social interaction, or sleep can all be detrimental to health. It is our continued need to respond or change to maintain homeostasis that increases the effects of stress (Figure 2-9, *A* to *D*).

STRESS

Our perception of a stressor is important. Anything we perceive as a threat, whether real or imagined, arouses fear or anxiety. How we respond is influenced by other conditions, some of which are under our control and some that are not. Our physical and mental health; hereditary predisposition and genetics; past experiences; current coping habits, both learned and inborn; diet; environment; and social support determine which stimuli are interpreted as stressors for each individual.

Hans Selye's groundbreaking work began in 1935 and was formalized in his book *The Stress of Life* published in 1956. Selye's research laid the foundation of current concepts about stress.

Selye called the body's response to stress the *general adaptation syndrome,* which he suggested be divided into three stages. The first stage is the alarm reaction, also called the fight-or-flight response, which is the body's initial reaction to the perceived stressor. The second stage is known as the resistance reaction, which, through the secretion of regulating hormones, allows the body to continue fighting a stressor long after the effects of the alarm reaction have dissipated. The third stage is exhaustion reaction, which takes place if the stress response continues without relief. General adaptation is a uniform, consistent general response to the perceived stimuli.

The word stress is currently used to refer to any stimulus that either directly or indirectly stimulates neurons of the hypothalamus to release corticotrophin-releasing hormone. The term *general-adaptation syndrome* is also often used to describe the way the body mobilizes different defense mechanisms when threatened by harmful (actual or perceived) stimuli. In generalized stress conditions the hypothalamus acts on the anterior pituitary gland to cause the release of adrenocorticotropic hormone, which in turn stimulates the adrenal cortex to secrete glucocorticoid. Glucocorticoids are a class of adrenal cortical hormones that work to protect our bodies against stress and aid in protein and carbohydrate metabolism. They also work to provide an antiinflammatory effect, assist in the release of amino acids from muscle, mobilize fatty acids from fat stores, increase the ability of skeletal muscles to maintain contraction and thus avoid fatigue, and increase adenosine triphosphate production.

In addition to causing glucocorticoid release, the adrenal medulla stimulates the release of epinephrine and norepinephrine to help the body in its response to stress. However, during periods of prolonged stress, continued release of these hormones may have harmful side effects, such as decreased immune response, lowered blood glucose levels, and altered protein and fat metabolism, which in turn decreases our resistance to stress. Therefore the continued releases of epinephrine and norepinephrine increase the possibility of high blood pressure, decreased digestion, reduced tissue repair, and more (Figure 2-10).

People who experience excessive or ongoing stress often express being overwhelmed by tension, anger, fear, and frustration, resulting in feelings of anxiety. This causes adrenaline levels to rise, blood pressure and heart rate to increase, and breathing to change. Overbreathing often results in overoxygenation of the blood, reducing carbon dioxide levels, which leads to the hyperventilation syndrome. This can be the beginning of panic attacks. Blood levels of glucose and fatty acids rise. This combination will eventually lead to plaque being laid down in the arteries and the development of coronary artery disease. Immune function becomes less effective, and the body is not as able to deal with pathogens or cancer cells. Often a decrease in memory and the ability to concentrate or problem solve occurs; susceptibility to infection increases; and complaints of stomach pain, heart palpitation, fatigue, and muscle aches are common. Sleep disorders and depression frequently accompany long-term stress. All these changes in our bodies are the result of prolonged stress.

Mood and behavior are affected by stress as well, and an ongoing interplay between physiologic and psychologic stress best described by the chicken and egg question of "which came first?" occurs. Certainly psychologic stress can result in physiologic response,

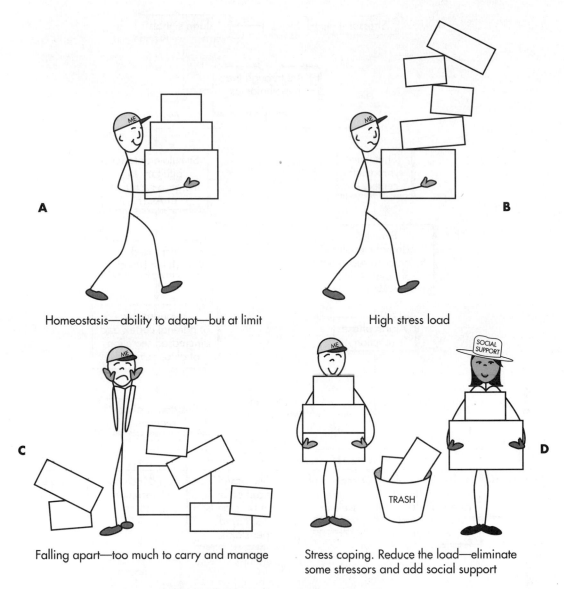

A Homeostasis—ability to adapt—but at limit

B High stress load

C Falling apart—too much to carry and manage

D Stress coping. Reduce the load—eliminate some stressors and add social support

It is not always the type of stress that causes problems, although some types of stress are more demanding than others. It is more the amount of the stress load and the need to balance many different things that cause breakdown. Many stressors cannot be easily altered, but the stress load can be managed through physical mechanisms such as exercise, diet, and relaxation methods that allow the body to better cope with those things that cannot be changed. The stress load can be lightened by eliminating those stressors possible and asking for help from social support such as family, friends and co-workers.

Activity:

In A, fill in the boxes with those stressors that you can manage. In B, again fill in the stressors from A, and add some additional stressors. In C, fill in the stressors you listed in B and add two more that would make the load too heavy. In D, identify the stressors that you can manage yourself. Write those in the boxes carried by the figure representing you. Identify two stressors that can be eliminated by putting them in the trash basket. Then identify two stressors that you can have someone help you with and write them in the boxes carried by the figure representing social support.

FIGURE 2-9 A to D, Stress load.

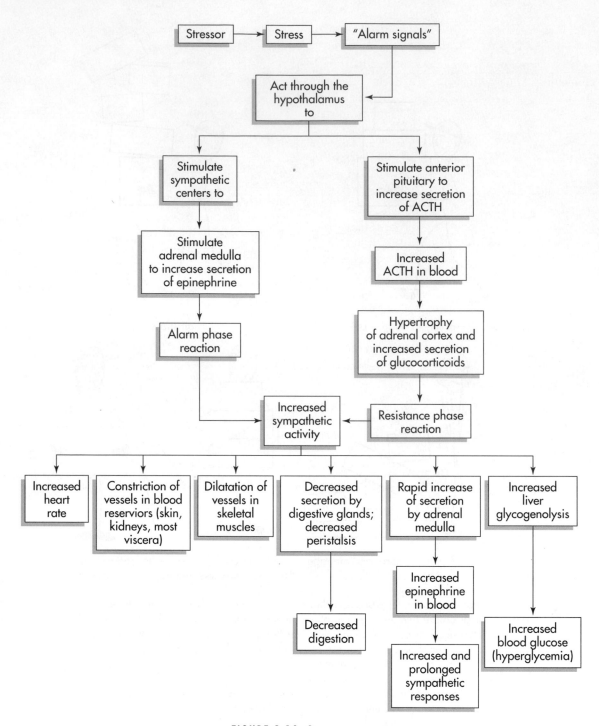

FIGURE 2-10 *Stress response.*

and the physiologic stress response alters perception, mood, thought processes, and behavior, thus creating psychologic stress.

When we see how many of our organs and glands are innervated by the autonomic nervous system, it is not surprising that there are such vast consequences to autonomic system disturbances. This is especially true of stress-induced diseases. A prolonged or excessive physiologic response to stress, the fight-or-flight response, can disrupt normal functioning—homeostasis—throughout the body. This reaction increases the strength and rate of the heartbeat, causes a rise in blood pressure, and results in hyperglycemia, pallor, coolness of skin, sweaty palms, and dry mouth. Water retention and increases in blood volume are caused by the increase in antidiuretic hormone and aldosterone secretion, which occurs as a result of stress.

Stress is considered a contributor or risk factor in many conditions. The following is a list of various areas susceptible to stress-related diseases, although the exact cause-and-effect relationship is often unclear:

Digestive tract—Diseases that may be either caused or aggravated by stress include gastritis, stomach and duodenal ulcers, ulcerative colitis, and irritable colon.

Reproductive organs—Stress-related problems include difficult conception or infertility, menstrual disorders or lack of menstrual periods in women, and impotence and premature ejaculation in men.

Bladder—A common stress response is sensitivity or irritability in the bladder, causing bladder urgency, bedwetting, or incontinence.

Brain—Many mental and emotional problems, among them anxiety, psychosis, and depression, may be triggered by stress.

Hair—Some forms of hair loss and baldness have been linked to high levels of stress.

Mouth—Sores, ulcers and oral lichen planus (thrush) often seem to develop under stress.

Lungs—Asthma symptoms often worsen under high levels of mental or emotional stress.

Heart—Heart rate disturbances and angina attacks often occur during or after periods of stress.

Muscles—Muscle tension and its associated pain are often the result of stress, as are an increase in muscle twitches and nervous tics. The muscular tremor of Parkinson's disease is also more marked at such times.

More and more people seek medical assistance to help sort out and identify stress-related symptoms. Because each of us responds to stress in very different ways, the possibility of an accurate diagnosis becomes difficult. This has led to frustration both with and by the health care systems. As more research is done in the area of stress coping, this situation is continuing to improve. Contemporary health care now recognizes excessive and long-term stress as an important and widespread cause of disease because stress disrupts homeostasis in numerous psychologic and physiologic control systems. Psychophysiology is the study of the interplay between psychologic and physiologic stressors and neuroimmunology, sometimes referred to as psychoneuroimmunology or the study of the mind-immunity link in uncovering the interaction of the mind/body connection.

Modern stress must be managed to support health. An increased openness, respect, and understanding of approaches, such as massage and other forms of bodywork along with acupuncture, meditation, and relaxation methods using breathing, biofeedback, music therapy, hypnosis, exercise, and other forms of movement therapy, exist as mechanisms that manage the stress response. Indigenous people's ancient health wisdom is now being understood through investigation by western scientific methods (Fritz, 1995).

Bodywork has been shown to reduce cortisol levels and decrease arousal of the sympathetic nervous system, resulting in reestablishment of homeostatic balance.

It is postulated that soft tissue and movement therapies introduce a different sort of stress into the system that the body can respond to and resolve through physiologic coping mechanisms. Because unresolved stress increases the intensity of the stress syndrome, the signals introduced by bodywork help reset the system, allowing for a more effective state of balance. Bodywork methods often have a pleasurable and comforting quality to them. They also can provide a soothing rhythmic pattern to which the recipient's body can entrain (organize and synchronize biologic rhythms). Bodywork is based on the premise of safe touch providing balanced sensory stimulation, which in turn supports health for its recipients.

Therefore soft tissue approaches can be an effective stress management tool. It is important to remember that the primary reason for the stress may require a multidisciplinary approach for resolution or effective long-term management, but soft tissue and movement modalities can play a part. Considering that it is the amount of stress instead of the type of stress coupled with a person's perception of the events, anything that can change the perception of threat to one of safety or reduce the intensity of the physical stress response is going to promote mechanisms of health. These supportive changes include effective sleep, reduction in pain perception, a sense of affiliation that supports effective social contact and support, and enhancement of the restorative and self-regulating process of the body.

The stress response and stress syndrome will be discussed throughout the text as it relates to each system studied. Because bodywork methods effectively deal with stress management, a thorough understanding of stress, stressors, and the stress response or syndrome is extremely important (Activity 2-7).

The Life Cycle

A human being is conceived by the joining of two cells, reinforcing the underlying concept of two opposites blending to make a whole. Cells multiply, divide, and differentiate, forming the organism. Birth brings forth an independent organism, which remains in a dependent functioning state while accelerated growth and development occur. The homeostatic mechanism of infants and young children are less regular because they are in the process of creating their bodies. From adolescence through middle adulthood we have the most efficient bodily func-

tions. Normal aging affects repair and replacement of the body's structural components. It is during the extremes of life, infancy and old age, when the body is presented its greatest challenges for homeostasis. Advancing age creates changes in cell number and ability to function effectively. Examples of decreased functional ability include muscle atrophy; loss of elasticity of the skin; and changes in the cardiovascular, respiratory, and skeletal systems. The term *atrophy* is used to describe the wasting effect of advancing age. In addition to structural atrophy the function of many physiologic control mechanisms also decreases and becomes less precise with advancing age. The aging process is cumulative, progressive, and natural.

Death can be thought of as the separation of structure (yin) and function (yang). In its purest form yang is totally immaterial and corresponds to pure

ACTIVITY 2-7

List three major stressors in your life:

Example   Losing car keys

Your Turn

1. _____

2. _____

3. _____

Now complete the following for each of the listed stressors:

When (the stressor) happens, I feel (What are the physical and emotional sensations experiences?). The result is (What do you do about the feelings?). What I could do to alleviate the stress response is (identify an activity that would restore homeostasis).

Example

When I lose my car keys, I feel very anxious and frustrated. My neck tenses up and I start to hyperventilate, which makes me feel light-headed, confused, and panicky. The result is that I begin to frantically look for my keys and start to

holler at anyone around. What I could do to alleviate the stress response is use a breathing method to reestablish the oxygen/carbon dioxide balance and reverse the hyperventilation.

Your Turn

Choose three different stressful situations and fill in the information.

When _____ happens:

I feel _____.

The result is _____.

What I could do to alleviate the stress response is _____.

When _____ happens:

I feel _____.

The result is _____.

What I could do to alleviate the stress response is _____.

When _____ happens:

I feel _____.

The result is _____

What I could do to alleviate the stress response is _____.

energy. Yin in its coarsest and most dense form is totally material and corresponds to matter. Yin and yang are essentially an expression of duality in time. Dying and gestation, death and birth are very similar processes. Metaphorically speaking, birth is anabolic and death is catabolic. The cycle of life is a balance of yin and yang: conception, gestation, birth, living, dying, and death.

Summary

In this chapter, we looked at homeostasis and factors influencing health and disease. Homeostasis consists of balancing mechanisms in constant communication with each other in a feedback loop system. Many factors can disrupt homeostasis, and yet in most situations the body is able to respond effectively and restore efficient functioning. We are equipped with the ability to deal with many different types of stressors. However, stress coping mechanisms can be overloaded with an accumulated heavy load of unresolved stress, which contributes to the development of disease and pain patterns. Many reasons exist for pain, and many types of pain and equally as many ways to manage pain exist. Acute pain can be a friend by alerting us to emergency situations. Even chronic pain can be a gauge by which to monitor the effectiveness of therapy and the return to health or as near health as possible. As stated, it is often the perception of a threat that makes the difference in the body's response to life events. Perception is something that can be altered with diligent work and awareness coupled with professional assistance when necessary. We are conceived, born, live, and die. As we travel through life, each event is equally important in the total experience of being. Physical, emotional, and spiritual health are our objectives.

WORKBOOK SECTION

1. Define homeostasis, self-regulatory mechanisms, and body rhythms in relationship to bodywork modalities and Oriental and Ayurvedic theories of health.

_____

_____

_____

_____

_____

_____

_____

2. Discuss and contrast the mechanisms of disease and health.

_____

_____

_____

_____

_____

_____

Define these terms:

1. Disease

_____

_____

2. Pathology

_____

_____

3. Etiology

_____

_____

4. Health

_____

_____

5. Pharmacology

_____

_____

6. Signs

_____

_____

7. Symptoms

_____

_____

8. Syndrome

_____

_____

9. Acute

_____

_____

10. Chronic

_____

_____

11. Subacute

_____

_____

12. Communicable diseases

_____

_____

13. Pathogenesis

_____

_____

14. Incubation

_____

_____

15. Convalescence

_____

_____

16. Remission

_____

_____

17. Carcinogens

_____

_____

18. Oncologist

_____

_____

19. Tissue repair

_____

_____

20. Regeneration

_____

_____

21. Replacement

_____

_____

EXERCISE

1. List sources that may disturb homeostasis.

_____

_____

_____

2. List the major risk factors in disease development.

_____

_____

_____

3. List the four primary signs of the inflammatory response.

_____

_____

4. Define pain and list the general and specific types of pain.

_____

_____

_____

_____

5. Identify viscerally referred pain patterns.

_____

_____

_____

_____

6. Explain phantom pain.

_____

_____

_____

7. List the factors influencing health.

_____

_____

_____

8. Identify factors contributing to the stress response and the body's response to stress.

_____

_____

_____

_____

_____

_____

_____

_____

_____

_____

_____

_____

9. List the stages in the cycle of life.

_____

_____

FILL IN THE BLANK

_____ (1) is the relatively constant state maintained by the physiology of the body. _____ (2) signals move toward a particular center or point of reference whereas _____ (3) signals move away from a particular center or point of reference.

_____ (4) are the internal, periodic timing of an organism generated within the body. _____ (5) is the synchronization of rhythms.

_____ (6) is the study of disease. _____ (7) is the study of all the factors involved in causing a disease.

Uncontrolled cell division is _____ (8) and can result in a _____ (9) or abnormal growth of new tissue called a tumor. A _____ (10) tumor is a contained and encapsulated neoplasm. _____ (11) is the reproduction of abnormal and undifferentiated cells that fail to mature into specialized cell types. _____ (12) is a nonencapsulated malignant cell mass that invades surrounding tissue. It has the devastating ability to break away from the primary tumor and form secondary cancer masses, called _____ (13)

_____ (14) is a protective response of the tissues to irritation or injury. The inflammatory response has four primary signs: heat, redness, swelling, and pain.

_____ (15) is an unpleasant complex, private, abstract experience. _____ (16) pain can be a symptom of a disease condition or a temporary aspect of medical treatment. It acts as a warning signal, activating the sympathetic nervous system. It is usually temporary, of sudden onset, and easily localized _____ (17) pain persists or recurs for indefinite periods, usually for more than 6 months. It frequently has an obscure onset, and the character and quality of the pain change over time. The pain is usually diffuse and poorly localized.

_____ (18) pain arises from stimulation of receptors in the skin, in which case it is called _____ (19) somatic pain, or from stimulation of receptors in skeletal muscles, joints, tendons, and fascia, in which case it is _____ (20) somatic pain. _____ (21) pain results from stimulation of receptors in the _____ (22) or internal organs.

_____ (23) pain is frequently experienced by people who have had a limb amputated and experience pain or other sensations in the extremity as if the limb were still there.

PROBLEM-SOLVING EXERCISE

Read the problem presented. There is no correct answer. Instead the exercise assists the student in the development of analysis and decision-making skills necessary in a professional practice.
1. Identify the facts presented in the information.
2. Identify the possibilities ("what if" statements) presented or develop your own possibilities that relate to the facts.
3. Evaluate each possibility in terms of the logical cause and effect and pros and cons.
4. Consider the feelings of the people involved.
5. Write each down in the space provided.
6. Develop your solution by answering the question posed.

PROBLEM

Supporting health is a lifetime commitment. Many factors encountered in day-to-day life threaten the homeostatic mechanism of the body. Not only are there inherent genetic strengths and weaknesses that may predispose us to disease but our learned behaviors also influence our perception of events and can determine whether we respond with survival fight-or-flight actions. Behavior is often determined by attempting to manage stress. Sometimes the behavior is resourceful, either bringing resolution to the situation or understanding that no answer to the problem exists and developing effective coping strategies. When this happens, people feel effective, empowered, and resourceful. On the other hand, if stress is managed with unresourceful behavior, such as the use of alcohol or temper tantrums, not only does the person feel out of control but those they interact with may also feel uncomfortable, helpless, or afraid. In general, people seem to respond to stress management better if they understand the physical, mental, and spiritual components that contribute to both health and a disruption in health. If more education were provided on these topics, maybe we could learn to better cope with what seems to be the increasing stress load in our societies. If the body were better understood, maybe we would take better care of it. Regardless, the inability to cope effectively with stress is becoming a major health concern, the result of which is renewed interest in drugless approaches to dealing with stress and pain management. This will likely create an environment in which bodywork methods are seen as important components in stress management programs.

QUESTION

What information would you need to become an effective educator about stress management methods?

The first response is provided as a guide to get you started. Fill in at least two more statements.

Facts:

1. Supporting health is a lifelong commitment.

2. _____

3. _____

Possibilities:

1. We could compromise our health by responding in ways that activate the fight-or-flight response.

2. _____

3. _____

Logical cause and effect:

1. The person may develop behaviors such as alcohol abuse.

2. _____

3. _____

Impact on people:

1. The person may feel out of control.

2. _____

3. _____

What information would you need to become an effective educator about stress management methods?

_____

_____

_____

_____

FURTHER STUDY

By use of a comprehensive anatomy and physiology text (see Works Consulted list at the back of this book), identify the chapters that pertain to the information presented in this chapter. As a study guide, locate the information presented in this text and elaborate by writing a paragraph of additional information on each of the following:

1. Feedback mechanism

_____

_____

_____

_____

_____

2. Tumor development and types

_____

_____

_____

_____

_____

3. Inflammatory response

_____

_____

_____

_____

_____

_____

4. Gate control theory of pain and Melzack and Wall

_____

_____

_____

_____

_____

5. Pain-spasm-pain cycle

_____

_____

_____

_____

_____

6. General adaptation syndrome and Hans Selye

_____

_____

_____

_____

7. Hyperventilation syndrome

_____

_____

_____

_____

8. Life cycle

_____

_____

_____

_____

_____

_____

Answer Key

1. Homeostasis is the relatively constant state maintained by the physiology of the body. Specific regulatory mechanisms constantly adjust and adapt our body systems to maintain homeostasis. The concept of balance—homeostasis—reflects the opposition of the yin/yang balance.

   In the ancient healing art of Ayurveda, an individual is made up of five primary elements. This model is similar to the five-element theory of the Oriental model. When any of these elements are present in the environment, they will in turn have an influence on us. Biologic systems have the ability to influence their own expression from moment to moment.

   When we genuinely experience positive emotional states, a tendency exists for the biologic rhythm to naturally oscillate together or entrain. In addition, the entrainment process can be facilitated with specific techniques that shift conscious attention to the breath, heart, and abdomen.

   Massage and other soft tissue approaches either support or stimulate homeostatic processes. Bodywork is generally nonspecific in that the stimulus disrupts the general existing homeostatic balance, requiring a response through the feedback mechanism. The objective is to reestablish homeostasis.

2. Disease is an abnormality in the functioning of the body that disrupts a person's physical, mental, or social well-being. Health is not a static condition but rather a condition of constant changes and adaptations to stress and stressors to maintain homeostasis. Health is the success of the organism to continuously and effectively adapt to change.

   Stress is any external or internal stimulus or substantial change in routine that causes the body to adapt. If a stress acts on the body, mechanisms attempt to counteract the effects of the stress and bring the condition back to normal

1. An abnormality in the functioning of the body, any part or system, especially when the abnormality threatens well-being
2. The study of disease
3. The study of the factors involved in causing a disease
4. The success of the organism to continuously and effectively adapt to change
5. The preparation, use, and action of prescription medications
6. Objective changes that can be seen or measured by someone other than the person
7. Subjective changes noticed or felt only by the person.
8. A group of signs and symptoms that identify a pathologic condition
9. A disease or process whose signs and symptoms develop quickly, last a short time, then disappear
10. Diseases or processes that develop slowly and last for a long time, sometimes for life
11. Diseases with characteristics between acute and chronic
12. Can be transmitted from one person to another
13. The pattern of the development of a disease
14. The latent stage in infectious diseases
15. The time when body functions return to normal and recovery occurs
16. A temporary or permanent reversal in chronic diseases
17. Chemicals that affect genetic activity in some way, causing abnormal cell reproduction
18. Doctor specializing in the treatment of cancer
19. New cells used for tissue repair are similar to those that they replace
20. The new cells in tissue repair are formed from connective tissue, resulting in a scar
21. The replacement of dead cells with living cells

EXERCISE

1. Genetic mechanisms, pathogenic organisms, tumors and cancer, physical and chemical agents, malnutrition, hypersensitivity, immunity, immune deficiency, inflammatory response, degeneration
2. Genetic factors, age, lifestyle, stress, environment, preexisting conditions
3. Heat, redness, pain, edema, or swelling
4. Pain is a complex, private, abstract experience, difficult to explain or describe. It has a physiologic, psychologic, and social aspect. Types of pain are acute pain, chronic pain, intractable pain, pricking or bright pain, burning pain, aching pain, deep pain, muscle pain, somatic pain, visceral pain, referred pain.
5. When pain is referred, it is usually to a structure that developed from the same embryonic segment or dermatome as the structure in which the pain originates.
6. A kind of pain frequently experienced by people who have had a limb amputated. It is suspected that phantom pain occurs because the remaining proximal portions of the sensory nerves that previously received impulses from the limb are being stimulated by the trauma of the amputation. Stimuli from these nerves are interpreted by the brain as coming from the nonexistent (phantom) limb.
7. Inherited and constitutional conditions, lifestyle, activity, rest, loving relationships, exercise, diet, empowering beliefs and attitudes, self-esteem, authentic personality, and freedom from self-hindering patterns.
8. Stressors are extreme stimuli—too much or to little of almost anything. The three stages of the general adaptation syndrome are the first stage of alarm, the fight-or-flight response, which is the body's initial reaction to the perceived stressor; the second stage, known as the resistance reaction that, through the secretion of regulating hormone, allows the body to continue fighting a stressor long after the effects of the alarm reaction have dissipated; third, the stage of exhaustion, if the stress response continues without relief. Unfortunately, during periods of prolonged stress, glucocorticosteroids may have harmful side effects that include decreased immune response, decreased blood glucose levels, altered protein and fat metabolism, decreased resistance to stress. Prolonged or frequent activation of the sympathetic division of the autonomic nervous style also results in increased likelihood of high blood pressure, decreased digestion, reduced tissue repair, and more.

   People experiencing excessive or ongoing accumulating stress are often overwhelmed by tension, anger, fear, and frustration. This results in feelings of anxiety. Adrenaline levels rise, blood pressure and heart rate increase, and breathing changes. Overbreathing often results in overoxygenation of the blood and the reduction of carbon dioxide levels, leading to hyperventilation syndrome. Panic attacks can result. Blood level of glucose and fatty acids rise. This combination over time leads to plaque being laid down in arteries and coronary artery disease developing. Immune function becomes less effective and the body is not as able to deal with pathogens or cancer cells. Often a decrease in memory and the ability to concentrate or problem solve exists; susceptibility to infection increases; and complaints of stomach pain, heart palpitations, fatigue, and muscle aches are common. Sleep disorders and depression frequently accompany long-term stress. Mood and behavior is affected.

9. Conception, gestation, birth, living, dying, and death

FILL IN THE BLANK

1. Homeostasis
2. Afferent
3. efferent
4. Biologic rhythms
5. Entrainment
6. Pathology
7. Etiology
8. hyperplasia
9. neoplasm
10. benign
11. Anaplasia
12. Cancer
13. metastasis
14. Inflammation
15. Pain
16. Acute
17. chronic
18. Somatic
19. superficial
20. deep
21. Visceral
22. viscera
23. Phantom

Chapter 3

Medical Terminology

CHAPTER OUTLINE

CHAPTER OBJECTIVES

After completing this chapter, the student should be able to perform the following:

1. Identify three word elements used in medical terms.
2. Combine word elements into medical terms.
3. Identify abbreviations used in health care and their meanings.
4. Use a charting method that incorporates a clinical reasoning/problem-solving model.
5. Define terms used to describe the positions of the body in relation to other body parts.
6. Identify terminology from an ancient Chinese healing model.

KEY TERMS

Acupuncture The practice of inserting needles in specific points on meridians, or channels, to stimulate or sedate energy flow to regulate or alter body function. A branch of Chinese medicine, it is the art and science of manipulating the flow of Qi, the basic life force, and Xue, the blood, body fluids, and nourishing essences. Western medicine uses it primarily to reduce pain. *Acupressure,* which uses digital pressure, follows the same Eastern principles.

Charting The process of keeping a written record of a client or patient. The most effective charting methods follow clinical reasoning, which emphasizes a problem-solving approach. Many systems of charting are used, but these models all have similar components: POMR (problem-oriented medical record) and SOAP (subjective, objective, analysis, and plan—the four parts of the written record).

Combining vowel A vowel added between two roots or a root and a suffix to make pronunciation of the word easier.

Disharmony Distortions in health that result when the functions or systems are neither balanced nor working at their optimum. In Chinese medicine, disharmony can be created by the Six Pernicious Influences or the Seven Emotions.

Prefix A word element added to the beginning of a root to change the meaning of the word.

Qi Also known as chi; it refers to the life force.

Root A word element that contains the basic meaning of the word.

The Seven Emotions The Oriental concept that joy, anger, fear, fright, sadness, worry, and grief are emotional responses that may trigger disharmony in the body, mind, or spirit under certain conditions.

The Six Pernicious Influences The Oriental concept that heat, cold, wind, dampness, dryness, and summer heat, which are natural climate changes, may induce disease under certain conditions.

Suffix A word element added to the end of a root to change the meaning of the word.

Tao An ancient philosophic concept that represents the whole and its parts as one and the same.

Word elements The parts of a word; the prefix, root, and suffix.

Yin/yang Yin and yang are terms used to describe polar relationships. Yin/yang refers to the dynamic balance between opposing forces and the continual process of creation and destruction. Yin/yang reflects the natural order and duality of the whole universe and everything in it, including the individual.

Professionals who use anatomy and physiology must have a standard terminology. Without a common language, health care practitioners cannot communicate. Professionals have an ethical responsibility to learn to communicate with their clients in a common language, to understand and communicate across disciplines with other health professionals, and to identify with language cross-culturally in order to appreciate a different perspective of the anatomic map of the body. This chapter introduces the student to the basic concepts necessary to enable her to communicate in generalized medical terms, to use a clinical reasoning approach in client care, and to consider a model of cross-cultural terminology.

The Language of Science and Medicine

Most scientific and medical terms are derived from Latin and Greek fundamental **word elements,** the commonly accepted language base. These elements are combined to form medical terms. A term can be interpreted easily by separating the word into its elements: prefix, root, and suffix.

Each of the following sections includes a list of some of the more common word elements. These lists are not meant to be all-encompassing, but they provide enough examples for you to gain a general understanding of most of the terms encountered by bodywork professionals.

PREFIXES

A **prefix** is an element placed at the beginning of a word to change the meaning of the word. A prefix cannot stand alone; it must be combined with another word element. A vowel, called a **combining vowel,** often is used to join word elements. The combining vowel most often used is *o,* but occasionally *i* or some other vowel is used. Table 3-1 presents a list of the more common prefixes and some examples of accompanying combining vowels. These prefixes will help you recognize and understand scientific and medical terminology.

ROOTS

The **root** (or stem) word element provides the fundamental meaning of the word. Roots are combined with prefixes and suffixes to form medical and scientific terms. In medicine, the root word often refers to a part of the body. As with prefixes, a combining vowel often is added when two roots are combined or

TABLE 3-1 COMMON PREFIXES AND THEIR MEANINGS

PREFIX	MEANING	PREFIX	MEANING	PREFIX	MEANING
a-, an-	Without or not	febr(i, o)-	Fever, boil	onc(o)-	Tumor, mass
ab-	Away from	fract-	Break, broken	ortho(o)-	Straight, erect, correct
acr(o)-	Extremity, tip	fund-	Base, bottom	osm(io, o)-	Smell, odor
ad-	Toward	gen-	Beginning, origin, produce	oxy-	Sharp, acute, acid
alba-	White	gluc-	Sweet, sugar, glucose	palp-	Touch, feel
ambi-	Both, on both sides	gyn(a, e, eco, o)-	Female	pan-	All
ana-	Upward, backward, excessive, through	hemi-	Half	para-	Abnormal, near
andr(o)-	Male	heter-	Other, different	path(o)-	Disease, suffering
ankyl(o)-	Crooked, fused, stiff	hol-	Whole, all	pept(o)-	Digestion
ante-	Before, forward	hom(eo,o)-	Unchanged, alike, same	per-	By, through
anti-	Against, opposed	hyg(ei, ie, io)-	Health	peri-	Around
audi-	Hear	hyper-	Excessive, too much, high	phag(e, o)-	Eat, consume
auto-	Self	hypo-	Under, decreased, less than normal	pharmaco-	Drugs, poison, medication
bi-	Double, two	iatr(o)-	Physician	physio-	Natural, physical agents
bio-	Life, living matter	idio-	Distinct, peculiar to the individual	poly-	Many, much
brach-	Short	immuno-	Protection	post-	After, behind
brady(o)-	Slow, short, dull	in-	In, into, within, not	pre-	Before, in front of, prior to
carcin(o)-	Cancer, malignant	infra-	Beneath	pro-	Before, in front of
cata-	Down, negative, under, against, lower	inter-	Between	pseudo-	False
caud-	Tail, inferior	intra-	Within	quadr(a, i)-	Four
cent(i)-	Hundred	intro-	Into, within	re-	Again
chron(i,o,us)-	Time, long time	iso-	Equal, like, identical	retro-	Backward
circum-	Around	juxta-	Adjoining, near to	schist(o)-	Split, divided
contra-	Against, opposite	kyph(o)-	Bend, hump	scler(o)-	Hard
counter-	Against, opposite	lact(o)-	Milk	semi-	Half
cry(mo,o)-	Cold	later(al, o)-	Side	sepsi-	Putrid, rotten
de-	Down, from, away from, not	leuk-	White	son(o)-	Sound
dext-	Right	levo-	Left	steno-	Contracted, narrow
di-	Two, double, twice	macro-	Large	strat(i)-	Layer
dia-	Across, through, apart	mal-	Bad, illness, disease	sub-	Under
dis-	Separation, away from	mega-	Large	super-	Above, over, excess
dys-	Bad, difficult, abnormal	micro-	Small	supra-	Above, over
ecto-	Outer, outside	mono-	One, single	therm-	Warm
en-	In, into, within	morph(o)-	Form, shape	tort(i, o)-	Twisted
endo-	Inner, inside	multi-	Many	tract-	Pull down
epi-	Over, on, upon	necr(o)-	Death, destruction, corpse	trans-	Across
eryth-	Red	neo-	New	ultr(a, o)-	Excessive, extreme, beyond
esthesi-	Sensation	noct(i, o)-	Night	uni-	One
etio-	Cause	non-	Not	zyg(o,us)-	Yoke, join, together
ex-	Out, out of, from, away from	olig-	Small, scanty		

Modified from Fritz S: *Mosby's fundamentals of therapeutic massage*, St Louis, 1995, Mosby.
* The vowels and vowel-consonant combinations in parentheses are combining vowels or combining elements.

TABLE 3-2 COMMON ROOT WORDS AND THEIR MEANINGS

ROOT (COMBINING VOWEL)	MEANING	ROOT (COMBINING VOWEL)	MEANING	ROOT (COMBINING VOWEL)	MEANING
abdomin(o)-	Abdomen	hemat(o)-	Blood	psych(o)-	Mind
aden(o)-	Gland	hepat(o)-	Liver	pulmo-	Lung
adren(o)-	Adrenal gland	hydr(o)-	Water	py(o)-	Pus
angi(o)-	Vessel	hyster(o)-	Uterus	rect(o)-	Rectum
arterio(o)-	Artery	ile(o)-, ili(o)-	Ileum	rhin(o)-	Nose
arthr(o)-	Joint	laryng(o)-	Larynx	salping(o)-	Eustachian tube, uterine tube
bronch(o)-	Bronchus, bronchi	mamm(o)-	Breast, mammary gland	splen(o)-	Spleen
card-, cardi(o)-	Heart	mast(o)-	Mammary gland, breast	sten(o)-	Narrow, constriction
cephal(o)-	Head	meno-	Menstruation	stern(o)-	Sternum
chondr(o)-	Cartilage	my(o)-	Muscle	stomat(o)-	Mouth
colo-	Colon	myel(o)-	Spinal cord, bone marrow	therm(o)-	Heat
cost(o)-	Rib	nephr(o)-	Kidney	thoraco-	Chest
crani(o)-	Skull	neur(o)-	Nerve	thromb(o)-	Clot, thrombus
cyan(o)-	Blue	ocul(o)-	Eye	thyr(o)-	Thyroid
cyst(o)-	Bladder, cyst	ophthalm(o)-	Eye	toxo-	Poison
cyt(o)-	Cell	orth(o)-	Straight, normal, correct	toxic(o)-	Poison, poisonous
derma-	Skin	oste(o)-	Bone	trache(o)-	Trachea
duoden(o)-	Duodenum	ot(o)-	Ear	uro-	Urine, urinary tract, urination
encephal(o)-	Brain	ped(o)-	Child, foot	urethr(o)-	Urethra
enter(o)-	Intestines	pharyng(o)-	Pharynx	urin(o)-	Urine
fibr(o)-	Fiber, fibrous	phleb(o)-	Vein	uter(o)-	Uterus
gastr(o)-	Stomach	pnea-	Breathing, respiration	vas(o)-	Blood vessel, vas deferens
gloss(o)-	Tongue	pneum(o)-	Lung, air, gas	ven(o)-	Vein
gyn-, gyne-, gyneco-	Woman	proct(o)-	Rectum	vertebr(o)-	Spine, vertebrae
hem-, hema-, hemo-,	Blood				

Modified from Fritz S: *Mosby's fundamentals of therapeutic massage,* St Louis, 1995, Mosby.

when a suffix is added to a root. The combining vowel usually is *o*, but occasionally it is *i*. Table 3-2 presents a list of some of the more common root words and their accompanying combining vowels.

SUFFIXES

A **suffix** is a word element that is added to the end of a root to change the meaning of the word. Suffixes cannot stand alone. In interpreting scientific terms, use the suffix as your starting point. Roots that end in a consonant require a combining vowel when adding a suffix. If the root ends with a vowel and the suffix begins with a vowel, the vowel at the end of the

root is deleted. Table 3-3 presents a list of some of the more common suffixes.

NOTE: The ability to use a medical dictionary is a necessary skill; it is amazing how much information can be found in a quality medical dictionary. The dictionary is the place to begin research or to clarify the meaning of a word or topic. With the condensed information gathered from the dictionary, the investigation can proceed. When selecting a medical dictionary, look for one that is encyclopedic and illustrated. Check the Appendix to see how expansive it is; it often contains a special section for medical terminology.

TABLE 3-3   COMMON SUFFIXES AND THEIR MEANINGS

SUFFIX	MEANING	SUFFIX	MEANING	SUFFIX	MEANING
-able	Capable of, suitable for	-graph	Diagram, recording instrument	-plasty	Surgical repair or reshaping
-ago	Disease	-graphy	Making a recording	-plegia	Paralysis
-algesia	Pain	-hood	State, quality of, condition	-pnea	To breathe
-algia	Pain	-iasis	Condition of	-porosis	Passage
-asis	Condition, usually abnormal	-ician	One skilled in, one who practices	-ptosis	Falling, sagging, dropping, down
-ase	Enzyme	-ism	Condition	-rrhage, -rrhagia	Excessive flow
-asis	State or condition of	-itis	Inflammation	-rrhea	Profuse flow, discharge
-cele	Hernia, herniation, pouching	-ity	Quality of, state of	-sclerosis	Dryness, hardness
-cide	Kill, causing death	-ive	Having power to, that which performs	-scoliosis	Curvature, crooked
-cule	Very small	-ize	To treat by a special method	-scope	Examination instrument
-cyte	Cell	-kinesis	Motion	-scopy	Examination using a scope
-dom	State of being	-lemma	Sheath, covering	-sepsis	Putrefaction
-duct	To lead, cause, tube, channel	-logy	The study of	-some	Body
-eal	Pertaining to	-lysis	Destruction of, decomposition	-stasis	Maintenance, maintaining a constant level
-ease	Condition	-malacia	Softening	-stenosis	Narrow, tighten, short, constrict
-ectasis	Dilatation, stretching	-megaly	Enlargement	-stomy, -ostomy	Creation of an opening
-ectomy	Excision, removal of	-oid	Form, like, resemble	-thymia	Thymus gland, mind, soul, emotions
-ema	Swelling, distention	-oma	Tumor	-tomy, -otomy	Incision, cutting into
-emesis (one of the few suffixes that can stand alone)	Vomiting	-opsy	View of	-tonia	Stretching, putting under tension
-emia	Blood condition	-osis	Condition	-trophic	Related to growth, development, or nutrition
-ferent	Bear, carry	-otomy	Cutting into	-ule	Little, small
-feron	To strike	-paresis	Paralysis	-uria	Condition of the urine
-form	Shape, structure	-pathy	Disease	-version	To turn
-genesis	Development, production, creation	-penia	Lack, deficiency	-vert	Turn
-genic	Producing, causing	-phasia	Speaking	-xenia	Strange, abnormal
-globin	Protein	-phobia	An exaggerated fear		
-gram	Record	-phylaxis	Protection		

Modified from Fritz S: *Mosby's fundamentals of therapeutic massage,* St Louis, 1995, Mosby.

Activity 3-1 gives you a chance to create some medical terms of your own.

ABBREVIATIONS

Abbreviations are shortened forms of words or phrases. They are used primarily in written communication to save time and space. Table 3-4 presents a list of some abbreviations. Most medical dictionaries have a more extensive list of accepted abbreviations. In charting and keeping records, if you are unsure if an abbreviation is acceptable, write the term out in full to ensure accuracy.

Activity 3-2 gives you a chance to put your knowledge of medical abbreviations into practice.

TABLE 3-4 COMMON ABBREVIATIONS AND THEIR MEANINGS

ABBREVIATION	MEANING	ABBREVIATION	MEANING	ABBREVIATION	MEANING
ABD	Abdomen	Dx	Diagnosis	OTC	Over the counter
ADL	Activities of daily living	ext	Extract	P	Pulse
ad lib	As desired	ft	Foot (or feet)	PA	Postural analysis
alt dieb	Every other day	fx	Fracture	PM, pm	Afternoon
alt hor	Alternate hours	GI	Gastrointestinal	PT	Physical therapy
alt noct	Alternate nights	GU	Genitourinary	Px	Prognosis
AM, am	Morning	h, hr	Hour	R	Respiration, right
a.m.a.	Against medical advice	H_2O	Water	R/O	Rule out
ANS	Autonomic nervous system	Hx	History	ROM	Range of motion
approx	Approximately	IBW	Ideal body weight	Rx	Prescription
as tol	As tolerated	ICT	Inflammation of connective tissue	SOB	Shortness of breath
BM	Bowel movement	id	The same	SP, spir	Spirit
BP	Blood pressure	L	Left, length, lumbar	Sym	Symmetric
Ca	Cancer	lig	Ligament	T	Temperature
CC	Chief complaint	M	Muscle, meter, myopia	TLC	Tender loving care
c/o	Complains of	ML	Midline	Tx	Treatment
CPR	Cardiopulmonary resuscitation	meds	Medications	URI	Upper respiratory infection
CSF	Cerebrospinal fluid	n	Normal	WD	Well developed
CVA	Cerebrovascular accident, stroke	NA	Nonapplicable	WN	Well nourished
DJD	Degenerative joint disease	OB	Obstetrics		
DM	Diabetes mellitus				

ACTIVITY 3-1

The beauty of medical terminology is that it allows new words to be created as needed. From the lists of prefixes, root words, and suffixes, make up five silly words and define them.

*Example oligorhinoscoliosis: oligo-*small; *rhino-*nose; *scoliosis-*curve

Your Turn

ACTIVITY 3-2

Using the abbreviations in Table 3-4, decipher the message below. (The answers can be found on p. 92.)

Your Turn

In the AM _____ evaluate Hx _____

and ADL _____. Use this information ad lib

_____ to CC _____

of GI _____ and ABD _____

meds _____. Use ROM _____

as tol _____ on the h _____

as PT _____ on the ft _____

to assist R_____. Monitor T _____

and P _____ in the PM _____

and provide H_2O _____ and TLC _____

as requested for OB _____ clients.

ACTIVITY 3-3

Using the list in Table 3-4, as well as lists from a medical dictionary and your own imagination, develop a key for abbreviations you plan to use the most.

Hint: Think in terms of symptoms, anatomic locations, methods and techniques, directional terms, body movement patterns, assessment, and referrals. As your learning progresses, you may want to expand this list.

Some examples have been provided to help you get started.

Example

SYMPTOMS

ACP: Acupuncture point
CFS: Chronic fatigue syndrome
HA: Headache
TP: Trigger point

Your Turn

Example

ANATOMIC LOCATIONS

L-5: Fifth lumbar
LB: Low Back
SI: Sacroiliac

Your Turn

Example

METHODS AND TECHNIQUES

CTM: Connective tissue massage
DP: Direct pressure
EB: Energy balance
MET: Muscle energy technique
MLD: Manual lymph drainage
SH: Self-help
STM: Soft tissue manipulation
XFF: Cross fiber friction

Your Turn

Example

DIRECTIONAL TERMS

ant: Anterior
L: Left
R: Right
sup: Superior

Your Turn

Example

BODY MOVEMENT PATTERNS

flex: Flexion
ROM: Range of motion
SB: Side bending

Your Turn

Example

ASSESSMENT

inter: Intermittent
PB: Pain behavior
WNL: Within normal limits

Your Turn

Example

REFERRALS

AP: Acupuncturist
DC: Doctor of chiropractic
MD: Medical doctor

Your Turn

Note that using too many abbreviations creates confusion. If you use abbreviations in charting, you should provide an abbreviation key with the clinical notes. Abbreviations are not universally understood, and a key ensures accurate interpretation of your notes by the client or a fellow health care professional (Activity 3-3).

Clinical Reasoning and Charting

Effective assessment, analysis, and decision making are essential to meeting the needs of each client. In attempting to individualize treatment, the practitioner often will find routines or recipe-type application of soft tissue and movement treatments of limited value or even ineffective, because clients' circumstances vary so widely. The mark of an experienced professional is skill in effective reasoning.

As the volume of knowledge grows and as soft tissue and movement treatments become part of the health care system, the practitioner will find it increasingly important to be able to think through an intervention process and justify the effectiveness of a therapeutic intervention. Bodywork practitioners must be able to gather information effectively, analyze the information and determine the type or appropriateness of a therapeutic intervention, and evaluate and justify the benefits derived from the intervention. This is a skill to be learned.

Charting is the process of keeping a written record of professional interactions. Effective charting is more than writing down what happened. It represents a clinical reasoning methodology that emphasizes a problem-solving approach to client care.

To clinically reason and chart effectively, a practitioner must have a comprehensive knowledge of medical terms, abbreviations, and anatomy and physiology in both balanced and altered states of functioning. *Assessment* procedures identify both deviations from the norm and effective functioning. *Information* obtained during the assessment serves as the basis for developing a care plan, identifying any contraindications to therapy, and evaluating the need for referral.

A commonly used method of charting is the problem-oriented medical record (POMR) as reflected in the process of subjective data, objective data, analysis, and plan (SOAP). In this method, the written account of the health assessment is divided into four parts for clarity and completeness.

Because the method is based on an analytic process, after one has been learned it can be relatively easily adapted to any other charting method. The key point is the ability to reason through a clinical situation rationally and comprehensively. A charting method can provide both a structure for and a record of the process.

Any problem-solving charting method must begin with a database, which is collected before the process of identifying the client's problems is actually begun. The database consists of all the information available that contributes to therapeutic interaction. It can be divided into two parts, which are created with information obtained from a history-taking interview with the client and other pertinent people, a physical assessment, prior records, and health care treatment orders.

The first part of the database, the history-taking interview, provides information about the client's health history and the reason for the visit, a descriptive profile of the client, a history of her current condition, a history of past illness and health, and a family illness history. It also contains an account of the client's current health practices.

The physical assessment makes up the second part of the database. The extent and depth of this assessment vary from setting to setting, practitioner to practitioner, and according to the client's situation. Practitioners of soft tissue and movement therapies generally use some sort of visual assessment process to look for bilateral symmetry and deviations. Functional assessment reveals restricted, exaggerated, painful, or otherwise altered movement patterns. Palpation is used to identify changes in tissue texture and temperature, to locate energy changes, and to identify areas of tenderness. Various manual tests may be used to distinguish soft tissue problems from muscle function or from other conditions, such as joint dysfunction.

After the information has been collected, it is analyzed. Problems are identified based on a conclusion or decision that results from examination, investigation, and analysis of the data collected. A problem is defined as anything that causes the client or care giver concern, including physical abnormalities, physiologic disturbances, and socioeconomic or spiritually based problems. A decision then is made on a care or treatment plan. Any action taken, its effectiveness, and the outcome are recorded progressively from session to session.

Not all therapeutic goals relate to problems. Clients commonly use soft tissue and movement therapies to maintain health, manage stress, and fulfill pleasure needs. The same analytic process is used to determine the methods that best meet the client's goals.

With the SOAP charting method, the following pattern is used:

S Subjective information from the client
O Objective data from inspection, palpation, and testing and a record of interventions performed
A Analysis or assessment of the subjective and objective data and analysis of the effectiveness of the intervention and action taken
P Plan, including the methodology for future intervention and the progress of the sessions

S and *O* are the data-collecting parts of the SOAP method, as shown above.

The *A*, or analysis, part of the SOAP method is perhaps the most complex of the four parts. Detailed steps in that process are presented below.

STEP 1

What are the facts?
What is considered normal or balanced function?
What has happened? *(Spell out events.)*
What caused the imbalance? *(Can it be identified?)*
What was done or is being done?
What has worked or not worked?

STEP 2

What are the possibilities? *(What could it all mean?)*
What does my intuition suggest?
What are the possible patterns of dysfunction?
What are the possible contributing factors?
What are possible interventions?
What might work?
What are other ways to look at the situation?
What do the data suggest?

STEP 3

What is the logical progression of the symptom pattern, contributing factors, and current behaviors?
What are the logical cause and effect of each intervention identified?
What are the pros and cons of each intervention suggested?
What are the consequences of not acting?
What are the consequences of acting?

STEP 4

For each intervention under consideration, what would be the impact on the people involved: the client, the practitioner, and other professionals working with the client?
How does each person involved feel about the possible interventions?
Is the practitioner within her scope of practice to work with such a situation?
Is the practitioner qualified to work with such a situation?
Does the practitioner feel confident to work with such a situation?
Does a feeling of cooperation and agreement exist among all parties involved?

The *P*, or plan, section of the SOAP method involves the development and implementation of a care or treatment plan. After the analysis has been completed, a decision must be made on what will be involved in the care or treatment plan. The plan is not an exact protocol set in stone, but rather a guideline. After the plan has been implemented, it is reevaluated and adjusted as necessary.

To summarize:

S and *O* are the facts and what was done.
A is the analysis of the data from *S* and *O* in terms of possibilities, logical cause and effect, consequences, and impact on the people involved.
P is the decision-making and implementation structure.

PRACTICAL APPLICATION

The ability to apply what is learned from the study of anatomy and physiology comes from the reasoning and problem-solving process. With this skill, the information acquired becomes alive and practical. Effective work with clients is a continual learning process of assessing, deciding on interventions, and analyzing effectiveness through evaluation of progress from session to session. Even in the most basic sessions, when the client's goals are pleasure and relaxation, decisions must be made on the best way to encourage the body to respond to meet the client's goals.

In order to use the information collected from the subjective and objective data, the practitioner must be able to analyze and make decisions about what the data mean and what patterns are represented in the whole person. Because of the amount of information involved and because most human difficulties are multidimensional, involving body, mind, and spirit, all areas must be addressed, although not necessarily by the same practitioner. Assessment and analysis may indicate a need to refer the client elsewhere or to use a team approach, working in a multidisciplinary cooperative effort to provide the best possible care for each client. Effective practice and ethical behavior require a practitioner to stay within the competencies of both a professionally defined scope of practice and a personal level of training, expertise, and experience.

Effective communication among client, practitioner, and fellow professionals serving the client is essential. A continuing written record provides the means for sharing information. The use of a model for information gathering and decision making such as POMR, SOAP, or a similar format is important. The terms of anatomy and physiology often become the common language base among health disciplines, and these terms also are relevant in cross-discipline and cross-cultural sharing of knowledge.

This textbook has been developed on a logical reasoning model. A model is a pattern to imitate. See if you can identify the reasoning model through the exercises and activities that encourage analysis and reasoning. Imitating a model is a good way to begin a learning process. After the student understands the model and can use it effectively, she can allow for variation as necessary to provide the best response to each set of circumstances. A model is a tool, not an absolute (Activity 3-4).

ACTIVITY 3-4

Synthesize the section just completed on charting and clinical reasoning by answering the following questions. A shortened version of the analysis process is provided for this activity. No particular answer is the correct one; instead, the exercise assists the student in the development of analysis and decision-making skills necessary in a professional practice. Each section has an example to help you get started.

STEP 1
1. What are the facts?
2. What has worked or not worked?

Example

1. Charting is written communication (fact).
2. In order to chart effectively, a practitioner needs a knowledge base of medical terms and abbreviations, and of anatomy and physiology (fact).

Your Turn

Give three more facts about charting and clinical reasoning.

STEP 2
1. What are the possibilities?
2. What does my intuition suggest?
3. What are other ways to look at the situation?
4. What do the data suggest?

Example

1. I may need to take a medical terminology class.
2. My instincts suggest that learning about assessment procedures is important.
3. I must be careful not to become too analytical.
4. The information suggests that further investigation of problem solving could be helpful.

Your Turn

Give three more possibilities.

STEP 3
1. What are the pros and cons?
2. What are the consequences of acting or not acting?

Example

1. The pros of charting include having a continuous log of progress.
2. A consequence of not charting would be a lack of information for reference or for other professionals.

Your Turn

Give three more consequences.

Continued

The General Structural Plan of the Body

When you look at a map, you see a plan for the layout of the map that is fairly universal. North usually is placed at the top. A legend identifies how many miles are indicated per inch, and symbols indicate types of roads and landmarks. So it is with the location of body areas. The map of the body begins with the body in the anatomic position (Figure 3-1).

The following information provides the basic knowledge needed to read the body map and give accurate descriptions to guide others around the body.

REGIONS OF THE BODY AND SURFACE ANATOMY

Regional terms are used to designate specific areas of the body (Activity 3-5). Carefully study the diagram and chart shown in Figure 3-2 and complete the exercise in Figure 3-3, *A* and *B*.

STRUCTURAL PLAN

The structural organization of the body follows a clear plan. All human beings have a vertebral column that supports the trunk and determines the central axis of the body. It also supports two body cavities: the dorsal cavity, which holds the brain inside the skull and the spinal cord in the vertebral column, and the ventral cavity, which is the combined thoracic, abdominal, and pelvic cavity (sometimes referred to as the abdominopelvic cavity). Human beings are bilaterally symmetric beings with left and right mirror images. Also, the body is segmented; this is most obvious in the vertebral column, ribs, and spinal cord. The body is designed as a tube within a tube. The digestive system is a tube that lies within the greater tube of the trunk (Figures 3-4 and 3-5).

Terms Related to the Structural Plan

Soma, somato: Root words that mean *the body*, as distinguished from *the mind*. Somatic organs and tissues are associated with the skin and skeleton (e.g., bone and skeletal muscles, extremities, body wall) and often can be controlled voluntarily.

Axial: Areas or organs along the central axis of the body, including the head, neck, trunk, brain, spinal cord, and abdominal organs.

Appendicular: The limbs, joined to the body as lateral appendages.

Torso, trunk: Structures related to the main part of the body, including the chest, abdomen, pelvis, and vertebral cavity. The head and limbs are attached to the trunk.

ACTIVITY 3-4—cont'd

STEP 4

1. What would be the effect on the people involved: client, practitioner, and other professionals working with the client? Does a feeling of cooperation and agreement exist among all parties?

Example

1. I would feel burdened with the paperwork and frustrated because of my spelling, but the client would feel a sense of caring.

Your Turn

Give three more effects on the people involved.

PLAN

Now that you have analyzed this information, write down your decisions on charting and problem solving and then develop an implementation plan based on that decision.

Example

I have come to the conclusion that charting is important and that I need to learn more about it. I want to explore methods other than SOAP. I will need to research charting procedures, and a logical place to begin would be nursing or psychologic charting systems. I will go to the library and check information on the computer about charting methods.

Your Turn

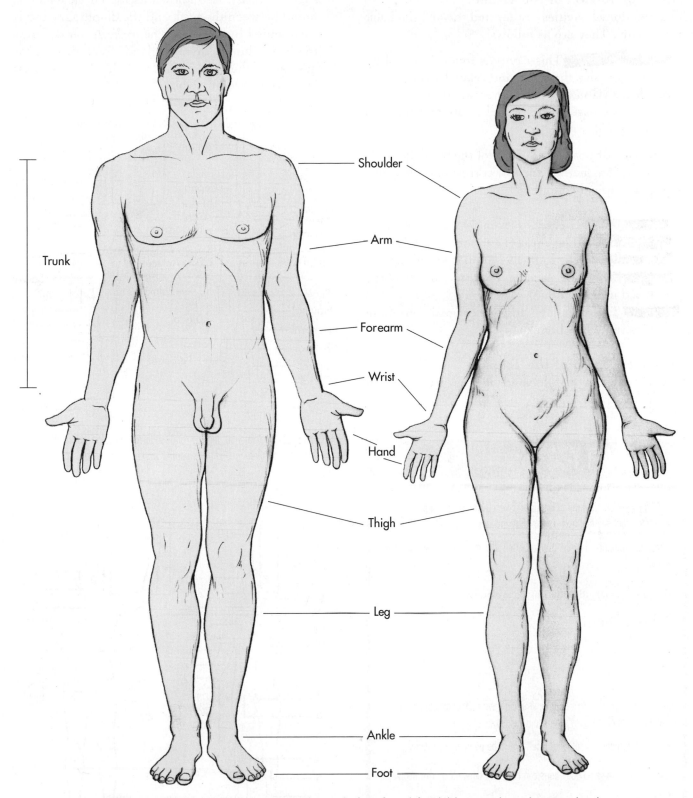

FIGURE 3-1 Anatomic position. The person is standing upright, facing forward, feet slightly separated, arms hanging at the sides with palms facing forward. Structures are named and their positions are described in this standard position. (From Mathers LH et al: *Clinical anatomy principles,* St Louis, 1996, Mosby.)

Posterior Region of the Trunk

The two dorsal cavities are located toward the back of the body. They are as follows:

The cranial cavity: This cavity is found in the skull and contains the brain and related structures.

The vertebral cavity: The vertebral cavity extends from the base of the cranial cavity and contains the spinal cord.

The back or posterior surface of the trunk is divided into regions named for the corresponding vertebrae in the spinal column.

Cervical region: The neck (seven cervical vertebrae)

Thoracic region: The chest (12 thoracic vertebrae)

Lumbar region: The loin (five lumbar vertebrae)

Sacral region: The sacrum (five sacral vertebrae fused into one bone)

Coccyx: The tailbone (four coccygeal vertebrae fused into one bone)

Anterior Region of the Trunk

Ventral cavities are located in the trunk. They include the following:

ACTIVITY 3-5

Stand in front of a mirror and identify each landmark and point of surface anatomy and body region. Say the words out loud.

Write one sentence describing what it felt like to be your own anatomy model.

Example I felt silly pointing at my body.

Your Turn

Repeat the exercise with a partner. Wearing a swimsuit or exercise wear that exposes more of the body's surface is helpful.

Write one sentence about what it felt like to be an anatomy model.

Example The same body parts can look very different on two people.

Your Turn

The thoracic cavity, also known as the chest, which is found between the neck and the diaphragm and is surrounded by the ribs. The *mediastinum* contains the heart, lungs, thymus gland, trachea, esophagus, and other structures and divides the chest into left and right parts.

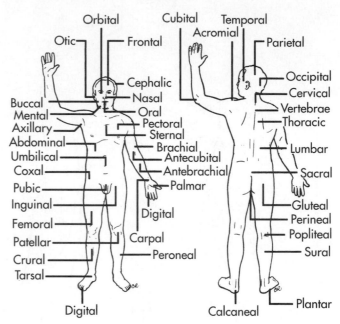

FIGURE 3-2 Anatomic regions and surface anatomy. (From Hinkle CZ: *Fundamentals of anatomy and movement: a workbook and guide,* St Louis, 1997, Mosby.)

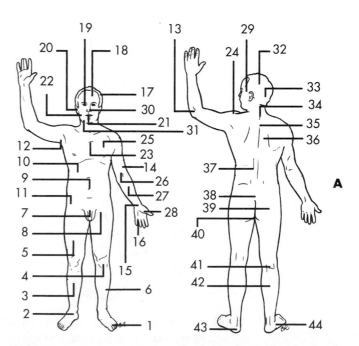

FIGURE 3-3 Anatomic region exercise. (**A,** From Fritz S: *Mosby's fundamentals of therapeutic massage,* St Louis, 1995, Mosby. **B,** From Hinkle CZ: *Fundamentals of anatomy and movement: a workbook and guide,* St Louis, 1997, Mosby.)

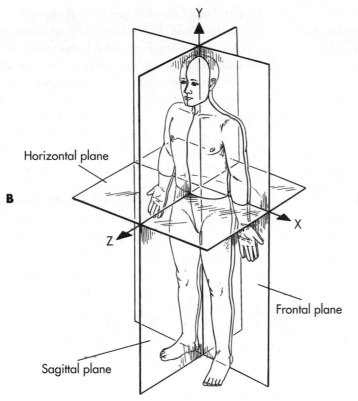

Horizontal plane

Frontal plane

Sagittal plane

Y

X

Z

B

FIGURE 3-3—cont'd For legend see opposite page.

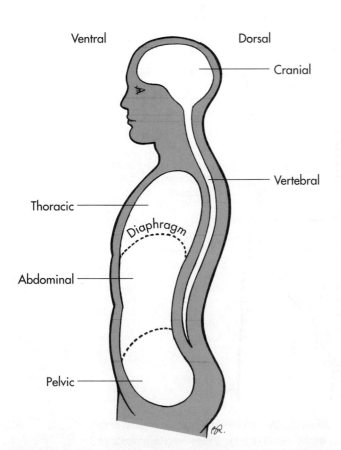

Ventral

Dorsal

Cranial

Vertebral

Thoracic

Diaphragm

Abdominal

Pelvic

FIGURE 3-4 Body cavities. (From Fritz S: *Mosby's fundamentals of therapeutic massage*, St Louis, 1995, Mosby.)

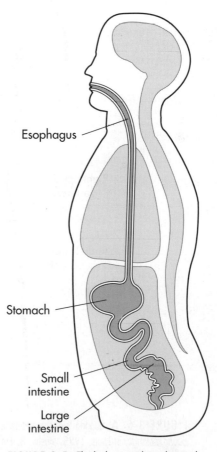

Esophagus

Stomach

Small intestine

Large intestine

FIGURE 3-5 The body as a tube within a tube.

The abdominal cavity, or the belly, which is located below the diaphragm and is enclosed within the abdominal muscles. It contains the liver, kidneys, spleen, pancreas, stomach, and intestines.

The pelvic cavity, which is found inferior to the abdomen, inside the pelvic bones. It contains a portion of the large intestine, the bladder, and the internal reproductive organs.

The *viscera* are internal organs of the thoracic, abdominal, and pelvic cavities that are considered to be under involuntary control.

Two types of membranes are associated with the regions of the trunk: *parietal membranes* line the body cavities and *visceral membranes* cover the visceral organs.

Abdominal Quadrants and Regions

The abdomen is divided into four quadrants and nine regions, the names of which are used to describe the location of body structures, pain, or discomfort. The *four quadrants* are the right upper quadrant, left upper quadrant, right lower quadrant, and left lower quadrant (Figure 3-6, *A*). The *nine regions* are the right hypochondriac, epigastric, left hypochondriac, right lumbar, umbilical, left lumbar, right iliac, hypogastric, and left iliac regions (Figure 3-6, *B*).

POSITIONS OF THE BODY

Anatomic position is a phrase used in Western terminology to describe the position of the body and the location of its regions and parts. The central axis of the body passes through the head and trunk.

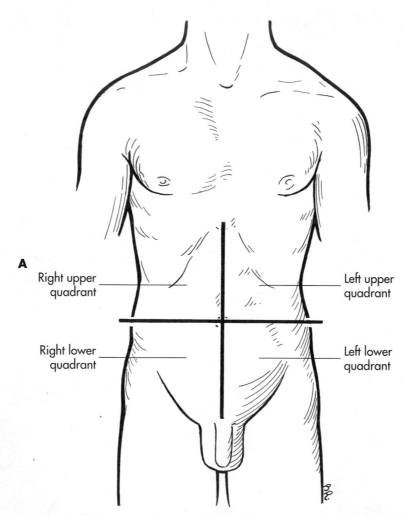

A

Right upper quadrant

Left upper quadrant

Right lower quadrant

Left lower quadrant

FIGURE 3-6 A, Quadrants of the abdomen. **B,** Anatomic abdominal regions. (**A,** From Fritz S: *Mosby's fundamentals of therapeutic massage,* St Louis, 1995, Mosby. **B,** From LaFleur-Brooks M: *Exploring medical language: a student-directed approach,* ed 3, St Louis, 1994, Mosby.)

Terms related to the position of the body include the following:

Anatomic position: Standing upright with the feet slightly apart, arms hanging at the sides, palms facing forward, thumbs outward (see Figure 3-1)

Erect position: Standing

Supine position: The body lies horizontally with the face up (Figure 3-7, *A*)

Prone position: The body lies horizontally with the face down (Figure 3-7, *B*)

Lateral recumbent position: The body lies horizontally either on the right or the left side (Figure 3-7, *C*)

BODY PLANES AND MOVEMENTS

The body can be divided into sections with imaginary lines and the various planes used to identify the areas created (Figure 3-8).

Movements are described as beginning in or returning to the anatomic position. Movement terms define the action as the body part passes through the various planes.

The sagittal plane is a vertical plane that divides the body into left and right. A midsagittal plane divides the body into equal left and right parts; a parasagittal plane divides it into unequal left and right parts.

The frontal (coronal) plane also runs vertically, but it divides the body into anterior and posterior (front and back) parts.

A transverse plane divides the body horizontally into two sections, described as superior (meaning above) and inferior (meaning below). The transverse plane runs perpendicular to the frontal and sagittal planes.

Movement

A movement that takes a part of the body forward from the anatomic position within a sagittal plane is called *flexion;* movement backward is called *extension.*

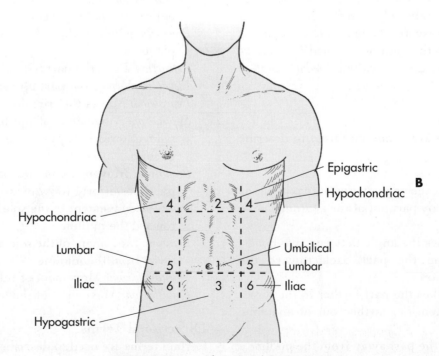

FIGURE 3-6—cont'd For legend see opposite page.

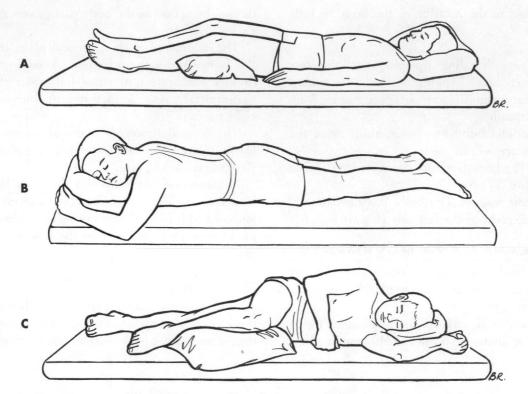

FIGURE 3-7   Positions of the body. **A,** Supine. **B,** Prone. **C,** Lateral recumbent. (From Fritz S: *Mosby's fundamentals of therapeutic massage,* St Louis, 1995, Mosby.)

Movements in a frontal plan that take a part of the body toward the midline are called *adduction;* movements away are called *abduction.* Lateral or side bending of the trunk also takes place in the frontal plane. A movement in a transverse plane that takes a part of the body away from the midline is called *lateral rotation;* movement inward is called *medial rotation* (Figure 3-9).

Movement Terms

The following terms are commonly used to describe movement:

Flexion: Decreases the angle between two bones as it moves the body part out of the anatomic position

Extension: Increases the angle between two bones, usually moving the part back toward the anatomic position

Hyperextension: Takes the part farther in the direction of the extension, farther out of anatomic position

Abduction: Moves the part away from the midline

Adduction: Moves the part toward the midline

Rotation: Partially turns or pivots the part in an arc around a central axis; may be medial or lateral

Circumduction: Turns or pivots the part through an entire arc, making a complete circle

Protraction: Pushes the part forward in a horizontal plane

Retraction: Pulls the part back in a horizontal plane

Elevation: Moves the part upward (superiorly)

Depression: Moves the part downward (inferiorly)

Supination: Movement of the hand that turns the palm anteriorly (upward), as in cupping a bowl of soup

Pronation: Movement of the hand that turns the palm posteriorly (downward)

Inversion: Movement of the sole of the foot inward, toward the midline

Eversion: Movement of the sole of the foot outward, away from the midline

Plantar flexion: Movement of the foot downward

Dorsiflexion: Movement of the foot upward

Directional Terms

Certain terms are used to describe the relationship of one body position to another (Figure 3-10). The fol-

Text continues on p. 80.

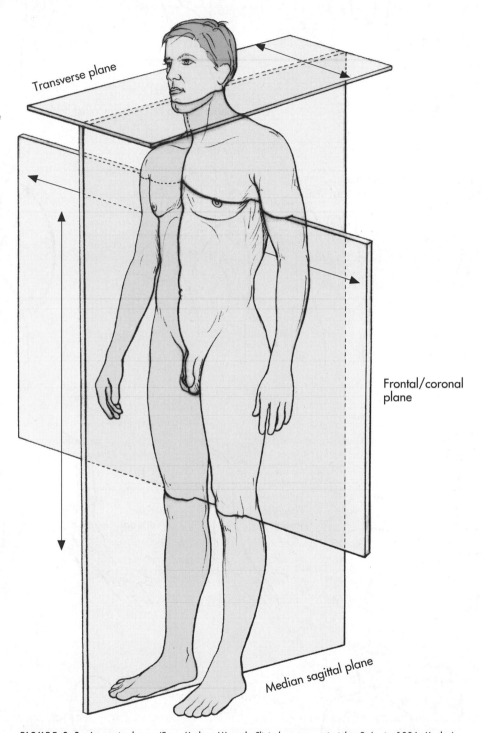

Transverse plane

Frontal/coronal plane

Median sagittal plane

FIGURE 3-8 Anatomic planes. (From Mathers LH et al: *Clinical anatomy principles,* St Louis, 1996, Mosby.)

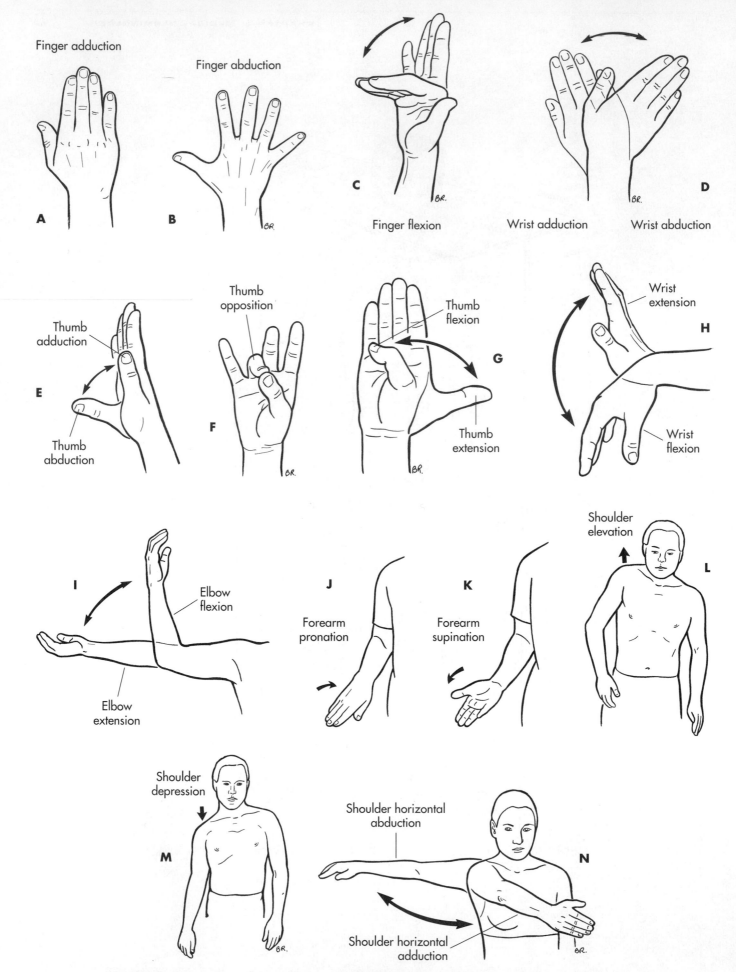

FIGURE 3-9 Body movements. (**A** through **CC,** From Fritz S: *Mosby's fundamentals of therapeutic massage,* St Louis, 1995, Mosby.)

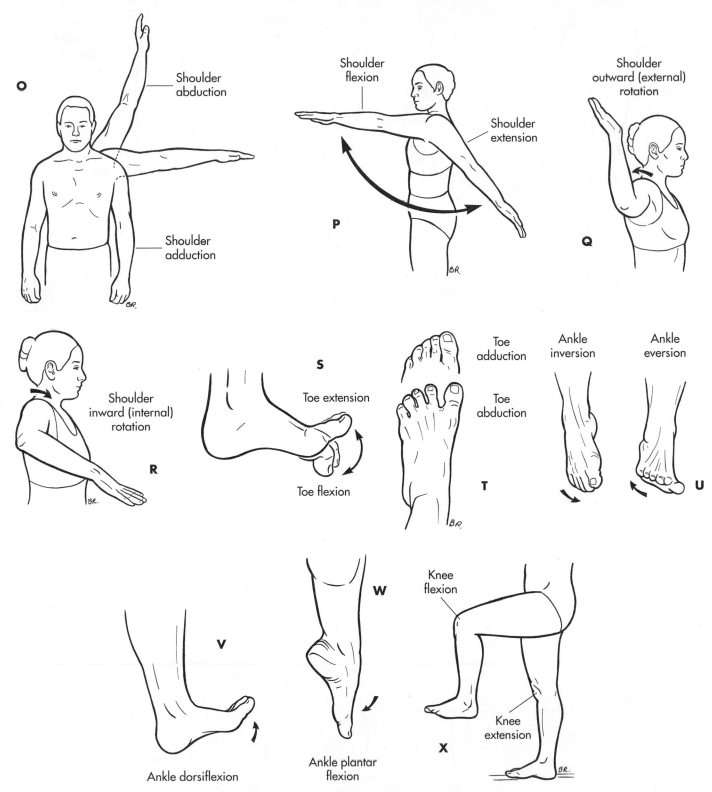

FIGURE 3-9—cont'd For legend see opposite page.

Continued

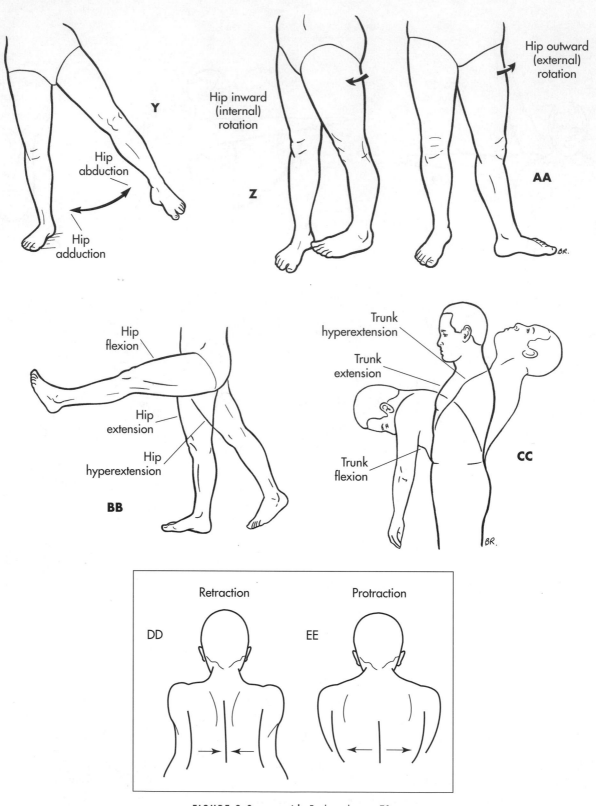

FIGURE 3-9—cont'd For legend see p. 70.

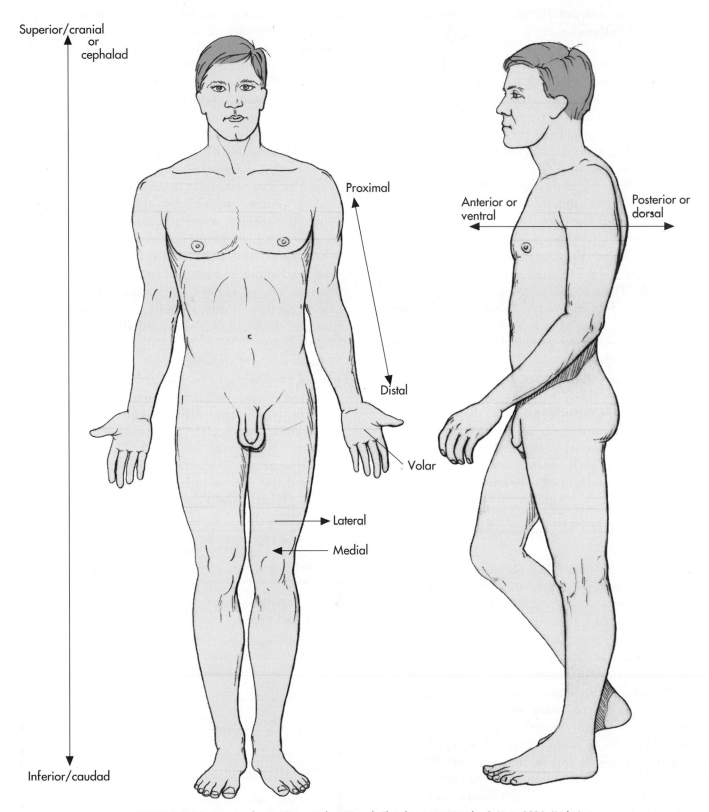

FIGURE 3-10 Directional terms. (From Mathers LH et al: *Clinical anatomy principles,* St Louis, 1996, Mosby.)

lowing directional terms, which are organized in pairs of opposites, are derived from some of the prefixes listed in this chapter:

Anterior (ventral): In front of or toward the front

Posterior (dorsal): Behind, in back, or in the rear

Proximal: Closer to the trunk or the point of origin

Distal: Situated away from the trunk or midline of the body; away from the origin

Lateral: On or to the side, outside, away from the midline

Medial: Relating to the middle, center, or midline

Ipsilateral: The same side

Contralateral: The opposite side

Superior: Higher than, or above

Inferior: Lower than, or below

Volar (palmar): The palm side of the hand

Plantar: The sole side of the foot

Varus: Ends bent inward; angulation of a part of the body inward toward the midline: ><

Valgus: Ends bent outward; for example, bent toward the wall: <>

Internal: An inside surface or the inside part of the body

External: The outside surface of the body

Deep: Inside or away from the surface

Superficial: Toward or on the surface

Dextral (dextro): Right

Sinistral (sinistro): Left; *levo* also is used for left

Ancient Healing Practices

Western science is a relatively new healing method, one that requires the practitioner to observe, measure concrete entities, accumulate data, and analyze findings in a clinical manner. Ancient approaches to healing also require observation, measurement, and accumulation and analysis of data, but in addition, they validate the importance of intuition.

Intuition is defined as knowing something without going through a conscious, problem-solving, rational process of thinking. According to researcher and scientist Hans Selye, nothing can be investigated or validated scientifically unless the researcher first has an idea—that is, uses intuition. And without validation, the chances for practical application are limited. Ancient or indigenous healing practices do not separate the body, mind, and spirit, as Western science does. Spiritual knowledge is knowledge based on intuition; that is, knowledge without material or con-

crete proof, and Western science until recently discounted anything that did not fit within the narrow boundaries of scientific validation. Today, technology and advances in research design are revealing the validity of the more subtle aspects of ancient healing wisdom. The gap between ancient and new knowledge is narrowing, and with this development comes the need to understand the terminologies involved in the different ways of describing the same thing.

The Chinese health system is based on continual accumulation of knowledge through centuries of experiential observation. It is similar to other cultural healing systems, which also endeavor to promote health by working toward homeostasis rather than by eliminating symptoms (a very Western approach). Watching as these older healing theories are "discovered" and explored and then become understood by Western science is exciting! As these systems move closer together in understanding, we all will benefit from the sharing and blending of all types of human knowledge.

As previously mentioned, the general structural plan of the body can be mapped out with standard descriptions and Western terminology. Each of the other healing systems also maps the body, using its own standards and terms, many of which are familiar to those who practice bodywork. These theories do not separate the body from the emotions, a fact reflected in the identification charts. Western mind/body medicine is developing along similar lines.

ACTIVITY 3-6

List three areas where ancient healing wisdom merges with current health practices.

Example Breathing rhythm patterns with biofeedback and relaxation training

Your Turn

1. _____

   _____

2. _____

   _____

3. _____

   _____

The Oriental perspective is based on the *meridian system*. Acupuncture points and the Five Element relationship system are used to identify and explain anatomy and physiologic functions.

The **yin/yang** concept, which was discussed in the previous chapter, is an excellent example of the Oriental perspective. In this chapter, we present more specific terminology for the Five Element theory and then provide a means of comparing and contrasting the language of the Oriental and Western systems (Activity 3-6).

POINTS AND MERIDIANS

In the past, treatments used to aid survival and recovery from trauma were mostly a matter of luck and chance. Some believe that, before the advent of pain-relieving drugs or treatments, a person would press, rub, or hit an affected part of the body to alle-

viate pain. Sometimes when a person was burned, bruised by a stone, or cut, preexisting pain would dissipate and healing would occur. The earliest concept of **acupuncture** was to stimulate a painful point by pressing on it, puncturing it, or burning it. The point was referred to as an Ah shi point, which loosely translates to "Ah, yes, that's where it hurts." In Western science this method of treatment can be explained by the gate control theory.

Healers identified specific points before they recognized any patterns. The mapping of points eventually developed into various healing systems. Meridians are a system of connecting points that affect a particular physiologic function. The actual tracts of each meridian were determined by plotting the various sensations that radiate above or below a point when it is pressed (Figure 3-11). In the past the points used most were those located below the elbow and the knee.

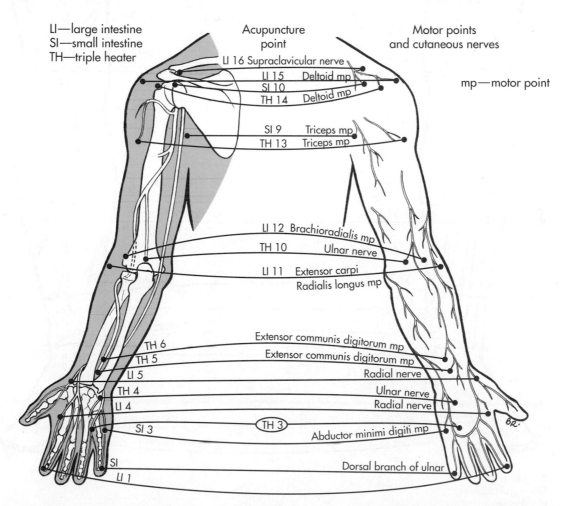

FIGURE 3-11 Typical location of meridians. Meridians tend to follow nerves. (From Fritz S: *Mosby's fundamentals of therapeutic massage,* St Louis, 1995, Mosby.)

Continued

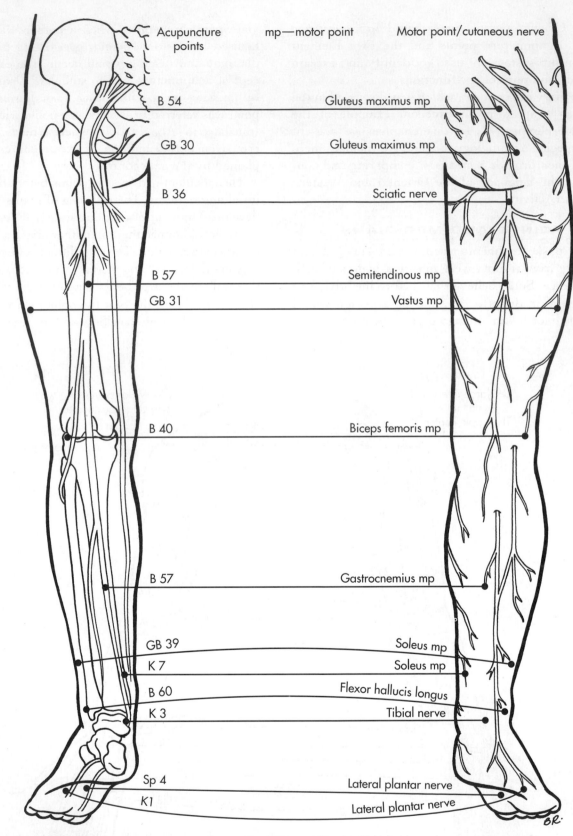

Acupuncture points

mp—motor point

Motor point/cutaneous nerve

B 54 — Gluteus maximus mp

GB 30 — Gluteus maximus mp

B 36 — Sciatic nerve

B 57 — Semitendinous mp

GB 31 — Vastus mp

B 40 — Biceps femoris mp

B 57 — Gastrocnemius mp

GB 39 — Soleus mp

K 7 — Soleus mp

B 60 — Flexor hallucis longus

K 3 — Tibial nerve

Sp 4 — Lateral plantar nerve

K1 — Lateral plantar nerve

B—bladder
GB—gallbladder
K—kidney
Sp—spleen

FIGURE 3-11—cont'd For legend see page 81.

In Western science, acupuncture points have been identified with various anatomic or physiologic locations or functions in the body. Most acupuncture points have been associated with the motor points of the nervous system. A *motor point* is the location where a nerve enters a muscle. Acupuncture points also correspond to Golgi tendon organs and muscle stretch receptors. These same acupuncture points have been shown to have an extremely close correlation to the trigger points and corresponding pain patterns described by Travell and Simons. A *trigger point* is a localized area of deep tenderness and increased tissue resistance. Pressure exerted on a trigger point causes referred pain in a predictable area (Figure 3-12). Ancient practitioners may have observed the referred pain pattern as they mapped the meridians. Pressure on acupuncture points also affects the levels of enkephalins and endorphins, pain- and mood-modulating chemicals in the body.

Point phenomena in the ancient and Western scientific systems have many commonalities; for example, they all share the following characteristics:

1. They are located in a palpable depression.
2. They are associated with a neurovascular formation consisting of free nerve endings, Golgi tendon receptors, spindle cells, pacinian corpuscles, and lymph or blood vessels that pass through the fascia.
3. They are located on the surface of A-Δ fiber afferent fast transmitting receptors sensitive to sharply pointed stimuli or heat. These points may correlate to the acupuncture points.
4. They have in place, deep to the A-Δ fibers in the same area, intramuscularly placed, C-afferent slow transmitting fibers, which are more sensitive to chemicals and may correlate to the trigger point.

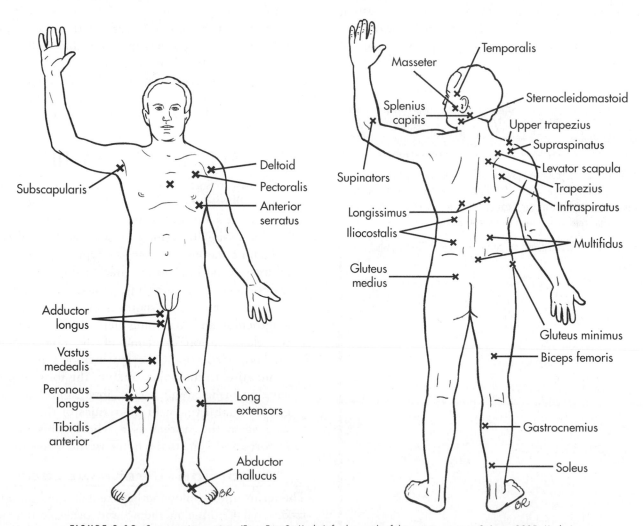

FIGURE 3-12 Common trigger points. (From Fritz S: *Mosby's fundamentals of therapeutic massage,* St Louis, 1995, Mosby.)

Mapping of 100 acupuncture points showed them to be located over large nerve trunks and cutaneous neurovascular bundles.

In less technical terms, points stimulated to create a body change are located in the same area on top of nerves (Activity 3-7). The more superficial nerves may be the acupuncture points, and the deeper nerves may be the trigger points (Chaitow, 1997) (Figure 3-13).

ORGAN RELATIONSHIPS

Unlike the Western concept of organs, Chinese medicine thinks in terms of organ systems, which comprise an organ and essences and fluids as they interact with the meridians. Ancient healing methods have always treated internal functions by external stimulation of the body, using methods such as acupuncture and massage. People have been using these techniques for centuries to help reestablish homeostasis within their bodies, adding to the belief that these practices must have some sort of consistent benefit to still be in existence. Current research has validated cutaneous/visceral connections as part of these processes.

ACTIVITY 3-7

Palpate one of your forearms and hands with moderate pressure, making sure you cover every inch. Whenever you find an Ah shi point, mark it with a washable marker. Compare the points you have identified on your arm and hand to the point charts in this chapter.

Draw a picture of your arm and the points located on it. Describe what you found.

Your Turn

As discussed in Chapter 2, nerve reflexes of internal organs manifest themselves in the surface areas of the body, showing up as referred pain patterns. The following are examples of other manifestations of nerve patterns that connect the internal organs with the surface:

Pain sensations felt on the skin may be referred by internal organs.
Muscular splinting may be noted over an area of internal disturbance.
The *autonomic nervous system* influences surface areas of the body.
Stimulus causes shifts in *endogenous chemicals* (those manufactured inside the body), which can affect organ function.

Theoretic discussion of the use of surface stimulation techniques to stimulate or balance internal organ function could explain the organ relationship of meridian and acupuncture points to specific internal physiology.

If the multitude of points described in the various health practices were mapped on the body, little space would be left. The case can be made that the entire body is a series of points. All this information can be used to reinforce the idea that events on the inside of the body affect the outside and vice versa.

PRACTICAL APPLICATION

Because trigger points are located in shortened muscle fibers, these fibers must be lengthened to the muscle's normal resting length and any connective tissue shortening must be addressed with stretching methods. Often the type of point being addressed is not clear; therefore, unless contraindicated, the shortened muscles should be restored to an appropriate resting length through lengthening and stretching methods. Regardless of the classification or name of the tender point, methods of soft tissue therapy include some sort of stimulation to the point, often in the form of pressure, to bring about a combined neurologic and chemical adjustment in the tissues of the area, as well as to the system as a whole. This method restores and adjusts the homeostatic mechanisms.

TRADITIONAL TERMINOLOGY

The terms in the following list are commonly used in traditional Chinese medicine and other indigenous Oriental healing systems:

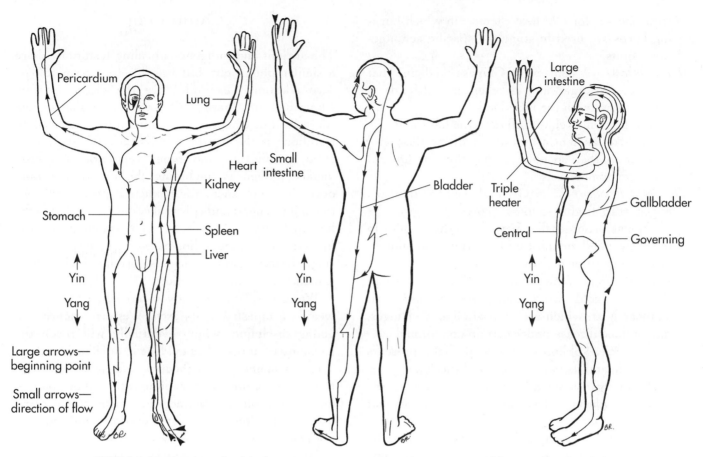

FIGURE 3-13 Comparison of traditional acupuncture points, motor points, and cutaneous nerves of the arm and leg. (From Fritz S: *Mosby's fundamentals of therapeutic massage,* St Louis, 1995, Mosby.)

Acupuncture—The practice of inserting needles in specific points on meridians, or channels, to stimulate or sedate energy flow to regulate or alter body function. A branch of Chinese medicine, it is the art and science of manipulating the flow of **Qi,** the basic life force, and Xue, the blood, body fluids, and nourishing essences. Western medicine uses it primarily to reduce pain. *Acupressure,* which uses digital pressure, follows the same Eastern principles

Cun—A method of measurement that uses a relative standard, usually the length of the second phalange of the second finger. It most often is applied in Oriental bodywork forms

Disharmony—Distortions in health that result when the functions or systems are neither balanced nor working at their optimum. In Chinese medicine, **disharmony** can be created by the **Six Pernicious Influences** or the **Seven Emotions**

Essential substances—The fluids, essences, and energies that maintain balance in the body, mind, and spirit. They include the Qi, or life force; Shen, or spirit; Jing, or essence; Xue, or blood fluids; and Jin-Ye, or fluids

Five Elements—The five basic processes or phases of a cycle that represent the inherent capabilities of change, which reflect yin and yang movements as observed in nature. The Five Elements are wood, fire, earth, metal, and water. When combined with the principles of Chinese medicine, they are used to determine the diagnosis and treatment of a dysfunction (see Figure 1-16)

Jing—The yin essence of life that nurtures growth, reproduction, and development

Jin-Ye, or jingye—Body fluids that warm and nourish the skin, muscles, joints, and brain (e.g., sweat, urine, mucus, saliva), as well as other secretions such as bile and gastric juice

Moxibustion—A form of heat therapy in which burning herbs are used to stimulate specific acupuncture points

Organ systems—A concept of Chinese medicine that describes an organ and its essences and fluids as they interact with the meridians

Qi—Also known as chi; it refers to the life force

Qi Gong—An ancient Chinese art of exercise and meditation that encourages the flow of Qi and supports homeostasis

The Seven Emotions—The Oriental concept that joy, anger, fear, fright, sadness, worry, and grief are emotional responses that may trigger disharmony in the body, mind, or spirit under certain conditions

Shen—The spirit or personality

The Six Pernicious Influences—The Oriental concept that heat, cold, wind, dampness, dryness, and summer heat, which are natural climate changes, may induce disease under certain conditions

Tao—An ancient philosophic concept that represents the whole and its parts as one and the same

Xue—Often translated as "blood," it refers to the blood and plasma, as well as other body fluids that transport Shen

Yin/yang—Yin and yang are terms used to describe polar relationships. Yin/yang refers to the dynamic balance between opposing forces and the continual process of creation and destruction. Yin/yang reflects the natural order of the whole universe and everything in it, including the individual (Cohen, 1996; Ding, 1990)

Summary

The ancient and indigenous healing traditions share a similar philosophy but use different terminology. Two additional examples are the chakra system (described in Chapter 6) and the dosha system (described in Chapter 2). Common to these healing traditions is the use of soft tissue methods; movement; meditation and inner reflection; exercise; dietary influences, including the use of naturally occurring substances for medicinal purposes; emotional influences; and spiritual connections that make human beings one with their environment and the universe. Often metaphor based on naturally occurring, observable phenomena is correlated with physical and psychologic function.

Western scientific study is no less colorful and weaves a tapestry of its own. Western science is a young discipline, which eventually will reach the harmony of approaches evident in ancient practices. Western methods and theories and ancient healing traditions are not in opposition; rather, they complement one another. Together they blend the learning and application of ancient wisdom and current understanding as we strive for homeostasis.

NOTE: It would be beneficial to have available various texts that describe Eastern and native perspectives on health. Those used in the development of this text, which are listed in the Works Consulted section at the end of this book, are a good place to begin.

WORKBOOK SECTION

1. List and define the three word elements used in medical terms.

_____

_____

_____

_____

_____

_____

2. Break the following words into their word elements and give the meaning of each element. Then define the word.

Antiseptic

_____

_____

_____

Contralateral

_____

_____

_____

Subaxillary

_____

_____

_____

Neurogenic

_____

_____

_____

Bradycardia

_____

_____

_____

Neuralgia

_____

_____

_____

Contraindication

_____

_____

_____

Periosteum

_____

_____

_____

Intracephalic

_____

_____

_____

Arthroplasty

_____

_____

_____

3. Give the meanings of the following abbreviations:

ADL:

_____

ad lib:

_____

a.m.a.:

_____

ANS:

_____

as tol:

_____

BP:

_____

CC:

_____

c/o:

_____

Dx:

_____

h (hr):

_____

H20:

_____

Hx:

_____

IBW:

_____

ICT:

_____

id:

_____

L:

_____

lig:

_____

M:

_____

ML:

_____

meds:

_____

n:

_____

NA:

_____

OTC:

_____

P:

_____

PA:

_____

PT:

_____

Px:

_____

R:

_____

R/O:

_____

ROM:

_____

Rx:

_____

SOB:

_____

SP, spir:

_____

Sym:

_____

T:

_____

TLC:

_____

Tx:

_____

WD:

_____

4. Define charting and explain the problem-solving model of charting.

_____

_____

_____

_____

_____

5. In what ways do the Oriental view and terminology act as a model for indigenous ancient healing practices? Compare the Oriental discipline with Western theory and terminology.

_____

_____

_____

_____

_____

_____

_____

_____

6. On the blank lines, write the terms used to describe the position of the body in relation to other body parts.

a. _____ In front of or toward the front of the body or body part

b. _____ Behind, in back of, or in the rear of the body or body part

c. _____ Situated away from the trunk or midline of the body; away from the origin

d. _____ On or to the side, outside, away from the midline

e. _____ Relating to the middle, center, or midline of the body

f. _____ Closer to the trunk or to the point of origin

g. _____ The same side

h. _____ The opposite side

i. _____ Toward the head

j. _____ Toward the tail

k. _____ Higher than, or above

l. _____ Lower than, or below

m. _____ The circumference, or an area away from the center

n. _____ The palm side of the hand; also called *palmar*

o. _____ The sole side of the foot

p. _____ Bent inward; angulation of a part of the body inward toward the midline

q. _____ Bent outward; bent toward the wall

r. _____ Right

s. _____ Left

t. _____ The inside surface or the inside part of the body

u. _____ The outside surface of the body

v. _____ Far beneath the surface

w. _____ Toward or on the surface

x. _____ The wall of a part of the body.

FILL IN THE BLANK

KEY TERMS

A (1) _____ is part of a word. A (2) _____ is placed at the beginning of a word to alter the meaning of the word. A vowel added between two roots or a root and a suffix to make pronunciation easier is a (3) _____. The (4) _____ word element contains the basic meaning of the word, and the (5) _____ is placed at the end of a root to change the meaning of the word. A shortened form of a word or phrase is an (6) _____. A (7) _____ is a written record of professional interactions representing a clinical reasoning methodology emphasizing a (8) _____ approach. The (9) _____ is a problem-oriented medical record, and (10) _____ is the acronym (subjective, objective, assessment/analysis, and plan) for the four parts of the written account of the health assessment.

(11) _____ is an ancient philosophic concept and orientation that sees the universe and each individual as one and the same. (12) _____ is the dynamic balance between opposing forces and the continual process of creation and destruction within the natural order of the universe and of each person's inner being. (13) _____ is the art and science of manipulating the flow of (14) _____, the basic life force. (15) _____ are the fluids, essences, and energies that keep the mind/body/spirit in balance. (16) _____ is the spirit. Moxibustion uses (17) _____ herbs placed on or near the body to stimulate specific acupuncture points. Unlike the Western concept of organs, Chinese medicine thinks in terms of an (18) _____ that includes the central organ and its interaction with the Essential Substances meridian.

(19) _____ is an ancient Chinese art of exercise and meditation that supports homeostasis. The Seven Emotions are (20) _____, _____, _____, _____, _____, _____, _____ . Heat, cold, wind, dampness, dryness, and summer heat are known as the (21) _____. The Seven Emotions and the Six Pernicious Influences are internal triggers of disharmony in (22) _____.

The (23) _____ are five basic processes or phases of a cycle that represent inherent capabilities of change. The Five Elements are (24) _____, _____, _____, _____, and _____.

A (25) _____ is a method of measurement using a relative standard of size and spacing on an individual, regardless of size or shape.

PROBLEM SOLVING

Analyze the following situation, using the problem-solving model, and complete the exercise at the end.

Agreement on terminology is an abiding issue in the sharing of information. Professionals often are speaking of the same process, methodology, or diagnosis but approaching it from a different cultural and language base. In one study, Mexican Americans refused medical treatment because their explanation of the disease process was discounted. If cultural differences were better understood, such problems might not arise. As researchers and health professionals take a serious look at ancient forms of healing and as more validity is given to noninvasive methods such as soft tissue and movement therapies, some sort of common language base must be found, or we will be unable to speak to one another. Consumers, meanwhile, will remain confused, unable to make informed decisions about the services they want to use. In all of these approaches, the body remains the same. Anatomy and physiology do not change.

In the following exercise, the first statement is provided as a guide. Fill in at least two more statements.

FACTS
1. Terminology is an abiding issue in the sharing of information.
2. _____
3. _____

POSSIBILITIES
1. Schools could teach more cross-cultural terminology.
2. _____
3. _____

LOGICAL CAUSE AND EFFECT
1. If schools expanded their curricula, more teachers and textbooks would be needed and the cost of education would rise.
2. _____
3. _____

EXPECTED IMPACT
1. People may find their spiritual belief systems challenged in the study of healing disciplines in which a spiritual practice has an intrinsic part, and they may feel uncomfortable with these philosophies.
2. _____
3. _____

What can you do as a professional to bridge the communication gap?

_____
_____
_____
_____
_____
_____
_____
_____
_____
_____
_____
_____
_____

FURTHER STUDY

1. In a comprehensive medical terminology text (see Works Consulted list at the end of this book), identify the chapters that pertain to the information presented in this chapter.
2. Do some research on one other ancient healing practice. Identify the major components of the discipline and correlate it to the Western model presented in this text. Pay particular attention to the following elements:

Healing practice

Soft tissue methods

Movement and exercise

Meditation and inner reflection

Dietary influences

Use of naturally occurring herbs for medicinal purposes

Emotional influences

Spiritual connections

Metaphor based on naturally occurring phenomenon

Correlation with Western scientific theories

Answer Key

1. *Prefix:* A word element added to the beginning of a root to change the meaning of the word.

   Suffix: A word element added to the end of a root to change the meaning of the word.

   Root: A word element that contains the basic meaning of the word.

2. *Anti*—against; *septic*—germs. Definition: Effective against germs.

   Contra—opposing; *lateral*—side. Definition: The opposite side.

   Sub—under; *axilla*—armpit. Definition: Under the armpit.

   Neur—nerve; *genic*—origin. Definition: Originating in the nerves.

   Brady—slow; *card*—heart; *ia-a* state or condition. Definition: Slow heartbeat.

   Neur—nerve; *algia*—pain. Definition: Nerve pain.

   Contra—opposing; *indication*—desired result. Definition: Opposite of the desired result.

   Peri—around; *oste*—bone. Definition: Around the bone. (Periosteum is a specialized membrane that surrounds bone.)

   Intra—within; *cephla*—head. Definition: Within the head.

   Arthro—joint; *plasty*—surgical repair. Definition: Reconstruction of a joint.

3. *ADL:* Activities of daily living

   ad lib: As desired

   a.m.a.: Against medical advice

   ANS: Autonomic nervous system

   as tol: As tolerated

   BP: Blood pressure

   CC: Chief complaint

   c/o: Complains of

   Dx: Diagnosis

   h (hr): Hour

   H_2O: Water

   Hx: History

   IBW: Ideal body weight

   ICT: Inflammation of connective tissue

   Id: The same

   L: Left; length; lumbar

   lig: Ligament

   M: Muscle; meter; myopia

   ML: Midline

   meds: Medications

   n: Normal

   NA: Nonapplicable

   OTC: Over the counter

   P: Pulse

   PA: Postural analysis

   PT: Physical therapy

   Px: Prognosis

   R: Respiration; right

   R/O: Rule out

   ROM: Range of motion

   Rx: Prescription

   SOB: Shortness of breath

   SP, spir: Spirit

   Sym: Symmetric

   T: Temperature

   TLC: Tender loving care

   Tx: Treatment

   WD: Well developed

4. Charting is the process of keeping a written record of professional interactions. SOAP (subjective, objective, assessment/analysis, and plan) is the mnemonic for the four parts of the written account of the health assessment. In a problem-solving model of charting, the practitioner collects a database before beginning the process of identifying the client's problems. The database contains all the subjective and objective information available that contributes to therapeutic intervention. Next, the information is analyzed. Each problem identified represents a conclusion or decision that arises from examination, investigation, and analysis of the data collected. A decision then is made about a plan of intervention. The plan needs to be implemented, reevaluated, and adjusted as necessary. The action taken, its effectiveness, and the outcome are recorded progressively from session to session.

5. Western science is a young discipline that uses the scientific methods of observation; it involves measuring concrete entities, accumulating data, and analyzing findings. Ancient approaches also require observation, measurement, and accumulation and analysis of data, but, in addition, they have validated the importance of intuition. Ancient or indigenous healing practices do not separate the body, mind, and spirit as does Western science. Most ancient healing systems are grounded in concepts similar to those presented in the Oriental model, mainly the idea of bringing the body into balance to promote health, rather than simply eliminating symptoms, as has been the method of the very young Western scientific approach. Western mind/body medicine is developing according to similar theories.

   Ancient methods reflect a common belief that internal functions can be affected by surface stimulation, such as in the application and rubbing in of ointments, the use of various types of massage and acupuncture, and the laying on of hands. In light of the accumulation of knowledge over eons, if these practices had not shown some sort of consistent benefit, they would not still be in effect. We now know that nerve reflexes of internal organs manifest themselves in the surface areas of the body.

   Common to these ancient and indigenous healing traditions is the use of soft tissue methods, movement, meditation and inner reflection, exercise, dietary influences and use of naturally occurring herbs for medicinal purposes, emotional influences and spiritual connections to help make human beings one with their environment and the universe. Metaphor based on naturally occurring phenomena that can be observed often is correlated with physical and psychologic function. Western scientific theories are not in opposition to these practices; rather, they actually are complementary.

6. a. Anterior or ventral
    b. Posterior or dorsal
    c. Distal
    d. Lateral
    e. Medial
    f. Proximal
    g. Ipsilateral
    h. Contralateral
    i. Cephalad
    j. Caudal
    k. Superior
    l. Inferior
    m. Peripheral
    n. Volar
    o. Plantar
    p. Varus
    q. Valgus
    r. Dextral
    s. Sinistral
    t. Internal
    u. External
    v. Deep
    w. Superficial
    x. Parietal

FILL IN THE BLANK

KEY TERMS

(1) word element
(2) prefix
(3) combining vowel
(4) root
(5) suffix
(6) abbreviation
(7) chart
(8) problem-solving approach
(9) POMR
(10) SOAP
(11) Tao
(12) Yin/yang
(13) Acupuncture
(14) Qi
(15) Essential Substances
(16) Shen
(17) burning
(18) Organ System
(19) Qi Gong
(20) Joy, anger, fear, fright, sadness, worry, grief
(21) Six Pernicious Influences
(22) Mind/body/spirit
(23) Five Elements
(24) Water, wood, fire, metal, earth
(25) Cun

ANSWERS TO ACTIVITY 3-1 ON P. 57

AM: Morning
Hx: History
ADL: Activities of daily living
ad lib: As desired
CC: Chief complaint
GI: Gastrointestinal
ABD: Abdomen
meds: Medications
ROM: Range of motion
as tol: As tolerated
h: Hour
PT: Physical therapy
ft: Foot (or feet)
R: Respiration
T: Temperature
P: Pulse
PM: Afternoon
H$_2$O: Water
TLC: Tender loving care
OB: Obstetrics

Section Two

Systems of Control

In the study of the way the body functions, it becomes evident that two systems, the nervous system and endocrine system, share in the coordination of body activities. These two systems of control are interdependent and unable to function effectively without each other.

After the mechanisms of control are understood, learning about the rest of the body becomes a matter of recognizing the structure of the pieces (anatomy) of each system functioning (physiology) under the direction of the control systems. Bodywork professionals often focus extensively on the musculoskeletal system. However, without the nervous system and endocrine system, the musculoskeletal system does not function. This section is presented before the study of the skeleton, joints, and muscles to establish the larger picture of the way the body—including movement—occurs.

The major benefits derived from soft tissue and movement therapies depend on reflex mechanisms and neurochemical feedback loops, all coordinated

COMPARISON OF NEWTONIAN PHYSICS AND QUANTUM MECHANICS

NEWTONIAN PHYSICS	QUANTUM MECHANICS
Can be pictured	Cannot be pictured
Based on ordinary sense perceptions	Based on systems not directly observable
Describes things, individual objects in space, and their changes in time	Describes statistical behavior of systems and groups
Predicts events	Predicts possibilities
Holds that we can observe something without changing it	Hold that we cannot observe something without changing it

through the nervous system and endocrine system. Function and structure have a circular relationship, each influencing the other.

Physics is the study of the way things work. Physicists ask the question "How does the world behave?" *Newtonian* principles were developed in a linear pathway (i.e., from an understanding that the world behaves in predictable ways of cause and effect). It would be Newtonian to believe that the nervous system and endocrine system tell the rest of the body what to do, and the parts respond in a predictable way. Usually this assumption is accurate but not always. *Quantum* principles look at the world in a more interactive way. Instead of predictable outcomes, decisions—at a subatomic to cosmic level—are being made constantly. Simply in the process of thinking, outcomes can be influenced in a multidimensional loop of events. It is much easier to view the world from a linear view and think that a specific nerve pathway, neurotransmitter, or hormone will always produce the same predictable response. However, the body does not always respond that way. Life is not always predictable and neither is physiology. Quantum theory exists from a *basis of tendency to exist or happen. Nothing is for sure.* The human potential to decide in terms of body, mind, and spirit is more circular and uncertain, harder to predict, and more elusive to learn. It is suggested then that the student proceed with fascination focused on possibilities as well as facts as the study of the functional aspect of the body is undertaken (see Table).

Even though these factors seem to be in opposition, they also reflect the duality of wholeness, which seems to be an accurate reflection of the way the body functions (Zukav, 1980; Dossy, 1982).

Certainly, as each of the other body systems is explored, it will be important to again review the effect of the control systems on specific structure and function. These chapters lay the foundation so that future study will be more than memorizing body parts and functions in a piece-by-piece approach. Instead, what is hoped to be accomplished is an appreciation of innate body intelligence and the orchestrated synchronized symphony conducted by the nervous and endocrine systems.

During the process of researching these chapters, it became apparent that the study of these important controlling mechanisms is a lifelong endeavor, and the authors concede that, particularly in this area, there is simply too much to know. Even the most comprehensive anatomy and physiology texts consulted resorted to choosing what to cover, recognizing that covering all the information in one general textbook is impossible. In addition, current research

ACTIVITY

In Chapters 1 through 3, many references have been made to the nervous system, in particular the autonomic nervous system, certain neurotransmitters, and the endocrine system. The interaction of both theory and application of bodywork modalities has been touched on. Review these three chapters and underline or highlight any references made to nerves, neurotransmitters, the autonomic nervous system (both sympathetic and parasympathetic divisions), hormones, and chemicals of the body.

List the chapter and page numbers where the information has been located.

is highly concentrated on these control systems. The information base is being expanded and altered almost daily. Whereas the study of the musculoskeletal system, cardiovascular system, and so forth is more stable because the bulk of the information concerns the anatomy, which is relatively static, the study of the nervous and endocrine systems is highly focused to the function of the body. This information is more likely to change and expand as researchers explore more deeply into the subtleties of neuroendocrine influences.

The information presented in these chapters is by no means an exhaustive study, and much important and interesting information has not been addressed. However, the student must begin somewhere in the learning process. Reference texts are an invaluable resource. We hope that the material will be of practical importance, both in understanding the mechanisms of effect for bodywork approaches and in understanding function and associated behavior from neuroendocrine influences.

As you completed the activities, did you notice the following in Chapter 1?

- The characteristics of life involve the movement of energy from one point to another.
- Subtle forms of energetic bodywork are based on electrical and chemical functions.
- Touch therapies stimulate sensory function of the skin.
- The storage and release of fat from adipose tissue is regulated by hormonal and nervous stimuli.
- Although not fully understood, the piezoelectric property of collagen produces some form of electrical influence.
- Nervous tissue is one of the four basic tissue types and is specifically developed to regulate and integrate body activity.

Did you notice the following in Chapter 2?

- The Vata dosha directs nerve impulses.
- The nervous system and endocrine system are the most important in maintaining homeostasis.
- Feedback loops are afferent and efferent information pathways traveled by nerve impulses or chemical hormone messengers. Each feedback loop consists of a sensory, integrating, and effector component from the nervous or endocrine system.
- Bodywork methods work through feedback loops.
- Body rhythms are influenced by the autonomic nervous system and endocrine system.
- Entrainment is coordinated by the nervous and endocrine systems.
- Pain and pain management are based on neurochemical mechanisms.

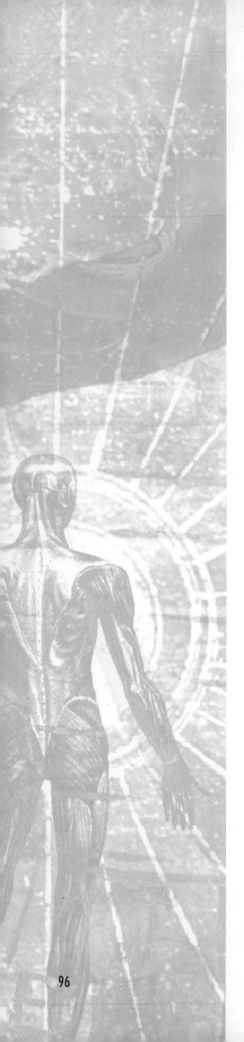

- The general adaptation syndrome response and effects of long-term stress are endocrine and autonomic nervous system events.
- Bodywork is a sensory stimulation approach that promotes mechanism of health and stress management.

Did you notice the following in Chapter 3?

- The dorsal body cavity houses the central nervous system.
- The point phenomenon in ancient healing practices is correlated to the nervous and endocrine systems.

Overview of the Nervous System and Endocrine System

The nervous system is the most complex of the body systems. It is made up of more than 110 billion nerve cells. It is divided into the central nervous system, composed of the brain, spinal cord, and coverings, and the peripheral nervous system, which includes the cranial nerves, spinal nerves, and ganglia. The peripheral nervous system is further divided into autonomic and somatic divisions. These subdivisions combine and communicate to innervate the somatic and visceral parts of the body. The somatic division is associated with the bones, muscles, and skin. The visceral or autonomic division is associated with the internal glands, organs, blood vessels, and mucous membranes. The autonomic nervous system (ANS) is further divided into two divisions. The sympathetic nervous system activates arousal responses and expends body resources in such a way to respond to emergency situations. The parasympathetic nervous system reverses the response of the sympathetic nervous system by returning the body to a nonalarm state and restoring body resources. The sympathetic division is considered the "flight, fight, fear" system. The parasympathetic ANS is connected to the "relaxation response." Much of the interaction between body and mind takes place through ANS activity. The concepts of yin and yang are reflected in the ANS, with parasympathetic functions relating to yin and sympathetic functions relating to yang (see color plate 3).

The basic structure of the nervous system is the neuron, or nerve cell. The nerve cell is an impulse-transmitting fiber connecting the central nervous system (CNS) with all parts of the body. Three basic types of neurons exist:

1. Afferent or sensory neurons that carry impulses to the CNS
2. Connecting or associative interneurons that transmit nerve impulses between neurons
3. Efferent or motor neurons that transmit impulses away from the CNS to the muscles, organs, and glands

Both the nervous and endocrine system transmit information from one part of the body to another, but they do it in different ways. The nervous system transmits information very rapidly, with a short duration of action by nerve impulse conducted from one body area to another. The endocrine system is a network of ductless glands and other structures that secrete chemicals called hormones directly into the bloodstream, affecting the function of specific target organs. The action of hormones is slower, with a longer duration of action than nerve impulses. Often it is the nervous system that initiates a response and the endocrine system that sustains it.

Both systems use chemicals. The nervous system uses neurotransmitters, and the endocrine system uses hormones. Many times these are the same chemicals. If the chemical is found in the synapses of the nervous system, it is a neurotransmitter. If the same chemical is found in the blood, it is a hormone. The influence of the nervous system regulates the endocrine system, and the endocrine system influences the nervous system, forming a feedback loop that increases or decreases activity for healthy function. The feedback system and autoregulation (maintenance of internal homeostasis) are interlinked in all body functions.

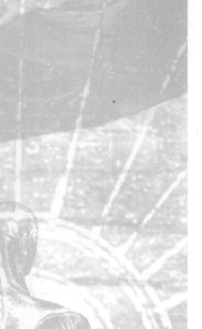

Chapter 4

Nervous System Basics and the Central Nervous System

KEY TERMS

Axon (AK-son) A single elongated projection from the nerve cell body that transmits impulses away from the cell body.

Brain The largest and most complex unit of the nervous system; it is responsible for perception, sensation, emotion, intellect, and action.

Brainstem The primitive portion of the brain; it contains centers for vital functions and reflex actions, such as vomiting, coughing, sneezing, posture, and basic movement patterns.

Central nervous system The brain and spinal cord and their coverings.

Cerebellum (sair-e-BELL-um) The second largest part of the brain; it is involved with balance, posture, coordination, and movements.

Cerebrospinal (sair-e-bro-SPY-nal) *fluid* A clear, colorless fluid that flows throughout the brain and around the spinal cord, cushioning and protecting these structures and maintaining proper pH balance.

Cerebrum (se-REE-brum) The largest of the brain divisions; it consists of two hemispheres that occupy the uppermost region of the cranium. The cerebrum receives, interprets, and associates incoming information with past memories, then transmits the appropriate motor response.

Dendrites (DEN-drites) Branching projections from the nerve cell body that carry signals to the cell body.

Gray matter Unmyelinated nervous tissue, particularly that found in the central nervous system.

Myelin (MY-e-lin) A white, fatty, insulating substance formed by the Schwann cells that surrounds some axons. Also produced in the central nervous system by oligodendrocytes.

Neurolemma (noo-ri-LEM-mah) The outer cell membrane of a Schwann cell that is essential in the regeneration of injured axons.

Neuroglia (noo-ROG-lee-ah) Specialized connective tissue cells that support, protect, and hold neurons together.

Neurons (NOO-rons) Nerve cells that conduct impulses.

Neurotransmitters (noo-ro-TRANS-mit-er) Chemical compounds that generate action potentials when released in the synapses from presynaptic cells.

Schwann (shwon) *cell* A specialized cell that forms myelin.

Spinal cord Portion of the central nervous system that exits the skull into the vertebral column. The two major functions of the spinal cord are to conduct nerve impulses and to be a center for spinal reflexes.

Synapse (SIN-aps) Spaces between neurons or between a neuron and an effector organ.

Tracts Collections of nerve fibers in the brain and spinal cord with a common function.

White matter Myelinated nerve fibers, particularly those found in brain and spinal tissue.

Nervous System Basics

NERVE CELL STRUCTURE

Two types of cells are found in the **central nervous system (CNS):** the **neurons,** or nerve cells that conduct impulses, and **neuroglia,** specialized connective tissue cells. The function of the neuron is to receive and transmit electrical signals to other neurons, muscles, or glands. The neuroglia (*glia* means glue) supports and protects neurons as it holds them together. In addition, neuroglia supports the tiny blood vessels (capillaries) in the brain.

Nerve cells consist of a cell body and its nerve fibers, the axons and dendrites. The cell body contains a nucleus and its organelles. The **dendrites,** which look like small hairs, are extensions of the cytoplasm of the cell. Their job is to carry signals to the cell body. The **axon** is an elongated projection that carries signals away from the cell body.

In the peripheral nervous system the neuroglia forms a protective sheath around the axons. It contains a fatty insulator called **myelin** produced by **Schwann cells.** The outer membrane is called the **neurilemma** and is also formed by Schwann cells. Small gaps between segments of the myelin sheath are called *nodes of Ranvier* and help speed the nerve impulses.

Neurons are identified by their functions. A *sensory neuron* conducts sensory signals to the CNS, whereas *motor neurons* conduct motor signals away from the CNS. *Association* or *interneurons* act as bridges in the CNS to conduct signals from one neuron to another (Figure 4-1).

NERVE FUNCTIONS

Let's examine a neuron to see the way nerve signals are sent through a healthy body.

When a neuron is at rest, the outside of its cell membrane is positively charged, whereas inside the charge is negative. This is called the *membrane potential.* It is created by the concentration of ions in the fluids in and around the cell. Excess sodium (Na^+) ions tend to concentrate in the extracellular fluid, and the cell membrane does not allow it to flow into the cell. A stimulus such as a pressure, light, temperature, or chemical change results in a very brief

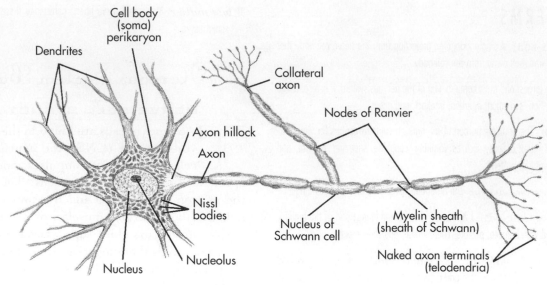

FIGURE 4-1   Neuron. (From Thompson JM et al: *Mosby's clinical nursing,* ed 4, St Louis, 1997, Mosby.)

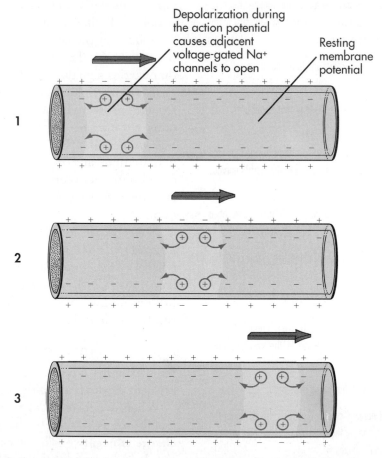

FIGURE 4-2   Conduction of the action potential. The reverse polarity characteristic of the peak of the action potential causes local current flow to adjacent regions of the membrane *(small arrows).* This stimulates voltage-gated Na+ channels to open and thus creates a new action potential. This cycle continues, producing wavelike conduction of the action potential from point to point along a nerve fiber. Adjacent regions of membrane behind the action potential do not polarize again because they are still in their refractory period. (From Thibodeau GA, Patton KT: *Anatomy and physiology,* ed 3, St Louis, 1996, Mosby.)

change in the charge of one segment of the neuron. This is called *depolarization*.

During this process the permeability of the cell membrane changes and the sodium ions are allowed into the neuron. The outside of that segment of the membrane becomes negative as it is *depolarized*, whereas the inside becomes positive. This is called the *action potential*. As this continues along the nerve fiber, the *nerve impulse* depolarizes the next section, causing it to reverse its charges while the previous segment returns to its original polarity or is *repolarized*; the outside again becomes positively charged and the inside becomes negatively charged. The term *excited* is used to describe the segment as it switches charges with the action potential, and the term *inhibited* describes the reversal of that action (Figure 4-2).

The *refractory period* is the very brief period after inhibition when the neuron recovers. The *absolute refractory period* is the time during which a neuron will not respond to any stimuli. This is followed by the *relative refractory period*, when the neuron will only respond to a very strong stimulus.

The path of the nerve impulse is different in myelinated and unmyelinated nerve fibers. The nerve impulse travels over the surface of the cell membrane when there is no myelination and excites one segment at a time. This results in a slowly transmitted signal. With myelinated fibers, the impulse jumps from a node of Ranvier to the next node. During this *saltatory conduction*, the speed of the moving signal is much faster (The term *saltate* means to dance, and it is used to describe the way this signal "dances" from one place to the next) (Figure 4-3).

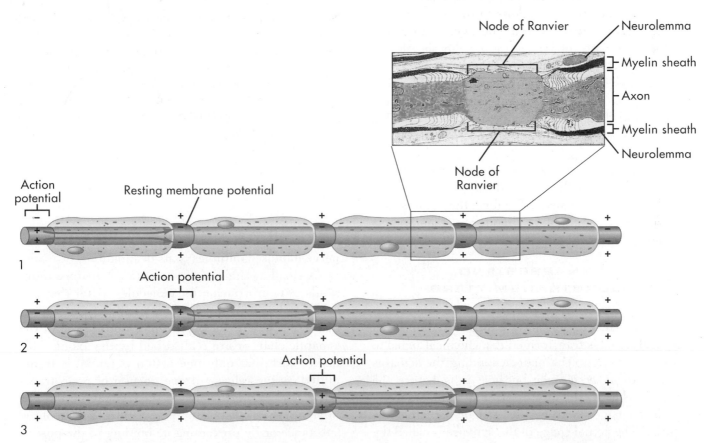

FIGURE 4-3 Saltatory conduction. This series of diagrams shows that the insulating nature of the myelin sheath prevents ion movement everywhere but at the nodes of Ranvier. The action potential at one node triggers current flow *(arrows)* across the myelin sheath to the next node, producing an action potential there. The action potential thus seems to "leap" rapidly from node to node. The inset is a transmission electron micrograph showing a node of Ranvier in a myelinated fiber. (From Thibodeau GA, Patton KT: *Anatomy and physiology,* ed 3, St Louis, 1996, Mosby; *inset,* courtesy Georg Thieme Verlag.)

🖐 PRACTICAL APPLICATION

Bodywork methods such as muscle energy techniques and proprioceptive neuromuscular facilitation use the aforementioned refractory period to their advantage. Muscles often resist lengthening by initiating a spasm. If the muscle is first contracted and then lengthened, it is less likely to spasm during the refractory period, and the muscle can be restored more easily to a more normal resting length. Because these periods are very short, gentle applications of lengthening procedures need to be used. Methods that generate any sort of strong stimuli, especially pain, must be avoided. If too strong a stimulus is introduced, instead of the muscle relaxing, it will be able to generate nerve impulses and contract, thus resisting any sort of lengthening or stretching methods.

Nerve Repair or Regeneration

If the cell body is damaged or separated, the neuron will die. If damage is only done to the axon and the neurilemma is not destroyed, the nerve can repair itself. At the point of injury, the myelin sheath and the distal portion of the axon degenerate. A tunnel is formed by the neurolemma from the point of injury to the original axon destination—another axon, muscle, or gland. This tunnel provides a path for the axon to follow as it regenerates. This process occurs in the peripheral nervous system.

Whereas oligodendrocytes are cells that produce myelin in the CNS, the myelin does not seem to form into the neurolemma needed to form the guiding tunnel from the area of injury. Therefore regeneration is extremely limited (Figure 4-4, *A to D*).

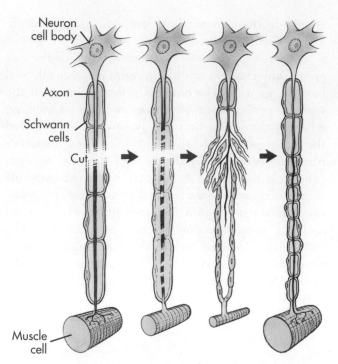

FIGURE 4-4 Repair of a peripheral nerve fiber. **A,** An injury results in a cut nerve. **B,** Immediately after the injury occurs, the distal portion of the axon degenerates as does its myelin sheath. **C,** The remaining neurolemma tunnel from the point of injury to the effector. New Schwann cells grow within this tunnel, maintaining a path for regrowth of the axon. Meanwhile, several growing axon "sprouts" appear. When one of these growing fibers reaches the tunnel, it increases its growth rate, growing as much as 3 to 5 mm per day. (The other sprouts eventually disappear.) **D,** The neuron's connection with the effector is reestablished. (From Thibodeau GA, Patton KT: *Anatomy and physiology,* ed 3, St Louis, 1996, Mosby.)

SYNAPSES AND NEUROTRANSMITTERS

The space or junction between two neurons or a neuron and an effector organ is called a **synapse.** An electrical signal is transformed to a chemical signal to cross the junction. The neuron sending the signal is referred to as *presynaptic* because it is before the synapse, whereas the neuron or muscle fiber receiving the signal would be *postsynaptic,* or after the synapse. The actual space in the synapse is called the *synaptic cleft* (Figure 4-5).

At the end of the axon of the presynaptic neuron, small sacs, or vesicles, are present that contain chemical compounds known as **neurotransmitters.** Once released, they cross the synaptic cleft and bind with or are absorbed by the postsynaptic neuron or mus-

cle. This generates another action potential, and the nerve impulse continues to its destination.

As small as the vesicles are, they can store thousands of neurotransmitter molecules. After they are released and their action completed, they are immediately broken down by enzymes, diffuse out of the synaptic cleft, or are reabsorbed by the axons. This makes sure that only one action potential is transmitted by the release of one portion of neurotransmitters. In certain instances, drugs may be used to interrupt the cycle by stopping the metabolism of the substance or by preventing its binding to the postsynaptic membrane.

Neurotransmitters regulate many of our body activities and senses. At present, more than 30 neurotransmitters have been identified, and it is suspected many more exist. When released into the bloodstream, these same chemicals are called *hormones.*

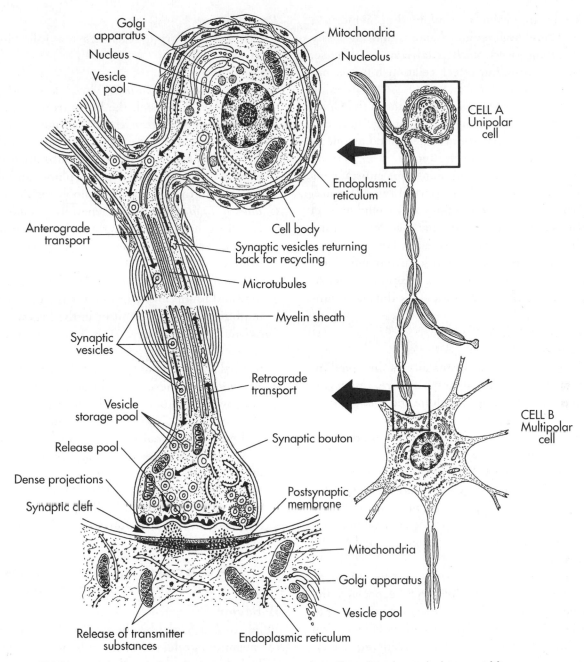

FIGURE 4-5 Functional relationship between two neurons in pathway. Electrical impulse travels along axon of first neuron to synapse. Chemical transmitter is secreted into synaptic space to depolarize membrane (dendrite or cell body) of the next neuron in pathway. (From Thompson JM et al: *Mosby's clinical nursing*, ed 4, St Louis, 1997, Mosby.)

Many of the known hormones are thought to work as neurotransmitters, implying a close link between the nervous system and endocrine activity.

To be classified as a neurotransmitter, a chemical must have certain characteristics. These include such things as being found in presynaptic vesicles, having the ability to be removed from the synaptic cleft, and being capable of stimulating a nerve impulse. The following is a list of some of the major neurotransmitters, their primary actions, and some of their locations:

Acetylcholine—Stimulates the skeletal muscles and primarily acts on the parasympathetic nervous system. It can stimulate or inhibit various organs, depending on the receptors to which it is bound.

Plentiful in the brain, it is involved in memory. A lack of acetylcholine has been found in many patients diagnosed with Alzheimer's disease, although a cause-and-effect relationship has not yet been established.

Serotonin — Usually works as an inhibitor in the CNS. It is synthesized into melatonin and affects our sleep and moods. Serotonin is described as one of the "feel-good" neurotransmitters.

Histamine — Considered a stimulant, this substance is released by the mast cells as part of the inflammatory process. It causes itching at a cellular level and also works as a vasodilator. Also found in the hypothalamus, it regulates body temperature, water balance, and plays a role in our emotions. Histamine also stimulates pain receptors to sensitize against further stimulation, as during a sunburn.

Catecholamines

Catecholamines are neurotransmitters involved in sleep, motor function, mood, and pleasure. Important endogenous catecholamines include the following:

Epinephrine — Can be a stimulant or inhibitor, depending on the type of receptor bound. It is found in several areas of the CNS and in the sympathetic divisions of the autonomic nervous system (ANS). It is also involved in "fight-or-flight" responses such as dilatation of blood vessels to the skeletal muscles. It is classified as a hormone when secreted by the adrenal gland.

Norepinephrine — Like epinephrine, it can excite or inhibit and is found in the CNS (especially the hypothalamus and limbic system) and the sympathetic division of the ANS. It causes constriction of skeletal blood vessels. It is considered a feel-good neurotransmitter and is involved in emotional responses. The release of norepinephrine is enhanced by amphetamines, whereas cocaine stops its removal from the synapses, so leftover norepinephrine continues to stimulate receptors.

Dopamine — Generally excitatory, it is found in the brain and ANS. A feel-good neurotransmitter, it is involved in emotions and moods and in the regulation of motor control and the executive functioning of the brain. Release is enhanced by L dopa and amphetamines. Deficiencies occur in Parkinson's disease, and it may be involved in schizophrenia.

Peptide group

The peptide group includes the following substances:

Endorphins and enkephalins — These are endogenous morphines that block the brain from feeling pain. Generally inhibitory, they are found in several regions of the CNS, retina, and intestinal tract. They inhibit pain by inhibiting substance P. Their effects are mimicked by morphine and heroin. They seem to play a part in mood regulation.

Glutamate (glutamic acid) — Generally excitatory and found in the CNS. Thought to be responsible for as much as 75% of the excitatory signals in the brain.

Gamma-aminobutyric acid (GABA) — Generally inhibitory and found in the brain, it is the most common inhibitory neurotransmitter in the brain.

Substance P — Excitatory. It is found in the brain, spinal cord, sensory pain pathways, and gastrointestinal tract. It transmits pain information.

Somatostatin — Generally inhibitory, it inhibits release of growth hormone; a gut-brain peptide.

Cholecystokinin (CCK) — Found in the brain, retina, and gastrointestinal tract, its function in the nervous system is uncertain. It may be related to feeding behavior; a gut-brain peptide.

Vasoactive intestinal peptide (VIP) — Found in the brain, some ANS and sensory fibers, retina, and gastrointestinal tract. Its function in the nervous system is uncertain.

THE BODY CHEMISTRY OF BEHAVIOR AND PAIN

Behavior

Behavior is affected by the type and amount of neurotransmitters released at the synaptic junction. Our daily behaviors such as those involved in pleasure, pain, and survival are determined by our chemistry. A pain behavior refers to the way we act when under the influence of pain. Too little or too much of any one neurotransmitter results in a behavior that takes extra effort to manage.

Depression may follow a block of the release of catecholamines, whereas anxiety is aggravated by an increase in these neurotransmitters. Current research involves study of the effect of serotonin on migraine headaches. Too much dopamine in the brain may result in hallucinations. This could cause mildly erratic behavior such as that displayed when we first fall in love or an extreme of schizophrenic behavior. Dopamine levels are thought to be involved in attention deficit hyperactivity disorders.

The presence of CCK and vasoactive intestinal peptide (VIP) in both the eye and the stomach indicates a connection between what we see and what we eat. These same neurotransmitters are in the brain. Could this suggest a connection between food, behavior, and emotions? Anyone who has emotional issues around food certainly would not deny that the food we eat changes the way we feel and influences the behavior connected with those emotions.

It is a matter of balance again. Neurotransmitters balance one another. Those that excite are usually paired with those that inhibit. An ongoing dynamic balance exists in this chemical soup, allowing for behavior that is resourceful for each situation encountered. In addition, we will behave in certain ways to increase or decrease levels of neurotransmitters or hormones (i.e., eating or not eating because we are depressed, exercising or not exercising because we are anxious). When medication is used to manage neurotransmitters, mood and behavior are affected.

The natural functions of the body allow for a wide range of behavior by continually adjusting the neurotransmitter and hormone balance. When neurochemical levels are held in more static ratio by medication, feelings, mood, and resultant behavior are held within the expected parameters. Medication alters the ability to have the highs and lows of emotional expression appropriate to daily circumstances. Compliance with taking psychotropic or mood-altering medication often is affected because people enjoy the edges of experiences where emotions are most intense. People sometimes miss the edges of their emotional selves and thus stop taking their medications, often with devastating results. Careful monitoring by the physician can minimize this situation, but it is also important to recognize that it exists. You have only to watch any television soap opera to see that there is little program content about day-to-day life in the midrange of emotional or behavioral expression. Seldom do we find ourselves caught up in stories about making the bed, changing the oil in the car, or going to the post office.

It seems that behavior is the outward manifestation of attempts at homeostasis, and we seek sensations that organize our brains. When behavior is effective in achieving some sort of balance, it will be reinforced. By observing behavior we can make educated guesses at the neurotransmitters involved. If the behavior is destructive, possibly other forms of behavior that are less detrimental can be introduced that result in similar neurotransmitter activity. It is important to recognize that repeated behavior is in some way accomplishing the goal of a form of homeostasis—including bizarre behavior such as drug addiction, excessive exercise, eating disorders, rage, thrill seeking, crisis orientation, and the deliberate creation of pain. An attempt to eliminate one form of behavior without replacing it with another way to achieve effective homeostasis will almost always result in failure and reversion to old behaviors. For example, substituting binge eating with movement and aerobic exercise may work because they operate from a similar neurotransmitter base. Eliminating binge eating without a substitute behavior leaves the client without a way to achieve chemical balance in his brain and body. Another common example is that eating chocolate affects serotonin (so does the consumption of potato chips, ice cream, and cookies)—a feel-good neurotransmitter—but so does massage and exercise. However, chocolate is faster, takes less energy, and it works. Although eating chocolate helps many people feel good, if eating chocolate is the only way someone can feel good, other problems can be generated. It is difficult to change a behavior from one that is quick and reliable to one that requires more effort.

The statements "moderation in all things" and "variety is the spice of life" are important and wise advice as far as brain chemistry is concerned. Sprinkled into this mix of expression are both the highs and lows of ecstasy and despair because these feelings are important as well. This ancient wisdom is found in most ancient healing practices. We will do best if we have many different ways to feel good. It is also important to understand what is causing us to feel bad. When we can respond deliberately with our behavior to generate appropriate feelings for the situation being faced instead of reacting and relying on only one type of behavior to meet our needs and cope, our neurotransmitters work for us instead of against us (Activity 4-1).

Pain

Pain is a protective device for the body and therefore important for survival. Pain is a complicated neurochemical event. Generally, the perception of pain

ACTIVITY 4-1

Understanding the neurochemical influence of behavior is important both to self-awareness and to clinical reasoning in the assessment and analysis process within the professional environment.

The following is an analysis of an event that resulted in a pattern of behavior.

1. Describe the event in factual terms.

   Example The hood on the car would not close, and I was late for an appointment.

2. Describe the emotions and feelings around the event.

   Example I became very frustrated and anxious because I could not drive the car with the hood unlatched.

3. Describe the behavior displayed.

   Example I tried to slam down the hood three or four times and then started to yell at the car.

4. Identify the possible neurotransmitters involved in the feelings and behavior.

   Example The catecholamines epinephrine and norepinephrine.

5. Indicate mode of action for the neurotransmitters—see pages 97-98.

   Example Epinephrine and norepinephrine: mostly excitatory, activating sympathetic arousal.

6. Correlate neurotransmitter with the feelings and behavior.

   Example I was anxious because I was late. Stress levels that increase sympathetic activity were high before I noticed the problems with the car. The increase in the catecholamines would produce or perpetuate the fight-or-flight behavior, resulting in my hitting the car and yelling.

7. Propose a balancing behavior to reset homeostasis and identify possible neurochemical interaction.

   Example I could have tightened all my muscles for a few seconds and then relaxed them and repeated this three or four times. This would simulate the activity of fighting or fleeing and use up some of the epinephrine. The goal would be to calm down.

Choose an event from your life in which you were unable to alter an inappropriate behavior pattern.

1. Describe the event in factual terms.

2. Describe the emotions and feelings around the event.

3. Describe the behavior displayed.

4. Identify the possible neurotransmitters involved in the feelings and behavior.

5. Indicate mode of action for the neurotransmitters—see pages 97-98.

6. Correlate the neurotransmitters with the feelings and behavior.

7. Propose a balancing behavior to reset homeostasis and identify possible neurochemical interaction.

occurs in the thalamus; interpretation of pain occurs in the cortex. A painful stimulus one day may not be painful the next. Pain results from a decision in the brain. Anesthetics, including alcohol and barbiturates, depress cortical neurons so that although the thalamus and other lower centers indicate pain, one "doesn't care" because pain perception is altered.

Drugs can interfere with the production of neurotransmitters or block the receptor sites of neurotransmitters. Aspirin interferes with the production of prostaglandin, which prevents it from sensitizing nerve endings.

During pregnancy, a woman's serotonin level gradually increases until it reaches its highest point at the time of delivery in preparation for birth pain. Some of the food cravings experienced during pregnancy may be due to the body's need to increase serotonin levels.

A pain-inhibiting system exists within the body. Receptors for opiates (e.g., morphine) are present along the pain pathway. Internal, or endogenous, opiates (e.g., endorphins, enkephalins) produced by the body block pain impulses in various portions of the pathway, probably as a protective device. The neurotransmitter substance P, secreted by pain fibers in the dorsal horns of the spinal cord, is blocked by enkephalins. Pain behavior is behavior that results from pain or perpetuates pain. Pain behavior is a brain chemistry event. Endorphins and enkephalins affect mood. A runner's high is an endorphin experience. Paradoxically, behavior that causes pain sufficient to increase endorphin and enkephalin activity can result in a pleasant change in mood. Many forms of touch and movement modalities can "hurt good," and the deliberate use of pain can actually be therapeutic. This too can become out of balance when one continually creates or seeks pain for the secondary (gain) pleasure. This complex behavior pattern usually requires professional counseling and support to shift to a more appropriate coping style.

The Central Nervous System

THE BRAIN

The **brain** is the largest and most complex unit of the nervous system (Figure 4-6). It is created from approximately 100 billion neurons packed together inside the skull. Besides its responsibility for our intellect, emotions, and actions, it interprets, regulates,

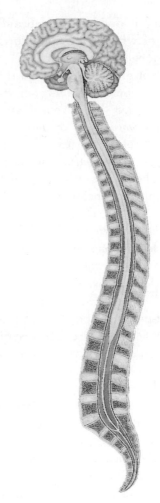

FIGURE 4-6 The central nervous system. (From Thibodeau GA, Patton KT: *Anatomy and physiology*, ed 3, St Louis, 1996, Mosby.)

and coordinates physiologic activities. Although it weighs an average of only 3 pounds, it makes up more than 97% of the nervous system. More than half of its weight comes from the neuroglia. With a composition of more than 85% water, the brain contains a higher percentage of fluid than our blood. The brain is divided into the cerebrum, cerebellum, and brainstem, which includes the diencephalon.

The Cerebrum
The **cerebrum,** also called the forebrain, is the largest portion of the brain. The major functions of the cerebrum are to receive sensory information, interpret it, associate it with past memories and experiences, then transmit the most appropriate motor impulse in response to the input. It is also involved in emotions and memories.

The cerebrum is divided into left and right hemispheres, each of which is divided further into five lobes. The surface of the cerebrum is covered by a very thin layer of gray matter called the *cerebral cortex*. Its gray color comes from its composition of dendrites and cell bodies. The cerebral cortex is formed into folds called *convolutions* or *gyri*, which increase the available area of the cortex. These folds are separated by creases called *sulci*. The deepest sulci are called *fissures*. The fissures can be used as landmarks when identifying and locating certain areas of the brain.

The *longitudinal fissure* divides the cerebrum into the right and left hemispheres. The central sulcus, also known as the *fissure of Rolando*, separates the frontal and parietal lobes. The lateral fissure, the *fissure of Sylvius*, lies above the temporal lobe and below the frontal and parietal lobes. A fifth lobe, the *insula*, lies deep in the lateral fissure. The occipital and parietal lobes are separated by the *parieto-occipital fissure*. The gyri are named for these fissures.

The left and right hemispheres each have motor control and receive sensory input from the opposite side of the body: the left hemisphere works with the right side of the body, and the right hemisphere works with the left side. A structure called the *corpus callosum* is located underneath the gray matter and functions to connect the left and right hemispheres. Because it is composed of myelinated axons, it is white. It is generally larger in women, which becomes clinically significant in the assessment of patterns of distribution of memory and functioning centers because they tend to be somewhat more random and less compartmentalized in the female brain. Some types of brain injury to these memory and function centers are able to be compensated far more easily by the female brain than by the more structured male brain pattern.

The rest of the cerebrum is composed of white matter. Areas of nerve cell bodies found in the cerebrum, known as *basal ganglia*, are small collections of gray matter that assist in coordination. The *limbic system* is also located on the interior of the cerebrum and is important in our emotional responses and sexual behavior. It is connected to the hypothalamus by the *fornix*, a band of fibers.

Brain dominance refers to the primary functioning hemisphere that specializes in language functions and linear thought processing. Most right-handed people have a dominant left hemisphere. More than 70% of left-handed people are also left-hemisphere

dominant. The right hemisphere, which is nondominant in most, concerns itself more with our creative and intuitive abilities and imagination. The left side of your brain works when you read this text, whereas the right jumps in when you daydream or wonder what all the information means.

Each side of the cerebral cortex is divided into five lobes, four of which are named for the skull bone lying over them:

Frontal lobe—The anterior portion of the cerebrum, the frontal lobe is positioned behind the frontal bone and contains the prefrontal cortex (governing personality, intellect, and cognition), premotor cortex (directing learned motor skills), and the precentral gyrus (managing motor control of muscles). This lobe is primarily responsible for control of the voluntary skeletal muscles and is active in moods and activities of problem solving that involve concentration and planning. An area known as *Broca's area* is found in the dominant hemisphere and controls the muscle movements involved in speech.

Parietal lobe—Located next to the parietal bones, this lobe contains the postcentral gyrus, which is the primary sensory area of the brain. This lobe receives and evaluates the sensory information of temperature, pressure, touch, taste, and pain. Its areas of association include speech, thought, and emotions.

Temporal lobe—Found below the lateral fissure, this lobe is next to the temporal bones. The temporal lobe is responsible for the reception and evaluation involved in hearing and smell. *Wernicke's area*, which is located in the superior portion of the gyrus of the dominant hemisphere, is involved in understanding language and transmits information to the Broca's area of the frontal lobe. Broca's area processes language information comprehended by Wernicke's area and relays it to the precentral gyrus. The areas of association combine complex sensory data such as from music and visual scenes into comprehensive patterns and form our memory.

Occipital lobe—Located just anterior to the occipital bone of the skull, this lobe is not separated from the other lobes. It is responsible for the mechanical control of eyesight and integration of visual input with other sensory experiences.

Insula, or Island of Reil—This fifth lobe is located under the lateral fissure. It is the part of the limbic system that gives us a feeling or impression of what is real, true, and important (Figure 4-7, *A* to *C*, and Table 4-1).

Integrative or associative functions of the cortex

Integrative or associative functions include all the activities that occur in the cerebrum after sensory signals are received and before motor responses are sent to where those signals originated. These responses include consciousness, emotions, memory, language, and learning mechanisms (Figure 4-8).

Consciousness. Consciousness is our awareness of the environment and our relationship to everyone and everything in that environment. Throughout the day there are degrees of normal changes in the levels of consciousness, from sleeping to wide awake. Consciousness depends on excitation of cortical neurons by impulses conducted from the reticular activating system. The reticular activating system (described on page 109) consists of centers in the brainstem that receive impulses from the spinal cord and relay them to the thalamus. The thalamus transmits the data to all parts of the cerebral cortex. Substances that stimulate the cerebrum, enhancing alertness, probably act by stimulating the reticular activating system.

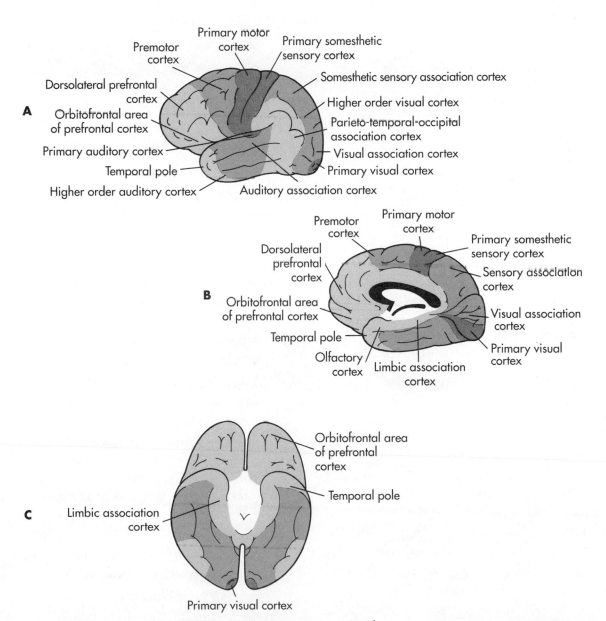

FIGURE 4-7 A to C, Functional organization of the cerebral cortex. (From Árnadóttir G: *The brain and behavior: assessing cortical dysfunction through activities of daily living,* St Louis, 1990, Mosby.)

TABLE 4-1 FUNCTIONS OF THE CEREBRAL CORTEX

FUNCTIONAL AREA	ANATOMIC AREA	FUNCTION AND PERFORMANCE COMPONENTS
FRONTAL LOBES		
Primary motor area	Precentral gyrus	Execution of movement
Secondary association area	Premotor cortex	Planning and programming of movement
		Sequencing, timing, and organization of movement
	Frontal eye field	Voluntary eye movements
	Broca's area in the left inferior frontal gyrus	Programming of motor speech
	Supplementary motor area	Intention of movement
Tertiary association area	Orbitofrontal and dorsolateral prefrontal cortex	Ideation
		Concept formation
		Abstract thought
		Intellectual functions
		Sequencing, timing, and organization of action and behavior
		Initiation and planning of action
		Judgment
		Insight
		Intention
		Attention
		Alertness
		Personality
		Working memory
		Emotion
PARIETAL LOBES		
Primary somesthetic sensory area	Postcentral gyrus	Fine touch sensation, proprioception, kinesthesia
Secondary somesthetic sensory association area	Superior parietal lobule	Coordination, integration, and refinement of sensory input
		Tactile localization and discrimination
		Stereognosis
Tertiary association area	Inferior parietal lobule	*Gnosis:* recognition of received tactile, visual, and auditory input
		Praxis: storage of programs or visuokinesthetic motor engrams necessary for motor sequences
		Body scheme: postural model of body, body parts, and their relation to the environment
		Spatial relations: processing related to depth, distance, spatial concepts, position in space, and differentiation of foreground from background
OCCIPITAL LOBES		
Primary visual sensory area	Calcarine fissure	Visual reception (from the opposite visual field)
Visual association area	Brodmann's areas 18 and 19	Synthesis and integration of visual information
		Perception of visuospatial relationships
		Formation of visual memory traces
		Prepositional construction of language comprehension and speech

Modified from Árnadóttir G: *The brain and behavior: assessing cortical dysfunction through activities of daily living,* St Louis, 1990, Mosby.

TABLE 4-1   FUNCTIONS OF THE CEREBRAL CORTEX—cont'd

FUNCTIONAL AREA	ANATOMIC AREA	FUNCTION AND PERFORMANCE COMPONENTS
TEMPORAL LOBES		
Primary auditory sensory area	Superior temporal gyrus	Auditory reception
Secondary association area	Superior and middle temporal gyri (Wernicke's area)	Language comprehension
		Sound modulation
		Perception of music
		Auditory memory
Tertiary association area	Temporal pole, parahippocampus	Long-term memory
		Learning of higher-order visual tasks and auditory patterns
		Emotion
		Motivation
		Personality
LIMBIC LOBES		
Tertiary association area	Orbitofrontal cortex in frontal lobe, temporal pole, and parahippocampus in the temporal lobe	Attention
	Cingulate gyrus in frontal and parietal lobes	Motivation
		Emotions
		Long-term memory

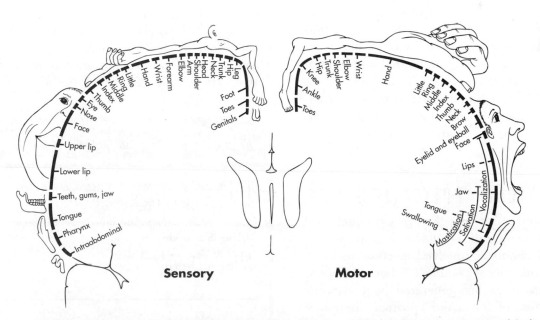

Sensory   **Motor**

FIGURE 4-8 Sensory and motor area representations of the brain. Surface area is largest for sensory interpretation of the face, lips, and fingers. Motor surface area is largest for the hands and face. (From Greenstein GM: *Clinical assessment of neuromuscu-loskeletal disorders,* St Louis, 1997, Mosby.)

Consciousness may be altered in many ways, including the use of medications or foods that change chemical processes, repetitive activities or sounds, and trance. For centuries, many cultures and religions have explored altered states of consciousness and used them readily in defensive actions, healing, and pain control. Meditation, tai chi, and yoga are examples of ancient methods used to achieve altered consciousness. We can create the same result with gardening, drawing, knitting, or playing a musical instrument. Any activity that uses a repetitive motion or sound will quiet or excite (depending on the speed of the rhythm) the nervous system through entrainment and alter the physiologic process of the body. An altered state of consciousness can also be achieved during a bodywork session by both the therapist and the client. When the altered state is achieved, it needs to be maintained for at least 15 minutes to best achieve therapeutic benefit.

Because of religious and political overtones, many people were hesitant in the past and still are hesitant to explore mystical imagery. Unconscious thought has been identified as a primary activity, whereas conscious thought is described as a secondary activity. States of "higher consciousness" refer to the primary activity that actually increases alertness and induces relaxation. Research has confirmed this to be a health-enhancing state.

Pleasure derived from the sense of well-being experienced by altered states of consciousness can be addictive. Various plants containing chemicals that alter consciousness have been used through the centuries in awareness rituals. Within the confines of cultural and religious ritual, the limited and judicial use of these plants was controlled. Today most, if not all, of the "old" discipline and structure is nonexistent, and drug abuse is contributing to the disempowerment of altered states of consciousness (Activity 4-2).

✍ PRACTICAL APPLICATION

Soft tissue and movement therapies interact with the cerebral cortex and reticular activating system, the same mechanisms involved in consciousness. Because of this, the sensations of altered states of consciousness often are generated by bodywork methods. Most of the major spiritual disciplines have a movement or positional aspect in their practices that contribute to the meditative states experienced by their participants. Some even incorporate touch, which enhances the experience.

Language. Language involves the perception of written and spoken words and the physical ability to speak and write. For 90% of the population, this takes place in the left hemisphere of the cerebrum in the frontal, parietal, and temporal lobes. The ability to apply labels to processes and subjects inside and outside the body is also tied to sensory systems.

Emotions. We experience and express our feelings and emotions through the limbic system of the brain. Located inside the cerebrum, it works in combination with other parts of the cerebral cortex. For most of us, the normal expressions of anger, pleasure, fear, and sorrow are under our control. Individuals whose limbic systems do not interact effectively with the cortex may have episodes of uncontrollable rage or other emotions.

Memory. Memory is the storing of information in the brain and is one of our major mental activities. There are two types of memory, short term (recent) and long term. *Short-term memory* is fragile, unstable, and disappears unless it is reinforced and transferred to long-term memory. The activities in this text are designed to assist in the transference of new data from short-term memory to long-term memory. *Long-term memory* can be retrieved days or even years after the initial event. The temporal lobes are involved with long-term memory. Long-term memory consists of some kind of structural traces called *engrams* in the cerebral cortex that involve protein synthesis and physical brain changes, resulting in permanent change in the synapses in a specific circuit of neurons. Repeated impulse conduction over a given neuronal circuit seems to produce the synaptic change. Many research findings indicate that the cerebrum's limbic system—the "emotional brain"—plays a key

ACTIVITY 4-2

How could you alter your state of consciousness in a health-enhancing way? Write down two methods.

Example Listen to gentle music for 15 minutes while rocking in a rocking chair.

Your Turn

_____

_____

_____

_____

role in memory also. Personal experience substantiates a relationship between emotion and memory. Highly emotional events seem to become stored immediately in long-term memory, indicating neurotransmitter involvement in memory structures.

✋ PRACTICAL APPLICATION

The key in long-term memory is repeated impulse. This text provides opportunities to repeat, in various forms, the same information to assist in the process of developing long-term memory. Learning strategies are often focused around circular learning, in which information continues to reappear, reinforcing the neurocircuit storing the memory.

Learning that takes place with excitement and enthusiasm or even tears and sorrow will be better remembered. Events that create tears of joy are some of the best remembered. Sometimes the memory takes the form of state-dependent memory. With *state-dependent memory* the engram cannot be accessed unless the consciousness state is similar to when the event occurred and was originally encoded. State-dependent memory can take many forms. Sometimes trauma beyond what the conscious centers can integrate is hidden in state-dependent memory.

Any form of therapy that can engage the consciousness state, such as hypnosis, biofeedback, or various forms of bodywork, may re-create the sequence of the consciousness state that holds the key to the memory structure, allowing it to surface. Depending on the person's coping skills, resources, support systems, and/or professional services available, this awareness of past experience can be a time of conscious understanding and integration of a part of a person's life. However, without the proper resources, this type of resurfacing of state-dependent memory can be devastating and extremely harmful.

Pleasure states are also encoded in state-dependent memory. The warm feelings such as being held or the feelings of exhilaration such as running in the wind on a beautiful spring day can be remembered and in a sense re-created with various forms of bodywork. These are health-enhancing states that support homeostasis.

Learning can be thought of as the best and simplest way to solve a problem. Anatomically and physiologically, learning is the use of multiple synaptic pathways to solve problems. Advanced learning takes place in the association areas of the cerebral cortex (some learning also takes place in the brainstem). Learning involves memory because it is the development of neural structures that remember the way to solve a problem. Solving problems supports survival. Learning can be thought of as conditioning. Pavlov's research identified some of the mechanisms of conditioning in which an external stimuli is connected to a natural occurrence in the body. With Pavlov, dogs were conditioned by a bell being rung at the same time as food was presented. Soon the dogs learned that the bell and food equaled the same thing. Then the sound of the bell alone stimulated digestion and eating behavior. This is behavioral conditioning. Conditioning can also be considered learned habit.

The process of learning is conscious, but after something has been integrated it often becomes unconscious—a habit. Some habits are beneficial and others no longer serve their original purpose. Breaking a habit is hard. Learning a new way to do something involves making the thought process go down a different road to get to a result. The body and learned memory tend to resist change, especially because learned behavior has such a strong component of primitive survival connected with it. In addition, it takes tremendous energy to change learned behavior, and the natural tendency of the body is to conserve energy. Unless the habit is causing us to expend resources in a detrimental way long enough to affect survival, it is difficult to rally the body's resources necessary to change the behavior.

Drugs affecting the cerebral cortex

Stimulants that affect the neurotransmitters and receptor sites of the cells in the cerebral cortex include caffeine, nicotine, amphetamines, and cocaine. Caffeine is a CNS stimulant that enhances the sense of alertness and diminishes the sense of fatigue and boredom. Nicotine first stimulates and then depresses the nervous system by affecting the release of norepinephrine and mimicking the action of acetylcholine. Amphetamines and cocaine stimulate the release of catecholamines (primarily norepinephrine and dopamine) from sympathetic neurons. Their effect on the CNS ranges from a feeling of well-being (euphoria) to psychosis.

Depressants (e.g., alcohol, narcotics, minor tranquilizers, barbiturates) act on the cerebral cortex by blocking norepinephrine and dopamine. The paradoxical effect of alcohol as a "stimulant" results from inhibiting learned behavior and releasing primitive biologic impulses from inhibitory control. Depressants are also anesthetics. The chain of action is as follows: The cortex is first depressed, then the more primitive centers (brainstem) are depressed as the dosage increases. Brainstem depression can result in death because respiration and cardiac function are slowed and eventually stop if the depression continues.

The hallucinogens include lysergic acid diethylamide (LSD), phencyclidine (PCP), peyote (mescaline) and marijuana (tetrahydrocannabinol, or THC). LSD blocks the neurotransmitter serotonin, and PCP blocks acetylcholine. These drugs seem to alter brain function by randomly stimulating and blocking neurotransmitters. A typical action would be that smell may be "seen," color may be "heard," and so forth. PCP is considered the most dangerous of the hallucinogens. It uncouples sensory pathways in the brain to produce a sensory deprivation syndrome, creating an increase in body strength accompanied by an acute schizophrenic reaction. Because of high fat solubility and the production of long-acting metabolites, PCP may remain in body tissues for months or even years, causing recurring episodes of violence and psychosis.

Physical dependency (addiction) means that when a drug is withdrawn, severe autonomic excitability occurs. The person thus requires the drug to feel "normal." It takes a period of time before the body reestablishes the ability to self-regulate without the drug.

Tolerance is seen with both stimulants and depressants. Tolerance means that larger doses of the drug are required for the same effect because the body has adjusted to the current dose. This makes amphetamines quite dangerous because physical dependency does not exist (thus no warning system), but tolerance does. Consequently, the person may approach the lethal dose without being aware of it.

Brainstem

The **brainstem** is considered the primitive portion of the brain and is divided into three main parts: the midbrain, pons, and medulla oblongata (see Figure 4-6). The diencephalon is often included as a fourth part. These areas are control centers for vital survival functions and reflex actions such as sneezing, coughing, vomiting, and balanced movements. Research shows that it is likely that the brainstem processes much of the sensory data generated by soft tissue and movement modalities.

Midbrain

The midbrain, or mesencephalon, is located in the middle of the brain, below the cerebrum and between the thalamus and the pons. It contains reflex centers for visual and auditory stimuli and correlates information about muscle tone and posture. The midbrain contains an important part of the reticular activating system.

Pons

The pons (pons varolii) is in the middle of the brainstem between the midbrain and the medulla. The pons assists in the coordinated patterns of breathing, eye movement, and facial expressions. It is involved in rapid eye movement (REM) sleep.

Medulla oblongata

The medulla or medulla oblongata connects the pons with the spinal cord. It is composed of white matter and the reticular formation, a network of white and gray matter. The fibers handle impulses to lower motor neurons. The fibers on one side of the medulla handle signals to the contralateral side. The medulla regulates our heartbeat, blood pressure, and breathing and reflex actions such as coughing or sneezing. Because it controls vital life functions, an injury or disease of the medulla is often fatal.

Diencephalon

The diencephalon is found between the cerebrum and midbrain and contains the thalamus, hypothalamus, pineal body, and other small structures. These structures perform various functions.

Thalamus. The thalamus is created from the gray matter of nerve cell bodies deep in the white matter of the cortex. It is a relay station from the sense organs to the cerebrum for all sensory input except smell. Signals from the reticular activating system are also sent through the thalamus to the cerebral cortex. The thalamus is associated with pain, temperature, crude touch, and reflex muscle coordination. It associates pleasant and unpleasant feelings with sensory input. The thalamus may act as a biooscillator involved with internal biorhythm entrainment.

Hypothalamus. The hypothalamus lies below the thalamus and above the pituitary gland. It regulates and coordinates functions such as heart rate, blood pressure, peristaltic actions, appetite and satiety, pleasure, temperature, and general coordination of ANS functions. It produces "releasing hormones" that affect pituitary gland hormones, which in turn influence important activities such as hunger, appetite, sleep cycles, wakefulness, sexual arousal, and water balance. It is an important link between the nervous and endocrine systems, which allows the mind to affect the body—the mind-body connection.

✋ PRACTICAL APPLICATION

The pleasure center deep inside the hypothalamus involves feel-good neurotransmitters and predisposes one to addictive behavior to feel good, alter mood, and so forth. Romantic love is a brain bath of norepinephrine and dopamine—both feel-good chemicals. Soft tissue and movement stimulation also influence the feel-good neurotransmitters. Substance abuse, including nicotine, alcohol, and caffeine, and behaviors such as extremes of eating, sex, gambling, exercise, thrill seeking, pain, violence, and crisis creating that have a potential for addictive behavior interact with feel-good neurotransmitters and hormones as well. Many psychotropic or mood-regulating medications act on the feel-good neurotransmitters. The use of chemicals or extreme behaviors to produce pleasure often depletes or inhibits the body's natural production of the chemicals, resulting in a big downslide after a big high. The extremes of pleasure and discomfort support addictive behavior.

Because soft tissue and movement modalities stimulate the release of the feel-good neurotransmitters and hormones, it has been shown that inclusion of these therapies supports the treatment of addictive behavior by replacing a destructive manner of mood alteration with a constructive, more moderate way to feel good. It is essential that the treatment of complex factors such as those found in addiction be monitored and dealt with in a multidisciplinary team approach.

Pineal body. The pineal body or gland is found on the dorsal side of the diencephalon. The pineal gland and its hormone *melatonin* are still a mystery. Approximately 30% of the pineal cells are magnetically sensitive and responsive to external magnetic patterns. It functions as an internal biologic clock that regulates daily activities (circadian rhythms), as well as yearly rhythms (circannual rhythms). Exposure to natural sunlight assists these functions. The pineal body needs darkness to convert serotonin to melatonin, which seems to be involved with sexual activity. Melatonin also triggers the pituitary gland to release luteinizing hormone, which affects sexual maturity and may be involved in puberty and menopause. Melatonin is involved in the sleep pattern.

Two of the best known sleep stages are slow-wave sleep and REM sleep. Sleep has stages from 1 through 4, with 4 being the deepest sleep. Slow-wave sleep produces slow-frequency, high-voltage brain waves and is associated with stages 2 and 3. It is almost entirely a dreamless part of the sleep pattern. At the deeper levels, the reticular activating system activity is depressed in the pons and medulla. REM sleep, on the other hand, is associated with dreaming. At intervals of 90 minutes or so, the closed eyes begin to move rapidly. Repeatedly waking a person at the beginning of REM sleep produces anxiety and irritability. If the person is then allowed to sleep, there is more than the usual REM sleep and dreaming for a few nights to "catch up." This is called *REM rebound.* Many medications, particularly sleeping pills and tranquilizers, suppress REM and stage 4 sleep. Stopping the drug may result in REM rebound, sometimes associated with nightmares. Therefore it is important to use medicines with minimal REM rebound when medication is necessary.

Reticular activating system

The reticular activating system (RAS) is a structural and functional part of the reticular formation in the brainstem. It maintains arousal levels in the cerebral cortex and alerts it to changes in homeostasis, thus keeping us awake and alert. Its importance in consciousness and the sleep state has already been discussed. It also helps regulate respiration, blood pressure, heart rate, endocrine secretion, and conditioned reflexes. Incoming stimuli are integrated by the reticular formation. Both epinephrine and amphetamines stimulate RAS conduction, whereas anesthesia and barbiturates depress conduction. Trauma or damage to the RAS can cause a person to become comatose.

✋ PRACTICAL APPLICATION

To maintain homeostasis, we need sufficient sleep for health and well-being. It is during this time of rest that most growth and repair of the body takes place. Disrupted sleep patterns are found in many chronic diseases. If it is possible for sleep to be restored to an effective pattern without the use of medications, often the body can better cope or even begin to heal a chronic problem over time. Many soft tissue and movement therapies are relaxing and conducive to supporting effective sleep patterns, providing benefit to the client and thus decreasing the effects of the chronic problem.

Cerebellum

The **cerebellum** is located in the posterior cranial fossa beneath the posterior portion of the cerebrum. It is the second largest part of the brain and consists of a cortex composed of gray matter and an inner portion composed of white matter. Like the cerebrum, it has sulci and gyri and contains two lateral hemispheres that are connected by the vermis. The cerebellum maintains balance and posture and, with proprioceptive input, coordinates everything from normal movements to the complex activities involved in dancing, gymnastics, and doing massage. The cerebellum, limbic system, and other relay centers of the brain have been shown to work on the same circuit. (Hooper, 1986).

PRACTICAL APPLICATION

Bodywork techniques that stimulate the cerebellum, such as rhythmic rocking, have a widespread influence. Rocking produces movement at the neck and head that influences our sense of equilibrium. It stimulates the balance mechanisms of the inner ear, including the vestibular nuclear complex and the labyrinthine righting reflexes, which work to keep our head level. This is also a bodywide effect, stimulating muscle contraction patterns that pass throughout the body. Pressure on the side of the body may stimulate the body's righting reflexes. A close relationship exists between the vestibular nerves and the cerebellum. This feedback information, which adjusts and coordinates movement, is relayed directly to the motor cortex and to the cerebellum. Methods that alter body positional sense and initiate specific movement patterns change sensory input from muscles, tendons, joints, and the skin. The output from the cerebellum goes to the motor cortex and brainstem. Stimulation of the cerebellum by altering muscle tone, position, and vestibular balance also stimulates the hypothalamus to adjust ANS functions and thus restore homeostasis.

Ventricles

Four fluid-filled chambers called ventricles are found within the brain—one in each of the cerebral hemispheres, one positioned just below and between them, and one at the attachment of the cerebrum and the brainstem. **Cerebrospinal fluid** (CSF) fills these ventricles, then passes through several small openings to the subarachnoid space. It circulates through the brain, around the spinal cord, and is returned to the venous system at the dural sinuses. CSF is continuously replenished from the fluid filtering out of the choroid plexus, a network of brain capillaries.

Classified as one of the body's circulating fluids, CSF is a colorless watery substance that flows throughout the brain and around the spinal cord, providing cushioning and protection. It maintains homeostasis of the brain environment, including pH balance (Figure 4-9).

Meninges

The brain and spinal cord are protected by the skull and spinal column. They also are surrounded by three membranes called the *meninges* (Figure 4-10). The dura mater is the outermost layer and is made up of a tough, white fibrous connective tissue membrane. It lines the cranial bones and covers the brain and spinal cord. Attachment points are at the foramen magnum, C1 to C3 and S2, and at the crista galli of the ethmoid bone; it hangs loosely in other areas. Portions of the dura mater line the fissures between the left and right hemispheres of both the cerebrum and cerebellum, between the cerebellum and the cerebrum, and cover the spinal nerve roots. Nerves and blood vessels run though the epidural space next to the dura mater.

The second layer is the arachnoid mater, a cobweb-like membrane containing many blood vessels. The third layer, the pia mater, is very thin and adheres directly to the brain and spinal cord. The meninges form three spaces that add additional cushioning and protection to the CNS. They are the following:

Epidural space—Found between skull and dura mater, it contains connective tissue, including fat.
Subdural space—Found between the dura mater and arachnoid membrane, it is filled with a cushioning serous fluid.
Subarachnoid space—Found between the arachnoid and pia mater, it contains the CSF.

PRACTICAL APPLICATION

Some methods of bodywork are thought to interact with the movement of the meninges, especially the dura mater, and affect the flow of CSF. In the CNS a rhythm known as the *cranial sacral impulse* can be observed and palpated.

The effect of bodywork on this rhythm is still under investigation, although entrainment meth-

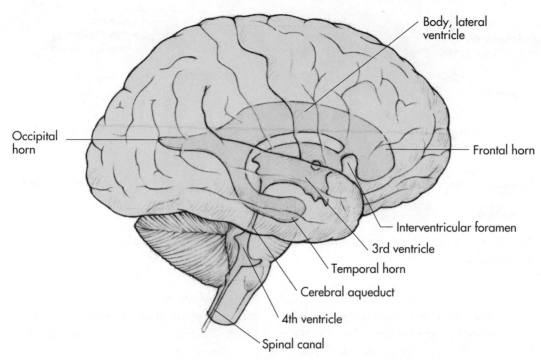

FIGURE 4-9 Ventricular system, lateral view. (From Mathers LH et al: *Clinical anatomy principles,* St Louis, 1996, Mosby.)

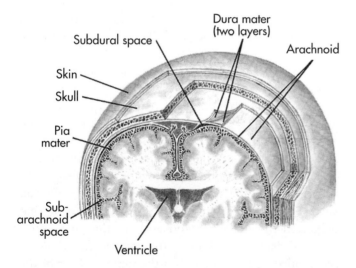

FIGURE 4-10 Meninges of brain. (From Thompson JM et al: *Mosby's clinical nursing,* ed 4, St Louis, 1997, Mosby.)

ods that synchronize the motions and rhythms of the body are credited with providing the most benefits. The application is to be done in a quiet, rhythmic manner by a quiet and focused practitioner that adds an additional external influence that allows the body rhythms to synchronize. When this is achieved, homeostatic mechanisms seem to operate more efficiently.

Vessels of the Brain

Blood is supplied to the brain through the middle cerebral arteries, which are a continuation of the internal carotid arteries, and the basilar artery. These are created from the two vertebrobasilar arteries. These three brain arteries are connected at the midbrain in the Circle of Willis, which is a check-and-balance system that provides for blood flow to the brain in case of blockage or damage to any of the three arteries. Blood is transported out of the brain by several veins and the dural sinuses, which drain into the internal jugular veins (Figure 4-11).

THE SPINAL CORD

The **spinal cord** is made of white and gray matter and is about 17 to 18 inches long in the average person. It begins at the base of the brainstem at the foramen magnum where it exits the skull. It continues through the vertebral column to the first and second lumbar vertebrae. At this point, the pia mater continues on as the filum terminale. It connects to the dura mater at S2, and they both end at the coccyx. Thirty-one pairs of spinal nerves connect the spinal cord and brain with the rest of the body as the peripheral nervous system.

The two main functions of the spinal cord are to conduct nerve impulses and be a center for spinal

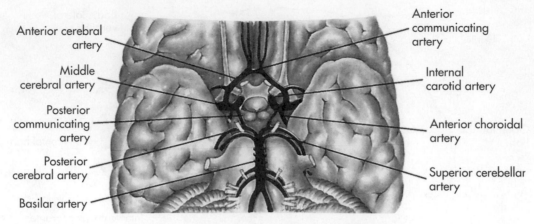

FIGURE 4-11 Anatomic diagram of circle of Willis. (From Thompson JM et al: *Mosby's clinical nursing,* ed 4, St Louis, 1997, Mosby.)

reflexes. The spinal cord is oval shaped and, like the brain, has fissures. The anterior fissure is deeper and wider than the posterior sulcus (Figure 4-12). On the outside of the spinal cord are pathways of **white matter** called **tracts,** created from the myelinated nerve fibers. They ascend to and descend from the brain. The ascending tracts conduct sensory impulses such as pain, touch, and temperature up from the spinal nerves through the spinal cord to the brain, whereas descending tracts conduct motor impulses from the brain down the cord to the spinal nerves. The functions of the axons in each tract are limited to one action such as transmitting specific touch and pain sensations.

The **gray matter** in the inside extends the length of the spinal cord. A cross section shows that it forms an H pattern. The dorsal portion of the H forms the dorsal horns and is composed of the cell bodies of association or interneurons. The anterior portion of the H forms the ventral horns, consisting of the cell bodies of motor nerves (Figure 4-13, *A* to *C*).

Sensory Ascending Tracts

Sensory receptors are found in the skin, muscles, and all organs. When stimulated by such things as touch, pain, and muscle action, they excite in response and initiate neural processes. The signals follow the nerve fibers from these receptors to the spinal cord, where they cross to the other side and ascend one of the sensory pathways or tracts to the thalamus, medulla, or cerebellum. In the brain the sensations are integrated into perceptions or filtered as unimportant. This sensory information is needed to help us maintain homeostasis.

Some of the most important sensory information for soft tissue and bodywork practitioners comes from sensory receptors and specifically proprioceptors that sense data concerning position and movement. Sensory fibers transmit signals about body position, deep touch or pressure, two-point discrimination, and vibration. The proprioceptors are located in muscles, tendons, ligaments, and joints.

Some proprioceptive signals initiate a response in the spinal cord; these are called *deep tendon reflex arcs.* Other fibers ascend the dorsal portion of the spinal cord, cross over in the medulla, and ascend to the thalamus and postcentral gyrus.

For a sensory signal to get from a sensory receptor to the brain, it passes through three different neurons. The first one, referred to as the primary, is a relay from the receptor to the brainstem or the spinal cord. This is part of the peripheral nervous system and will be discussed in detail in the next chapter.

The second neuron extends from the brainstem or spinal cord to the thalamus. The secondary neuron synapses with the tertiary (or third) neuron that begins in the thalamus and ends in the postcentral gyrus of the parietal lobe of the cortex. The axons of these third neurons make up the white matter of the cerebrum, referred to as the internal capsule, whereas the dendrites and cell bodies make up the gray matter of the cerebral cortex. The actual crossing of sensory signals from the left to the right side takes place mostly in the secondary neurons before they enter the thalamus.

Motor Descending Tracts

Motor tracts transmit information regarding adaptive responses to sensory experiences concerned with gross movements, posture, and fine motor skills. One of the main motor tracts is the pyramidal or corticospinal tract, which ties in to the voluntary motor

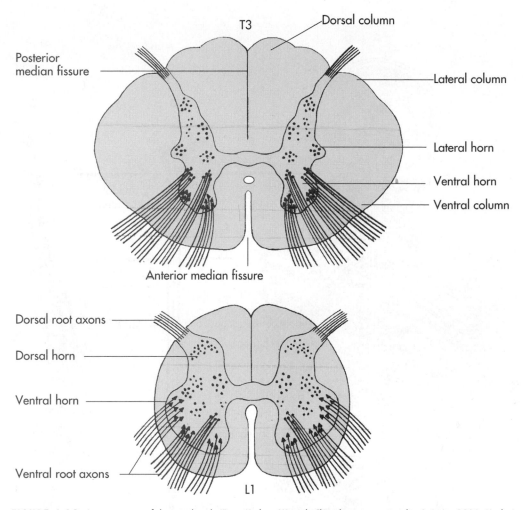

FIGURE 4-12 Inner structure of the spinal cord. (From Mathers LH et al: *Clinical anatomy principles,* St Louis, 1996, Mosby.)

system. The fibers begin in the cortex at the precentral gyrus and descend to the medulla, where they cross to the opposite side of the spinal cord. From here they descend through the lateral corticospinal tract to the motor neurons of the skeletal muscles. The pyramidal fibers handle both voluntary and reflex signals to the muscles.

For signals to get from the CNS to the muscles, they use the somatic motor pathways. For signals that begin in the brain, following the "wiring" of the somatic motor pathway may be very difficult. It is much simpler to identify the pathways for reflex signals that begin in the spinal cord. Spinal reflexes are centered in the gray matter of the spinal cord; these actions will be discussed in Chapter 5 because they directly involve the peripheral nervous system. We will limit our exploration here to the nonreflex actions.

One important rule to remember is the final common path principle. Each motor unit within a muscle receives impulses that are conducted along a single motor neuron that begins in the anterior gray horn of

the spinal cord. This principle is important to health care providers who are exploring muscle dysfunction and its relationship to spinal cord injuries. By identifying a muscle dysfunction, common relationship to the spinal nerve can also be surmised. The common path principle does not hold for the neurons from the cerebrum to the motor neurons in the spinal cord.

There are five main motor tracts in the spinal cord:

1. Lateral corticospinal tracts—These deal with our voluntary movements, especially the contraction of small groups of muscles such as those in the hands and feet. They affect muscles on the opposite sides of body from the cerebral cortex.
2. Anterior or ventral corticospinal tracts—These deal with the same lateral tracts, but the muscles are on the same side of the body as the cortex.
3. Lateral reticulospinal tracts—These transmit facilitatory impulses from the medulla through the anterior horn motor neurons to skeletal

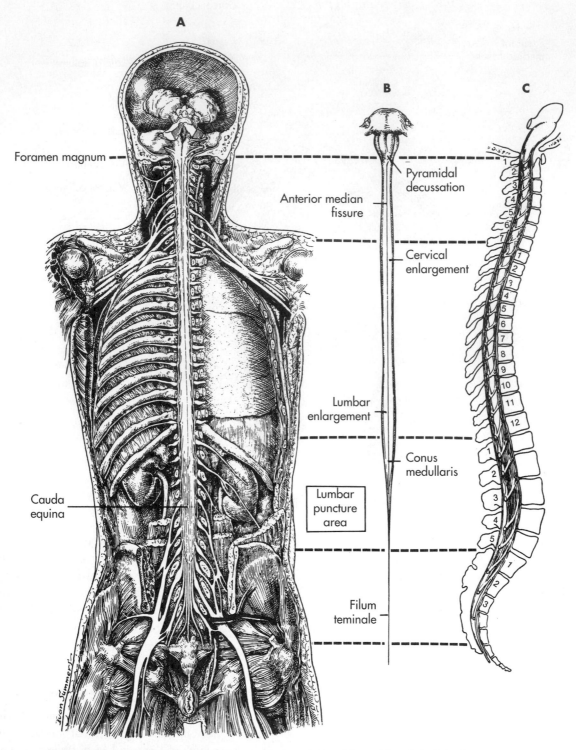

FIGURE 4-13 A, Posterior surface of a spinal cord within a vertebral canal dissected from the back. **B,** The way the anterior surface of the same spinal cord would look after removal of dura, arachnoid, and spinal nerves. **C,** Spinal cord exposed from the lateral direction, showing the way in which the cord ends at about the L1-L2 level and spinal nerves travel progressively longer distances in the cauda equina to reach their exits from the vertebral canal. (From Nolte J: *The human brain: an introduction to its functional anatomy,* ed 3, St Louis, 1993, Mosby.)

muscles that handle muscle tone and extensor reflexes.

4. Medial reticulospinal tracts—These carry mainly inhibitory impulses from the pons through the anterior horn motor neurons to skeletal muscles that deal with muscle tone and extensor reflexes.

5. Rubrospinal tracts—These transmit impulses that coordinate body movements and maintenance of posture.

The term *pyramidal tracts* refers to the lateral and anterior corticospinal tracts. The neurons from the cerebral cortex cross through the pyramid areas of the medulla. Here most of them cross to the other side and descend the spinal cord. The rest of the neurons extend through the pyramid areas and continue down the same side of the spinal cord. The pyramidal neurons are referred to as the upper motor neurons. When they reach their termination point in the gray matter of the spinal cord, they connect to lower motor neurons, which innervate the muscles. Most of these connections involve an additional synapse with an interneuron.

The *extrapyramidal tracts* are composed of the lateral and medial reticulospinal and rubrospinal tracts, none of which enter the medullar pyramid areas. They relay motor signals through the cerebrum, thalamus, brainstem, and cerebellum to the gray matter of the spinal cord. At this point, most synapse with interneurons, which then synapse with the lower motor neurons. It should be noted that both facilitating and inhibiting signals are sent through these motor neurons.

Injuries to the upper and lower motor neurons result in very different responses in the skeletal muscles. When upper motor neurons are damaged or destroyed through trauma or disease, the result is usually an increase in rigidity and an exaggerated response to reflexes. This is referred to as spastic paralysis. Injuries to the lower motor neurons result in a lack of signal to the muscles, causing absence of movement. This is known as flaccid paralysis (Figure 4-14).

PRACTICAL APPLICATION

The disability or dysfunction caused by brain and spinal cord injuries is determined by the region and function of the area affected. The prognosis for trauma to the motor neurons is often difficult to identify. The use of soft tissue work and other

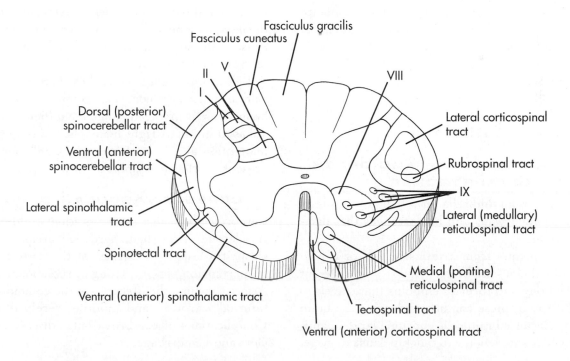

Ascending tracts (sensory)   **Descending tracts (motor)**

FIGURE 4-14 Ascending and descending tracts. (From Greenstein GM: *Clinical assessment of neuromusculoskeletal disorders,* St Louis, 1997, Mosby.

forms of movement therapies seems to be most beneficial when it is part of the whole health care picture. It is difficult for specific recommendations regarding bodywork to be given solely on the basis of the location of damage because of the body's compensation through rerouting of the interrupted signals. This is why clinical reasoning methods are so important. The ability to process a situation and determine the best intervention methods to be used is essential to the successful bodywork professional.

For example, spastic paralysis is the result of upper motor neuron injuries. A client with upper motor neuron injuries will have spastic paralysis of the muscles in the affected region. Voluntary control over movements is lost, and limbs may need to be restrained to prevent involuntary movement at inappropriate times. Usually less muscle atrophy is present, and lymph and blood flow continues because of the working of the muscles. The preferred modalities, when applied to each individual case, can moderate some of the random spasms and keep the soft tissues more supple and the joints more mobile, resulting in less rigidity in the muscles. With lower motor neuron difficulties, the muscles atrophy and actions and reflexes are slow, limited, or nonexistent. Massage and joint movement may be able to replace the mechanical pumping action of normal muscle contraction and assist in moving the blood and lymph. In addition, keeping the soft tissue pliable may lessen any contractures (Activity 4-3).

Pathology

CEREBROVASCULAR ACCIDENTS (CVA)/STROKES

CVA or stroke is an umbrella term that covers disorders such as aneurysms and hemorrhages that damage brain tissue.

Ulcerated plaque from arteriosclerosis or a portion of a blood clot may break away from a different part of the body and form an embolus that travels to the brain. Any of these conditions deprive the brain of oxygen. Because brain cells consume large quantities of oxygen, any deficit can quickly cause damage.

Stroke Types

A transient ischemic attack (TIA) is a "prestroke" condition that mimics a stroke. It resolves in less than 24 hours. In some cases when the deficit lasts longer than 24 hours and then clears completely, it is termed a reversible neurologic deficit, a residual ischemic neurologic deficit.

The signs of a TIA are transient blindness in one eye, aphasia, numbness or weakness of the hand or foot, slurred speech, dizziness, ataxia, syncope, and numbness around the lips. The signs may only last a few minutes and then disappear. They are often ignored. It is important to know the basic signs of TIA and refer the client immediately because a TIA is frequently a warning of a major stroke.

When a stroke occurs, an artery in the brain is occluded or closed off from a blood clot called a thrombus. A stroke lasts longer than 24 hours. The location and duration that the blood flow is cut off determines the damage caused by the stroke. The following deficits may occur:

Hemiparesis — Partial motor deficit on one side of the body
Quadriplegia — Total motor deficit of both arms and legs; usually seen in trauma
Sensory losses — Pain, temperature, vibration, and so forth

The limbs are initially flaccid (relaxed). Later they become spastic (contracted). It is common to see the forearm in flexion and the leg in extension because of the unequal innervation of extensors and flexors. The cause of the spasticity is thought to be loss of control of lower motor neurons.

Behavioral changes caused by damage in the association areas of the cortex are often present. If the left hemisphere is involved, language difficulties (such as aphasia) occur. A right hemisphere stroke produces inattention and lack of concern. Confusion may be present if either hemisphere is affected.

CEREBROVASCULAR DISEASE

Cerebrovascular disease is a gradual buildup of arteriosclerotic (thickened, hardened areas of reduced elasticity) lesions in arteries of the neck and brain. Hypertension is a strong predisposing factor. Arteries commonly affected are the common carotid, internal carotid, and middle cerebral arteries. Complications of cerebrovascular disease are blood clots and hemorrhage.

ANEURYSM

An aneurysm is a weakening and bulging of an artery. If the artery breaks, bleeding and complica-

ACTIVITY 4-3

Remember—there is no cookbook approach to therapeutic intervention or the application of soft tissue and bodywork modalities. It is truly an artful science in which a practitioner must be able to think rationally and trust intuition. Refer to Chapter 3 and review the steps involved in clinical reasoning. Then come up with a *hypothetical (made up) treatment plan* for both an upper neuron and lower neuron spinal cord injury.

Fill in at least three statements in each category. An example is given to get you started.

UPPER NEURON INJURY

What are the facts?

Example Client has spasm in the legs with the left leg affected more than the right leg.

Your Turn

1. _____
2. _____
3. _____

What is considered normal or balanced function?

Example Voluntary control over muscle activity

Your Turn

1. _____
2. _____
3. _____

What has happened?

Example Client was in a car accident.

Your Turn

1. _____
2. _____
3. _____

What caused the imbalance?

Example A spinal cord compression

Your Turn

1. _____
2. _____
3. _____

What was done or is being done?

Example Client is in rehabilitation.

Your Turn

1. _____
2. _____
3. _____

What has worked or not worked?

Example Client has not responded well to physical therapy methods applied to decrease spasm in the left leg.

Your Turn

1. _____
2. _____
3. _____

What are the possible patterns of dysfunction?

Example Overdependence on function in the right arm may be part of the pattern with reflex tension.

Your Turn

1. _____
2. _____
3. _____

What are the possible contributing factors?

Example The angle of the way the client is sitting in the wheelchair may be increasing reflex signals to the spinal cord for the left leg.

Your Turn

1. _____
2. _____
3. _____

What are other ways to look at the situation?

Example Maybe it would help to recommend that the client consult an acupuncturist.

Your Turn

1. _____
2. _____
3. _____

After the analysis is complete, look carefully at the facts and effects of the injury. Outline a possible treatment care plan.

Continued

Example Massage to be used in an attempt to reduce tension in the left leg by stimulation of reflexes, either directly through the left leg or indirectly by working with the arms. Client sessions scheduled biweekly with daily self-care program. Tracking to see whether the situation improves, stays static, or continues to worsen over a 4-week period. Will suggest that positioning in the chair be changed often by the care giver to see whether that decreases symptoms. Will continue to encourage the client to have the chair evaluated for proper positioning. Reevaluation of the above interventions in 4 weeks. If no benefit is received, then referral will be made.

Your Turn
Come up with your own hypothetical case (make it up).

LOWER NEURON INJURY
What are the facts?

1. _____

2. _____

3. _____

What is considered normal or balanced function?

1. _____

2. _____

3. _____

What has happened?

1. _____

2. _____

3. _____

What caused the imbalance?

1. _____

2. _____

3. _____

What was done or is being done?

1. _____

2. _____

3. _____

What has worked or not worked?

1. _____

2. _____

3. _____

What are the possible patterns of dysfunction?

1. _____

2. _____

3. _____

What are the possible contributing factors?

1. _____

2. _____

3. _____

What are other ways to look at the situation?

1. _____

2. _____

3. _____

What do the data suggest?

1. _____

2. _____

3. _____

What is the logical progression of the symptom pattern, contributing factors, and current behaviors?

1. _____

2. _____

3. _____

What is the sequence for possible treatment care plan development?

1. _____

2. _____

3. _____

After the analysis is complete, look carefully at the facts and effects of the injury. The plan then needs to be implemented, reevaluated, and adjusted as necessary. Come up with your own hypothetical case (make it up).

NOTE—This is a difficult activity. It is suggested that you return to it periodically through your studies to help gain a more complete interpretation of the clinical reasoning process.

tions can be fatal. Sometimes the rupture is preceded by a series of small leaks producing transient headache and neck stiffness. These symptoms are common in many other conditions, as well as with normal stress. This is why it is important to have a qualified medical professional rule out more serious conditions before assuming that symptoms are minor or only stress related.

INDICATIONS **CONTRAINDICATIONS**

For Soft Tissue and Movement Therapies

Soft tissue and movement therapies in a supervised setting can be supportive during rehabilitation. These methods are effective in the management of discomfort caused by the functioning portions of the body working extra hard to compensate for nonfunctioning areas. Stress management is an important part of the long-term management of these conditions. Because anticoagulants are often used to prevent further CVA or TIA, care needs to be taken with soft tissue methods used so that bruising does not occur during therapy. Careful attention needs to be paid to any symptom of thrombosis, and the type of bodywork used should not place heavy pressure over vulnerable vessels to avoid the possible movement of an embolism.

CENTRAL NERVOUS SYSTEM TRAUMA

A sudden blow to the head or intense shaking of the head may or may not involve a fracture. The fracture itself is usually not important; more significant is the possibility of intracranial bleeding or brain swelling (edema). Trauma to the tissues of the brain and surrounding structures and a change in pressure or fluid concentration is of significance to any trauma regarding the CNS.

A *concussion* is a brain trauma that may be mild, moderate, or severe. Symptoms of mild concussions include brief loss of consciousness or a state of confusion. A headache and vomiting may follow the episode. In most cases, complete recovery occurs in a matter of a few days to a week, although in rare cases recovery may be more lengthy.

With moderate to severe concussions a brain *contusion*, or bruise, may cause swelling of the brain tissues. This is common in trauma known as closed head injuries. Prolonged unconsciousness and problems with vasomotor and respiratory functions may be present. On waking the person may exhibit behavioral and personality changes, amnesia, and motor and sensory disturbances. The prognosis can range from complete recovery to continued deterioration. Because the amount of internal injury may not be immediately recognizable, it is important that any head injury should be watched carefully and referred to a medical professional if any loss of consciousness takes place or any of the aforementioned symptoms appear.

Intracranial bleeding, called *intracerebral hemorrhage*, may occur within brain tissue. When the bleeding occurs between the dura and arachnoid, it is called a *subdural hematoma;* when the bleeding is located between the skull and dura, it is referred to as an *epidural hematoma.*

Cerebral palsy is a general term for brain damage that takes place before, during, or shortly after birth. Damage may involve the whole brain but is usually limited to the pyramidal tracts, which results in motor function disturbance. The most common symptoms include muscle spasticity (especially in the feet, legs, and hands), impaired speech, vision, hearing or tactile sensations, and seizures. Impaired intellectual function may or may not result.

INDICATIONS **CONTRAINDICATIONS**

For Soft Tissue and Movement Therapies

Soft tissue and movement therapies are an effective part of a supervised comprehensive care program. Massage and other forms of bodywork can help manage secondary muscle tension resulting from the alteration of posture and the use of equipment such as wheelchairs, braces, and crutches.

SEIZURE

Seizures or convulsions are defined as a sudden involuntary series of muscle contractions. The most common group of seizure disorders is referred to as epilepsy, which occurs when the nerve cells of the cerebral cortex send out uncontrolled signals. In many cases the cause of the neuron stimulation is unknown, but known precipitating factors include heredity factors, trauma to the head, stroke, brain tumor, and infections.

Minor seizures are known as petit mal and may not include actual spasms of the skeletal muscles. Usually seen in children, these petit mal seizures are typified by a moment of blankness. Major seizures, known as grand mal, begin with an aura or sensation such as a taste, smell, or feeling. The person usually has involuntary spasms or continuous tension in the skeletal muscles and loss of consciousness. A sense of confusion and a desire to sleep are common aftereffects.

Most forms of epilepsy can be controlled by the use of antiseizure medication, most commonly phenobarbital and phenytoin (Dilantin). The side effects of the medications can include headache, muscle tension, nervousness, joint pain, and sleeping difficulties.

INDICATIONS CONTRAINDICATIONS

For Soft Tissue and Movement Therapies

The side effects of medications may be decreased by the application of bodywork techniques. Bodyworkers must remember that any exaggerated or increased symptoms should be referred to the prescribing physician.

TUMORS

It is very rare that a brain tumor develops from a neuron because neurons do not divide. Most tumors are formed from the neuroglia, tissues of the membranes, and the blood vessels found in and around the brain. The tumors are usually started by the cells of malignant tumors that begin elsewhere in the body, often in the breasts of women and the lungs of men.

Most tumors that develop in the brain are benign. Because no space is available for them to expand, they compress the brain and its supporting tissues, sometimes with fatal results. That is why surgical removal is indicated whenever possible.

Signs and symptoms of tumor-caused compression are as follows:

- The loss of sensory or motor function, mainly on one side of the body
- Personality changes, behavior changes, or both
- Headaches
- Awkward movement or gait (ataxia)

INDICATIONS CONTRAINDICATIONS

For Soft Tissue and Movement Therapies

It is important to recognize the signs and symptoms of a possible brain compression and refer the client for diagnosis. During rehabilitation from surgery, soft tissue work can be used both as supportive care and in any compensation patterns from brain damage that results from surgery.

DEGENERATIVE DISORDERS

A variety of degenerative diseases referred to as dementia are organic mental disorders caused by such things as chemical imbalance, endocrine dysfunctions, and trauma to the brain. These can result in the destruction of brain neurons. As the degeneration progresses, symptoms such as memory loss, decreased attention span, diminished intellectual capacity, and loss of control of personality or behavior are often observed.

Alzheimer's disease is a type of dementia in which the brain degenerates, resulting in judgment errors, memory difficulties, and a tendency to become confused. Neuronal tangles and plaque found in brain tissue contain amyloid, a pathologic insoluble starch-like protein. Neurons essential for memory are particularly vulnerable to this degenerative process. The current theory is that Alzheimer's disease is somehow genetically determined by amyloid B, which is regulated by a gene located in chromosome 21.

INDICATIONS CONTRAINDICATIONS

For Soft Tissue and Movement Therapies

The degeneration of Alzheimer's disease may be slowed with therapeutic intervention and medication. Studies indicate that sensory stimulation modalities such as rhythmic bodywork and movement may provide both calming and orienting influences.

SCHIZOPHRENIA

Schizophrenia is the most common mental disorder. It includes a large group of psychotic disorders characterized by gross distortion of reality; disturbances of language and communication; withdrawal from social interaction; and disorganization and fragmentation of thought, perception, and emotional reaction. No single cause has been identified, but increased dopamine activity in parts of the brain are strongly indicated. A diagnosis of schizophrenia requires the exclusion of other disorders. Management of chronic schizophrenia requires expert multidisciplinary support along with psychopharmacologic and long-term psychosocial intervention.

As previously stated, schizophrenia is associated with increased dopamine levels in the brain. The symptoms are helped with medications that block or reduce the release of dopamine at the synapses. Large amounts of cocaine and some amphetamines associated with the increase of dopamine often mimic schizophrenic behaviors in otherwise "normally" behaved persons.

DEPRESSION

Depression is associated with a decrease in the neurotransmitters norepinephrine, serotonin, and dopamine. Affected persons can often be helped with medications such as amphetamines that inhibit the reuptake of norepinephrine and monoamine oxidase inhibitors that reduce the breakdown of norepinephrine. A class of medications known as serotonin uptake inhibitors is often helpful in the management of depression.

TREMORS

Tremors are involuntary muscle twitches. They may be minor and occur in a tired muscle or exaggerated in conditions such as St. Vitus' dance, Huntington's chorea, or Parkinson's disease. They are not a form of epilepsy, although they originate in the CNS.

Parkinson's Disease

In Parkinson's disease the neurons that release the neurotransmitter dopamine in the brain degenerate, thus slowing or stopping its release. Parkinson's disease occurs mainly in the elderly; the symptoms include rigidity of the muscles of the limbs, tremors while the person is at rest, a shuffling gait, and a masklike face.

Pharmacologic intervention includes the use of L-dopa (levodopa), the precursor of dopamine; amantadine (Symmetrel), which releases dopamine at the synapse; and bentropine (Cogentin) and trihexyphenidyl (Artane), both of which are anticholinergic drugs

Chorea

Chorea results from the degeneration of neurons in the basal ganglia. The affected person's normal voluntary movements are replaced with involuntary dancelike motions. The most common forms are St. Vitus' dance and Huntington's chorea, a hereditary disease that also includes a form of dementia.

INDICATIONS CONTRAINDICATIONS

For Soft Tissue and Movement Therapies

Soft tissue and movement modalities are supportive in a multidisciplinary treatment of depression because serotonin, among other neurotransmitters, is influenced by such methods. Because bodywork has been shown to increase dopamine activity, its use is indicated in the management of Parkinson's disease. In addition, secondary muscle tension can be effectively managed with methods such as massage therapy and other forms of soft tissue manipulation.

INFECTIOUS DISEASE

Most CNS infections are bacterial or viral infections. Infections of the brain are called *encephalitis*. When the meninges are affected, it is called *meningitis*. The two diseases may appear separately or together. Both have symptoms of fever, nausea, and vomiting. Encephalitis may affect motor function, cause seizures, and cause behavioral and mood changes. Meningitis, found mainly in the subarachnoid fluid, adds stiffness of the neck to its symptom list. As with other infections, the primary treatment for viral infection is support for general immune function, with antibiotics given for a bacterial infection.

Myelitis is an infection of the spinal cord and/or brainstem. In the past the poliomyelitis virus was the most common infection. Its symptoms affect motor and sensory functions. Because most forms of myelitis result from viruses, treatment supports the body while the immune functions resolve the problem.

INDICATIONS CONTRAINDICATIONS

For Soft Tissue and Movement Therapies

Infectious processes are contraindicated for soft tissue and movement intervention unless closely supervised by appropriate medical personnel. Refer unusual or unexplained stiff neck for diagnosis.

HEADACHE

Headaches can be caused by stress, muscle tension, chemical imbalance, circulatory and sinus disorders, or tumors.

Migraine headache pain is believed to be caused by dilatation of the cranial vessels. The pain is knife-like, throbbing, and unilateral. Any visual distortion (e.g., flashing lights) is believed to be caused by vasoconstriction preceding the vasodilation and pain.

Cluster headaches come in "clusters" on one side of the head, with remissions and recurrence lasting for long periods. They usually occur at night and are associated with other symptoms such as red eyes and sinus drainage.

Medications used to treat headaches are usually nonsteroidal analgesics such as aspirin, but migraines may not respond to medication after the headache begins. Migraines may sometimes be prevented by the medication ergotamine (a vasoconstrictor) or other vasoconstricting medication. The judicious use of caffeine may reduce migraine symptoms.

INDICATIONS CONTRAINDICATIONS

For Soft Tissue and Movement Therapies

Massage and other forms of soft tissue therapy are effective in the treatment of muscle tension headache but much less so with migraine or cluster headaches. Soft tissue therapy can relieve secondary muscle tension headache caused by the pain of the primary headache. Headache is often stress induced. Stress management in all forms is usually indicated in chronic headache conditions.

SPINAL CORD INJURY

Injuries to the spinal cord can result in a number of neurologic problems. Studies of blood flow and metabolism indicate that spinal cord injury involves not only direct neuronal trauma but also direct and delayed vascular trauma. The most frequently injured sites are at the most mobile segments of the spine such as the cervicothoracic (C7-T1) and the thoracolumbar junctions (T12-L1-4). About 40% of spinal cord injuries result in complete function interruption. The balance of the injuries result in the impairment or destruction of certain sensory and motor functions.

INDICATIONS CONTRAINDICATIONS

For Soft Tissue and Movement Therapies

Soft tissue and movement therapies are an effective part of a comprehensive supervised rehabilitation and long-term care program. Massage and other forms of bodywork can help manage secondary muscle tension resulting from the alteration of posture and the use of equipment such as wheelchairs, braces, and crutches. Specifically focused massage can help manage difficulties with bowel paralysis.

Summary

This chapter has focused on nervous system basics and the components and functions of the CNS. Behavior and the nervous system are linked in the feedback loop pattern. Consciousness is a function of the CNS. Soft tissue and movement modalities are supportive, maintaining health of the CNS. Pathologic conditions of the CNS disrupt many types of body functions, and bodywork methods can provide support in coping with many of these dysfunctions.

WORKBOOK SECTION

1. List the parts of the neuron.

   _____

   _____

   _____

2. Explain the function of the nerve cell.

   _____

   _____

   _____

3. Describe neurotransmitter functions and list the major neurotransmitters.

   _____

   _____

   _____

   _____

4. Relate brain chemistry to behavior.

   _____

   _____

   _____

   _____

5. Define the major parts and functions of the CNS.

   _____

   _____

   _____

   _____

6. Describe consciousness and altered states of consciousness.

   _____

   _____

   _____

   _____

7. Explain the process of memory and learning.

   _____

   _____

   _____

   _____

8. Describe common pathologic conditions of the CNS.

   _____

   _____

   _____

   _____

9. List the drugs that influence the CNS.

   _____

   _____

   _____

   _____

10. Explain the influence of bodywork methods on the CNS.

   _____

   _____

FILL IN THE BLANK

The CNS consists of the brain and _____ (1).

_____ (2) are nerve cells that conduct impulses.

Neuroglia is specialized _____ (3) cells that support, protect, and hold neurons together. _____ (4) are branching projections from the nerve cell body. Axons are _____ (5) elongated projections from the nerve cell body. _____ (6) is the outer cell membrane of a Schwann cell that plays an essential part in the _____ (7) of injured axons.

White matter is _____ (8) nerve fibers. Gray matter is formed by nerve cell bodies in the CNS that are _____ (9). Neurotransmitters are chemical transmitters released in the _____ (10) from presynaptic cells. A synapse is a _____ (11) between neurons.

The _____ (12) is the largest and most complex unit of the nervous system and is responsible for perception, sensation, emotion, and intellect. The _____ (13) is the largest of the brain divisions and occupies the uppermost region of the cranium. It consists of two _____ (14). The cerebrum is covered by a thin layer of gray matter called the _____ (15) that is formed into folds called convolutions or _____ (16). These folds are separated by creases called _____ (17). Underneath the gray matter is the _____ (18) made up of complicated pathways of myelinated axons called white matter that connect the gray matter of the left and right hemispheres.

The _____ (19) of the cerebral cortex is the anterior area positioned behind the frontal bone. Its major function is to control the voluntary skeletal muscles in an area called the _____ (20) and is active in functions of problem solving involving concentration and planning. The _____ (21) is located next to the parietal bones of the skull and contains the _____ (22), which is the sensory area of the brain and functions with the sensory data reporting of temperature, pressure, touch, and pain. The _____ (23) is positioned next to the temporal bones. The temporal lobe is responsible for the sensory functions of _____ (24) and _____ (25). The occipital lobe is located just anterior to the occipital bone of the skull and is responsible for the control of _____ (26).

The _____ (27) is a group of structures located on the interior of the cerebrum that plays an important role in arousal and emotional responses, endocrine and autonomic responses, and sexual behavior. The _____ (28) is the second largest part of the brain and is involved with _____ (29). The brainstem contains centers for _____ (30) function connected with _____ (31), as well as vomiting, coughing, and sneezing; posture; and basic movement patterns. Located in the _____ (32) are the thalamus, hypothalamus, and pineal gland. The _____ (33) is associated with pain, temperature, touch sensations, crude sensation, and muscular coordination.

The _____ (34) controls the pituitary gland by producing "releasing hormones" and is the temperature center, the sexual center, the thirst and hunger center, and the rage and fear center. The pineal body gland appears to act as a _____ (35) regulating circadian rhythms. The midbrain or _____ (36) is located between the thalamus and the pons and contains centers for visual and auditory reflexes and correlating information about muscle tone and posture, as well as visual reflexes. Nerve fibers entering on one side of the _____ (37) cross and exit the other side;

therefore one side of the brain controls the opposite side of the body. The _____ (38) regulates heartbeat, blood pressure, breathing, coughing, sneezing, swallowing, and vomiting.

The CNS is surrounded by three membranes called the _____ (39). _____ (40) is a clear, colorless fluid that flows throughout the brain and around the _____ (41), cushioning and protecting these structures.

The spinal cord is the portion of the CNS that exits the skull into the _____ (42). The two major functions of the spinal cord are to conduct nerve impulses and to be a center for _____ (43). _____ (44) are collections of nerve fibers in the CNS having a common function.

EXERCISE

For the illustration of a neuron pictured below, fill in the blanks for each part indicated by a letter, then color each part.

A. _____

B. _____ _____

C. _____

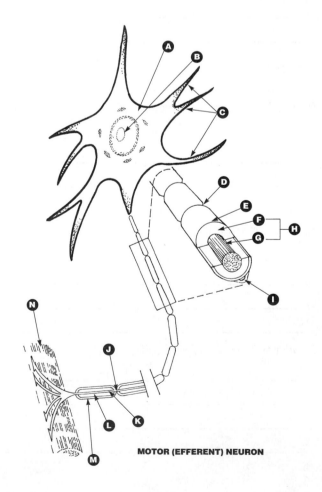

MOTOR (EFFERENT) NEURON

D. _____

E. _____

F. _____

G. _____

H. _____

I. _____

J. _____

K. _____

L. _____

M. _____

N. _____

PROBLEM-SOLVING EXERCISE

Read the problem presented. There is no correct answer. Instead, the exercise assists the student in the development of analysis and decision-making skills necessary in a professional practice.

1. Identify the facts presented in the information.
2. Identify the possibilities ("what if" statements) presented or develop your own possibilities that relate to the facts.
3. Evaluate each possibility in terms of the logical cause and effect and pros and cons.
4. Consider the feelings of the people involved.
5. Write each down in the space provided.
6. Develop your solution by answering the question posed.

PROBLEM

It is obvious that behavior influences the CNS. It seems important that a person engages in pleasure-seeking activity that stimulates the feel-good neurotransmitters. Connected with this process is the drive for altered states of consciousness. Today's world places many demands on individuals. Most of these demands are performance based. Time becomes a rare commodity. When this is the case for an individual, the structure for satisfying pleasure needs decreases. Could this situation support the search for quick methods to affect neurotransmitters? Ancient meditative processes and touch and movement therapies, including exercise, are time consuming. Maybe people do not do what they know is beneficial because these methods are cumbersome to integrate into a busy lifestyle. How does one balance the need for pleasure, excitement, calm, joy, sadness, love, companionship, and so forth with the time necessary to procure such experiences? One wonders if this current situation is not responsible, at least in part, for extreme behavior and the use of chemicals to create the internal chemical response that satisfies these needs in a fast and reliable way, regardless of how destructive the long-term consequences may be.

QUESTION

What do soft tissue and movement therapies have to offer to satisfy pleasure needs, and how does one efficiently integrate these methods into a busy schedule or begin to justify the time necessary to use the important approaches to CNS health?

FACTS

1. Behavior influences the CNS.

2. _____

3. _____

POSSIBILITIES

1. People may not take the time to fulfill pleasure needs.

2. _____

3. _____

LOGICAL CAUSE AND EFFECT

1. Not taking time to fulfill pleasure needs would seem to produce extreme behavior resulting in addictive actions.

2. _____

3. _____

IMPACT ON PEOPLE

1. People may feel helpless because they do not understand why they do something that initially felt good but ultimately hurts them.

2. _____

3. _____

What do soft tissue and movement therapies have to offer to satisfy pleasure needs, and how does one efficiently integrate these methods into a busy schedule or begin to justify the time necessary to use the important approaches to CNS health?

_____

_____

_____

_____

PROFESSIONAL APPLICATION

What additional knowledge base would one need to work in CVA rehabilitation and long-term care using soft tissue and movement therapies? Where might a practitioner find this information and get additional training?

_____

_____

_____

_____

FURTHER STUDY

Using a comprehensive anatomy and physiology text (see Works Consulted list at the back of this book), identify chapters pertaining to the information presented in this chapter. Locate the information presented in this text and then elaborate by writing a paragraph of additional information on each of the following.

Nerve cell regeneration:

_____

_____

_____

_____

Neurotransmitters:

_____

_____

_____

_____

Memory:

_____

_____

_____

_____

Difference in the male and female brain:

_____

_____

_____

_____

Differences in dominant and nondominant cerebral hemisphere functions:

_____

_____

_____

_____

Brainstem function in relationship to survival behavior:

_____

_____

_____

_____

Reticular activating system:

_____

_____

_____

_____

Spinal cord tracts:

_____

_____

_____

_____

Answer Key

1. Neuroglia, dendrites, axon, neurolemma.
2. A nerve impulse is a self-perpetuating wave of electrical energy that travels along the surface of a neuron's plasma membrane. Nerve impulses have to be initiated by a stimulus that changes the neuron's environment. A neuron is said to be excited when a stimulus triggers the opening of additional Na^+ channels, allowing the membrane potential to move toward zero. Inhibition occurs when the stimulus triggers the opening of additional K^+ channels, increasing the membrane potential. The electrical disturbance stimulates a similar change in the next section of membrane, resulting in a nerve impulse traveling in one direction along the neuron's surface.

   After a local area of a neuron's membrane has been stimulated and a nerve impulse has been generated, it resists restimulation and will not respond to a stimulus no matter how strong. This is called the refractory period.

   In myelinated fibers, action potentials in the membrane only occur at the nodes of Ranvier. If the traveling impulse encounters a section of membrane covered with insulating myelin, it jumps over the myelin, resulting in faster transmission than is possible in nonmyelinated sections.
3. Neurotransmitters are chemical compounds that regulate many body activities and states. Neurotransmitter effects may be excitatory, by increasing activity, or inhibitory, by decreasing an activity.

   Chemical synapses occur at presynaptic cells that release chemical transmitters called *neurotransmitters* across a tiny gap to the postsynaptic cell. The plasma membrane of a postsynaptic neuron has protein molecules that serve as receptors for the neurotransmitters. When a nerve impulse reaches a synaptic knob, thousands of neurotransmitter molecules flow into the synaptic cleft and bind to specific receptors, generating an action potential. The neurotransmitter's action is quickly terminated by either neurotransmitter molecules being transported back into the synaptic knob or metabolized into inactive compounds. Many drugs act by disturbing the termination phase.

   The major neurotransmitters are acetylcholine, serotonin, histamine, epinephrine, norepinephrine, and dopamine (endorphins); and glutamate, or glutamic acid, gamma-aminobutyric acid, or GABA, substance P, somatostatin, cholecystokinin, or CCK, and vasoactive intestinal peptide, or VIP (enkephalins).
4. A change in neurotransmitter concentrations at various synapses will cause a change in behavior. Both mental illness behaviors and much of our daily behavior, especially pain, pleasure, and survival behavior, are determined by brain chemistry. An ongoing dynamic balance in this chemical soup allows for resourceful behavior for each situation we encounter. In addition, we behave in certain ways to increase or decrease levels of neurotransmitters or hormones. When medication is used to manage neurotransmitters, mood and behavior are affected. Repeated behavior is in some way accomplishing the goal of a form of homeostasis—even bizarre behavior such as drug addiction, excessive exercise, eating disorders, rage, thrill seeking, crisis orientation, and pain behavior. Pain

behavior is also a brain chemistry event. Pain becomes a decision in the brain. A pain-inhibiting system exists in the body. Internal, or endogenous, opiates (endorphins, enkephalins) produced by the body block pain impulses in various portions of the pathway, probably as a protective device. The neurotransmitter substance P is blocked by enkephalins. Endorphins and enkephalins also affect mood.

5. The brain is the center for interpreting, regulating, integrating, and coordinating physiologic functions. It is divided into the following major segments.

The cerebrum—the major functions of the cerebrum are as follows:

Interpretation of sensory information received from the eyes, ears, nose, taste, tactile, and other sensory structures of the body

Transmitting motor impulses that initiate voluntary movements and some involuntary movements in response to sensory data

Association functions that allow learning, reasoning, recall, language, and consciousness

The brainstem—contains centers for vital functions connected with survival, as well as vomiting, coughing, and sneezing; posture; and basic movement patterns; houses cranial nerves. Located in the brainstem are the thalamus, hypothalamus, and pineal gland

The midbrain or mesencephalon—contains centers for visual and auditory reflexes and correlating information about muscle tone and posture, as well as visual reflexes; contains cranial nerve nuclei, an important part of the reticular activating system

The pons (pons varolii)—located between the midbrain and the medulla; functions in the rhythmic discharge of the respiratory center of the medulla, chewing, facial expressions, and eye movement; contains cranial nerve nuclei and important centers for REM sleep

The medulla or medulla oblongata—connects the pons and spinal cord. The functions of the medulla include the following:

Cardiac center: regulates heartbeat

Vasomotor center: regulates blood pressure

Respiratory center: regulates breathing

Other functions include coughing, sneezing, swallowing, and vomiting

Cerebellum—located in the posterior cranial fossa of the skull; second largest segment of the brain; contains centers for balance, equilibrium, muscular coordination, posture, and balance; controls subconscious movements of skeletal muscle, input from proprioceptors, feedback loops, posture, future positioning; regulates sensations of anger and pleasure

The reticular formation and the reticular activating system—primitive inner core of the spinal cord and brainstem involved in the regulation of respiration, blood pressure, heart rate, endocrine secretion, conditioned reflexes, learning, and consciousness

The meninges—three membranes called the *meninges:* the dura mater, arachnoid, the pia; three spaces are developed by the meninges:

Epidural space between skull and dural matter

Subdural space between dura and arachnoid

Subarachnoid space between arachnoid and pia that ends at the vertebral level

Vessels of the brain—internal carotid system and the vertebrobasilar artery connect (anastomose) at the midbrain as the Circle of Willis, ensuring blood flow to the brain despite occlusion of either the carotid or basilar arteries; venous drainage from the brain is by several veins, as well as the dural sinuses, spaces in the dura that drain to the internal jugular veins

Spinal cord—conduct nerve impulses and to be a center for spinal reflexes; 31 pairs of peripheral spinal nerves connect the spinal cord and brain with all areas of the body

The white matter on the outside of the spinal cord is made up of myelinated nerve fibers called *tracts* that ascend to and descend from the brain. Ascending tracts conduct impulses up the spinal cord to the brain, transmitting pain, temperature, and positional information. Descending tracts conduct impulses from the brain down the cord, sending effector information to muscles and glands. The gray matter on the inside of the spinal cord forms an H pattern.

6. Consciousness is the awareness of the environment and the relationship of ourselves to those in that environment. Consciousness depends on excitation of cortical neurons by impulses conducted from the reticular activating system, which relays them to the thalamus. The thalamus transmits the data to all parts of the cerebral cortex. Drugs that stimulate the cerebrum enhancing alertness probably act by stimulating the reticular activating system.

People of various cultures have explored altered states of consciousness for centuries. Many ways of altering consciousness exist. Meditation produces a state of higher consciousness typified by both relaxation and alertness. Meditation is simply a highly focused peaceful state, usually in a calm environment, produced by synchronizing the breath and other body rhythms. Pleasure behavior derived from the sense of well-being experienced by altered states of consciousness can be addictive, and the associated behavior to achieve the pleasure state can be detrimental if excessive.

7. Memory is the storing of information in the brain and is one of our major mental activities. There are two types of memory, short term (recent) and long term. Highly emotional events seem to immediately become stored in long-term memory, indicating neurotransmitter involvement in memory structures.

The key in long-term memory is repeated impulse. Learning strategies are often focused around circular learning where information continues to reappear reinforcing the neurocircuit storing the memory.

Learning in a basic and primitive sense can be thought of as the best and simplest way to solve a problem. Anatomically and physiologically, learning is the use of multiple synaptic pathways to solve problems. Advanced learning takes place in the association areas of the cerebral cortex (some learning also takes place in the brainstem). Learning requires memory and is the development of neural structures that remember the way to solve a problem. Solving problems supports survival. Learning can be thought of as conditioning. Conditioning can also be considered learned habit. The process of learning is conscious, but after something has been integrated often it becomes unconscious.

8. CVA, or stroke, is an umbrella term that covers disorders such as aneurysms and blood clots and hemorrhages. When a stroke occurs, an artery in the brain is occluded or closed off from a blood clot called a *thrombus.*

An aneurysm is a weakening and bulging of an artery.

A blood clot may break away from a different part of the body and travel to the brain.

CNS trauma may occur when a concussion causes a brief loss of consciousness or a state of confusion after a head injury. A contusion is a bruise of the brain. Intracranial bleeding is called *intracerebral hemorrhage* or *hematoma.*

Cerebral palsy is a general term for brain damage before, during, or shortly after birth.

Seizure in epilepsy is characterized by an abrupt alteration in brain function, ranging from a mild behavior change to a general convulsion.

Primary tumors form from the neuroglia, membrane tissues, and blood vessels associated with the neuron. Most brain tumors do not originate in the brain. They are metastatic from malignant tumors elsewhere in the body.

Spinal cord injury can result in a number of neurologic deficits.

9. The stimulants are caffeine, nicotine, the amphetamines, and cocaine. The depressants are alcohol, narcotics, minor tranquilizers, and barbiturates. The hallucinogens are LSD, PCP, peyote, and marijuana.

10. Soft tissue and movement therapies provide stimulation to the CNS, causing the brain and spinal cord to respond. Neurotransmitters are also affected.

FILL IN THE BLANK

1. spinal cord
2. Neurons
3. connective tissue
4. Dendrites
5. single
6. neurolemma
7. regeneration
8. myelinated
9. unmyelinated
10. synapses
11. junction
12. brain
13. cerebrum
14. hemispheres
15. cerebral cortex
16. gyri
17. sulci
18. corpus callosum
19. frontal lobe
20. precentral gyrus
21. parietal lobe
22. postcentral gyrus
23. temporal lobe
24. hearing
25. smell
26. eyesight
27. limbic system
28. cerebellum
29. movement
30. vital
31. survival
32. brainstem
33. thalamus
34. hypothalamus
35. biologic clock
36. mesencephalon
37. pons
38. medulla
39. meninges
40. cerebrospinal fluid
41. spinal cord
42. vertebral column
43. spinal reflexes
44. Tracts

EXERCISE

A. Cell body
B. Nucleus
C. Dendrites
D. Node of Ranvier
E. Neurolemma
F. Myelin sheath
G. Axon
H. Nerve fiber
I. Nucleus of Schwann cell
J. Node of Ranvier
K. Axon
L. Myelin sheath
M. Neurolemma
N. Neuromuscular junction

Chapter 5

The Peripheral Nervous System

CHAPTER OUTLINE

Basics of the Peripheral Nervous System
Nerves
Cranial nerves
Spinal nerves
Nerve plexuses
Cervical plexus
Brachial plexus
Lumbar plexus
Sacral plexus
Injury
Dermatomes
Myotomes
Reflex mechanisms
Sensory receptors
Reflex arc
Stretch reflex
Tendon reflex
The autonomic nervous system
Sympathetic structure and function
Parasympathetic structure and function
Adrenergic stimulation
Medications that affect the autonomic nervous
system
A-adrenergic blockers (α-blockers)
B-adrenergic medications
B-adrenergic blockers (β-blockers)
Parasympathetic blockers
Sympathomimetic medications
Eastern/Western connection

The Four Basic Senses
Hearing
Vision
Taste
Smell

Pathologic Conditions of the Peripheral Nervous System
> Entrapment and compression
> Nerve root compression
> Disk herniation
> Bell's palsy
> Guillain-Barré syndrome
> Herpes
> Demyelination disease
> Neurotransmitter-based disorders
>> *Depression*
>> *Anxiety states*
> Neuropathy
> Headache
> Vertigo

Summary

KEY TERMS

Afferent (AF-fer-ent) *nerves (sensory nerves)* Nerves that link sensory receptors with the central nervous system (CNS) and transmit sensory information.

Autonomic (aw-toe-NOM-ik) *nervous system* A division of the peripheral nervous system composed of nerves that connect the CNS to the glands, heart, and smooth muscles to maintain the internal body environment.

Cranial nerves Twelve pairs of nerves that originate from the olfactory bulbs, thalamus, visual cortex, and brainstem. They transmit information to and from the sense organs of the face and the muscles of the face, neck, and upper shoulders.

Dermatome (DER-mah-tohm) A cutaneous (skin) section supplied by a single spinal nerve.

Efferent (EF-fer-ent) *nerves (motor nerves)* Nerves that link the CNS to the effectors outside the CNS and transmit motor impulses.

Free nerve endings Sensory receptors that detect itch and tickle sensations.

Mechanical receptors Sensory receptors that detect changes in pressure, movement, temperature, or other mechanical forces.

Mixed nerves Nerves that contain both sensory and motor axons.

Myotome (MY-o-tohm) A skeletal muscle or group of skeletal muscles that receives motor axons from a particular spinal nerve.

Nerve A bundle of axons or dendrites or both.

Nociceptors (no-se-SEP-tors) Sensory receptors that detect painful or intense stimuli.

Parasympathetic nervous system The energy conservation and restorative system associated with what commonly is called the *relaxation response.*

Peripheral (pe-RIF-er-al) *nervous system (PNS)* The system of somatic and autonomic neurons outside the CNS. The PNS comprises the afferent (sensory) division and the efferent (motor) division.

Plexus (PLEK-sus) A network of intertwining nerves that innervates a particular region of the body.

Proprioceptors (pro-pree-o-SEP-tors) Sensory receptors that provide the body with information about position, movement, muscle tension, joint activity, and equilibrium.

Reflex An automatic, involuntary reaction to a stimulus.

Somatic (so-MA-tik) *nervous system* A system of nerves that keeps the body in balance with its external environment by transmitting impulses between the CNS, skeletal muscles, and skin.

Spinal nerves Thirty-one pairs of mixed nerves, originating in the spinal cord and emerging from the vertebral column, that make sensation and movement possible.

Sympathetic nervous system The part of the autonomic nervous system that provides for most of the body's active function; when the body is under stress, the sympathetic nervous system predominates with fight-or-flight responses.

Thermal receptors Sensory receptors that detect changes in temperature.

Basics of the Peripheral Nervous System

The **peripheral nervous system** comprises the motor nerves, sensory nerves, and ganglia outside the brain and spinal cord. The system consists of 12 pairs of cranial nerves and 31 pairs of spinal nerves, as well as their various branches in the body.

Sensory, or **afferent,** peripheral nerves transmit information to the central nervous system; motor, or **efferent,** peripheral nerves carry impulses from the brain back to the body. The two signals usually travel together in one nerve, with some fibers serving as sensory transmitters and others as motor transmitters. At the spinal cord the fibers separate into a posterior sensory root and an anterior motor root.

Fibers that innervate the body wall are called *somatic* fibers. Those that supply the internal organs are called *visceral* fibers.

The **autonomic nervous system** is made up of the peripheral nerves involved in regulating cardiovascular, respiratory, endocrine, and other automatic body functions.

✋ PRACTICAL APPLICATION

Stimulation of the peripheral nervous system (PNS) and the responses elicited by this stimulation constitute one of the main physiologic modes by which soft tissue and movement therapies benefit the client. Those who practice these therapies must thoroughly understand the anatomy and physiology of the PNS and comprehend the way soft tissue and movement methods interact with the PNS.

NERVES

A **nerve** is a bundle of axons or dendrites or both. Nerves may be of the motor, sensory, or mixed type. *Motor nerves* innervate or provide action, whereas *sensory nerves* transmit input from sensory receptors. **Mixed nerves** contain both sensory and motor fibers. A delicate connective tissue covering known as the *endoneurium* surrounds and holds each nerve fiber. A group of nerve fibers is called a *fasciculus*, and each fasciculus is surrounded by a sheath of connective tissue, called the *perineurium* (Figure 5-1).

Cranial Nerves

Twelve pairs of **cranial nerves** enter (sensory) or leave (motor) the olfactory bulbs, thalamus, visual cortex, and brainstem. They are identified both by Roman numerals (according to their order from the front to the back of the brain) and by names (which refer to their function or distribution) (Figure 5-2; Table 5-1).

Disorders of the cranial nerves can arise from a stroke or tumor or from trauma. The resulting change in action may help locate the lesion because a lack of function may indicate damage to the nerve associated with that function. For example, the accessory nerves (XI) affect the trapezius and sternocleidomastoid muscles. Dysfunction in either of these muscles may be an indication of involvement of this nerve.

✋ PRACTICAL APPLICATION

The distribution of the vagus nerve affects many visceral functions. Massage has been shown to support vagus nerve function, especially in premature babies, resulting in better development (particularly in weight gain) and fewer developmental problems.

Spinal Nerves

Thirty-one pairs of **spinal nerves** originate in the spinal cord and emerge from the vertebral column. All contain sensory and motor fibers in the same nerve (forming a mixed nerve), making both sensation and movement possible. The nerve path generally follows the path of the arteries. Each nerve attaches to the spinal cord by way of two short roots on each side, one in front and one in back. The *anterior*, or *ventral*, root is motor; the fibers originate in the ventral horn cells and innervate skeletal muscles. The *posterior*, or *dorsal*, root is sensory; the fibers originate in the sensory receptors and travel to the dorsal roots of the spinal cord. The dorsal root of each spinal nerve is recognized by a swelling, known as the *dorsal root ganglion*, which contains the cell bodies of the sensory neurons.

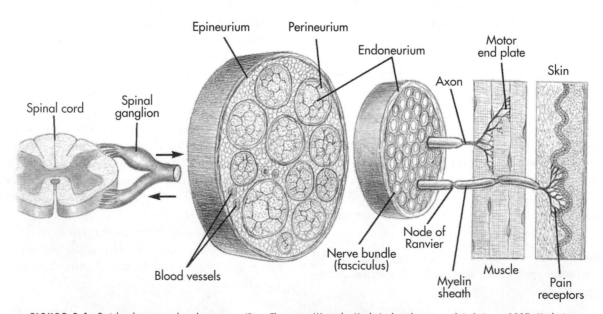

FIGURE 5-1 Peripheral nerve trunk and coverings. (From Thompson JM et al.: *Mosby's clinical nursing*, ed 4, St Louis, 1997, Mosby.)

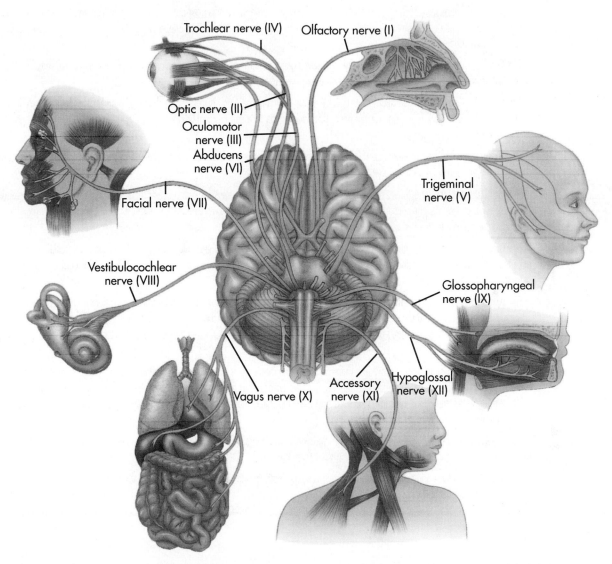

FIGURE 5-2 Cranial nerves. Ventral surface of the brain, showing the attachments of the cranial nerves. (From Thibodeau GA, Patton KT: *Anatomy and physiology,* ed 3, St Louis, 1996, Mosby.)

TABLE 5-1 CRANIAL NERVES

CRANIAL NERVE	DESCRIPTION
I	The *olfactory nerves* are sensory and transmit information about taste and smell from the nasal cavity to the cerebrum (into the olfactory bulb of the forebrain).
II	The *optic nerves* are sensory and transmit information about clarity and field of vision from the retina to the midbrain of the cerebrum via the thalamus.
III	The *oculomotor nerves* are both sensory and motor. The sensory portion transmits information about eye movement. The motor portion originates in the midbrain and controls all external eye muscles (except the superior oblique and lateral rectus muscles) as well as pupil contraction and relaxation.
IV	The *trochlear nerves* comprise mainly motor nerves, which begin in the midbrain. They innervate the superior oblique eye muscles. The few sensory neurons provide proprioceptive information about eye movement.
V	The *trigeminal nerves* arise in the pons. The motor neurons innervate the muscles involved in chewing. The sensory neurons carry information about sensations and proprioception for the head, face, skin of the face and mucosal linings, eyelids, and tongue. The trigeminal nerves are the largest of the cranial nerves.
VI	The *abducens nerves* arise in the pons. The motor neurons innervate the lateral rectus eye muscle (an eye abductor). The sensory neurons provide proprioceptive information about eye movement.
VII	The *facial nerves* have motor fibers that arise in the pons and innervate the muscles that produce facial expression as well as the glands that release tears and saliva. The sensory fibers carry information about taste to the cerebral cortex. Some of the fibers also relay proprioceptive information about the face and scalp.
VIII	The *vestibulocochlear nerves* are sensory and are divided into two branches. The vestibular branch begins in the semicircular canals of the ear and carries signals for equilibrium to the pons, medulla, and cerebellum. The cochlear branch arises in the organ of Corti and carries impulses for hearing to the pons and medulla.
IX	The *glossopharyngeal nerves* contain both sensory and motor neurons. The sensory fibers extend to the medulla from the pharynx and the tongue; they are concerned primarily with taste. Another sensory fiber extends from the carotid sinus in the internal carotid artery; it aids in the control of respiration and blood pressure. The motor neurons arise in the medulla and affect saliva production, swallowing, and the gag reflex.
X	The *vagus nerves* contain both sensory and motor neurons. The motor fibers originate in the medulla and carry signals that control the muscles involved in swallowing and speaking. Other motor fibers terminate in the muscles of the digestive and respiratory tracts and in the heart. The sensory fibers arise from the same structures that the motor fibers innervate and carry information about sensations and proprioception of these organs.
XI	The *accessory nerves* arise in the medulla and are primarily motor neurons for speaking, turning the head, and moving the shoulders. The few sensory neurons relay proprioceptive information from these muscles.
XII	The *hypoglossal nerves* originate in the medulla and contain mostly motor neurons, which innervate the tongue and throat. A few sensory neurons carry proprioceptive information from the tongue.

Spinal nerves are identified by a letter and a number, which refer to their segment of attachment to the spinal cord (Figure 5-3; Box 5-1).

NERVE PLEXUSES

Most of the spinal nerves, except those that emerge from T2 to T12, converge in small groups to form an intersecting network known as a nerve **plexus**. Each plexus contains fibers that innervate a specific region of the body. Overlap of nerve function prevents total loss of function if just one of the nerves in the group is damaged. The four major plexuses are the cervical, brachial, lumbar, and sacral plexuses.

Cervical Plexus

The cervical plexus, formed from nerves C1 to C4 and part of C5, consists of sensory distribution from the head, front of the neck, and upper part of the shoulders, as well as motor impulses to many neck and shoulder muscles and the diaphragm (Figure 5-4).

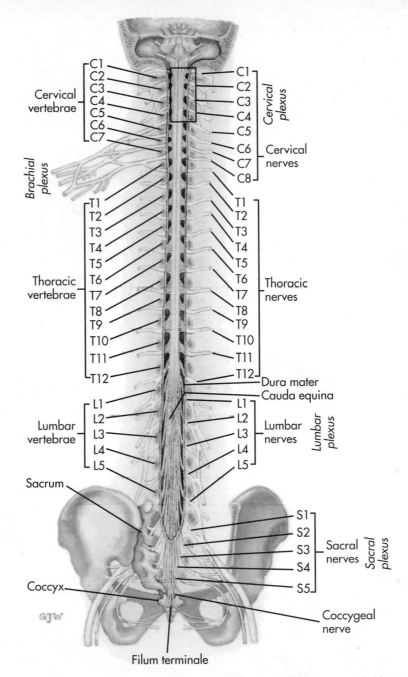

FIGURE 5-3 Spinal nerves. Each of 31 pairs of spinal nerves exits the spinal cavity from the intervertebral foramina. Notice that after leaving the spinal cavity, many of the spinal nerves interconnect to form networks, called *plexuses*. (From Chipps EM, Clanin NJ, Campbell VG: *Neurologic disorders,* St Louis, 1992, Mosby.)

Cervical plexus

Brachial plexus

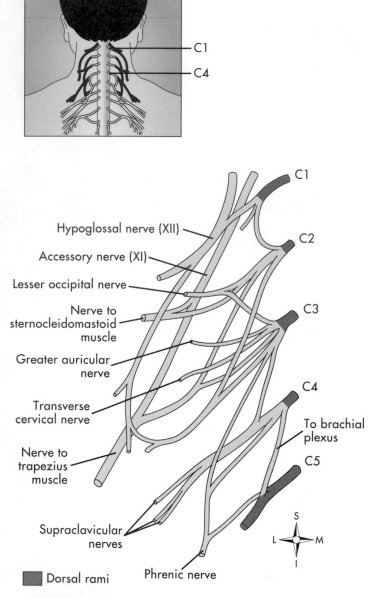

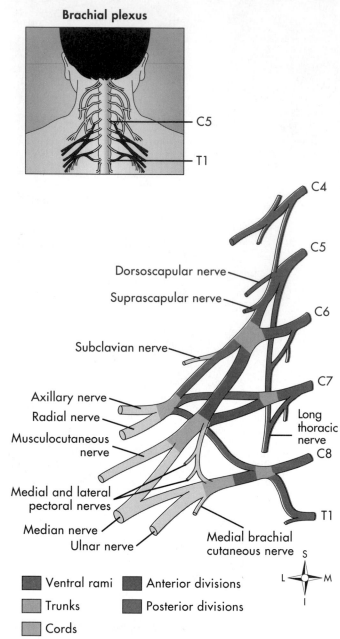

FIGURE 5-4 Cervical plexus. Ventral rami of the first four cervical spinal nerves (C1 through C4) exchange fibers in this plexus found deep within the neck. Notice that some fibers from C5 also enter this plexus to form a portion of the phrenic nerve. (From Thibodeau GA, Patton KT: *Anatomy and physiology,* ed 3, St Louis, 1996, Mosby.)

FIGURE 5-5 Brachial plexus. From the five rami, C5 through T1, the plexus forms three trunks. Each trunk subdivides into an anterior and a posterior division. The divisional branches reorganize into three cords, and the cords give rise to the individual nerves that exit this plexus. (From Thibodeau GA, Patton KT: *Anatomy and physiology,* ed 3, St Louis,1996, Mosby.)

NERVE	INNERVATION
Ansa cervicalis	Hyoid muscles
Lesser occipital	Skin behind and above the ear
Greater auricular	Skin in front of, below, and over the ear and parotid glands
Transverse cervical	Skin on the anterior portion of the neck
Phrenic	Diaphragm
Supraclavicular	Skin on the shoulders and upper portion of the chest
Segmental branches	Deep neck muscles, mid-scalenes, and levator scapula muscle

Brachial Plexus

The brachial plexus, formed from nerves C5 through T1, is organized into three divisions: the superior, middle, and inferior trunk. These divisions supply the skin and muscles of the upper limbs (Figure 5-5).

NERVE	INNERVATION
Dorsoscapular	Superficial muscles of the scapula
Long thoracic	Serratus anterior muscle
Subclavian	Subclavius muscle
Suprascapular	Infraspinatus and supraspinatus muscles
Musculocutaneous	Biceps, brachialis and coracobrachialis muscles, and skin
Subscapular	Subscapularis and teres major muscles
Median	Forearm flexors and palmar surface of the skin of the thumb, index, and middle fingers.
Thoracodorsal	Latissimus dorsi muscle
Pectorals	Pectoralis major and minor muscles
Axillary	Deltoid and teres minor muscles and skin
Radial	Triceps and forearm extensors, skin of the forearm and hand, and dorsal surface of the thumb, index, and middle fingers
Medial cutaneous	Skin of the arm
Ulnar	Muscles of the hand and skin of the ring and baby fingers

Thoracic nerves that are not part of the brachial plexus are the motor nerves to the intercostal muscles and sensory nerves from the skin of the thorax.

The lumbar and sacral nerves combine to form the lumbosacral plexus (Figure 5-6). We present them separately.

Lumbar Plexus

The lumbar plexus is composed of nerves L1 to L4.

NERVE	INNERVATION
Iliohypogastric	Abdominal muscles and skin of the abdomen and buttocks
Ilioinguinal	Abdominal muscles and skin of the external genitalia
Genitofemoral	Skin of the external genitalia and inguinal region
Lateral femoral cutaneous	Skin of the thigh (except the medial portion)
Femoral	Hip flexors and extensors and skin of the medial and anterior thigh and medial leg and foot
Obturator	Adductor muscles, skin of the medial thigh

Sacral Plexus

The sacral plexus is created from nerves L5 to S3.

NERVE	INNERVATION
Sciatic	Leg and foot muscles; the skin of the foot divides into the tibial and peroneal nerves at the popliteal fossa
Gluteal	Buttocks and tensor fasciae latae muscle
Nerves to hip rotators	Piriformis, quadratus femoris, obturator internus, superior and inferior gemellus
Posterior femoral cutaneous	Skin of the buttocks, perineum, back of the thigh, and leg
Pudendal	Muscles and skin of the perineum (may be considered in the coccygeal plexus)

INJURY

Injury to the sensory portion of any spinal nerve causes loss of sensation (anesthesia) in the innervated area; injury to the motor portion results in flaccid paralysis of the muscles of that area (Activity 5-1). For example, damage to the radial nerve (C5-C8) at the forearm results in anesthesia of the dorsal portion of the first three fingers and paralysis of the hand and finger extensors. This causes a condition known as wrist drop.

DERMATOMES

A **dermatome** is a section of skin that is supplied by a single spinal nerve. Dermatomes are identified by the number of the nerve. Although Figure 5-7 shows a clear boundary for each cutaneous segment, the nerve supplies in adjoining dermatomal segments overlap. Knowing the dermatome pattern enables a clinician to locate injuries in the spinal cord and spinal nerves. A correlation can be seen between dermatome patterns and the pathway of meridians.

MYOTOMES

A skeletal muscle or group of muscles that receives motor axons from a single spinal nerve is known as a **myotome**. As with dermatomes, the boundaries of myotomes are not always exact; some muscle groups may be innervated by motor axons from more than one spinal nerve. Figure 5-8 shows which spinal

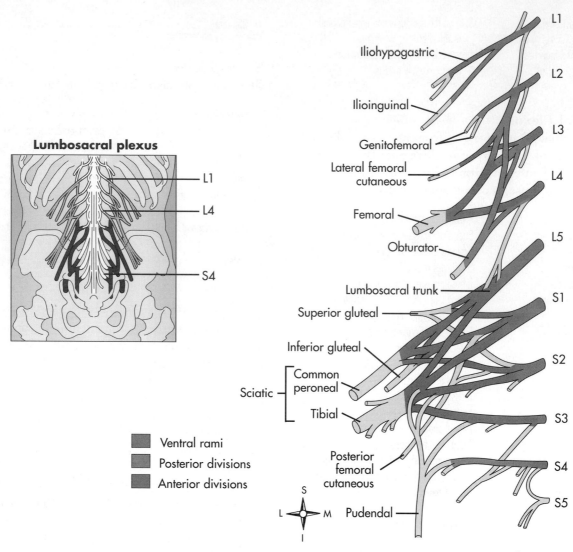

Lumbosacral plexus

L1
L4
S4

Iliohypogastric
Ilioinguinal
Genitofemoral
Lateral femoral cutaneous
Femoral
Obturator
Lumbosacral trunk
Superior gluteal
Inferior gluteal
Sciatic {
Common peroneal
Tibial
Posterior femoral cutaneous
Pudendal

L1
L2
L3
L4
L5
S1
S2
S3
S4
S5

Ventral rami
Posterior divisions
Anterior divisions

S
L — M
I

FIGURE 5-6 Lumbosacral plexus. The lumbosacral plexus is formed by the combination of the lumbar and the sacral plexuses, as shown in the inset. Notice that the ventral rami split into anterior and posterior divisions before reorganizing into the individual nerves that exit this plexus. (From Thibodeau GA, Patton KT: *Anatomy and physiology,* ed 3, St Louis, 1996, Mosby.)

nerves innervate the skeletal muscles that produce the movements indicated by arrows.

REFLEX MECHANISMS

A nerve **reflex** is an involuntary action. As a result of the "wiring" of the body, a simple activity that stimulates a few receptors can involve many neurons going to and from muscles and glands. A brief action such as bumping the "funny bone" (the ulnar nerve) requires many neurons. Some conduct signals to and from the spinal cord to prompt withdrawal of the arm; others carry signals to and from the brain, letting us know when to yell "Ow!" and stimulating tears.

Involuntary reflexes involve receptors, neurons, interneurons, and the spinal cord. Conditioned learned reflexes also involve the brain. Almost every reflex is polysynaptic, meaning that many synapses are crossed during the internal reflex signaling. Breaking down these complex patterns often is difficult but can be a clinical necessity if we are to understand the automatic and sometimes perpetuating responses of both functional and dysfunctional reflex patterns that interact in the body's continual attempt to maintain homeostasis.

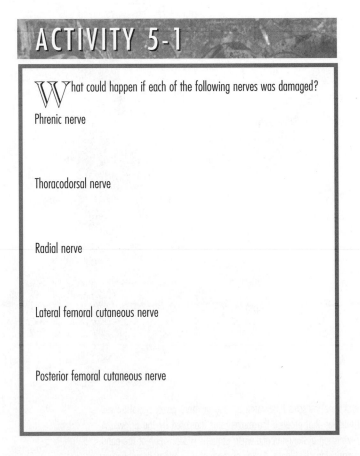

ACTIVITY 5-1

What could happen if each of the following nerves was damaged?

Phrenic nerve

Thoracodorsal nerve

Radial nerve

Lateral femoral cutaneous nerve

Posterior femoral cutaneous nerve

SENSORY RECEPTORS

Our bodies contain many different types of receptors located in various areas. Receptors on the outside of our bodies are called *exteroceptors* and are stimulated by actions or changes in our external environment. Two examples would be our eyes and ears. Changes in our internal environment stimulate the *visceroceptors*, or *interoceptors*. These receptors receive signals monitoring such factors as blood pressure and hunger. In and around the muscles and joints of our body are the **proprioceptors**, which are affected by changes in position, movement, and tension (Figure 5-9).

Most of the time we are not aware of the subtle changes that stimulate sensory receptors or of the adaptations that result from these changes. These natural reflexes, processed in the brainstem or portions of the spinal cord, not only affect our physical response but also the behavior that may result. We can train ourselves to be aware of the stimuli and purposefully adapt our responses; this is called a *conditioned reflex*. These learned behaviors are present in our daily actions such as tying our shoes and are highlighted in forms of sports training and conditioning. We can learn to shoot a basketball or throw a baseball or swing a golf club. After the basic skills have been mastered, we don't have to think about most of the actions; these are conditioned reflexive patterns. Personal habits such as nail biting or eating while watching television are also conditioned reflexive patterns, and these habits may be hard to break after they become reflexive.

When a sensory receptor is stimulated by an appropriate stimulus, an impulse is sent to the central nervous system, where the information is processed. Sensory receptors adapt by becoming less sensitive to a stimulus, and they reduce the number of signals sent, or stop altogether, even if the stimulus is still present. If this did not happen, we would never get used to things such as clothing because the nervous system constantly would be made aware of the sensations and would be unable to sort through what is important to respond to and what isn't. Some forms of minimal brain damage or learning difficulties that involve difficulty focusing or attending to sensory input seem to be perpetuated by a diminished capacity for sensory adaptation. Some of the receptors, especially those associated with pressure and touch, adapt quickly; such receptors play a major role in signaling changes in a particular sensation. Other receptors, such as those that detect pain and body position, adapt slowly and signal information about

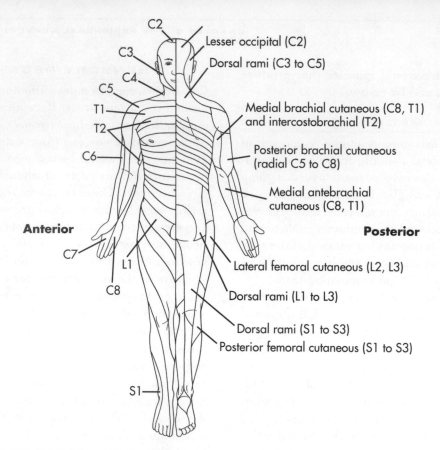

FIGURE 5-7 Dermatomal map (anterior view) and cutaneous nerve distribution (posterior view) of the human body. (From Greenstein GM: *Clinical assessment of neuromusculoskeletal disorders, St Louis, 1997, Mosby.*)

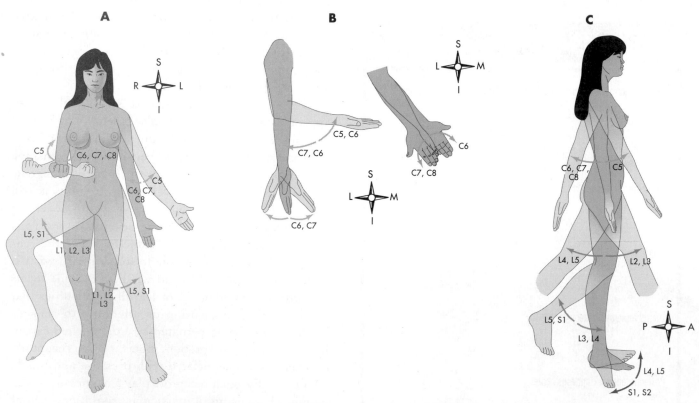

FIGURE 5-8 Myotomes and body movement. Myotomes are skeletal muscles innervated by one or more given spinal nerves. These examples show which spinal nerves innervate the skeletal muscles that produce the movements indicated by the arrows. **A,** Rotation and abduction/adduction of the arm and hip. **B,** Flexion/extension of the hand and wrist; pronation/supination of the hand. **C,** Flexion/extension/hyperextension of the arm, hip, and knee; dorsiflexion and plantar flexion of the foot. **C,** Cervical spinal nerves; *L,* Lumbar spinal nerves; *S,* Sacral spinal nerves; *T,* Thoracic spinal nerves. (From Thibodeau GA, Patton KT: *Anatomy and physiology,* ed 3, St Louis, 1996, Mosby.)

steady states of the body. Numerous sensory structures are classified as **mechanical receptors**. Some of them are listed below:

Mechanoreceptors—These structures detect changes in pressure, movement, temperature, or other mechanical forces.

Pacinian (lamellated) corpuscles—This type of corpuscle senses brief touch, pressure, and high-frequency vibrations. Located in the submucosal, subcutaneous, and connective tissue of the hands, feet, genitals, joints, and other structures, they respond to most forms of rapidly changing mechanical stimulation.

Meissner's corpuscles—Meissner's corpuscles are touch receptors found in the hairless portions of the skin, mainly on the palms, fingertips, and soles of the feet, as well as on the eyelids, lips, tongue, and genitals. They can identify both the exact location of touch (known as discriminative touch) and the initial onset of touch, as well as low-frequency vibration, and they adapt quickly.

Hair root (root hair) plexuses—This type of plexus is a network of dendrites that surrounds hair follicles. Hair root plexuses are stimulated by subtle hair movements such as those caused by light touch or a soft breeze. They respond and adapt quickly.

Ruffini's end organs—These structures are touch and pressure receptors located in the deeper areas of hairy portions of our skin and in our joints. They recognize both heavy and continuous touch and pressure sensations.

Merkel's disks—Merkel's disks are a type of mechanoreceptor and can be found in hairless portions of the skin. They function in discriminative touch.

Free nerve endings—Structures that detect temperature are known as **thermal receptors** (thermoreceptors). One type detects warmth, and another type senses the lack of warmth, or coolness. The brain compares this information to help identify what we would perceive as hot, warm, cool, or cold. The dorsal side of the hand has many thermal receptors and is ideally suited for identifying temperature. It is commonly used by care givers to check a child for fever. A clinician can use the dorsal side of the hand to assess for warm areas on the body. Free nerve endings also detect itch and tickle sensations.

Nociceptors—Specific free nerve endings that detect painful stimuli. Overstimulation of any of the

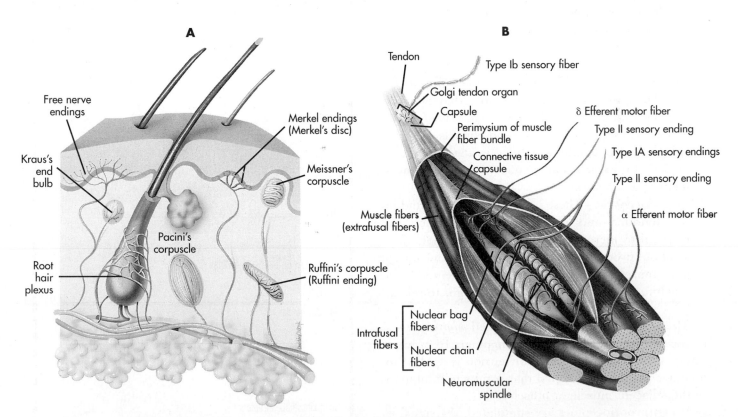

FIGURE 5-9 Somatic sensory receptors. **A,** Exteroceptors. **B,** Proprioceptors. (From Thibodeau GA, Patton KT: *Anatomy and physiology*, ed 3, St Louis, 1996, Mosby.)

thermal receptors can signal pain as a protective response.

Mechanical receptors that provide us with information about position and movement are called *proprioceptors*. Balance is achieved with input from muscle tension, joint position, and the relative movement of each of our parts as well as of the whole body. Because proprioceptors adapt slowly to sensations, they tend to signal the central nervous system (CNS) over longer periods. These signals are received by the motor control centers in the brain, which coordinate normal muscle actions and patterns of movement. Some signals elicit a response when the signal reaches the spinal cord; these are called *reflexes*. Reflexes have a faster response time and allow the body to prevent injury by withdrawing or changing position to compensate for the additional stress. Some of these reflexes persist even when injury or disease affects the spinal cord.

Some mechanical receptors also work as joint proprioceptors. Ruffini's end organs (referred to as type II cutaneous mechanoreceptors), which are located in the joint capsule, monitor joint pressure. Pacinian corpuscles, also found in the joint capsule and surrounding connective tissue, respond to pressure in and to the muscles as well as to pain in the joint itself. They also monitor joint acceleration.

The following are proprioceptors:

Muscles spindles (neuromuscular spindles) — Muscle spindles are located primarily in the belly of the muscle. They are stretch receptors that monitor and respond both to sudden and excessive lengthening. These same fibers send signals via the spinal cord that inhibit actions in the antagonist muscle (the muscle that creates the opposite movement of an action).

Golgi tendon organs — These fibers, which are found in the tendons and musculotendinous junctions, respond to increases in tension. The signals they send out produce a slight stimulation to the antagonist muscle; return responses are prevented from reaching the signaling muscle, causing it to relax.

The ligaments have receptors called *joint kinesthetic receptors* that work in a similar manner. To prevent injury when excessive strain or tension is applied to a joint, they initiate a signal that results in inhibition of the adjacent muscle or muscles.

When proprioceptors are stimulated, the signal is processed and interpreted as a spinal reflex in the somatic reflex arcs (Activity 5-2). A feedback loop works to protect the muscles and joint from injury. If the demand on either could cause injury, the result often is pain, weakness, or muscle relaxation.

PRACTICAL APPLICATION

Soft tissue and movement therapies introduce stimulation through touch, pressure, vibration, and movement, causing sensory receptors to respond. Input from the sensory systems plays a role in controlling motor functions by stimulating spinal reflex mechanisms. Almost all forms of

ACTIVITY 5-2

Depending on the modality being studied, highly successful soft tissue and movement treatments in some way stimulate many if not all of the various sensory receptors. For each receptor given, identify a technique and explain the way it stimulates the receptor. An example is given to get you started.

Example Pacinian (lamellated) corpuscles

Use of a mechanical vibrator to stimulate high-frequency vibrations

Your Turn

Meissner's corpuscles

Hair root plexuses

Ruffini's end organs

Merkel's disks

Thermal receptors

Nociceptors or free nerve endings

Muscle spindles

Golgi tendon organs

Joint kinesthetic receptors

bodywork use some aspect of touch that stimulates the various touch receptors found in the skin. Methods that use light touch stimulate root hair plexuses, free nerve endings, Merkel's disks, Meissner's corpuscles, and Ruffini's end organs. Techniques such as compression; deep, gliding strokes; and joint movement stimulate the pressure receptors such as the pacinian corpuscles. The rapid, repetitive sensory signals of vibration and percussion techniques directly influence the corpuscles of touch and the pacinian corpuscles. Movement affects *all* the proprioceptors.

REFLEX ARC

A *reflex* is a fast, automatic response to a stimulus that helps to maintain homeostasis. A *reflex arc* is the pathway that the nerve impulse follows from the receptor through sensory neurons to the spinal cord (or brain), back through motor neurons to the effector of the action. Association neurons between the sensory and motor neurons help connect the signal pathway for its most efficient routing. The effector is either a muscle that contracts or a gland that secretes. The response is classified as somatic with a skeletal muscle contraction and autonomic (visceral) with a glandular secretion or contraction of a smooth or cardiac muscle.

The *somatic reflexes* most often stimulated by soft tissue and movement therapies are the stretch reflex, tendon reflex, flexor reflex, and crossed extensor reflex. Autonomic reflexes are discussed later.

The simplest form of reflex results from a monosynaptic (one synapse) and ipsilateral (one-sided) reflex arc. It begins with the stimulation of a receptor, which sends out a nerve impulse via an afferent (sensory) neuron. The signal travels to the brain or spinal cord and synapses with an efferent (motor) neuron. The only true monosynaptic reflex is a deep tendon reflex (DTR), which involves just sensory and motor neurons. DTRs are important because they can be used to evaluate the sensory nerve, a portion of the spinal cord, the motor nerve, and the muscle or muscles supplied by the nerve. To evaluate the reflex, a physician or trained medical professional uses a device to tap the tendon, which stimulates the receptor in the tendon. The impulse travels along the sensory nerve to the spinal cord, where it synapses with motor neurons and continues along the motor axon, signaling the muscle to contract. A defect at any point in this arc interferes with the reflex contraction of the muscle.

The following are important deep tendon reflexes:

The *biceps* and *triceps reflexes* help in the evaluation of spinal cord levels C5 and C6, the brachial plexus, and the biceps and triceps muscles.

The *patellar reflex* (the knee-jerk reflex) helps in the evaluation of spinal cord level L4, the lumbar plexus, the femoral nerve, and the quadriceps muscle.

The *Achilles reflex* (the ankle-jerk reflex) helps in the evaluation of spinal cord level S1, the sacral plexus, and the gastrocnemius and soleus muscles. The result of such an evaluation would be abnormal, for example, if the stimulus (tendon tapping) were accompanied by low back pain that radiated to the leg and foot; this could indicate a slipped disk at the level of L5-S1.

✋ PRACTICAL APPLICATION

Reflex patterns can be used during bodywork to make muscles contract. This could be done to stimulate a weakened muscle or assist lengthening and stretching by stimulating a muscle to contract, which would inhibit any action in its antagonist and thus allow the muscle to relax.

Stretch Reflex

The *stretch reflex* is a protective contraction that results when a muscle is suddenly or intensely stretched. Not to be confused with the action of slow stretching or lengthening, it is a homeostatic mechanism that prevents muscle trauma in response to a stretch. The muscle spindles initiate a nerve impulse that travels to the posterior root of the spinal nerve and into the spinal cord. A nerve impulse is then conducted back to the same muscle. When the impulse reaches the muscle, the action potential is generated, which causes the muscle to contract. This contraction prevents the muscle spindle from initiating any more nerve impulses. The stretch reflex itself is *monosynaptic* (one synapse); however, the response becomes a *polysynaptic* (many synapses) reflex arc as association neurons in the spinal cord relay the impulses to motor neurons for synergistic muscles, causing them to contract. Other association neurons interrupt the signal to the antagonist muscles or muscle, allowing it to relax.

Reciprocal innervation is the "wiring" of our circuitry that prevents injury and allows for coordinated actions by allowing the signal for contraction of one muscle to continue while interrupting the signal to its opposing muscle. Reciprocal inhibition is the "action" or "lack of action" that results from this process. During a bodywork session, reciprocal inhibition often is used as preparation for stretching, to avoid stimulating the stretch reflex and thus prevent muscle spasm. Because muscles operate in groups, this stretch reflex coordinates the various contractions and relaxation as well as the stabilization and balance we need to move effectively, if not always gracefully.

PRACTICAL APPLICATION

Bodywork methods can make use of the stretch reflex to normalize weakened muscle patterns by stretching the muscles just to the point of initiating the reflex. The response would be for the muscle to begin contracting. The result is restoration of a more normal strength pattern in the muscle. An awareness of this reflex response is important in all methods intended to lengthen and relax the muscles to their more normal resting length. In these instances, the stretch reflex must be avoided. As a caution, it is not uncommon for stretch reflexes to become hyperactive, resulting in increased muscle tension. This may occur in the leg muscles after a fall when the muscles were quickly and extensively stretched. The stretch reflex may become more sensitive. In muscles in which this has happened, cramping may be more common.

Tendon Reflex

Also known as the inverse stretch reflex, the tendon reflex is a feedback mechanism that controls muscle tension by allowing for muscle relaxation. Golgi tendon organs detect and respond to changes in muscle tension. As the tension increases, often because of an increase in a muscle contraction, these sensors initiate a signal that follows the sensory neuron to the spinal cord. Association neurons inhibit any signal from returning to the same muscle while other neurons continue allowing a signal to reach the antagonist via motor neurons. This causes a slight contraction in the antagonist, which allows the prime mover to relax since no impulse is available to generate the action potential.

NOTE: In some medical texts, the term *tendon reflex* is used to describe a reflex action initiated by tapping a tendon rather than by stretching the muscle belly (which may be called a *muscle reflex* even if the result

is the same for both). The student needs to be aware that such references describe the stimulus and not the resulting reflex action.

PRACTICAL APPLICATION

The most common bodywork technique used to stimulate the tendon reflex is postisometric relaxation. A muscle is contracted against a resisting force, which increases the tension in the tendon. If the load or stimulation is sufficiently strong, initiating the tendon reflex results in relaxation of the muscle. During the relaxation phase, the muscle can be lengthened, stretched, or both more easily. This technique increases tension at the tendon by introducing contraction in the muscle, usually the result of active participation.

The stretch reflex and tendon reflex are simple examples of the way our bodies are programmed to maintain homeostasis. In our normal actions, these reflexes usually are activated for full-body responses instead of isolated muscle groups. The *flexor (withdrawal) reflex* and the *crossed-extensor reflex* are polysynaptic reflex arcs that work with larger areas and the whole body.

The flexor reflex begins with stimulation of the sensory receptor, often by something painful such as stepping on a pin or contact with a noxious stimulus such as a hot flame. The signal travels to the spinal cord, crosses association neurons (as in the tendon reflex), and returns to the muscles involved. This muscle contracts in order to withdraw; simultaneously, the signals have been sent to other muscles on the same limb to do likewise. For example, if you step on a pin with your left foot, your left anterior tibialis muscle, quadriceps (rectus femoris), and psoas contract. The antagonist muscles, including the gastrocnemius, soleus, hamstrings, and gluteus maximus, are inhibited from acting (remember the way in which the association neurons can block signals), thus allowing the entire leg to remove itself from the stimuli.

The crossed-extensor reflex works in coordination with the flexor reflex. When the initial signal reaches the spinal cord, not only does it travel to the flexor muscles on the same side of the body to allow the limb to withdraw, it also crosses the spinal cord and travels to the extensor muscles to maintain balance. This action starts contraction of the right gastrocnemius, soleus, hamstrings, and gluteus maximus, while inhibiting the action of the right anterior tibialis, quadriceps, and psoas. The muscles of the torso and arms also can be stimulated or inhibited through this reflex for complete balance if needed.

This reflex action explains why a tension pattern in one part of our body can be seen in other areas. The extensive pathways that the signals follow are called *contralateral reflex arcs*. The initial stimulus given in the example above was pain, but the body can respond in a similar fashion to other stimuli. If you are standing and begin to walk by lifting your right foot off the floor, the signal of loss of balance begins this process, allowing the right leg and left arm to swing forward (flexing), and the left leg and right arm to keep the body steady (extending). This reflex interaction is known as gait. The withdrawal reflexes are very powerful, taking precedence over all other concurrent reflex actions.

PRACTICAL APPLICATION

Most benefits derived from movement therapies result from a resetting of tension patterns caused by reflex actions, especially those that begin as a result of a fall or trauma, repetitive movement, or maintenance of a fixed position. The practitioner who understands the interactive patterns can use corrective bodywork procedures to resolve or support these actions. Because of the crossed-extensor reflex, the limbs on one side of the body can be deliberately stimulated to affect the limbs on the opposite side of the body. For example, if the goal is relaxation of the flexors of a lower limb, stimulating the extensors of the upper limb on the opposite side produces reciprocal innervation in the thigh flexors, resulting in this relaxation response.

Many of these types of patterns can be puzzled out by thinking in terms of reflex patterns. By effective application of these reflex arcs, a therapist can affect any neuromuscular area of the somatic system without even touching that area; this is very beneficial for very sensitive areas that are in pain or areas that are difficult to reach, such as the deep muscles of the axilla or groin (Activity 5-3). Reflex patterns are also responsible for many compensatory body patterns found in relation to posture. Imagine that a person suddenly stumbles when walking. The crossed-extensor reflexes, via contralateral reflex arcs, respond to restore balance. The body's attempt to stay upright by avoid-ing the fall may result in a chain reaction of muscle tension and relaxation adjustments throughout the body, which can develop into postural distortion over time if the situation continues. The body may readjust muscle tension patterns, and neuromuscular feedback loops may become confused. The resulting skeletal muscle pathologic conditions can lead to discomfort and postural distortion from uneven muscle contraction and relaxation patterns. Touch and movement therapies often can reset these unproductive reflex patterns. Resetting of reflex communication patterns may result in a return of more efficient and coordinated movement patterns.

The effects produced by soft tissue and movement therapies depend heavily on the reflex mechanism. The effectiveness of the particular techniques depends on how efficiently the receptors for these reflexes are stimulated. The receptor being targeted must be reached with the appropriate technique and level of intensity so that the reflex stimulated is allowed to function in the appropriate manner. Fast- and slow-acting receptors, light- and deep-touch receptors, and so on are stimulated by different durations and levels of intensity of touch and movement. The practitioner must understand what type of message is to be sent to the CNS to be processed. Treatment methods will not produce the desired benefit if the wrong signal is sent.

Touch and movement are considered stimuli because they constitute a change in the environment. When the body is called on to restore homeostasis, problematic nerve transmission pathways often can be overridden and a more effective pattern established. The student will find it worthwhile to learn the body's receptor language and explore the reflex patterns initiated by the various forms of stimuli to override these nonproductive transmissions. The more this information is incorporated into practical applications, the more effective the therapeutic intervention will be.

THE AUTONOMIC NERVOUS SYSTEM

We have been discussing the somatic division of the peripheral nervous system and its feedback loops that provide for voluntary and reflexive control of our skeletal muscles. The actions of the smooth muscles and glands are under the control of the autonomic nervous system (ANS), another division of the peripheral nervous system (PNS). As in the somatic PNS, information from sensory receptors is sent to the brain, which in turn relays the most effective effector response to maintain homeostasis. The sensors are located in areas such as the smooth muscles, blood vessels, lungs, and glands. Motor neurons carry the signals to these same organs to prompt an increase or decrease in the rate of our heartbeat, breathing, or digestive processes or to initiate glandular secretion. The system is called involuntary because its actions normally are outside conscious control.

The ANS is divided into the sympathetic and parasympathetic divisions. In general, the **sympathetic nervous system** tends to stimulate and functions primarily when the body is under stress. The **parasympathetic nervous system**, which usually diminishes or inhibits actions, tends to work most often under normal body conditions or when energy conservation is needed.

Our skeletal muscles are innervated by neurons that either carry a signal to contract or carry no signal at all, which causes the muscles to relax. The ANS has a different form of control. Most of the

ACTIVITY 5-3

Try to determine three upper and lower body interactions based on the withdrawal and contralateral reflex arc. An example is provided to get you started. Pay attention to the patterns and movements, not the specific names and functions of muscles.

Example Lower body situation: Tight calf on the left

Possible interactions:
Weak dorsiflexors on the left; tight dorsiflexors on the right
Weak calf on the right
Weak hip flexors on the left; tight hip flexors on the right
Tight hip extensors on the left; weak hip extensors on the right
Weak arm flexors on the left; tight arm flexors on the right
Tight arm extensors on the left; weak arm extensors on the right
Weak neck extensors; tight neck flexors
Weak abdominals
Tight back extensors

Your Turn

1. _____
_____
_____
_____
_____
_____
_____
_____
_____

2. _____
_____
_____
_____
_____
_____
_____
_____
_____
_____
_____

3. _____
_____
_____
_____
_____
_____
_____
_____
_____

organs contain neurons from both the sympathetic and parasympathetic divisions; this is called *dual innervation.* By constantly receiving signals from both divisions, the body can maintain or quickly restore homeostasis because the organs can be stimulated or inhibited rapidly. This form of autonomic antagonism is another example of the duality of wholeness discussed earlier in this text. If sympathetic impulses tend to stimulate an effector, parasympathetic impulses tend to inhibit it. These types of antagonistic activity give precise control, just like having an accelerator and a brake on a car.

For example, moment-to-moment regulation of blood pressure involves continuously changing sympathetic and parasympathetic signals to the heart. The regulation comes from centers in the brainstem that "turn up" or "turn down" each type of input to keep blood pressure constant as the body changes position or activity.

Another major difference is that in the ANS, two neurons are relayed from the brainstem or spinal cord to the organ, gland, or smooth muscle innervated. The first neuron synapses with the second, and the second synapses with the receptor. In the sympathetic nervous system, the synapse, or ganglion, is located near the spinal cord. In the parasympathetic system, the ganglion is near or at the receptor organ, gland, or muscle. The neurotransmitter released at the ganglionic synapse near the spinal cord is acetylcholine (ACh), just as in the **somatic nervous system**. At the postganglionic synapse to the organs, different neurotransmitters are involved. In the sympathetic postganglionic synapse, norepinephrine is released, except in the adrenal medulla, where epinephrine and only some norepinephrine is released. The benefit of epinephrine in the blood is that it reinforces and prolongs the effect of norepinephrine. ACh is found in the parasympathetic postganglionic synapse (Figure 5-10).

SYMPATHETIC STRUCTURE AND FUNCTION

The sympathetic nervous system begins in the spinal cord, where the neurons exit between the levels of T1 to L2. Because of this location, it often is referred to as the thoracolumbar division. The sympathetic ganglia found near the spinal cord are connected by collateral tissues and form a chain. This interconnected chain allows for many different sources of input of sympathetic activity to each of the effectors, thus producing more sympathetic activity with very little input. The preganglionic neurons are short and end in this chain; the postganglionic neurons are much longer and end at the effector organs.

The major function of the sympathetic nervous system primarily involves the emergency response. The signals sent out allow the body to be more prepared for an increase in the intensity of activities that require increased metabolism, higher blood sugar levels, a stronger heartbeat, and dilated bronchi, allowing for more oxygen to the lungs and faster exhalation of carbon dioxide. During this function, the blood is rerouted from the digestive system to the muscles so that they can respond to the increased stress.

Whether the stimulus is physical or psychologic or whether the threat is real or imagined, all our responses are set into action immediately. Dr. Walter B. Cannon described this group of sympathetic responses as the "fight-or-flight" reaction. These responses are normal and healthy in times of stress. However, chronic exposure to stress or perceived threats to our well-being can affect our health adversely. They can lead to dysfunction of sympathetic effectors and perhaps even to the dysfunction of the ANS itself. Excessive sympathetic output causes most of the stress-related diseases physicians encounter. Problems with headaches, gastrointestinal difficulties, high blood pressure, anxiety, muscle tension and aches, and sexual dysfunction all can be related to excessive sympathetic stimulation.

We think of the aforementioned functions as life preserving because they can be used to remove us from dangerous situations and keep us active in self-preservation. But the sympathetic system also is active during many of our normal functions. Dual innervation allows the sympathetic system to oppose the effects of the parasympathetic system, providing balance and maintaining homeostasis. Also of importance is the fact that smooth muscles in the walls of the blood vessels are innervated only by sympathetic fibers, which maintain the tone of the muscles of the arteries, resulting in proper blood pressure whether we are active or at rest. This is another example of general homeostatic balance.

PARASYMPATHETIC STRUCTURE AND FUNCTION

The parasympathetic nervous system is referred to as the *craniosacral division* because of the location of its

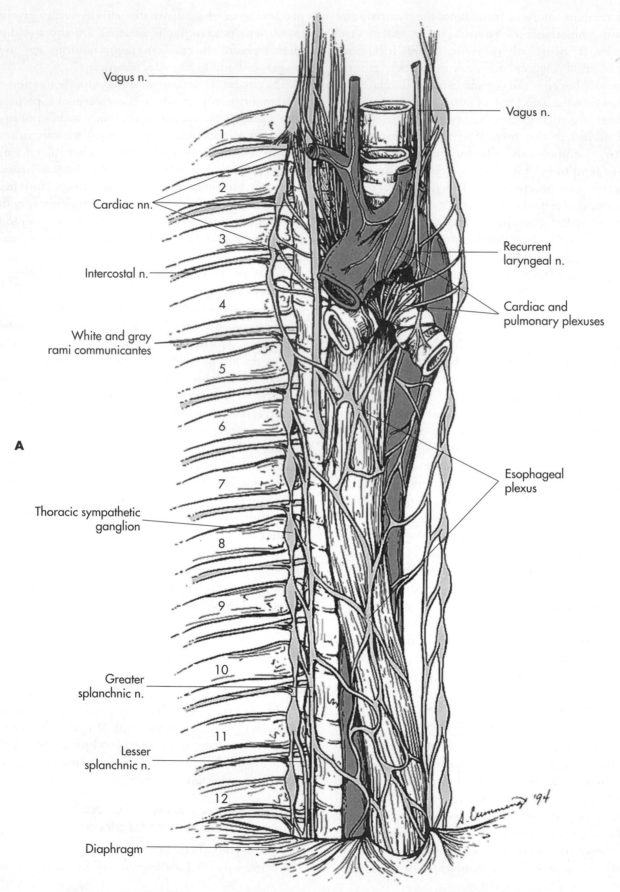

FIGURE 5-10 Sympathetic trunk. **A,** Above the diaphragm. **B,** Below the diaphragm. (From Cramer GD, Darby SA: *Basic and clinical anatomy of the spine, spinal cord, and ANS,* St Louis, 1995, Mosby.)

nerves. Parasympathetic fibers leave the CNS through cranial nerves, including the oculomotor, facial, glossopharyngeal, and vagus nerves, as well as at the sacrum and some pelvic nerves. The three long preganglionic neurons that innervate the pupil and the salivary and lacrimal glands end outside the actual organs. The rest of the preganglionic neurons end at the walls of the organ, with the short postganglionic fibers entering the organ. This is the opposite of the sympathetic division, in which the neurons end just before the organ.

The parasympathetic system generally functions as

the energy conservation system, which allows our body to rest and restore itself after emergency responses. The result is a relaxation response. To maintain balance with the sympathetic division, the parasympathetic system is dominant under nonstressful conditions; this means that during nonstressful times, more impulses to the effectors are received by parasympathetic fibers than by sympathetic fibers.

The parasympathetic system is active in regulating digestion and digestive processes, slowing the heart rate, and constricting eye muscles to focus on near vision. In addition, it increases glandular secretions,

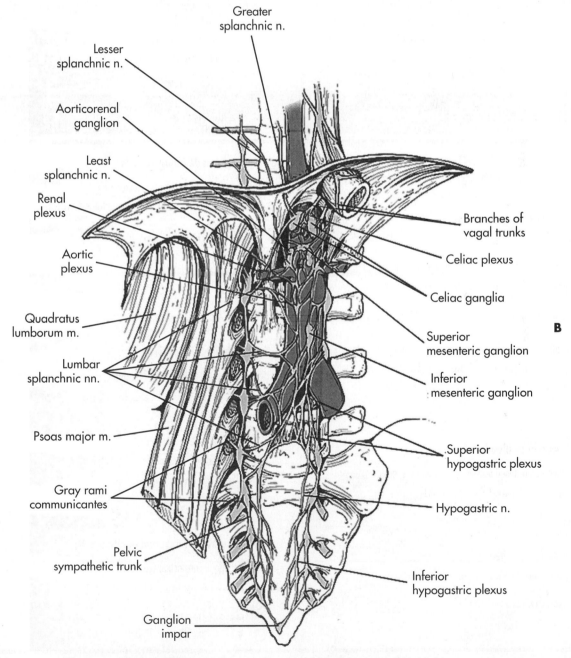

FIGURE 5-10—cont'd   For legend, see opposite page.

constricts the bronchioles in the lungs, and slows breathing. Parasympathetic stimulation of the nerves to the internal and external genitalia in both males and females causes vasodilatation in the clitoris and labia minora and erection in the penis.

Reactions to parasympathetic stimulation are highly localized and tend to counteract the adrenergic effects of the sympathetic system (Activity 5-4). Learning one system usually is simpler, because the other is the opposite. Memorizing the fight-or-flight response seems to be the more practical way. These responses make fighting or fleeing possible; for example, pupillary dilatation to improve vision, faster heart rate for increased cardiac output, bronchodilatation to improve breathing, and slowing of digestive responses to reduce interference with fight or flight (Figure 5-11).

ADRENERGIC STIMULATION

The term *adrenergic* is used to describe stimulation of the sympathetic nervous system that causes release of epinephrine and similar neurotransmitters and hormones. Stimulation of the sympathetic nervous system can either excite or inhibit the smooth muscles, depending on the receptors in the organ involved. Receptors are divided into two major groups: (α-receptors, which respond to norepinephrine and certain blocking substances, and (β-receptors, which respond to epinephrine and similar blocking substances. Each of these groups can be divided again, into α_1 and α_2, and β_1 and β_2, which better classifies the generalized responses they produce.

When α-receptors are stimulated, they cause dilatation of the pupils and constriction of the smooth mus-

ACTIVITY 5-4

After reviewing the effects of both sympathetic and parasympathetic stimulation, identify a sensation, body function, daily activity, or behavior influenced by the ANS. An example is given to get you started.

Cardiovascular System

Cardiac muscle

Sympathetic—Increased rate and strength of contraction (β-receptors)

Example Feeling that the heart is pounding

Your Turn

Parasympathetic—Decreased rate of strength of contraction

Example Possible lower blood pressure; may feel washed out or fatigued

Your Turn

Smooth muscle of blood vessels

Sympathetic—Skin, blood vessels: constriction (α-receptors)

Example Hands and feet get cold

Your Turn

Parasympathetic—No effect

Example Hands and feet get warmer

Your Turn

Skeletal muscle blood vessels

Sympathetic—Dilatation (β-receptors)

Example Feels as if the body wants to move and is restless

Your Turn

Parasympathetic—No effect

Example Increased ability to sit still

Your Turn

Abdominal blood vessels

Sympathetic—Constriction (α-receptors)

Example Stomach seems in a knot

Your Turn

Parasympathetic—No effect

Example Stomach seems relaxed

Your Turn

Blood vessels of external genitals

Sympathetic—Constriction (α-receptors)

Example May not feel sexual

Your Turn

ACTIVITY 5-4—cont'd

Parasympathetic—Dilatation of blood vessels, causing erectile tissues to engorge

Example May have sexual thoughts

Your Turn

Smooth Muscle of Hollow Organs and Sphincters

Bronchioles

Sympathetic—Dilatation (β-receptors)

Example May feel like can't get enough air

Your Turn

Parasympathetic—Constriction

Example Breathing may get slower

Your Turn

Digestive tract, except sphincters

Sympathetic—Decreased peristalsis (β-receptors)

Example May be constipated

Your Turn

Parasympathetic—Increased peristalsis

Example May digest food better

Your Turn

Digestive tract sphincters

Sympathetic—Constriction (β-receptors)

Example May be constipated

Your Turn

Parasympathetic-Relaxation

Example May have more frequent bowel movements

Your Turn

Urinary bladder

Sympathetic—Relaxation (β-receptors)

Example Can go long periods without urinating

Your Turn

Parasympathetic—Contraction

Example May need to urinate after period of relaxation

Your Turn

Urinary sphincters

Sympathetic—Constriction (α-receptors)

Example May have difficulty urinating

Your Turn

Parasympathetic—Relaxation

Example May leak urine when coughing

Your Turn

Eye

Iris

Sympathetic—Contraction of radial muscle; dilated pupil

Example May need sunglasses even in moderate lighting

Your Turn

Parasympathetic—Contraction of circular muscle; constricted pupil

Example Frequently finds lighting too dim

Your Turn

Ciliary

Sympathetic—Relaxation; accommodates for far vision

Example May find newspaper harder to read

Your Turn

Parasympathetic—Contraction; accommodates for near vision

Example May not be able to read road signs

Your Turn

Glands

Sweat

Sympathetic—Increased sweat (neurotransmitter, acetylcholine)

Example Sweaty palms when nervous

Your Turn

Continued

ACTIVITY 5-4—cont'd

Parasympathetic—No effect

Example Dry palms when relaxed

Your Turn

Lacrimal

Sympathetic—No effect

Example Has difficulty crying when anxious

Your Turn

Parasympathetic—Increased secretion of tears

Example May cry more easily at a heart-warming movie

Your Turn

Digestive (e.g., salivary, gastric)

Sympathetic—Decreased secretion of saliva and gastric secretions

Example Finds food harder to swallow when anxious

Your Turn

Parasympathetic—Increased secretion of saliva

Example May drool when relaxed

Your Turn

Pancreas (including islets)

Sympathetic—Decreased secretion

Example May have indigestion

Your Turn

Parasympathetic—Increased secretion of pancreatic juice and insulin

Example May be prone to hypoglycemia

Your Turn

Liver

Sympathetic—Increased glycogenolysis or conversion of glycogen to glucose (β-receptors); increased blood sugar level

Example May feel a sugar high when excited

Your Turn

Parasympathetic—No effect

Example Mood stays more even

Your Turn

Adrenal medulla

Sympathetic—Increased epinephrine secretion

Example May have exaggerated response to conflict

Your Turn

Parasympathetic—No effect

Example Stays calm in confused environment

Your Turn

Hairs (Pilomotor Muscles)

Sympathetic—Contraction produces goose pimples, or piloerection (α-receptors)

Example May become more aware of the movement of people because of increased sensitivity to air movement

Your Turn

Parasympathetic—No effect

Example Less aware of people entering a room

Your Turn

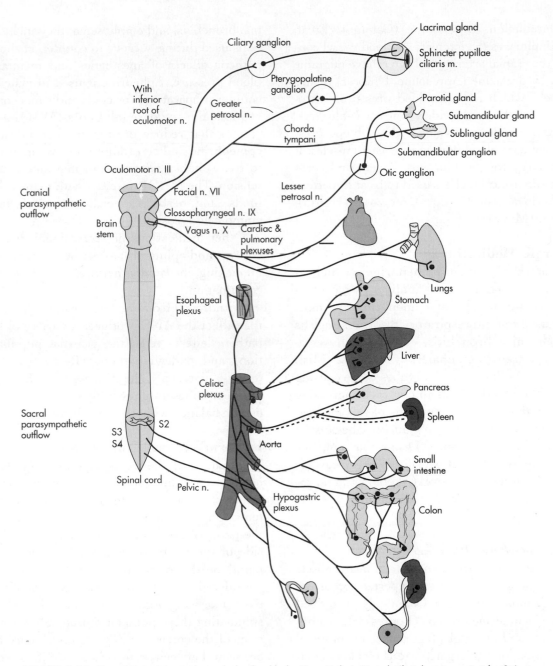

FIGURE 5-11 Parasympathetic innervation to the head and body. (From Mathers LH et al: *Clinical anatomy principles,* St Louis, 1996, Mosby.)

cles and blood vessels. Stimulation of β_1-receptors, which are found mainly in the heart, results in an increase in the force and rate of heart muscle contraction; β_2-receptors, located in the lungs, cause relaxation of the bronchial muscles, resulting in bronchodilatation.

MEDICATIONS THAT AFFECT THE AUTONOMIC NERVOUS SYSTEM

Certain groups of medications bind to or join with α- and β-receptors, thereby enhancing or blocking the receptor sites for the binding of norepinephrine, acetylcholine, or other neurotransmitters and hormones. The effects determine the medication used to modify ANS function. The major problem with many of these medications is the side effects, which range from tachycardia to constipation.

α-Adrenergic Blockers (α-Blockers)

α-adrenergic blockers bind to receptors and thus prevent norepinephrine from binding, causing a decrease in blood vessel tone; this lowers blood pressure and increases circulation. Ergotamine (Cafergot, Ercaf, Wigrane) diminishes the intensity of blood vessel contraction in the cranial arteries and can relieve migraine headaches. Hydralazine (Apresoline, Unipres) dilates blood vessels, which reduces blood pressure. Nitroglycerin, one of the most widely known α-blockers, rapidly dilates arteries and veins, reduces blood pressure, and increases blood flow to the heart muscles. It is used primarily for patients with angina and coronary artery disease α-blockers used to treat hypertension include doxazosin (Cardura), terazosin (Hytrin), and prazosin (Minipress).

β-Adrenergic Medications

Medications that include epinephrine (which is either a β_1 or a β_2 agonist) or that affect β_2-receptors by enhancing the uptake of epinephrine are most commonly used to treat respiratory disorders such as asthma, chronic bronchitis, and emphysema. Epinephrine-adrenaline inhalers (Bronkaid Mist, Primatene Mist) dilate bronchial tubes while causing the walls of the blood vessels to contract, increasing blood flow to the lungs. Other forms of this medication are used as eye drops for glaucoma because it reduces internal eye pressure. Drugs that enhance epinephrine uptake without causing as many cardiac side effects include pirbuterol (Maxair), metaproterenol (Alupent, Metaprel), and albuterol (Proventil, Ventolin).

β-adrenergic blockers (B-blockers)

β-blockers diminish the force and rate of heart muscle contractions and are used to treat hypertension, irregular heart rhythms, and angina. Commonly prescribed medications include metoprolol (Lopressor), penbutolol (Levatol) and atenolol (Tenormin). Propranolol (Inderal) and nadolol (Corgard) are β-blockers commonly used to treat hypertension and migraines.

Parasympathetic Blockers

Many of the alkaloid medications are anticholinergic and block the uptake of acetylcholine. Because of its bronchodilatory effect, atropine (Atrovent) is used to treat chronic bronchitis and emphysema, as well as some forms of asthma.

Sympathomimetic Medications

Chemical substances that mimic the effect of or increase the uptake of norepinephrine are called sympathomimetic, because they imitate sympathetic stimulation. Besides the bronchodilators used to treat asth-

ma, bronchitis, and emphysema, they include medications used during surgery to counteract the parasympathetic effects of anesthetics and maintain normal blood pressure. Ephedrine is used in many over-the-counter preparations for colds and sinus congestion.

Monamine oxidase inhibitors (MAOIs) are medications that reduce or stop the breakdown of norepinephrine and serotonin; they commonly are used to treat phobias, depression, migraines, and hypertension. The MAOIs interact with many other drugs, foods, and herbs, especially those containing the amino acid tyrosine.

Other medications or recreational drugs such as codeine and opium also affect norepinephrine use by mimicking the sympathetic effect. A side effect is constipation.

Withdrawal from medications or other substances that affect the ANS produces a variety of both sympathetic effects (e.g., tachycardia, pupillary dilatation) and parasympathetic effects (e.g., increased tearing, diarrhea). The distress of withdrawal symptoms continues until the body is able to restore homeostatic balance without the substance.

Eastern/Western Connection

The ganglia of the parasympathetic system tend to occupy the same areas traditionally identified as chakras, or energy centers, by Eastern meridian systems. The sympathetic chain ganglia follow one of the paths of the bladder meridian, located on either side of the vertebral column. Specific acupuncture points on this meridian, called back-shu points, are considered to be the locations where qi of the respective yin or yang organs is assimilated. Techniques for stimulating these points are used to relieve dysfunctions of the corresponding organs. A correlation can be seen between sympathetic ANS function and these important organ points in the Eastern meridian system (Figure 5-12; Table 5-2).

⬛ PRACTICAL APPLICATION

Bodywork modalities seem initially to stimulate sympathetic functions. Homeostatic mechanisms then work to increase restorative parasympathetic functions as needed. Point holding methods such as acupressure, reflexology, or the dry needling of acupuncture release the body's own pain killers and mood-altering chemicals from the entire endorphin class. These chemicals stimulate the parasympathetic responses of relaxation and contentment. Acupressure is a specific pinpoint compression over motor points and other areas of neurovascular concentration. These specific points and areas are the focal meeting of superficial nerves in the sagittal plane, superficial nerves or plexuses, and muscle tendon junctions at the Golgi tendons. These areas, where nerves are close to the surface of the body, correspond with the traditional acupuncture points. Acupressure produces

sympathetic inhibition. Acupuncture probably works by taking advantage of the body's natural inhibitory influences such as endorphins and enkephalin that normally can block pain pathways. For example, researchers have established that sensory pain fibers release the neurotransmitter known as substance P, which increases the transmission of pain impulses. Enkephalin blocks the release of substance P, inhibiting pain trans-

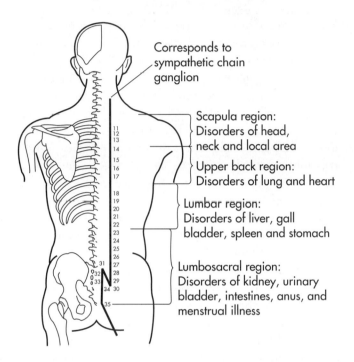

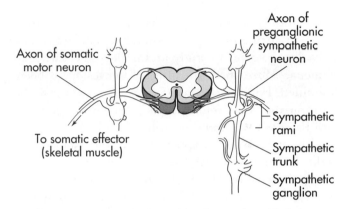

FIGURE 5-12 Comparison of sympathetic chain ganglia and back-shu points. (Modified from Li D: *Acupuncture meridian theory and acupuncture points,* San Francisco, 1990, China Books and Periodicals.)

TABLE 5-2 BACK-SHU POINTS OF INTERNAL ORGANS

ZANGFU ORGANS	BACK-SHU POINTS	LOCATIONS
Lung	Feishu (U.B. 13)	1.5 Cun* lateral to lower border of T3
Pericardium	Jueyinshu (U.B. 14)	1.5 Cun lateral to lower border of T4
Heart	Xinshu (U.B. 15)	1.5 Cun lateral to lower border of T5
Liver	Ganshu (U.B. 18)	1.5 Cun lateral to lower border of T9
Gallbladder	Danshu (U.B. 19)	1.5 Cun lateral to lower border of T10
Spleen	Pishu (U.B. 20)	1.5 Cun lateral to lower border of T11
Stomach	Weishu (U.B. 21)	1.5 Cun lateral to lower border of T12
Sanjiao	Sanjiaoshu (U.B. 22)	1.5 Cun lateral to lower border of L1
Kidney	Shenshu (U.B. 23)	1.5 Cun lateral to lower border of L2
Large intestine	Dachangshu (U.B. 25)	1.5 Cun lateral to lower border of L3
Small intestine	Xiaochangshu (U.B. 27)	1.5 Cun lateral to lower border of L4
Urinary bladder	Pangguangshu (U.B. 28)	1.5 Cun lateral to lower border of L5

Modified from Ding Li: *Acupuncture meridian theory and acupuncture points,* San Francisco, 1990, China Books and Periodicals.
*Cun is a method of measurement that uses a relative standard, usually the length of the second phalange of the second finger.

mission to the brain. The effects of these and other neurotransmitters may validate the use of sensory stimulation methods to treat pain and anxiety.

Research over the past 20 years has identified the crucial role the ANS plays in stress-related disorders. This research also has validated the effectiveness of many ancient healing, cultural, and spiritual practices that serve to bring the ANS under voluntary control, bringing conscious control to homeostatic processes (Activity 5-5).

The Four Basic Senses

With all the possibilities of sensory stimulation, compartmentalizing the types of stimuli and our responses makes it easier to study and understand the phenomena. More than 20 different senses have been identified. For our purposes, we will focus our study here on the basic four special senses we encounter and use daily. In addition to touch, which was covered earlier in this chapter, the primary senses are sight, hearing, taste, and smell. Many of us learned about these senses back in school. Research brings more new information about the way senses work,

the way they are processed in our brains, and the way they interact to enhance our lives.

The processes of sensation involve taking in the constantly received mechanical, chemical, and thermal energy forms with our sensory receptors, modifying or enhancing them, transforming them into electrical signals, and sending that information to the brain to be processed and associated with previous experiences.

HEARING

Sounds are vibrations created by mechanical methods that are turned into recognizable patterns of electrical energy in our nervous system. These vibrations can travel through air, water, or solid substances.

The brain can recognize immense variations in pitch, volume, and tone. When several sounds reach the ear, they are all transferred to the hair cells. The lower-frequency signals are given priority when transmitted as electrical signals to the brain; thus a slow, deep, even voice is the best one to use when we really want to be heard.

Our sense of hearing is well-developed even at birth. Newborns can identify the direction of a voice and turn in response. Only in the past decade has investigation been conducted into the fetus's ability to hear or sense sound carried through the amniotic fluid. Research indicates that the fetus does respond to sound.

Vibrations in the air are taken in by the external ear, called the *auricle, or pinna,* and funneled into the external auditory meatus, which leads to the middle ear (Figure 5-13). Inside the middle ear, the sounds reach the *tympanic membrane,* or eardrum. As the eardrum vibrates in response, it pulls on the *ossicles* to amplify the sounds. These three bones of the middle ear work together. The motion is transferred to the hammer, which hits the anvil, which pulls on the stapes, or stirrup. This bone rests on the *oval window,* a membrane at the beginning of the inner ear. The *eustachian* (auditory) *tube* connects the middle ear with the throat and equalizes pressure between the middle ear and the outside air. Any imbalance in pressure can cause pain and distort or muffle sounds. Activities that open this tube (e.g., yawning, swallowing, or chewing) often can relieve the pressure.

Sound waves leave the middle ear and travel to the inner ear, where the *cochlea,* named for its shape as a spiral shell, is the center of our hearing. The inner ear has three canals. The outer two carry the amplified vibrations. The sound waves travel through a thin membrane to the middle canal, the organ of Corti. In

ACTIVITY 5-5

Identify a control process you use to influence both the sympathetic and parasympathetic divisions of the ANS and explain the way it works. An example is provided to get you started.

Example

Sympathetic—Brisk walking for 30 minutes in the morning: The fast pace activates the sympathetic functions and helps wake me up and give me energy for the day.

Parasympathetic—Eating a bowl of cereal before bed: Signaling digestion also helps make me sleepy.

Your Turn

Sympathetic

Parasympathetic

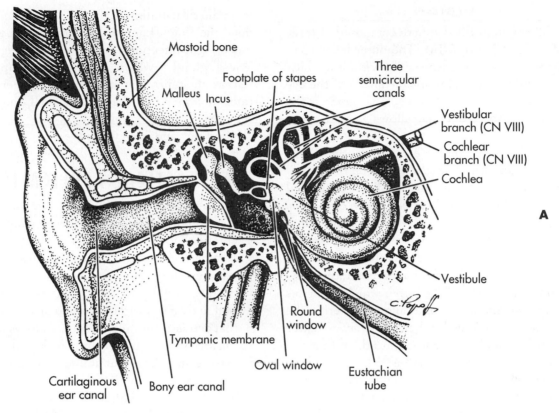

FIGURE 5-13 **A,** External auditory canal, middle ear, and inner ear. (From Barkauskas VH et al: *Health and physical assessment,* ed 2, St Louis, 1998, Mosby.)

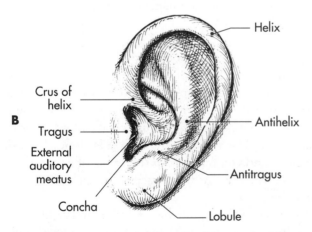

FIGURE 5-13—cont'd **B,** Structures of the external ear (pinna).

this region, fluid-filled circular ducts are positioned at right angles to each other, and each duct contains hair cells embedded in a gelatinous substance. These specialized receptor cells respond to vibrations and motion. As we move, the directional hair cells transfer information about our head position and speed of movement. All this sensory information is trans-

formed into electrical signals, which are carried to the brain by the auditory nerve.

If this proprioceptive mechanism is disrupted, the result often is vertigo, or balance problems. If the disruption goes undetected or untreated, the erroneous sensory information can contribute to anxiety and panic disorders.

PRACTICAL APPLICATION

Any movement activity, especially those that cause head movements that affect the inner ear, shifts the perception of balance in the somatic system, thus altering muscle tension patterns. Many of the benefits of movement therapies are derived indirectly, through the therapies' effect on the inner ear balance system.

Rhythmic rocking is used universally to calm infants, children, and adults because it interacts with balance mechanisms that influence the ANS to initiate parasympathetic functions. The rocking chair can be a lifelong calming companion in our hectic world.

VISION

The eyeball is a fluid-filled sphere composed of three layers of tissue (Figure 5-14). The outer layer comprises the sclera and the cornea. The *sclera* is a white, fibrous structure that maintains the shape of the eye and protects the inner structures. The *cornea* is the clear portion in the front that allows light to enter the eye.

In the middle layer of the eyeball are the ciliary body, choroid, and iris. The *ciliary body*, on the anterior portion, contains smooth muscles that are attached to the lens by ligaments. The *choroid*, which covers the posterior of the sclera, is filled with capillaries that nourish the eye. The cells of the choroid contain melanin and absorb light as it enters the eye. The *iris*, the colored portion of the eye, contains smooth muscles. It controls the size of the pupil, which increases or decreases the amount of light allowed to enter the eye. Vision is produced when light rays enter through the lens and are focused onto the retina.

The inner layer of the eyeball is the *retina*, which contains photoreceptor cells and neurons. The *rods*, which are concentrated on the outer edges of the retina, take in information about the levels of lightness and darkness. They are responsible for recognizing shapes and patterns and providing contrast. *Cones*, which are concentrated at the fovea, or center, of the retina, help us identify color and brightness. We can see colors that range from red to purple. Both rods and cones receive the mechanical signals, transform them into chemical substances, and create an electrical signal that is sent to the brain via the optic nerve. The optic nerve is created from association neurons in the retina. The point where they exit the eye is called the *optic disk*, or blind spot, because it has no photoreceptors.

Vision signals are organized and processed in our cerebral cortex. Information received from the left and right eyes stays separate until it converges in the visual cortex. Signals received when we are not paying attention to any specific item are sent to the posterior parietal cortex for processing. Anything we focus on is sent to the visual cortex. Items that reflect a change in the environment cause a signal to be sent to the frontal lobe. These three areas of the brain (cerebral cortex, visual cortex, and parietal cortex) all work to process and coordinate visual information.

The eyeball is protected by the skull within cavities known as *orbits*. Movement of the eyeball is controlled by six muscles. Eyelids and eyelashes close over the eyes for protection, to block light, and to maintain distribution of fluid. The *lacrimal glands* produce the fluids known as tears that keep our eyes moist, fight infections, and remove foreign particles. These glands, which are located supralaterally, release their product into the eye, where it evaporates or drains into the nasolacrimal duct, alongside the nose. This explains why the nose becomes "stuffed up" and runs when we cry.

▥ PRACTICAL APPLICATION

Both visual orientation and eye movement are very important in posture mechanisms. Visual orientation aids in posture by confirming sensations coming from proprioceptive senses in the body's muscles and joints. The combination of proprioceptive, visual, and inner ear (vestibular) information activates various posture or righting reflexes that activate muscular responses to regain balance. Disturbance of the vestibular, visual, or proprioceptive impulses that initiate these reflexes may cause equilibrium disturbances, nausea, vomiting, muscle tension patterns, and other symptoms. Some forms of movement methods use various eye positions as part of the intervention protocol. The effectiveness of these methods depends partly on the visual orientation aspects of posture.

TASTE

Taste is one of the more complex of our senses. Separating taste from smell is difficult. Specific areas on the tongue correspond to four distinct tastes: sweet, sour, salty, and bitter. Molecules of food bind to receptor sites on the tongue, cheeks, and floor of the mouth. The rest of our tasting is done through our nose and combines with the sense of smell. (You can confirm this by holding your nose and tasting something.)

On average, an adult has more than 10,000 taste buds, but as we age, our taste buds, which usually last about 10 days, are not replaced as frequently. This may explain why older adults are much less sensitive to taste than younger persons. Most of the nerve fibers that carry taste information to the brain can carry information about more than one taste, although they are mainly sensitive to just one and usually are classified as such.

Our individual preferences for certain tastes may be due to cultural differences or genetics. We can be much more or much less sensitive to certain tastes, making them either something we love or something

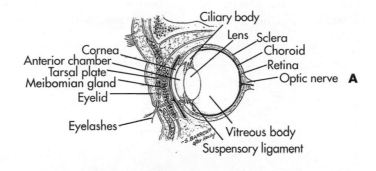

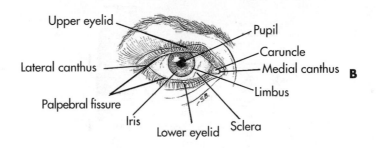

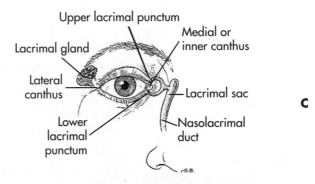

FIGURE 5-14 A, Structures of the eyelid and globe of the eye. B, Anterior view of the eye. C, Lacrimal system. (From Barkauskas VH et al: *Health and physical assessment,* ed 2, St Louis, 1998, Mosby.)

extremely unpleasant. For most of us, bitter tastes are the most easily identified. This may be due to the fact that most of the poisonous substances around us are bitter.

⬛ PRACTICAL APPLICATION

Many ancient healing practices use taste as part of their diagnostic and treatment criteria. During the assessment process, information is gathered on the foods eaten and what types of taste predominates as an indication of the imbalance. The taste of a person's secretions, such as sweat, also is considered; current medical practice considers this criterion a possible indicator of a pathologic condition.

SMELL

The actual activity of olfaction, or smell, involves chemical receptors found in the roof of the nasal cavity (Figure 5-15). As an odor makes contact, chemi-

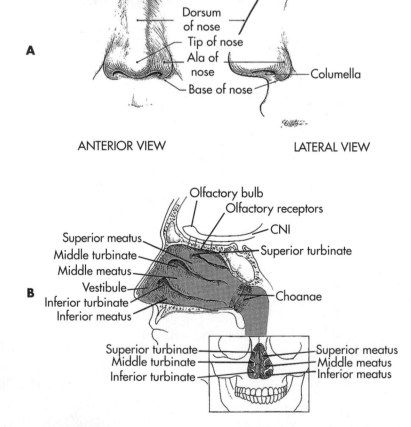

ANTERIOR VIEW   **LATERAL VIEW**

FIGURE 5-15 A, External structure of the nose. **B,** Lateral view of the left nasal cavity. (From Barkauskas VH et al: *Health and physical assessment,* ed 2, St Louis, 1998, Mosby.)

cal signals are transformed into electrical signals and transmitted to the temporal lobes of the brain. The smell centers in the brain are connected with the limbic system and thus have an emotional and a behavioral impact. If the nasal passages are blocked, both the senses of smell and taste are affected.

Unlike with our other senses, smells are hard to imagine. We can picture a scene, remember a soothing voice, and conjure up a taste that makes our mouth water. But most of us have difficulty imagining a smell. Smell also is the hardest sense to describe to another person.

The sense of smell is a very primitive sense that does not translate well to methods of human communication. For our ancestors, it was a main lifesaving sense. Today it still alerts us to dangers. The sense of smell is considered primitive because it deals with our unconscious, animal-like behaviors and experiences, and elicits gut-level emotions. The nerves from the nose end in the olfactory bulb in the limbic area of the brain, the portion of the brain that also controls much of our autonomic, involuntary actions. The more civilized we become, the more we attempt to cover up our body smells and what they mean. Each of us has a unique body odor that changes in response to our emotions. It is true that we can smell fear, danger, anger, and sexual arousal, and we can smell a friend. Past memories, associated with déjà vu, are elicited most with our sense of smell. Much of the information we received from smells helps integrate other information being processed at the same time.

⬛✋ PRACTICAL APPLICATION

Smell therapies, such as aromatherapy, can be used deliberately to influence our physiology and moods. Scents used as the trigger to conditioned learning can be very helpful in establishing a method of reaching a more desirable state of homeostatic balance. Application involves connecting a smell to a particular state of consciousness, be it a relaxed state or a state of focused arousal. While the person is in the conscious state, they also smell a scent of their choosing. If this is done consistently, the two will become connected in the body. Eventually the smell alone will be able to elicit the state of consciousness. This type of conditioned behavior is beneficial in the management of pain and anxiety.

Pathologic Conditions of the Peripheral Nervous System

ENTRAPMENT AND COMPRESSION

Technically, entrapment and compression are different. Entrapment results when soft tissue (e.g., muscles, ligaments) exerts inappropriate pressure on nerves; compression occurs when hard tissue (e.g., bone) exerts inappropriate pressure on nerves. Regardless of what is impinging (pressing) on the nerve, the symptoms are similar; however, the therapeutic intervention is different. Soft tissue approaches are beneficial in entrapment but less so with compression.

Tissues that can bind and impinge on nerves are the skin, fascia, muscles, ligaments, and bones. Spastic muscles and shortened connective tissue (fascia) often impinge on both major and minor nerves, causing discomfort. Because of the body's structural arrangement, these impingements often occur at major nerve plexuses. The specific nerve root, trunk, or division affected determines the condition, producing such disorders as thoracic outlet syndrome, sciatica, and carpal tunnel syndrome.

If the cervical plexus is being impinged on, the person most likely will have headaches, neck pain, and breathing difficulties. The muscles most responsible for pressure on the cervical plexus are the suboccipital and sternocleidomastoid muscles. Shortened connective tissue at the cranial base also will press on these nerves. The cervical plexus is formed by the ventral rami of the upper four cervical nerves. The phrenic nerve is part of this plexus. It innervates the diaphragm. Any disruption to this nerve will affect breathing. Many cutaneous (skin) branches of the cervical plexus transmit sensory impulses from the skin of the neck, ear area, and shoulder. The motor branches innervate muscles of the anterior neck. Impingement causes pain in these areas.

The brachial plexus is situated partly in the neck and partly in the axilla. It consists of virtually all the nerves that innervate the upper limb. Any imbalance that increases pressure on this complex of nerves can result pain in the shoulder, chest, arm, wrist, and hand. The muscles most often responsible for impingement on the brachial plexus are the scalenes, pectoralis minor, and subclavius muscles. The muscles of the arm also occasionally impinge on branches of the brachial plexus. Brachial plexus impingement is responsible for thoracic outlet symptoms, which often are misdiagnosed as carpal tunnel syndrome. Whiplash injury often causes impingement on the brachial plexus.

Carpal tunnel syndrome is caused by compression of the median nerve as it passes under the transverse carpal ligament at the palmar aspect of the wrist. This often is seen in postmenopausal women, but it also is found in conditions in which fluid retention causes swelling of the hand and wrist. The syndrome is common in workers who use their hands in repetitive movements, usually because of inflammation that results in compression on the nerve. The symptoms are palmar pain and numbness in the first three digits. Sometimes surgically opening the transverse carpal ligament can help relieve the pain.

Impingment on the lumbar plexus gives rise to low back discomfort, which is marked by a beltlike distribution of pain and pain in the lower abdomen, genitals, thigh, and medial lower leg. The main muscles that impinge on the lumbar plexus are the quadratus lumborum and the psoas muscles. Shortening of the lumbar dorsal fascia exaggerates a lordosis and can cause vertebral impingement on the lumbar plexus.

The sacral plexus has about a dozen named branches. About half of these serve the buttock and lower limb; the others innervate pelvic structures. The main branch is the sciatic nerve. Impingement on this nerve by the piriformis muscle gives rise to sciatica. Shortened ligaments that stabilize the sacroiliac joint can affect the sacral plexus. Pressure on the sacral plexus can cause pain in the gluteals, leg, genitals, and foot.

INDICATIONS CONTRAINDICATIONS

For Soft Tissue and Movement Therapies

Various forms of soft tissue therapy reduce muscle spasm, lengthen shortened muscles, and soften and stretch connective tissue, restoring a more normal space around the nerve and alleviating impingement. When bodywork is combined with other appropriate methods, surgery is seldom necessary. If it is performed, adhesions must be managed appropriately to prevent reentrapment of the nerve in the future. This is accomplished by maintaining soft tissue suppleness around the healing surgical area and, as healing progresses, extending the soft tissue methods to deal with the forming scar more directly. Before any work is done near the site of a recent incision, the physician's approval must be obtained. In general, work close

to the surgical area can begin after the stitches have been removed and all inflammation is gone. Direct work on a new scar usually is safe 8 to 12 weeks into the healing period.

NERVE ROOT COMPRESSION

Many different conditions can result in compression of the nerve root, including tumors, subluxation of vertebrae, and muscle spasms. Disk degeneration is a common cause. As the degeneration progresses and the fluid content of the disk decreases, the disk becomes narrower. As a result, the amount of space between vertebrae declines. Because spinal nerves exit and enter in the spaces between the vertebrae, this situation increases the likelihood of nerve root compression. This most commonly happens in the areas where the spine moves the most: C6-C7, T12-L1, L3-L4, and L5-S1. The result is radiating nerve pain, often associated with protective and stabilizing muscle spasm or weakness, or both.

DISK HERNIATION

Disk herniation occurs when the fibrocartilage surrounding the intervertebral disk ruptures, releasing the nucleus pulposus, which cushions the vertebrae above and below. The resultant pressure on spinal nerve roots may cause pain and damage the surrounding nerves. This condition most often occurs in the lumbar region and involves the L4 or L5 disk and L5 or S1 nerve roots. This particular back pain radiates from the gluteal area down the lateral side or back of the thigh to the leg or foot. Often caused by back strain or injury, it occasionally is precipitated by coughing or sneezing.

The symptoms of herniation are similar to those produced by a compressed disk but often more severe. In extreme cases, surgical intervention (laminectomy) may be necessary; however, more conservative measures usually are attempted first. Conservative treatment consists of rest, exercise, and other methods, including bodywork to reduce spasm. Traction can be beneficial.

INDICATIONS CONTRAINDICATIONS

For Soft Tissue and Movement Therapies

Various forms of bodywork are important in the management of the muscle spasm and pain associated with the aforementioned conditions. The student must remember that the muscle spasms serve a stabilizing and protective function. Without some protective spasm, the nerve could be further damaged, but too much muscle spasm increases the discomfort. Therapeutic intervention seeks to reduce pain and excessive tension and restore moderate mobility while allowing for the resourceful compensation produced by the muscle tension pattern. Because low back pain is a common disorder, the practitioner must be familiar with its etiology and treatment protocols.

BELL'S PALSY

Bell's palsy causes partial or total paralysis of the facial muscles on one side as the result of inflammation or injury to the seventh cranial nerve. The exact cause of the inflammation is unknown, but current research suggests a reactivation of the herpes simplex virus as one of the probable causes. Mechanical causes include bone spurs, tumors, or temporomandibular joint (TMJ) disorders. Bell's palsy also is found in people affected by diabetes and Lyme disease. The facial nerve swells and is compressed in its narrow course through the temporal bone. The primary method of treatment is administration of oral steroids. The condition usually resolves and normal functioning returns within 6 weeks.

GUILLAIN-BARRÉ SYNDROME

Guillain-Barré syndrome, or infectious polyneuritis, may occur 1 or 2 months after a viral infection. Lymphocytes and macrophages invade the myelin sheath, causing partial demyelination. The person develops tingling in the hands or feet, and motor weakness, and a decrease in DTRs; mild sensory loss ensues. Paralysis usually begins in the legs and moves upward. Facial weakness is common and may appear as Bell's palsy. Sometimes respiratory support must be given. Most people recover in a few weeks.

HERPES

Herpes zoster, or shingles, is a self-limiting viral disease in which groups of vesicles (fluid-filled blisters) appear along a cutaneous nerve distribution, usually on one side of the trunk. Pain occurs before the rash is visible. The varicella-zoster virus, a member of the Herpesvirus family, is the same virus that causes chickenpox. Some researchers believe that after infection, the virus remains in the body in an inactive state in dorsal root ganglia. Primary treatment consists of administration of an analgesic and the antiviral medication acyclovir (Zovirax).

The herpes simplex virus, which is categorized as type I or type II, causes contagious, chronic viral infections that produce painful, fluid-filled blisters on the skin and mucous membranes. Outbreaks of these types seem to be related to stress. Acyclovir can control the symptoms and accelerate healing but does not destroy the virus or cure the infection. Herpes virus lies dormant in the nerve between outbreaks.

INDICATIONS CONTRAINDICATIONS

For Soft Tissue and Movement Therapies

Bodywork approaches for infectious disease can be supportive and can reduce stress. Soft tissue and movement therapies can help control the number of recurrent outbreaks by managing stress, especially in recurring viral conditions. Universal precautions are to be followed with any contagious disease. The patient's total stress load is an important factor. When a person is immunocompromised to the extent that she is susceptible to viral and bacterial disease, the stress load is greater. Keep in mind that many forms of soft tissue and movement treatments are stress producing in a therapeutic sense. The intensity and duration of any therapeutic intervention must be gauged so that the body's demand to adapt does not overtax an already stressed system, aggravating the condition. The "less-is-more" philosophy of intervention, which calls for shorter, more frequent interventions, often is indicated.

DEMYELINATION DISEASE

Multiple sclerosis (MS) is a disease of autoimmune or viral etiology (or both) in which myelin degenerates in random areas of the central nervous system. Hard, plaquelike lesions replace the destroyed myelin, and affected areas are invaded by inflammatory cells. As the myelin around the axons is lost, nerve conduction is impaired, and weakness, diminished coordination, gait difficulties, incontinence, vision problems, and speech disturbances occur. MS is a chronic condition with periodic remissions, because the axon is preserved even though the myelin degenerates. Relapse shows some indication of being stress responsive. MS should not be confused with amyotrophic lateral sclerosis (ALS), which involves degeneration of motor neurons.

INDICATIONS CONTRAINDICATIONS

For Soft Tissue and Movement Therapies

Soft tissue and movement therapies can be an effective part of a comprehensive, long-term care program. Stress management also is an important component of an overall care program for any chronic disease. Massage and other forms of body-work can help manage secondary muscle tension caused by the alteration of posture and the use of equipment such as wheelchairs, braces, and crutches. As previously mentioned, because therapeutic massage produces some stress, the intensity and duration of any therapeutic intervention must be gauged so as not to aggravate the condition.

NEUROTRANSMITTER-BASED DISORDERS

Depression

Depression is one of the more common causes of physical complaints that are a manifestation of underlying psychiatric illness. Many forms of depression respond to medications that increase norepinephrine, dopamine, or serotonin in certain synapses in particular areas of the brain. Imipramine (Tofranil), amitriptyline (Elavil), fluoxetine (Prozac), and phenelzine (Nardil) are examples of these types of drugs. Although primarily considered a CNS disease, dysfunction can be linked to synaptic transmission as the peripheral nervous system delivers information to the CNS.

INDICATIONS CONTRAINDICATIONS

For Soft Tissue and Movement Therapies

Soft tissue and movement therapies have the effect of increasing the availability of the aforementioned neurotransmitters and as such can play an important part in the care program for depression. Aerobic exercise is another important component in depression management. These methods use the peripheral nervous system as the point of access.

Anxiety States

Anxiety states are classified into two basic types. The first type, endogenous anxiety, is a biochemical phenomenon usually unrelated to environmental stimuli. Panic disorder, involving hyperventilation and other breathing difficulties, heart palpitations, chest pain, dizziness, sweating, and feelings of impending doom, is an example of this type. An increase in the activity of the neurotransmitters γ-aminobutyric acid (GABA), epinephrine, and norepinephrine is implicated. Imipramine, MAOIs, and alprazolam have proven moderately effective in treating panic disorder.

Hyperventilation syndrome may be an underlying factor in anxiety, resulting in a change in body chemistry that alters the feedback loop mechanisms.

Restrictions in the soft tissue or the bony structures of the thorax may interfere with appropriate breathing, predisposing a person to hyperventilation. Bodywork can be effective in restoring more balanced function and supporting appropriate breathing. Thus breathing retraining may be an important factor in managing anxiety. Additional information on hyperventilation syndrome is presented in Chapter 12.

The second basic anxiety type is reactive, or exogenous, anxiety, which is prompted by an anxiety-provoking stimulus such as specific events, situations, relationships, or conflicts. Management of this type of anxiety requires dealing with the precipitating difficulties directly or improving mechanisms and skills for coping with environmental or social problems. Making changes in the stressful situation, resolving smoldering conflicts, using relaxation methods, and cognitive restructuring of the client's views of the situation are all helpful. Professional counseling often is beneficial. Other helpful measures include avoiding caffeine, getting regular exercise, eating a healthy diet, and generally gaining control of those things we can control ourselves. Diazepam-type medications such as Valium are useful in short-term management of this type of anxiety.

Both types of anxiety can be thought of as activation of the sympathetic autonomic nervous system. With endogenous anxiety, a faulty internal feedback system results in the panic attack. With exogenous anxiety, the tendency for responding with fight-or-flight behavior is present, but some sort of inhibition of those feelings is in place. What occurs is a fight-or-flight response without the appropriate expression; it therefore internalizes as anxiety.

INDICATIONS CONTRAINDICATIONS

For Soft Tissue and Movement Therapies

Soft tissue and movement therapies often are very effective as part of a comprehensive management strategy dealing with anxiety symptoms.

NEUROPATHY

Neuropathy is the inflammation or degeneration of the peripheral nerves. *Neuralgia* is severe nerve pain caused by a variety of noninflammatory disorders of the nervous system. *Neuritis* is the inflammation of a nerve.

Diabetic neuropathy is caused by the ketoacidosis and hypoglycemic reaction of diabetes as they affect the myelin covering of the neuron. This condition is a painful and severe complication of diabetes for which effective control measures are limited. One such pain-control measure is hyperstimulation analgesia, which interrupts the pain.

Trigeminal neuralgia (tic douloureux) causes sudden, severe pain in the jaw area on one side of the face. Often the pain is caused by chewing or simply by touching the face. The cause is unknown. One hypothesis is that the condition is related to a viral infection of the upper portion of the trigeminal nerve. The analgesic carbamazepine (Tegretol) can be effective in some cases, although surgical intervention sometimes is necessary. Extreme caution should be exercised if any form of therapy is to be performed in this area.

INDICATIONS CONTRAINDICATIONS

For Soft Tissue and Movement Therapies

Nerve pain is difficult to manage. It does not respond well to analgesics and often is intractable. Soft tissue and movement therapies, because of their interface with the nervous system, may provide short-term, symptomatic pain relief through shifts in neurotransmitters and stimulation of alternate nerve pathways, resulting in hyperstimulation analgesia. Any therapy that increases mood-elevating and pain-modulating mechanisms makes coping with nerve pain somewhat easier for short periods.

HEADACHE

Headache is a common symptom with a multitude of causes. Because the brain has no sensory innervation, headaches do not originate in the brain. The pain of a headache is produced by pressure on the sensory nerves, vessels, or meninges or the muscle-tendon-bone unit.

A tension or muscle contraction headache is the most common type. Tension headaches are believed to be caused by a muscle-tendon strain at the origin of the trapezius and deep neck muscles at the occipital bone or at the origin of the frontalis muscle on the frontal bone (occipital or frontal headaches). Tension headache also can originate in the TMJ muscle complex. Connective tissue structures that support the head may be implicated in headache if they are shortened and pull the head into nerves, creating pain. Conversely, if connective tissue support structures are lax and fail to support the neck and head, nerve structures may be compressed as well.

Most headaches are treated with nonsteroidal antiinflammatory drugs (NSAIDs) such as aspirin or ibuprofen.

INDICATIONS CONTRAINDICATIONS

For Soft Tissue and Movement Therapies

Massage and other forms of soft tissue therapy are effective in the treatment of muscle tension headaches. Because headaches often are stress induced, stress management in all forms usually is indicated in chronic headache conditions.

VERTIGO

Vertigo is the sensation that the body or environment is spinning or swaying. It can occur when disturbances occur in the inner ear balance mechanism or between the visual-vestibular balance mechanisms. The most common type of vertigo is called benign paroxysmal positional vertigo, or BPPV. This condition occurs when otolith particles stimulate movement sensations that do not actually exist. Muscle tension, nausea, and mood disturbances, particularly anxiety, can result.

INDICATIONS CONTRAINDICATIONS

For Soft Tissue and Movement Therapies

Movement therapies can either help or aggravate vertigo; therefore care must be taken to design an individual therapeutic program based on the client's history. Bodywork methods can deal effectively with muscle tension and diminish anxiety and nausea, but the benefit is temporary because the symptoms return with a recurrence of vertigo.

Summary

In this chapter, we studied the peripheral nervous system, its components and the names of its many parts. Important information about reflexes and sensory receptors was presented because these portions of the peripheral nervous system function directly with soft tissue and movement therapies.

The role of the autonomic nervous system, the body/mind connection, and the perspectives of Eastern and Western thought were reinforced.

The four basic senses were discussed briefly, and soft tissue and movement therapies were related to specific functions of the peripheral nervous system. A student of soft tissue and movement therapies would do well to learn this particular material thoroughly, because these therapies work so closely with the peripheral nervous system. Such an understanding can only benefit the clients we strive to serve.

WORKBOOK SECTION

1. Define the peripheral nervous system.

_____

_____

2. List the components of the peripheral nervous system.

_____

_____

3. List the cranial nerves and describe the general function of each.

_____

_____

_____

_____

_____

_____

_____

_____

_____

_____

_____

_____

_____

4. List and describe the spinal nerves.

_____

_____

_____

_____

5. Identify the four nerve plexuses.

_____

_____

_____

_____

6. Compare and contrast a dermatome and a myotome.

_____

_____

_____

_____

_____

_____

7. Explain reflex mechanisms and sensory receptor reflex arcs and their relationship to soft tissue and movement therapies.

_____

_____

_____

_____

_____

_____

_____

_____

8. Identify the two divisions of the autonomic nervous system.

_____

9. List and compare the functions of the sympathetic and parasympathetic nervous systems.

_____

_____

_____

_____

_____

_____

_____

_____

_____

_____

10. List the major drugs that affect the ANS.

_____

_____

_____

_____

_____

_____

_____

11. Describe the Eastern/Western connection as it relates to autonomic nervous system functions.

_____

_____

_____

_____

_____

_____

_____

_____

12. Describe the four basic senses discussed in this chapter.

_____

_____

_____

_____

_____

_____

_____

13. List at least 12 of the various pathologic conditions of the peripheral nervous system.

1. _____

2. _____

3. _____

4. _____

5. _____

6. _____

7. _____

8. _____

9. _____

10. _____

11. _____

12. _____

14. Explain the way soft tissue and movement therapies support health in the peripheral nervous system.

_____

_____

_____

_____

FILL IN THE BLANK

The _____ (1) consists of neurons outside the CNS. The _____ (2) (sensory) division consists of nerves that link sensory receptors with the CNS. The efferent, or _____ (3), division consists of nerves that link the CNS to the effectors outside the CNS. The _____ (4) nervous system is made up of nerves that act to keep the body in balance with its external environment by transmitting impulses between the CNS and the skeletal muscles and skin. The _____ (5) nervous system connects the CNS to the glands, heart, and smooth muscles to maintain the _____ (6) body environment. The _____ (7) nervous system functions when the body is under stress, producing fight-or-flight responses. The _____ (8) nervous system functions under normal body conditions and is the energy conservation and restorative system, associated with what commonly is called the _____ (9) response. A nerve is a group of _____ (10) nerve fibers, or axons, wrapped together. Twelve pairs of _____ (11) originate from the olfactory bulbs, thalamus, visual cortex, and brainstem. Thirty-one pairs of _____ (12) originate in the spinal cord and emerge from the vertebral column. _____ (13) nerves make both sensation and movement possible.

A _____ (14) is a network of intertwining nerves that innervates a particular region of the body. The four nerve plexuses are the _____ (15) plexus, the _____ (16) plexus, the _____ (17) plexus, and the _____ (18) plexus.

A _____(19) is a cutaneous (skin) section supplied by a single spinal nerve. A _____(20) is a skeletal muscle or group of muscles that receives motor axons from a given spinal nerve.

_____(21) receptors are sensory receptors that detect changes in pressure, movement, or temperature or other mechanical forces.

_____(22) receptors are sensory receptors that detect changes in temperature. _____(23) are sensory receptors that detect painful stimuli. _____(24) are sensory receptors that provide the body with information about position, movement, muscle tension, joint activity, and equilibrium.

A reflex in the physiologic or functional unit of nerve function is a (an) _____(25) action. The _____(26) reflex results when stretching of a muscle elicits a protective contraction of that same muscle. The tendon reflex operates as a feedback mechanism to control muscle _____(27) by causing muscle relaxation. The flexor (withdrawal) and crossed extensor reflexes are _____(28) reflex arcs. When these reflexes are stimulated, an entire area on one side of the body (_____)(29) or specific areas on both sides of the body (_____)(30) are affected.

The four basic senses discussed are _____(31), _____(32), _____(33), and _____(34).

PROBLEM SOLVING

Read the problem presented. There is no correct answer; rather, the exercise is intended to assist the student in developing the analytic and decision-making skills necessary in a professional practice.

1. Identify the facts presented in the information.
2. Identify the possibilities presented ("what if" statements) or develop your own possibilities.
3. Evaluate each possibility in terms of the logical cause and effect and pros and cons.
4. Consider the feelings of the people involved.
5. Write each down in the space provided.
6. Develop your solution by answering the question posed.

PROBLEM

Most soft tissue and movement therapies are beneficial because of a direct interaction with the peripheral nervous system. The sensory mechanisms of the peripheral nervous system are the communication link with the rest of the body's systems and functions. Research is demonstrating the beneficial effects of these therapies on the somatic nervous system, primarily through reflex arcs and dermatome and myotome patterns, coupled with the interaction with the ANS. Some difficulty may arise because various approaches have emerged within soft tissue and movement therapies based on specific protocols developed by very gifted practitioners and teachers over the course of centuries. At the time the particular approach was developed, science may not yet have been able to identify the underling physiology. Consequently, many forms of soft tissue and moment therapy have developed along individual paths, and they work because of the same physiologic reasons. This does not discount the uniqueness and value of any one particular approach. However, confusion results with many different methods working through the same basic anatomy and physiology with slight variations in style and different terminology bases. Professionals in soft tissue and movement therapies often may not realize that they are talking about the same thing. If we have some difficulty understanding each other, then how much more confusing it is for professionals outside the touch and movement therapy discipline. Explaining treatment methods in terms of anatomy and physiology may help, because this language base is more universally understood. Such an effort could give rise to an agreement and understanding of the overlap of methods, especially in terms of the peripheral nervous system interaction.

QUESTION

How would you explain the benefit of soft tissue and movement therapies in terms of the peripheral nervous system? Examples are provided to get you started. Fill in at least two more statements.

FACTS

1. Touch and movement therapies are not always explained in terms of anatomy and physiology.

2. _____

3. _____

POSSIBILITIES

1. Professionals may not be able to share information effectively.

2. _____

3. _____

LOGICAL CAUSE AND EFFECT

1. Appropriate referral between professionals would not happen from lack of information.

2. _____

3. _____

POSSIBLE IMPACT

1. Professionals may feel frustrated when they discover that they were talking about the same thing all along.

2. _____

3. _____

How would you explain the benefit of touch and movement therapies in terms of the PNS?

_____

_____

_____

_____

_____

_____

_____

FURTHER STUDY

Using a comprehensive anatomy and physiology text (see the Works Consulted list at the back of this book), identify chapters that pertain to the information presented in this chapter. Locate the information presented in this text and then elaborate on it by writing a paragraph of additional information on each of the following topics.

Nerve distribution patterns for the four nerve plexuses

_____

_____

_____

_____

_____

_____

_____

_____

_____

Reflex mechanisms

_____

_____

_____

_____

_____

_____

_____

_____

ANS and the body/mind influence

_____

_____

_____

_____

_____

_____

_____

_____

_____

_____

Taste

_____

_____

_____

_____

_____

_____

_____

_____

_____

Smell

_____

_____

_____

_____

_____

_____

_____

_____

Hearing

_____

_____

_____

_____

_____

_____

_____

Vision

_____

_____

_____

_____

_____

_____

_____

_____

PROFESSIONAL APPLICATION

Groups of people with a common need or interest are sometimes referred to as populations. When considering touch and movement therapies, certain populations need different types of approaches. Working with an athlete on balancing reflex patterns is somewhat different from working with a person who has cerebral palsy who wants a similar outcome. Nerve entrapment in the elderly is common, but this condition also is common in repetitive work environments. Interaction with anxious clients is different from interaction with someone who is depressed, even though therapeutic intervention focuses on the ANS. The approaches will be similar, yet different. Identify a pathologic condition listed in this chapter and develop two hypothetical treatment plans for the condition with two different populations. After you have done this, identify the differences and similarities in theories and the practical applications of the methods.

_____

_____

_____

_____

_____

_____

_____

_____

_____

_____

_____

_____

_____

_____

_____

Answer Key

1. The peripheral nervous system (PNS) is made up of neurons outside the central nervous system (CNS).
2. Nerves are peripheral nerve fibers or axons wrapped together. They include afferent or sensory nerves, efferent or motor nerves, and the somatic and autonomic nervous system.
3. *Cranial nerve I*—The olfactory nerves are sensory and transmit taste and smell information directly to the cerebrum.

   Cranial nerve II—The optic nerves are sensory and transmit visual information (e.g., visual acuity, pupillary reaction, visual fields) to the thalamus.

   Cranial nerve III—The oculomotor nerves are both sensory and motor nerves; they originate in the midbrain and transmit information about eye movement.

   Cranial nerve IV—The trochlear nerves arise in the midbrain and are composed primarily of motor nerves that contain few sensory neurons. These nerves innervate the muscles of the eyeball.

   Cranial nerve V—The trigeminal nerves arise in the pons and contain sensory neurons for the head, face, skin of the face, and corneas; they also contain motor neurons for mastication (chewing).

   Cranial nerve VI—The abducens nerves arise in the pons and contain numerous motor neurons that innervate eye muscles; they also have sensory neurons that provide information about eye movement.

   Cranial nerve VII—The facial nerves arise in the pons and contain sensory neurons for taste and motor neurons for facial expression, tear production, and salivation.

   Cranial nerve VIII—The vestibulocochlear (acoustic or auditory) nerves arise in the pons and are sensory nerves for hearing and equilibrium.

   Cranial nerve IX—The glossopharyngeal nerves arise in the medulla; they contain sensory neurons for taste and motor neurons for saliva production, swallowing, and the gag reflex.

   Cranial nerve X—The vagus nerves arise in the medulla, with some motor axons originating in the pons. They contain sensory neurons for the pharynx, larynx, trachea, heart, carotid body, lungs, bronchi, esophagus, stomach, small intestine, and gallbladder. Motor neurons carry impulses to the pharyngeal and laryngeal muscles, where they control swallowing and thoracic and abdominal viscera;

they also carry impulses to the heart and other body organs, where they control the heart rate and other visceral activities. Most motor fibers of the vagus nerves are autonomic (parasympathetic) fibers.

Cranial nerve XI—The accessory nerves arise in the medulla and contain mainly motor neurons for speaking, turning the head, and moving the shoulders (they supply the larynx, pharynx, trapezius muscles, and sternocleidomastoid muscles).

Cranial nerve XII—The hypoglossal nerves arise in the medulla and contain mostly motor neurons, which innervate the tongue and throat.

4. Thirty-one pairs of mixed spinal nerves originate in the spinal cord and emerge from the vertebral column, making both sensation and movement possible. Each spinal nerve attaches to the spinal cord by means of two short roots. The dorsal root is sensory, and the ventral root is motor.

5. The cervical plexus, brachial plexus, lumbar plexus, and sacral plexus; nerves T2 through T12 do not form a plexus

6. A dermatome is a cutaneous (skin) section supplied by a single spinal nerve. A myotome is a skeletal muscle or group of skeletal muscles that receives motor axons from a particular spinal nerve. The dermatomes and myotomes are distributions of spinal nerves; however, dermatomes relate to skin function, and myotomes relate to muscle function.

7. Input from sensory systems plays a role in the control of motor functions by stimulating spinal reflex mechanisms. Soft tissue and movement therapies introduce touch, pressure, vibration, and positional stimuli, causing sensory neurons to respond. Most benefits derived from movement therapies result from a resetting of reflex patterns that may be disrupted by a fall, trauma, repetitive movement, or fixed position. Because of the crossed-extensor reflex, the limbs on one side of the body can be stimulated deliberately to affect the limbs on the opposite side. Reflex patterns are also responsible for many compensatory body patterns found in relation to posture. Soft tissue and movement therapies depend heavily on the reflex mechanism; the effectiveness of the techniques depends on how efficiently the receptors for these reflexes are stimulated. The receptor being targeted must be reached with the appropriate technique and intensity so that the reflex stimulated can function in the appropriate manner. The practitioner must understand the type of message to be sent to the CNS for processing.

8. Sympathetic and parasympathetic

9. Sympathetic stimulation; neurotransmitter is usually norepinephrine; adrenergic
Parasympathetic stimulation; neurotransmitter is acetylcholine; cholinergic

CARDIOVASCULAR SYSTEM
Cardiac muscle
Sympathetic: Increased rate and strength of contraction (β-receptors)
Parasympathetic: Decreased rate and strength of contraction

Smooth muscle of blood vessels
Sympathetic: Skin blood vessels—constriction (α-receptors)
Parasympathetic: No effect

Skeletal muscle blood vessels
Sympathetic: Dilatation (β-receptors)
Parasympathetic: No effect

Abdominal blood vessels
Sympathetic: Constriction (α-receptors)
Parasympathetic: No effect

Blood vessels of external genitals
Sympathetic: Constriction (α-receptors)
Parasympathetic: Dilatation of blood vessels, causing erectile tissues to engorge

SMOOTH MUSCLE OF HOLLOW ORGANS AND SPHINCTERS
Bronchioles
Sympathetic: Dilatation (β-receptors)
Parasympathetic: Constriction

Digestive tract (except sphincters)
Sympathetic: Decreased peristalsis (β-receptors)
Parasympathetic: Increased peristalsis

Sphincters of digestive tract
Sympathetic: Constriction (α-receptors)
Parasympathetic: Relaxation

Urinary bladder
Sympathetic: Relaxation (β-receptors)
Parasympathetic: Contraction

Urinary sphincters
Sympathetic: Constriction (α-receptors)
Parasympathetic: Relaxation

EYE
Iris
Sympathetic: Contraction of radial muscle; dilated pupil
Parasympathetic: Contraction of circular muscle; constricted pupil

Ciliary
Sympathetic: Relaxation; accommodates for far vision
Parasympathetic: Contraction; accommodates for near vision

GLANDS
Sweat
Sympathetic: Increased sweat (neurotransmitter, acetylcholine)
Parasympathetic: No effect

Lacrimal
Sympathetic: No effect
Parasympathetic: Increased secretion of tears

Digestive (e.g., salivary, gastric)
Sympathetic: Decreased secretion of saliva and gastric secretions
Parasympathetic: Increased secretion of saliva

Pancreas (including islets)
Sympathetic: Decreased secretion
Parasympathetic: Increased secretion of pancreatic juice and insulin

Liver
Sympathetic: Increased glycogenolysis (conversion of glycogen to glucose) (β-receptors); increased blood sugar level
Parasympathetic: No effect

Adrenal medulla
Sympathetic: Increased epinephrine secretion
Parasympathetic: No effect

Hairs (pilomotor muscles)
Sympathetic: Contraction produces goose pimples, or piloerection (α-receptors)
Parasympathetic: No effect

10. Epinephrine is both a β_1- and β_2-agonist; examples are metaproterenol (Metaprel, Alupent), pirbuterol (Maxair), and albuterol (Ventolin). β-blocking agents such as propranolol (Inderal), metoprolol (Lopressor), and nadolol (Corgard) are useful in the treatment of cardiac arrhythmias, angina, and hypertension. Opiates have a sympathetic effect (sympathomimetic action) on the gastrointestinal tract and cause constipation.

11. Autonomic parasympathetic ganglia tend to occupy the same areas traditionally identified as chakras, or energy centers. The sympathetic chain ganglia follow one of the paths of the bladder meridian.

   Point holding, such as acupressure, reflexology, or dry needling of acupuncture, releases the body's own pain killers and mood-altering chemicals from the entire endorphin class. These chemicals stimulate the parasympathetic responses of relaxation and contentment. Acupressure is a specific pinpoint compression over motor points of the body at the focal meeting of superficial nerves in the sagittal plane, superficial nerves or plexuses, and the muscle-tendon junction at the Golgi tendons. These areas where nerves are close to the surface of the body correspond to the traditional acupuncture points. Acupressure produces sympathetic inhibition. Acupuncture probably works by taking advantage of the body's natural inhibitory influences that normally can block pain pathways. Research over the past 20 years has identified the crucial role the ANS plays in stress-related disorders. This research has validated ancient healing, cultural, and spiritual practices that bring the ANS under voluntary control and as such bring conscious control to homeostatic processes.

12. Taste: The four primary taste sensations are sweet, sour, salty, and bitter. Most chemical receptors for the sense of taste are located on the tongue; a few are located in the cheeks and on the floor of the mouth.

   Smell: Also called olfaction, this sense relies on chemical receptors located in the roof of the nasal cavity. Smell centers are interconnected with the limbic system and therefore have emotional and behavior implications.

   Hearing: The ear is a complex of three structures, all of which are necessary to effect the process of hearing.

   Vision: The eyes, the organs of vision, are contained within protective bony cavities of the skull, called orbits. The eye perceives light in the form of colors ranging from violet to red. Six small muscles attached to each eye effect movement.

13. Nerve root compression, disk herniation, Bell's palsy, Guillain-Barré syndrome (infectious polyneuritis), herpes zoster (shingles), herpes type I and II, MS, depression, anxiety, entrapment and compression, neuropathy, trigeminal neuralgia (tic douloureux), headache from muscle tension, and vertigo

14. All bodywork methods are based on the peripheral nervous system. The effects on the ANS are related directly to stress, as are the effects on the somatic nervous system function of posture and movement. By encouraging balance in this system, health is supported.

FILL IN THE BLANK

1. peripheral nervous system
2. afferent
3. motor
4. somatic
5. autonomic
6. internal
7. sympathetic
8. parasympathetic
9. relaxation
10. peripheral
11. cranial nerves
12. spinal nerves
13. Mixed
14. plexus
15. cervical
16. brachial
17. lumbar
18. sacral
19. dermatome
20. myotome
21. Mechanical
22. Thermal
23. Nociceptors
24. Proprioceptors
25. involuntary
26. stretch
27. tension
28. polysynaptic
29. withdrawal reflex
30. crossed-extensor reflex
31. taste
32. smell
33. hearing
34. vision

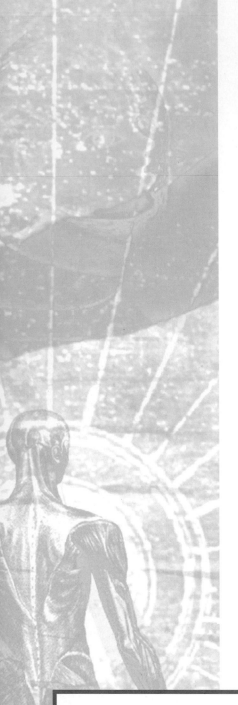

The Endocrine System

CHAPTER OUTLINE

CHAPTER OBJECTIVES

After completing this chapter, the student should be able to perform the following:

- List the traditional endocrine glands.
- Define endocrine tissues and give examples.
- Describe the functions of hormones.
- Explain the difference between hormones and neurotransmitters.
- Describe hypersecretion and hyposecretion pathologic conditions of the endocrine system.

KEY TERMS

Endocrine gland (EN-doe-krin) A ductless gland that secretes hormones directly into the bloodstream.

Endorphins (en-DOR-fin) Peptide hormones that mainly work like morphine to suppress pain. They influence mood, producing a mild euphoric feeling such as is seen in runner's high.

Exocrine gland (EK-so-krin) A gland that secretes its hormones through ducts directly into specific areas. They are part of the endocrine system.

Half-life The amount of time required for half of a hormone to be eliminated from the bloodstream.

Hypersecretion The excessive release of a hormone.

Hyposecretion The insufficient release of a hormone.

Negative feedback system A control mechanism that provides a stimulus to decrease a function, like a fire alarm, that causes a series of reactions that work to reduce the fire.

Tropic (or trophic) hormones Hormones produced by the endocrine glands that affect other endocrine glands.

The endocrine system works in partnership with the nervous system to maintain homeostasis in the body. In this capacity the endocrine system is primarily involved with physiologic function. Functional aspects of hormone molecules include the mobilization of body defenses against stressors; maintenance of electrolyte, water, and nutrient balance of the blood; and regulation of cellular metabolism and energy balance. Not only are hormones of the endocrine system involved with maintaining homeostasis, they also direct the creation of our very form (such as our size, shape, and sexual characteristics). The major form processes controlled and integrated by hormones are reproduction, growth, and development. Therefore hormonal pathology affects function, as does the nervous system, and it can also affect form.

The **endocrine glands** are ductless glands that secrete hormones directly into the bloodstream or diffuse into nearby tissues (Figure 6-1). In contrast, **exocrine glands**, or glands with ducts, such as salivary and sweat glands, secrete their products directly into ducts that open to specific areas.

The endocrine glands of the body include the pituitary, thyroid, parathyroid, adrenal, pineal, and thymus glands. In addition, several organs of the body such as the pancreas, ovaries, and testes contain areas of endocrine tissues that produce hormones as well as exocrine products. The hypothalamus, considered part of the nervous system, also produces and releases hormones. It can thus be considered a neuroendocrine organ.

The endocrine glands have important implications in the Eastern chakra system. The chakra system is a mapping of energy centers with interesting anatomic correlations to the autonomic nervous system plexus and functional aspects interrelated with the endocrine gland functions. Many Eastern healing traditions (e.g., Ayurvedic, Tibetan) work from this knowledge base, just as many Oriental healing philosophies were developed around the meridian system.

The body of knowledge of the chakra system is expansive and not inconsistent with Western scientific thought. Just as the meridian system sees anatomy and physiology as an interrelated system encompassing emotional and spiritual energy conjoined with the major organs, the chakra system represents similar patterns in relationship to the endocrine functions. As various endocrine functions are described, the related chakra pattern will also be presented (Leadbetter, 1927) (Figure 6-2).

New research in endocrinology continues to discover endocrine tissues that are separate from the traditional endocrine glands. It is now known that the heart and intestinal mucous membranes secrete hormones. The concept of tissue hormones or hormone-like substances such as the prostaglandins has altered and expanded the idea of hormones being carried throughout the blood to distant sites in the body. Instead of affecting distant sites in the body by being carried by the blood, prostaglandins have a much more local effect in surrounding tissue.

Endocrine functions are typically regulated by negative feedback systems. Pathologic conditions are mainly found with hyposecretion (not enough) and hypersecretion (too much). This pattern should now seem familiar as the elegance of the body shows itself in repetition of basic patterns.

In the previous chapters, we learned that a chemical found in the synapse is called a *neurotransmitter*. When the same chemical is found in the bloodstream or tissue, it is a hormone. Neurotransmitters act on adjacent cells, whereas hormones may travel long distances in the body before they reach their target cells. The main differences between the endocrine

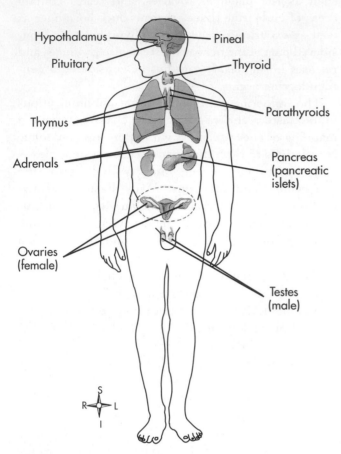

FIGURE 6-1 Locations of the major endocrine glands. (From Thibodeau GA, Patton KT: *Anatomy and physiology,* ed 3, St Louis, 1996, Mosby.)

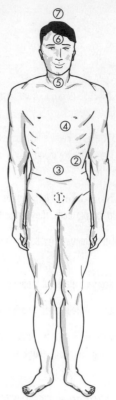

	English Name	Sanskrit Name	Situation
1	Root of basic chakra	Mūlādhāra	At the base of the spine
2	Spleen or splenic	*	Over the spleen
3	Naval or umbilical chakra	Manipūra	At the naval, over the solar plexus
4	Heart or cardiac chakra	Anāhata	Over the heart
5	Throat or laryngeal chakra	Vishudda	At the front of the throat
6	Brow or frontal chakra	Ājnā	In the space between the eyebrows
7	Crown or coronal chakra	Sahasrāra	On the top of the head

FIGURE 6-2 Name and location of major chakras. (Modified from Leadbeater CW: *The chakras,* Wheaton, Ill., 1927, Quest Books.)

ACTIVITY 6-1

List three situations in which you believe that nervous system control is most effective and explain why. An example is given.

Example While we are driving, a car stops suddenly in front of us. Normal reflexes activate our muscles to step on the brake. The nervous system's quick response and short duration is sufficient to handle this situation.

1. _____
   _____
   _____

2. _____
   _____
   _____

3. _____
   _____
   _____

List three situations in which you believe endocrine system control would be most effective and explain why. An example is given.

Example Sledding in the cold for a couple of hours. The longer effect of hormones better supports the increase in heat production required to maintain body temperature.

1. _____
   _____
   _____

2. _____
   _____
   _____

3. _____
   _____
   _____

system and the nervous system control are speed and duration of effect. The nervous system is fast acting with a short duration of effect, whereas the endocrine system is slow acting with a long duration of effect. This offers a balance of control, with the nervous system responding quickly and the endocrine system taking over to sustain a response (Activity 6-1).

Hormones

Hormones are derived from amino acids or steroids. Hormones exert their effect on target organs and cells at very low blood levels. The concentration of a hormone in the blood is determined by the rate of release and the speed of inactivation and removal from the body. The influence of a hormone in the blood can range from seconds to 30 minutes. The term **half-life** is used to describe the time required for half of the hormone to be eliminated from the bloodstream. After this occurs, the effect is slowed. A very large variation in time is required for hormones to generate noticeable influences in the body or on behavior. Some hormones promote target organ responses almost immediately such as the effect of epinephrine on the heart. In contrast, steroid hormones such as testosterone and estrogen may require hours or days for their effects to be seen.

Hormones are secreted by endocrine glands and other specialized cells into the bloodstream to bind to specific receptors on or in their target cells. In a "lock-and-key" mechanism, hormones will bind only to receptor molecules that "fit" them exactly. Any cell with one or more receptors for a particular hormone is said to be a target of that hormone. Cells usually have many different types of receptors, so they can be target cells for many different hormones (Figure 6-3).

Each different hormone-receptor interaction produces different regulatory changes within the target cell. Hormones bring about their characteristic effects on the normal cellular processes of target cells by increasing or decreasing the rate of those cell processes.

Even though the diffusion of a hormone is usually system-wide through the blood, the effects are more specific because of the specificity of the target cells in organs and tissues. Ancient healing practices speak often of internal communication mechanisms and identify the blood as an important life-giving force. Today, what science calls hormones seem representative of this ancient wisdom (Activity 6-2).

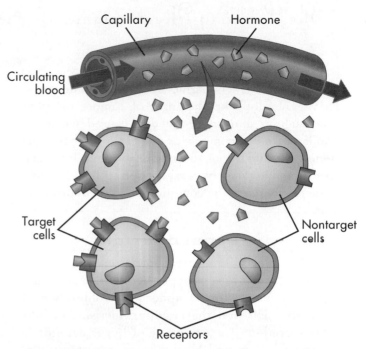

FIGURE 6-3 The target cell concept. A hormone acts only on cells that have receptors specific to that hormone because the shape of the receptor determines which hormones can react with it. This is an example of the lock-and-key model of biochemical reactions. (From Thibodeau GA, Patton KT: *Anatomy and physiology,* ed 3, St Louis, 1996, Mosby.)

ACTIVITY 6-2

Before we go any further in this chapter, do the following. In 1 minute, list as many physiologic processes influenced by hormones as you can. Come back at the end of the chapter and compare your "before-and-after" knowledge.

Example Pregnancy

Your Turn

The Primary Mechanisms of Endocrine Disease

Diseases of the endocrine system are numerous. They generally take the form of tumors or other abnormalities and are frequently caused when the glands secrete too much or too little of their hormones. Production of too much hormone by a diseased gland is called **hypersecretion**. If too little hormone is produced, the condition is called **hyposecretion.**

HYPERSECRETION

Any of several different mechanisms may be responsible for a given case of hypersecretion. Tumors are often responsible for an abnormal proliferation of endocrine cells and the resulting increase in hormone secretion. Another cause of hypersecretion is autoimmunity caused by the immune system functioning abnormally. A further possible cause of hypersecretion of a hormone is a failure of the feedback mechanisms that regulate secretion of a particular hormone.

HYPOSECRETION

Various mechanisms have been shown to cause hyposecretion of hormones. Although most tumors cause oversecretion of a hormone, they can cause a gland to undersecrete its hormone(s). Tissue death, caused by a blockage or other failure of blood supply, can also cause a gland to reduce its hormonal output. Still another way in which a gland may reduce its secretion below normal levels is through abnormal operation of regulatory feedback loops. An example of this is hyposecretion of testosterone and gonadotropic hormones in men who abuse anabolic steroids. Men who take testosterone steroids increase their blood concentration of this hormone above set point levels. The body responds to this high concentration by reducing its own output of testosterone and gonadotropins. This may lead to sterility and other complications.

Abnormalities of immune function may also cause hyposecretion. An autoimmune attack on glandular tissue sometimes has the effect of reducing hormone output. Some endocrinologists theorize that autoimmune destruction of pancreatic islet cells, perhaps in combination with viral and genetic mechanisms, is a "culprit" in many cases of type I (insulin-dependent) diabetes mellitus.

ACTIVITY 6-3

List three causes of hypersecretion:

1. _____
2. _____
3. _____

List three causes of hyposecretion:

1. _____
2. _____
3. _____

In recent research many types of hyposecretion disorders have been shown to be caused by insensitivity of the target cells to pituitary tropic hormones rather than from actual hyposecretion. **Tropic hormones** target other endocrine glands, stimulate their growth, and promote their function (Activity 6-3).

THREE ADDITIONAL TYPES OF DISORDERS OF THE ENDOCRINE SYSTEM

1. Some cancers can produce hormonelike substances that cause endocrine syndromes.
2. An abnormal decrease in the number of hormone receptors on target cells, thus blocking their action
3. Abnormal metabolic response to the hormone-receptor complex by the target cell

The Hypothalamus

The hypothalamus is the link in the body/mind and nerve/endocrine function. During stress, the hypothalamus translates nerve impulses into hormone secretions by endocrine glands. The hypothalamus exerts its primary influence over the pituitary gland, which in turn controls other endocrine glands with tropic hormones. This is accomplished through releasing or inhibiting hormones that affect the secretion of pituitary hormones. Psychosocial dwarfism, failure-to-thrive syndrome, and delayed tissue healing, all resulting from stress, emotional disorders, and deprivation, are a result of suppression of the hypothalamic release of growth hormone-releasing hormone (GH-RH). GH-RH suppresses the secretion of growth hormone from the pituitary gland.

✋ PRACTICAL APPLICATION

Soft tissue and movement therapies provide the hypothalamus with the stimulation needed to function efficiently. It is as if a "touch" hunger needs to be fed to maintain homeostasis. It is important that the body be able to deal with its individual stress load in an effective way. That is why stress management systems are so important. If we analyze ancient healing practices and spiritual wisdom made concrete through ritual, it is easy to see similarities to current recommendations for stress management programs.

Because isolation is a recognized problem with many, even within social groups (lonely in a crowd?), many types of professionals are concerned about the quality of physical, emotional, and spiritual health for those without touch interactions. Psychosocial influences on hypothalamic function reflect the importance of resourceful contact with fellow human beings or loving pets. Even caring for plants has been shown to increase the sense of well-being for some. We seem to be preconditioned to need others to be healthy. On a professional level, practitioners using a primary modality of touch can offer important health-restoring interventions and act in a preventive mode for those at risk from touch deprivation (Activity 6-4).

Endocrine Glands, Tissues, and Hormones

THE PITUITARY GLAND

The pituitary gland, or hypophysis, is located in the head at about eye level. It "hangs down" from the hypothalamus and sits in the sella turcica, a recessed area in the sphenoid bone. About the size of a peanut, it has an anterior lobe and a posterior lobe. The posterior lobe is not a true endocrine gland because it only stores and releases hormones but doesn't synthesize them. According to tradition, the pituitary

ACTIVITY 6-4

First, identify a current stress management program and briefly describe the process.

Then describe a ritual process with which you are familiar. Compare the two processes. Two examples are provided to get you started.

Example

1. Current stress management programs often use a combined method of sitting quietly and concentrating on the number *1* while repeating the word *one* slowly over and over.

   Ancient meditative practices used seated positions while chanting a mantra, sound, or phrase slowly over and over.

   Comparison: both use repetitive patterns and static positions to reduce stress responses.

2. Current practices of therapeutic massage use oil lubricants to rub the soft tissues of the body.

   Many ancient religious practices use anointing or rubbing with oil as part of a healing or purification ritual.

   Comparison: both use the application of oil and rubbing.

Your Turn

Current practice:

Ancient practice:

Comparison:

gland and its regulating counterpart the hypothalamus are related to the crown or brow chakra with primary functions of integration of energetic patterns and realization of the total self.

The pituitary gland secretes hormones that regulate growth, fluid balance, lactation, and childbirth. It is the main source of **tropic hormones,** hormones that have a stimulating effect on other endocrine glands. The pituitary gland is regulated through releasing and inhibiting hormones from the hypothalamus. The negative-feedback mechanism acts on the hypothalamus and not directly on the pituitary gland. (A negative feedback system provides a stimulus to decrease a function.) The terms *primary* and *secondary* are used to refer to target organ problems versus problems in other organs that affect the target gland. For example, primary hyperthyroidism means that the cause is in the thyroid gland. Secondary hyperthyroidism refers to the pituitary gland and its influence on the thyroid gland.

The larger anterior lobe secretes six major hormones, and the posterior lobe secretes two major hormones.

Anterior Pituitary Hormones
Growth hormone or somatotropin (GH)
Growth hormone (GH), or somatotropin, stimulates most body cells to increase in size and divide. The major target organs are bones and muscles. In the adult the response of GH is the repair and rebuilding of tissues. GH follows a circadian cycle, with the highest levels occurring during evening sleep, primarily delta-level sleep. GH releases stored fat and raises blood glucose concentrations to provide us with energy. It is also triggered for release during exercise and periods of stress. As we age, the total amount secreted declines daily.

GH release can be inhibited by emotional deprivation, excessive blood sugar, and high blood fat levels. Disruption in the sleep pattern will interfere with GH functions as well. GH disturbances are often implicated in chronic pain disorders such as fibromyalgia.

🖐 PRACTICAL APPLICATION

GH stimulates the production of fibroblasts, mast cells, ground substance, and collagen fibers, and is essential in healing wounds. Because GH is most active during delta-wave sleep, and the sleep pattern is usually disrupted in fibromyalgia and other pain and fatigue syndromes, the body may have problems with cellular repair. Given this premise, it has been suggested that a disrupted sleep pattern may be one of the primary causes of fatigue and pain syndromes.

Soft tissue and movement therapies have been shown through research to have a beneficial influence on the development of a restful sleep pattern, thus enabling the body to better restore and heal itself.

Thyroid-stimulating hormone (TSH)—a tropic hormone
Thyroid-stimulating hormone (TSH) promotes and maintains the growth and development of the thyroid gland and controls the release of thyroid hormones in a negative feedback system. Production of TSH is often increased in response to cold temperature.

🖐 PRACTICAL APPLICATION

A licensed medical professional may recommend hydrotherapy or the use of water for therapeutic intervention to encourage the production of TSH if hyposecretion is a concern. Cold has an effect on the hypothalamus, resulting in the release of TSH. Typical applications include standing in cold water or alternating hot and cold water baths or showers. Whenever cold is used therapeutically, the body needs to be warm first. Before using standing cold water, first warm the feet in warm foot bath. With alternating hot and cold baths or showers, begin with a warm water application for 5 to 15 minutes, then add cold applications, starting with 15 to 30 seconds, gradually increasing to up to 5 minutes. Start the entire cold process with tepid water and gradually, over days or even weeks, reduce the temperature and duration of the cold water application. These methods are contraindicated in conditions in which a hypersensitivity to cold such as Raynaud's disease exists.

Adrenocorticotropic hormone (ACTH) —a tropic hormone
Adrenocorticotropic hormone (ACTH) promotes and maintains normal growth and development of the adrenal cortex by stimulating the release of glucocorticoids and androgens. Androgens are hormones such as testosterone that produce secondary male characteristics. Stress, mild-to-moderate fevers, and hypoglycemia can increase the amount of ACTH secreted.

✋ PRACTICAL APPLICATION

Stress encountered over a long period generates abnormal glucocorticoid effects on the body, which are responsible for some diseases. It is known that glucocorticoids suppress the immune system. Any modality that reduces the effects of stress, including soft tissue and movement therapies, promotes appropriate levels of ACTH and thus brings the immune system back in balance.

Follicle-stimulating hormone (FSH)—a tropic hormone

Follicle-stimulating hormone (FSH) in the female stimulates the growth and maturation of ovarian follicles, which contain eggs. It also stimulates the secretion of estrogen; in the male it stimulates sperm production.

Luteinizing hormone (LH)—a tropic hormone

In women, luteinizing hormone (LH) causes ovulation (the release of the mature egg) and stimulates progesterone production in the ovaries. In men, LH stimulates the production and secretion of testosterone in the testes.

Prolactin (PRL)

Although found in both men and women, prolactin primarily works in two areas of a woman's body. First, in combination with other hormones, it plays a part in breast development. Second, it initiates milk production when stimulated by the central nervous system.

Melanocyte-stimulating hormone (MSH)

Melanocyte-stimulating hormone (MSH) acts on the pigment cells in the skin and the adrenal glands. The exact function is uncertain. One theory suggests that MSH, ACTH, and other hormones that darken the skin control pigmentation of normal skin.

Posterior Pituitary Hormones

Posterior pituitary hormones are made by hypothalamic neurons and stored in the posterior pituitary gland.

Oxytocin

Oxytocin stimulates smooth muscle contraction, especially in the uterus. It is released in large quantities just before a woman gives birth. This is part of a positive feedback cycle that ends when the child is born. Pitocin is synthetic oxytocin used mainly to induce labor in women. Oxytocin stimulates the milk letdown response, which causes the breast ducts to contract and release milk. Oxytocin may also be implicated in bonding behavior or feelings of belonging to another as occurs between a parent and child. When increased sympathetic activity releases epinephrine, which inhibits oxytocin, problems in lactation and bonding may occur. Oxytocin is found in both men and nonpregnant women as well as pregnant and postpartal women. It is suggested that the role of this hormone in men may be to support pair bonding between couples and to enhance parental behavior.

✋ PRACTICAL APPLICATION

Research has shown that massage, both giving and receiving, reduces sympathetic arousal. This enhances the effects of oxytocin, supporting lactation and bonding between infants and parents. Research has also shown that pleasurable rhythmic skin stimulation increases levels of oxytocin. This could explain some of the feelings of connectedness that occur between the client and practitioner when these type of methods are used.

Antidiuretic hormone (ADH)

Also known as vasopressin, antidiuretic hormone (ADH) stimulates the kidneys to remove water from urine and release it into the bloodstream. Its release is stimulated by pain, anxiety, nicotine, tranquilizers, and low blood pressure. The release of ADH is inhibited by alcohol, so the amount of urine produced is increased. Because it can cause arterioles to contract, it increases blood pressure, which is beneficial during hemorrhaging. It can decrease the rate of perspiration, thus helping a person who is dehydrated.

✋ PRACTICAL APPLICATION

The use of soft tissue and movement therapies that reduce the perception of pain and anxiety indirectly interact with the release of ADH, possibly supporting a more effective homeostasis function.

PATHOLOGY

In gigantism and acromegaly, the pituitary gland produces excessive growth hormone. The term *gigantism* is used to refer to the condition if it begins in infancy or early childhood. It results in excessive growth of the entire body. Acromegaly is an abnormal condition that happens in adults, in which the excess hormone thickens bones and enlarges organs. In secondary Cushing's disease the pituitary gland produces excessive ACTH, resulting in increased production of steroids by the adrenal gland. The symptoms include increased fat on the face and between the shoulder blades, thinning of bones and skin, and bruising. Treatment of gigantism, acromegaly, and secondary Cushing's disease includes surgery or radiation therapy. If a pituitary tumor is present, drug therapy with somatostatin is usually the treatment of choice.

Height deficiencies may be caused by decreased GH production and insufficient tropic hormones. In

ACTIVITY 6-5

If the pituitary hormones were represented by cartoon characters, what would each one be? Create and draw a cartoon character or other figure in the appropriate space or find a picture of one and paste it in the space to represent each pituitary hormone.

Growth hormone (GH)

Thyroid-stimulating hormone (TSH)

Adrenocorticotropic hormone (ACTH)

Follicle-stimulating hormone (FSH)

Luteinizing hormone (LH)

Prolactin (PRL)

Oxytocin (OT)

Antidiuretic hormone (ADH)

pituitary deficiency a decrease exists in all pituitary hormones, which results in the loss of target organ hormones, specifically adrenal steroids, thyroxin, and the gonadotropins. Dwarfism can be the result. Dwarfism in children is treated by administration of synthetic GH and, if necessary, replacement of thyroid, adrenal, and sex steroid hormones.

In diabetes insipidus (not to be confused with diabetes mellitus) the amount of vasopressin released by the pituitary gland is decreased. It is often caused by scarring or damage from head injuries. The ability of the water in urine to be reabsorbed decreases, and urine output increases, sometimes up to 20 L/day. Maintaining an adequate fluid intake may control mild cases, but in others treatment with a synthetic form of vasopressin has proven effective. If diabetes insipidus is caused by the kidney's inability to respond to vasopressin, reducing salt intake and taking medications focused on kidney function is the normal treatment. In rare cases in which diabetes insipidus is caused by a tumor, radiation therapy, surgery, or both are indicated (Activity 6-5).

THE THYROID GLAND

The thyroid gland lies on the trachea below the thyroid cartilage. It consists of a right and left lobe connected by a bridge (isthmus), resulting in a butterfly shape. The gland is heavier in women than in men. The thyroid and parathyroid glands are related to the Eastern energy chakra of the throat whose function is communication and creativity in a balanced function.

The thyroid gland regulates metabolism in the body by maintaining an adequate amount of oxygen consumption at the cellular level. Its two principal hormones are thyroxine (T_4) and triiodothyronine (T_3). TSH from the pituitary gland stimulates these hormones, and iodine is necessary for their synthesis. A third hormone, calcitonin, inhibits bone reabsorption by limiting the rate at which calcium is released from bone tissue to plasma. This, in turn, reduces the blood calcium level and counters the effect of the parathyroid hormones.

Pathology
Hyperthyroidism

Hyperthyroidism, or thyrotoxicosis, is the second most common endocrine disorder after diabetes mellitus. It affects mostly women. The most common cause is autoimmune dysfunctions. Symptoms include increased metabolic rate, excessive sweating, weight loss even with increased food intake, fatigue, nervousness, loose stools, tachycardia, warm moist skin, hand tremor, and hyperactivity. Hyperthyroidism mimics manic-depressive psychosis and is almost always accompanied by a goiter. (NOTE: A goiter, which is an enlarged thyroid gland, may be found in hyperfunction, hypofunction, or normal thyroid function.) Plummer's disease, or toxic nodular goiter, is another form of hyperthyroidism.

The symptoms of Grave's disease include an enlarged thyroid gland and abnormal eyeball protrusion, called *exophthalmos*. It is a result of excess fluid behind the eye and may not diminish even after treatment. Grave's disease runs in families, is associated with autoimmune problems, and is most common in women between the ages of 20 and 40. Treatments include thyroidectomy, the use of antithyroid medications such as propylthiouracil (blocks iodine from being incorporated into thyroxin), or the use of radioactive iodine, which shrinks (destroys) the thyroid gland without affecting other tissues.

Hypothyroidism

Hypothyroidism can be a result of treatment for hyperthyroidism by radioactive iodine, overdose of antithyroid medication, or partial or complete thyroidectomy. The next most common causes are autoimmune dysfunction and a decrease in thyroid-releasing hormone from the hypothalamus. Symptoms include weakness, fatigue, lower metabolic rate, constipation, hoarseness, bradycardia, skin dryness, weight gain (often resulting in obesity), sluggishness, and slowed mental function sometimes with psychotic behavior. Again, a goiter is often present. Mild hypothyroidism is common in perimenopausal women between the ages of 35 and 45. Because of this, thyroid function should be checked as part of the routine health care of women. Hypothyroidism responds well to oral medication.

If thyroid hormones are absent in the fetus or during infancy, the result can be cretinism, a condition that results in mental retardation and dwarfism. Hashimoto's disease is an autoimmune hypothyroid disorder. It is hereditary, found mainly in women ages 30 to 50, and causes tissue changes in the thyroid gland itself. Myxedema is the most severe form of this, causing many of the previously mentioned symptoms as well as swelling of the face, hands, and feet.

A summary of the major effects and disturbances of T_3 and T_4 thyroid hormones on the body can be found in Table 6-1.

TABLE 6-1 NORMAL VERSUS MAJOR EFFECTS AND DISTURBANCES OF T_3 AND T_4 THYROID HORMONES ON THE BODY

NORMAL FUNCTION	HYPOSECRETION	HYPERSECRETION
Maintains basal metabolic rate (BMR) and temperature regulation to promote appropriate oxygen consumption and production of heat and energy; enhances effects of catecholamines and sympathetic nervous system activity	Can result in BMR less than normal with a decreased body temperature, cold intolerance, decreased appetite, weight gain, muscle and joint pain, decreased sensitivity to catecholamines, and general slowed state; low thyroid function mimics many disease symptoms and should be checked when any of the above symptoms are experienced	Can result in BMR greater than normal with an increase in body temperature; heat intolerance; appetite; weight loss; sensitivity to catecholamines, which may lead to hypertension (high blood pressure); mood changes; and anxiety-type symptoms
Promotes appropriate carbohydrate/lipid/protein metabolism and glucose catabolism, mobilizes fats, essential for protein synthesis; enhances liver secretion of cholesterol	Can result in decreased glucose metabolism, elevated cholesterol and triglyceride levels in the blood, decreased protein synthesis, and edema	Can result in enhanced catabolism of glucose and fats, weight loss, increased protein catabolism, and loss of muscle mass
Promotes development of the nervous system in the fetus and infant, as well as normal adult nervous system function	Can result in slowed brain development in the infant with retardation and mental dulling, depression, paresthesias, memory impairment, listlessness, and hypoactive reflexes in the adult	Can result in irritability, restlessness, insomnia, overresponsiveness to environmental stimuli, bulging eyes (exophthalmos), personality change
Promotes functioning of the heart	Can result in decreased efficiency of the pumping action of the heart, slow heart rate, and low blood pressure	Can result in rapid heart rate, high blood pressure, and if prolonged, can lead to heart failure
Promotes normal muscular development, tone, and function	Can result in sluggish muscle action, muscle cramps, and myalgia	Can result in muscle atrophy and weakness
Promotes growth and maturation of the skeleton	Can result in growth retardation, skeletal malabsorption, retention of child's body proportions in adults, and joint pain in the adult	Can result in excessive skeletal growth initially, followed by early epiphyseal closure and short stature in children; adults experience demineralization of skeleton
Promotes gastrointestinal (GI) motility and tone and increases secretion of digestive juices	Can result in depressed GI motility and tone and increased secretion of digestive juices	Can result in excessive GI motility, diarrhea, and loss of appetite
Promotes female reproductive ability and normal lactation	Can result in depressed ovarian function, sterility, and depressed lactation	Can result in depressed ovarian function in females and impotence in males
Promotes secretory activity of skin	Can result in skin that is pale, thick, and dry; facial edema; coarse and thin hair; and hard and thick nails	Can result in skin that is flushed, thin, and moist; may produce thin and soft hair and nails

ACTIVITY 6-6

List three thyroid dysfunction symptoms that may cause a client to seek bodywork modalities. Examples are provided to get you started.

Example Nervousness, fatigue, constipation

Your Turn

1. _____

2. _____

3. _____

INDICATIONS CONTRAINDICATIONS

For Soft Tissue and Movement Therapies

Some studies suggest that mild cases of hypothyroidism respond to cold water hydrotherapy and moderate aerobic exercise. Thyroid-stimulating hormone is triggered for release by exposure to cold.

Bodywork may be beneficial in the management of symptoms of both hyperthyroidism and hypothyroidism. Because thyroid conditions can go undiagnosed as a result of the symptoms being common to many stress-related conditions, it is important to refer clients for medical assessment to rule out thyroid dysfunction when they have any hyperthyroid or hypothyroid symptom patterns (Activity 6-6).

THE PARATHYROID GLANDS

The parathyroid glands are made up of four round, pea-sized bodies located on the posterior surface of the thyroid lobes. Their hormone, parathormone (PTH), when combined with vitamin D decreases the amount of calcium excreted, causes the release of calcium from bone, and absorbs more calcium from the gastrointestinal tract, resulting in an increase in blood levels of calcium and phosphorus.

Pathology

An excess of parathormone causes too much calcium to be removed from bone, resulting in weak bones. A deficiency of parathormone can cause hypocalcemic tetany, the symptoms of which include loss of sensation, muscle twitches, uncontrolled spasm, and convulsion.

In hypoparathyroidism the levels of calcium in both blood and urine are less than normal, frequently resulting in spasms of skeletal muscles. Moderate-to-mild deficiency can result in neuromuscular excitability that could be misdiagnosed as simple muscle tension. Anxiety may result as well. It is important to rule out hypoparathyroidism in cases of unresolved anxiety and muscle tension. Emergency treatment of tetany caused by hypoparathyroidism is an injection of calcium chloride. For maintenance therapy, calcium and vitamin D supplements are used.

In primary hyperparathyroidism, usually resulting from a benign tumor, levels of calcium are increased in blood and urine. In secondary hyperparathyroidism, resulting mostly from kidney disease, blood calcium is decreased and urine calcium is increased. The frequency of hyperparathyroidism is much more common than hypoparathyroidism and seems to be on the increase.

INDICATIONS CONTRAINDICATIONS

For Soft Tissue and Movement Therapies

The symptoms of hyperparathyroidism include mild-to-severe skeletal pain; osteoporosis may result as well. The client may seek body therapies for these conditions and care must be taken by bodyworkers to provide the appropriate referral to determine the underlying cause of the problem.

THE PANCREAS

The pancreas is a long, slender gland located behind the stomach. In Eastern philosophies, it is related to the solar plexus chakra located at the thoracolumbar junction and navel. This chakra functions with willpower and awareness of emotion.

The pancreas is both an exocrine and endocrine gland. Although its enzymes aid in digestion, our focus will be on its hormone production. Islands of cells called the islets of Langerhans are interspersed within the exocrine gland tissues. These islets produce the hormones insulin and glucagon. Two other hormones are secreted in small amounts: somatostatin inhibits the release of all islet hormones, and amylin acts as an antagonist to insulin.

The beta cells of the islets of Langerhans secrete the hormone insulin, which lowers blood glucose levels by transporting glucose into cells to be used for energy. Insulin binds to the cells and allows glucose and potassium to be transported across the cell membrane. Although insulin receptors are present on most cell membranes, only our muscle, connective tissue, and white blood cells need it for glucose transport. However, glucose is readily available to the liver, brain, and kidneys no matter what our blood insulin levels. Insulin removes glucose from blood, making it available for cellular activity.

Insulin

Insulin is released when levels of blood sugar, amino acids, and fatty acids rise. Insulin secretion is also affected by other hormones, including ACTH, growth hormone, epinephrine, thyroxin, and glucocorticoids. Because these hormones necessitate response from muscles, the demand for energy is increased thus energy is supplied from insulin secretion. Fluctuations in blood sugar during experiences of stress put additional strain on the body because the body often does not actually need increased amount of energy.

Glucagon

Alpha cells of the islets of Langerhans secrete the hormone glucagon, which increases blood glucose, the opposite of insulin response. These cells are stimulated by growth hormones and are a part of the feedback loop in hypoglycemia. Both high protein intake and exercise raise the amount of amino acids in the blood, which also increases glucagon secretion. This happens by requiring the liver to speed up the conversion of glycogen to glucose, as well as creating glucose from fatty acids, lactic acid, and amino acids. Blood levels of glucose increase but do not enter the cells, so cellular levels of glucose decrease.

Pathology

Hyperfunction

A high insulin level is occasionally caused by a benign tumor. More commonly, it is seen in a diabetic client who takes insulin without eating properly. This results in what is known as an insulin reaction, which means the body is flooded with insulin. Glucose enters the cells at an increased rate and the blood glucose level falls, causing hypoglycemia (low blood sugar). When the brain is deprived of glucose, confusion and weakness result. Hypoglycemia may be caused by a deficient production of glucagon.

True hypoglycemia is rare. More common is reactive hypoglycemia, a diet-induced condition that can be balanced by eating a balanced diet on a regular schedule.

Hypofunction

Diabetes. The disorder known as diabetes mellitus is the result of the pancreas either not producing enough insulin or totally stopping insulin production. Because glucose is not absorbed by the cells, the amount in the bloodstream is elevated (hyperglycemia). Glucose is a powerful diuretic, so as glucose enters urine, it is accompanied by water. As it flows through the kidneys, some of the excess is released in the urine (glycosuria). This causes many of the first symptoms of diabetes, such as dehydration, increased thirst (polydipsia), increased urination (polyuria), and an increased appetite (polyphagia).

When the body is unable to use glucose, fats are used for energy. The breakdown in fats results in the formation of ketones (ketoacids) as by-products, increasing body acidity and causing ketoacidosis. In severe instances the combination of dehydration, high blood sugar, and acidosis may depress the cerebral cortex to the point of coma. This metabolic acidosis stimulates the respiratory center to increase the breathing rate.

There are two types of diabetes mellitus. Type I, or insulin-dependent diabetes, is usually severe and occurs at a young age. Symptoms develop quickly, with ketoacidosis often the first manifestation. Ketoacidosis is treated with saline, bicarbonate, potassium and insulin. A controlled diet and the daily use of insulin are the most common long-term treatments.

Type II, or non–insulin-dependent diabetes, is usually milder and in most cases begins in adults. Heredity and obesity are important contributing factors. Symptoms include dehydration, increased thirst and appetite, frequent urination, reduced resistance to infection, blurred vision, and fatigue. These symptoms most often develop over a period of years. Treatment usually begins with dietary changes, such as those recommended by the American Diabetes Association (ADA). An exercise program is implemented to control weight and increase general fitness. Weight loss is an important first step because fewer insulin receptors are present and they become less sensitive to insulin in an overweight person. Oral medications, including chlorpropamide (Diabinese) or tolbutamide (Orinase), reduce blood sugar levels. Insulin may be used if blood sugar levels remain high but is not necessarily a permanent form of treatment.

Complications of diabetes can include vascular disease because diabetes increases the development of arteriosclerosis. High glucose levels also raise the chances of infection because they provide a good medium for bacterial growth. Other complications include kidney disease, heart attacks (diabetics have twice the average), eye problems (diabetic retinopathy), impotence in men, and loss of menstrual cycles in women. Gangrene of the feet in diabetic clients accounts for more amputations of the feet than any other condition, including trauma. Treatment for the complications of diabetes include meticulous attention to the hygiene of the feet and an exercise program for weight loss and fitness. Diabetic neuropathy is a painful and difficult-to-manage condition resulting from peripheral nerve damage; it is more severe with type I diabetes because the nerve damage results from the ketoacidosis. (Ketoacidosis is not seen as often in those with type II diabetes.)

INDICATIONS CONTRAINDICATIONS

For Soft Tissue and Movement Therapies

A general stress management program is supportive in the management of diabetes. Soft tissue and movement therapies can be an integral part of such a program. It is important when working with the diabetic client that bodywork be a part of an overall treatment program with medical supervision. Careful observation of the feet during massage supports a hygiene program. Referral for immediate medical care should be made for any noted tissue changes. In pain management of diabetic neuropathy, using bodywork approaches as part of a supervised program can prove beneficial for short-term reduction of pain symptoms (Activity 6-7).

THE ADRENAL GLANDS

We have two adrenal glands, one on top of each of our kidneys. Each gland consists of an inner portion called the *medulla* and an outer layer called the *cortex*. The adrenal glands are related to the root or basic chakra center located at the base of the spine and focused to functions of survival and grounding.

Adrenal Medulla

The tissue structure of the adrenal medulla is similar to nerve tissue and functions as part of the sympathetic nervous system. It secretes two catecholamines, epinephrine (sometimes called *adrenaline*) and norepinephrine (or noradrenaline). They are the hormones active in the sympathetic

ACTIVITY 6-7

Identify a reason why soft tissue and movement therapies can be beneficial as part of a total diabetes management program. Justify your position using the clinical reasoning model.

Example

Statement: Soft tissue and movement therapies support weight loss programs.

1. What are the facts?

Weight loss and changes in diet result in chemical changes in the body. Mood-elevating chemicals that are generated from high sugar/fat foods are substantially reduced in a diabetic diet.

Soft tissue and movement therapies increase the "feel-good" chemicals in the body.

2. What are the possibilities?

Soft tissue and movement therapies can act as a substitute for food to provide stimulation for mood elevation.

3. What are the pros and cons? What are the consequences of not acting (not doing bodywork)? What are the consequences of acting (doing bodywork)?

Positive consequences include pleasure sensations that do not contribute to the diabetic problem. Negative consequences include the cost and inconvenience that may prevent easy implementation of these methods into a person's lifestyle.

4. What would be the impact on the people involved: client, practitioner, and other professionals working with the client?

The person would feel cared for and supported during the weight loss program by receiving the personal attention from a professional during a time in which he may feel deprived.

Your Turn

Statement:

1. What are the facts?

2. What are the possibilities?

3. What are the pros and cons? What are the consequences of not acting? What are the consequences of acting?

4. What would be the impact on the people involved: client, practitioner, and other professionals working with the client?

"fight-or-flight" or alarm response to stress. Epinephrine has its primary influence on the heart, causing an increase in heart rate, whereas norepinephrine has a greater effect on peripheral vasoconstriction, which raises blood pressure. The hormones produced by the adrenal medulla prolong and intensify the activity begun by the sympathetic nervous system neurons. The hypothalamus, the adrenal medulla, and the adrenal cortex are linked and interdependent in the management of the stress response. When stress-producing events are unresolved within about 15 minutes (Selye's alarm phase) a more prolonged stress-coping pattern of the adrenocortical responses are activated by these symptoms (Selye's resistance phase). Over the long term, if epinephrine and norepinephrine remain elevated, they perpetuate predisposing factors for stress-related disease.

✋ PRACTICAL APPLICATION

Bodywork methods have been shown to help dissipate the concentration of adrenal medulla hormones, reducing their detrimental effects in the body. Because the effects of catecholamines dissipate within a short time, the usual goal for soft tissue and movement therapies is to support the body in a return to homeostasis and prevent a recurrence of the excessive alarm response so that the body can remain in a steady state of homeostasis. The general application in a typical 1-hour session is to work with more vigorous methods for the first 15 minutes to use up the catecholamines, then begin to transition the work to trigger and support the relaxation response of parasympathetic function over the next 45 minutes.

Because the major repair and energy-resorting mechanisms of the body are supported most effectively in the parasympathetic pattern and because most energy is expended and tissue damage created during fight-or-flight activity, we can begin to see the wisdom in supporting parasympathetic function to allow sufficient time for restoration and repair of the body. A general rule of thumb is that for every 15 minutes of catecholamine-generated sympathetic activity, the body will require about 45 minutes of parasympathetic balancing time. In a "healthy," well-balanced person, sympathetic activities account for 25% of daily actions, with parasympathetic restorative actions making up another 25%. The other 50% of the time is taken up with activities that use sympathetic and parasym-

pathetic functions together. It is suggested that this seldom happens, and the ratio is often reversed. Dysfunction occurs when sympathetic activity dominates, often because of lifestyle demands. Over time the body cannot provide enough restorative action, and homeostatic balance is disrupted. Again, it seems that many of the healing rituals of old were based on supporting parasympathetic activity and providing effective outlets for the fight-or-flight hormones of the adrenal glands. The use of sweat lodges, ceremonial bathing, quiet reflection, chanting, dancing, feasting, and other such activities are seen as effective ways to dissipate the fight-or-flight hormones while promoting restorative functions (Activity 6-8).

ACTIVITY 6-8

Design a personal 15-minute sympathetic activity sequence.

Then design a personal 45-minute parasympathetic relaxation sequence.

Example

15-minute sympathetic activity sequence: I will go to the recreation center and spend 5 minutes on the track and 10 minutes on the stair-climbing machine.

45-minute parasympathetic relaxation sequence: I will spend 15 minutes doing slow stretching combined with coordinated breathing. I will take a 15-minute hot bath, and I will read inspirational and heart-warming stories for 15 minutes.

Your Turn

Design a personal 15-minute sympathetic activity sequence:

Design a personal 45-minute parasympathetic relaxation sequence:

Adrenal Cortex

The adrenal cortex secretes three major corticosteroid hormones that are derived from cholesterol. These hormones—cortisol, aldosterone, and the gonadocorticoids—are stimulated for release by ACTH from the pituitary gland, which receives its messages from the hypothalamus. The adrenal cortex hormones are involved with metabolism of most body cells. Without a functioning adrenal cortex, a person could die from excessive stress and its effects.

Cortisol

Hydrocortisone, or cortisol, is the main glucocorticoid (glucose-producing steroid). It is secreted in very small amounts. If the body does not have sufficient supplies of fat or glycogen stored to use for energy, cortisol synthesizes certain amino acids into glucose (gluconeogenesis), causing a rise in blood sugar. Cortisol also converts starches into glycogen in the liver if there are not enough carbohydrates for the body to use.

Cortisol secretion is stimulated by eating and activity. It seems to follow daily biologic rhythm patterns. Peak cortisol levels occur shortly after waking, whereas the lowest levels are reached just as the sleep cycle begins. High levels of cortisol in the blood may disrupt the sleep cycle. Any situation that produces acute stress will increase blood levels of cortisol, and the sympathetic nervous system will override any inhibitory effects in feedback loop regulation. This results in a rise in blood levels of glucose, fatty acids, and amino acids—all caused by cortisol. Levels of stress are often measured by cortisol levels, and research in stress-management methods often uses cortisol as a measurement criterion, with a drop indicating a reduction in the stress response. Cortisol contains antiinflammatory agents that limit the amount of substances released during the inflammation response. Cortisol slows wound healing as a result of a decreased rate of connective tissue regeneration. Excessively high levels of cortisol, especially over a long period, can cause such symptoms as a decrease in cartilage and bone formation; inhibition of the inflammatory response, which reduces normal signals for tissue repair; depression of the activity of the immune system; and promotion of detrimental changes in cardiovascular, neural, and gastrointestinal function.

It is important to remember the idea of balance. The body needs glucocorticoids for normal function to achieve homeostasis. Excessive stress and use of steroids as pharmacologic agents may lead to the disruption of this homeostasis.

✋ PRACTICAL APPLICATION

Studies show that massage reduces cortisol levels and therefore promotes such activities as improved sleep, better digestion, increased immune function, and improved tissue repair. Other forms of relaxation, including moderate aerobic exercise and slow stretching methods such as yoga, show similar results. It seems that the most effective interventions are rhythmic, with a duration of 15 to 60 minutes producing the best results. Because the effects wear off within a 24-hour period, some sort of relaxation method needs to be done every day to best support well-being.

Aldosterone

Aldosterone is a mineralocorticoid, a sodium- and potassium-regulating steroid. It causes the kidneys to reabsorb more sodium and water and excrete more potassium and hydrogen. Although aldosterone is necessary for our survival, excessive amounts lead to sodium and water retention accompanied by elevation of potassium ions and in some instances alteration of the acid-base balance of blood. Under excessive stress the hypothalamus secretes corticotrophin-releasing hormone (CRH). ACTH blood levels rise and trigger an increase in aldosterone secretion. The increase in blood volume and blood pressure that results helps ensure adequate delivery of nutrients and respiratory gases during the stressful period.

✋ PRACTICAL APPLICATION

The release of aldosterone, although effective when the body is expending physical energy such as required in actual fighting behavior, increases the likelihood of stress-induced disease such as high blood pressure when the energy expenditure is less than the physiologic response. This happens often as people try to deal with increased emotional and mental stress without physical activity involvement. Aerobic activity and moderate weight resistance exercises are helpful in managing this situation, balancing emotional and mental activity (Activity 6-9).

ACTIVITY 6-9

Outline the progression of the adrenal hormone patterns in response to a stress that lasts 24 hours. Identify the stressor, the hormones involved, the possible duration of effect, and the possible results.

Example

Situation: Parent worried about adolescent child who comes home 2 hours late.

1. Anger—first 15 minutes—epinephrine and norepinephrine—results in increase in fight-or-flight response and increased sympathetic activity.

2. Worry—next 30 minutes—with increase in anxiety, still supporting continuance of catecholamine response.

3. Increased worry—next 60 minutes—shift to cortisol release, resulting in inability to sleep.

4. Recurring anger—15 minutes—epinephrine and norepinephrine with aldosterone increase—results in increased fight-or-flight response and increased sympathetic activity with raise in blood pressure because of increasing fluid levels of blood.

5. Child comes home and is met by a very angry and worried parent.

6. Inability of parent to sleep rest of night because of increased cortisol levels.

7. Fatigue next day with irritability and dull headache caused by effects of increased cortisol and aldosterone levels.

8. Because of increased cortisol and aldosterone levels, parent has suppressed immune function and catches a cold 3 days later.

Your Turn

Situation:

Response pattern:

Gonadocorticoids

Although most of the sex hormones are produced in the ovaries and testes, the adrenal glands also produce similar male and female sex steroids called *gonadocorticoids*. Estrogen, progesterone, and the male androgens are secreted in both sexes, with androgens predominating. This hormone secretion is significant in the fetus and during early puberty. The effect of the adrenal sex hormones increases as we age and hormone production in the gonads decreases. This effect can be seen in the use of adrenal estrogen in postmenopausal women when ovarian function decreases.

✋ PRACTICAL APPLICATION

Healthy functioning adrenal glands support successful aging. As gonadocorticoids secreted by the gonads decline, the secretion of these hormones from strong and healthy adrenal glands supports the body in vitality well into the aging process.

Care of the adrenal glands is the same as care for the whole body. Effective stress management, adequate exercise and rest, fresh air, sunshine, proper nutrition, good social support, and a feeling of purpose in life all contribute to this care. Is it possible that the ageless quality of sages, elders, gurus, and others considered as the old ones of wisdom is due, in part, to the care they took of their adrenal glands?

Pathology

In Cushing's syndrome, corticosteroid levels in the blood and urine are elevated, specifically cortisol and urinary 17-hydroxycorticosteroids, both of which are excretory products of cortisol. The usual cause of Cushing's disease is taking large doses of corticosteroid drugs for long periods. When the cause is primary Cushing's disease, ACTH is low. ACTH is high in secondary Cushing's disease. Usually caused by a pituitary tumor, it is referred to as Cushing's disease instead of syndrome. In both cases, symptoms include fat accumulation, edema, hyperglycemia, muscle weakness, suppressed immunity, osteoporosis, acne, and increased facial hair. Diabetes mellitus can be brought on during Cushing's disease and can develop into a chronic condition.

Conn's syndrome, caused by an adrenal tumor, is primary hyperaldosteronism. In very rare cases, if caused by a nonspecific enlargement of the adrenal glands, it is referred to as aldosteronism. Levels of aldosterone and sodium are elevated in plasma and urine, and potassium is decreased. Symptoms include headache, tingling and weakness in the limbs, increased thirst, fatigue, hypertension, and increase in urine volume, especially at night.

Addison's disease shows low plasma cortisol, low sodium, and high potassium levels (all opposite of Cushing's disease). Urinary 17-hydroxycorticosteroids and blood glucose levels are low. Primary Addison's disease shows a high ACTH level (with no cortisol to oppose ACTH). Secondary Addison's disease shows a low ACTH level because of nonstimulation of the adrenal gland by the pituitary gland. Symptoms include weakness, decreased endurance, increased pigmentation of the skin and mucous membranes, anorexia, dehydration, weight loss, intestinal disturbances, anxiety, depression (or similar emotional distress), and decreased tolerance to cold. The onset is usually gradual and may be mistaken as general stress symptoms. This can be a life-threatening condition, and proper diagnosis is essential for appropriate treatment.

INDICATIONS CONTRAINDICATIONS

For Soft Tissue and Movement Therapies

After these conditions are diagnosed, stress management can be an important part of ongoing therapeutic management.

Pharmacologic use of synthetic adrenocorticosteroids (corticosteroids, steroids)

Synthetic steroids are primarily used to decrease the effects of inflammation. They do this by reducing both capillary dilatation and permeability. Steroids also prevent the release of vasoactive substances such as histamine and kinins. Allergic disorders such as asthma, reactions to bee stings, contact dermatitis, drug reactions, hay fever, and hives are treated with steroids. They are also used in arthritis, bursitis, and autoimmune disorders, including lupus erythematosus and rheumatoid arthritis. Steroids have been shown to be useful in the treatment of leukemia, multiple myeloma, Crohn's disease, ulcerative colitis, kidney failure, infections, and skin disorders.

Common side effects seen with the use of synthetic steroids include such diverse symptoms as mood changes, insomnia, high blood pressure, increased susceptibility to infection, glaucoma, headache, reduced wound healing, sweating, fragile skin, vertigo, stunted growth in children, osteoporosis, and an increased risk of bone breakage.

It is dangerous to use steroids for extended periods without reevaluation. Periodic decreases in dosage are often necessary, but dosages must never be altered or stopped except by licensed medical practitioners. It is necessary to wean gradually from large doses of steroids because they suppress the pituitary gland and ACTH by negative feedback. When ACTH is suppressed, the adrenal glands do not function. When steroid treatment is stopped, sometimes the adrenal glands do not rebound to a functioning mode, and the person may lapse into Addison's disease. A side effect of oral steroid therapy is gastrointestinal bleeding. Protection of the stomach lining with cimetidine (Tagamet) is often necessary when oral steroids are used.

INDICATIONS CONTRAINDICATIONS

For Soft Tissue and Movement Therapies

Some forms of bodywork may be used to manage some of the side effects from synthetic steroids. However, bodywork methods such as frictioning that may cause inflammation should be avoided when a person is taking synthetic adrenocorticosteroids. Massage is also contraindicated directly over areas of injected steroids used to treat localized inflammation such as bursitis because it is important for the steroid to remain in the localized tissues (Activity 6-10).

ACTIVITY 6-10

Develop a list of at least three indications and contraindications for integrating soft tissue and movement therapies in combination with synthetic pharmacologic steroid use.

Example

Indications: Beneficial to sleep
Contraindications: Heavy compressive force on bones

Your Turn

Indications:

1. _____

2. _____

3. _____

Contraindications:

1. _____

2. _____

3. _____

THE TESTES AND OVARIES

The male and female gonads are located in the pelvic cavity and produce sex hormones identical to those of the adrenal cortex. Because this is their primary function, they secrete larger amounts than the adrenal cortex and, in the female, secrete them in a very cyclic manner to regulate the menstrual cycle, support pregnancy, and prepare for lactation.

The testes and ovaries are related to the root chakra located at the base of the lumbar vertebrae in the lower abdomen near the genitals and womb. The function of this chakra is desire, pleasure, sexuality, and procreation, with the attraction of opposites.

The two primary female sex hormones are estrogen and progesterone. Male sex hormones are called *androgens*. The main male sex hormone is testosterone. All help develop and maintain primary sexual characteristics. Sexual behavior, male and female brain development, and gender influences have been directly linked to concentrations of these hormones. Testosterone has an effect on the sex drive (libido) for both men and women. Sex hormones influence biologic function and behavior throughout life. Males and females are most similar in the beginning and end of life, with the greatest differences from puberty to mid-life (the reproductive years), when these hormones are more active.

These sex hormones have other effects on the body. Estrogen, progesterone, and androgens affect epithelial and connective tissue and circulation. Continuing research concerning the sex hormones secreted by the adrenal glands indicates functions of these hormones other than reproduction. It is known that testosterone, along with other androgens, influences hair growth and distribution of hair in both men and women. Androgens also affect the skin and are a factor in acne development.

Androgens and estrogens exert their major influence at puberty. Androgens in particular stimulate growth and maturation of bone, cartilage, and muscle. Low levels of estrogens promote growth, whereas high levels inhibit growth. Beyond puberty, androgens increase hemoglobin levels, whereas estrogen protects against bone loss and epidermal tissue atrophy. Estrogen can also be synthesized by adipose tissue, which converts naturally occurring androgens.

Besides the primary sex hormones, the ovaries produce relaxin, a hormone that relaxes and dilates the cervix near the end of pregnancy and relaxes pelvic and pubic ligaments to prepare for delivery. The ovaries also produce inhibin, the hormone that inhibits FSH and LH after ovulation and during pregnancy. The testes produce inhibin, which controls sperm production.

THE PINEAL GLAND

The pineal is a tiny gland inside the brain within the diencephalon and surrounded by pia mater. All the functions of this gland have not been identified. To add to the gland's mysticism, it is located in the position of the "third eye" in many Eastern philosophies. It is related to either the crown or brow chakra, depending on the Eastern discipline. The functions of this chakra area are concerned with inner sight or awareness.

Serotonin, norepinephrine, dopamine, histamine, and other neurotransmitters and hormones have been identified from this gland, but its major function seems to be to secrete melatonin. The gland is light sensitive and is involved with regulating the rhythmic patterns of the body. The pineal gland also produces a hormone that stimulates secretion of aldosterone by the adrenal cortex.

It has long been known that many body rhythms move in step with one another or are entrained. Body temperature, pulse, hormone concentrations, and the sleep-wake cycles seem to follow the same "beat" over approximately a 24-hour period. Many of these rhythms are activated by the influences of light on the biologic clock of the hypothalamus. Melatonin secretion is inhibited when light reaches the eyes and enhanced during darkness. Light produces melatonin-mediated effects on reproductive, eating, and sleeping patterns. People are influenced by light intensity, spectrum (color mixture), and timing (day/night or seasonal changes).

Such conditions as illness, drug use, jet travel, alteration of eating pattern, weather changes, changing to the night shift, or other disruptions in the sleep/wake cycle can throw these rhythms out of sync. When these rhythms are disrupted, we experience mood changes, the immune function is affected, digestion is altered, and the entire homeostatic balance is unsettled. Researchers have identified a relatively common emotional disorder called seasonal affective disorder (SAD) in which mood swings are grossly exaggerated. As the days grow shorter each fall, people with SAD become irritable, anxious, sleepy, and socially withdrawn. Their appetite becomes insatiable; they crave carbohydrates and gain weight readily. Phototherapy, the use of very bright lights, for up to 2 hours daily reversed these symptoms in nearly 90% of people studied and was more effective than the use of antidepressant drugs in the research. When people stopped receiving phototherapy or were given melatonin, their symptoms returned as quickly as they had lifted, indicating that melatonin may be a key to seasonal mood changes also.

Symptoms of SAD are virtually identical to those of individuals with carbohydrate-craving obesity (CCO) and premenstrual syndrome (PMS), except that CCO sufferers are affected daily and PMS sufferers are affected monthly. Phototherapy relieves PMS symptoms in some women according to some research.

People who work all night exhibit reversed melatonin secretion patterns. When they are exposed to light during the night, no hormone is released; during daytime sleeping hours, high levels of melatonin are secreted. If these people are awakened from sleep and exposed to bright light, their melatonin levels drop. The same sort of melatonin inversion occurs in those who fly from coast to coast. This causes sleep patterns to be disrupted. Anything that disrupts sleep will eventually cause widespread stress in the body.

People have worshipped the sun since the earliest times. Many ancient healing rituals were timed with the rising or setting of the sun. The cycles of the moon are also important in biologic rhythm regulation. Some native traditions refer to the menstrual cycle as the moon time because women would usually menstruate during the full moon. The word lunatic is derived from lunar or the moon because tradition has attributed increased emotional behavior on the full moon.

Not only are we deficient in natural light we are also dark starved. The drastic increase in insomnia and disruptive sleep patterns has been influenced by exposure to artificial light well beyond the natural cycle. Our bodies are out of touch with the natural rhythms they were designed to follow, which places more stress on our systems. Artificial lights do not provide the full spectrum of sunlight. Incandescent bulbs used in homes primarily provide red wavelengths, whereas fluorescent bulbs used in many businesses and schools provide yellow-green wavelengths. Animals exposed for long periods to artificial lighting exhibit reproductive abnormalities and an enhanced susceptibility to cancer. Could it be that some of us are unknowingly experiencing the same effects?

Scientists are just now beginning to understand the reasons for these effects, and as they do, they are increasingly distressed about windowless offices, restricted and artificial illumination of work areas, and the growing number of institutionalized and isolated individuals who rarely feel the energy of the sun, the natural rhythm of the moon, or the quieting enveloping of the dark.

PRACTICAL APPLICATION

Effective sleep patterns can be supported by relaxation methods, including soft tissue and movement therapies. Sleep patterns can be reestablished by adhering to a bedtime and wake-time schedule. It seems important to sleep in the dark and experience adequate natural light during the day. Moderate exercise during the day and a gentle stretching program before retiring is beneficial. Eating on a regular schedule also reinforces the rhythm pattern (Activity 6-11).

ACTIVITY 6-11

Develop a daily schedule that supports biologic rhythms, particularly those mediated by the pineal gland. Carry this schedule from wake-up to bedtime.

Example

5:30 AM—Wake up
5:45 AM—Quiet mediation
6:00 AM—Exercise outside in rising sun
7:30 AM—Breakfast

Your Turn

THE THYMUS

The thymus gland is located deep to the sternum and mediastinum of the thorax and between the lungs at the level of T4 or T5. Often considered part of the lymphatic system and identified as the master gland of the immune system, it does have endocrine secretions. Its hormones are thymopoietin, thymic humoral factor (THF), thymic factor (TF), and thymosin. These hormones function in the growth and development of T cell lymphocytes of the immune system. The thymus is relatively large in children, providing some evidence that its production of hormones may slow down with the aging process.

The thymus is located in the general region of the heart and is related to the heart and spleen chakras with the functions of love, compassion, and transformation in Eastern doctrine.

OTHER ENDOCRINE TISSUES

Endocrine glands are not the only tissues that secrete hormones. Numerous cells and tissues throughout the brain, gut, and cardiovascular system produce hormones as well. As an example, the placenta is an endocrine gland. The following are a few of the major hormones produced throughout the body.

Endorphins

Endorphins belong to a family of peptide hormones that have many different effects, but especially work like morphine to suppress pain. They are synthesized in the brain, primarily in the anterior lobe of the pituitary, and bind to receptors in the brain that increase pain thresholds. Endorphins appear to enhance the release of thyroid-releasing hormone from the hypothalamus and also influence the neurosecretion of vasopressin, ACTH, and growth hormone. Endorphins influence mood, producing a mild euphoric feeling such as that seen in runner's high. They also help control body temperature; assist with memory and learning; and help regulate sex hormones that control puberty, sex drive, and reproduction. Endorphins are a factor in mental illness, especially schizophrenia and depression.

ACTIVITY 6-12

Review all the hormone functions described in this chapter and make an intuitive choice by picking the one gland you believe needs the most consideration in the support of your personal homeostasis and endocrine health. Justify the choice. After this choice, design a support program for yourself that includes a form of soft tissue and movement therapy.

Example

Thyroid—The idea that the thyroid is linked to communication and creativity intrigues me because a large part of my day is involved in communicating to teach others. Also, the link to metabolism and oxygen consumption seems relevant to my busy lifestyle. Because osteoporosis is a concern and healthy thyroid function supports proper bone density, it would serve me to support my thyroid function.

Program—The hypothalamus stimulates thyroid function in response to cold. As a program to support thyroid function, I could first take a warm shower in the morning and then turn the water to a cold shower. I could seek out a polarity practitioner and work on balancing my throat chakra. I could also increase my exercise walking pace to support oxygen delivery to the cells. Investigation of nutritional support for the thyroid along with a sound diet would be appropriate.

Your Turn
Gland—

Program—

PRACTICAL APPLICATION

Research has shown that massage and acupuncture stimulate the release of endorphins, supporting the use of these methods in pain management.

Atrial Natriuretic Factor (ANH)

Besides its obvious function, the heart is part of the endocrine system. Specific cells located in the right atrium produce atrial natriuretic hormone. As the fibers are stretched when blood returns to the heart, the hormone is released. It works like a calcium channel blocker, inhibiting aldosterone secretion, thus lowering blood pressure by increasing the amount of water excreted. It also inhibits the release of ADH, resulting in the same effect.

Erythropoietin

If oxygen levels in the body decrease, erythropoietin is produced in the kidneys and stimulates the production of red blood cells in the bone marrow.

Insulin-like Growth Factor (IGF-I)

Insulin-like growth factor (IGF-I) is produced primarily in the liver and looks like the insulin molecule. It is released in response to growth hormone. IGF-I stimulates the growth in target cells of insulin and matrix production in cartilage and fibroblast growth in connective tissue; it also synthesizes lipids and glycogen in adipose tissue.

Gastrointestinal Hormones

Gastrointestinal (GI) hormones were the first hormones discovered. They are produced in the mucosa of the GI tract and released when food is present to help regulate digestion. Although many types are produced, a brief overview of three of the most prominent follows.

Gastrin is produced in the mucosal cells of the stomach and duodenum and stimulates the release of hydrochloric acid and pepsin from the stomach. *Secretin,* produced by the small intestine, stimulates the release of pancreatic digestive enzymes. *Cholecystokinin (CCK)* is produced in the mucosa of the intestine and secreted into the bloodstream. It controls digestion on the basis of the amount of food located in the GI tract. CCK causes the release of bile from the gallbladder, stimulates the pancreas to release its digestive enzymes, and inhibits the secretion of stomach enzymes.

Tissue Hormones

Unlike most hormones that travel to distant target cells, most of the tissue hormones work in the vicinity of or on the exact organs where they are found. These local hormones are called *prostaglandins* (PGs) and are a group of about 14 unsaturated fatty acid hormones. PGs are important and extremely powerful substances found in a wide variety of tissues. They play an important role in communication and control of many body functions but do not meet the definition of a typical hormone. PGs are very specific, highly concentrated, and the shortest acting of the naturally occurring biologic compounds. They are important in overall endocrine regulation and vascular, metabolic, GI, reproductive, respiratory, and inflammatory functions.

PGs and histamines are released during inflammation, resulting in vasodilation and pain. Aspirin and other antiinflammatory agents act as analgesics by inhibiting the synthesis of PGs. Aspirin also acts as an anticoagulant by preventing the release of the PGs that cause platelet clumping (Activity 6-12).

Summary

Endocrine functions coordinate most body functions in concert with the nervous system. The nervous system functions as the yang portion, working quickly, expending energy, and responding to demand, whereas the endocrine system functions as the yin, sustaining, coordinating, and restoring physiologic function. The wisdom of ancient healing arts combines with the concreteness of scientific understanding to validate the wonder of human form and function. These two systems of control (the nervous system and the endocrine system) provide the organic basis for the healing mysteries. As our understanding increases, it is likely that more of the knowledge found in Eastern and Western healing traditions; ancient and future thought; and body, mind, and spirit will blend into our understanding.

WORKBOOK SECTION

1. What are the traditional endocrine glands?

    _____

    _____

    _____

    _____

2. What are endocrine tissues? Give examples.

    _____

    _____

    _____

    _____

3. What are the functions of hormones?

    _____

    _____

    _____

    _____

    _____

4. What is the difference between hormones and neurotransmitters?

    _____

    _____

    _____

    _____

5. Briefly describe hypersecretion and its causes.

    _____

    _____

    _____

    _____

6. Briefly describe hyposecretion and its causes.

    _____

    _____

    _____

    _____

FILL IN THE BLANK

The main differences between endocrine system and nervous system control are speed and duration of effect. The nervous system is _____ (1) with a _____ (2) duration of effect, whereas the endocrine system is _____ (3) with a _____ (4) duration of effect.

The concentration of a _____ (5) in the blood is determined by the rate of release and the speed of inactivation and removal from the body. The term _____ (6) is used to describe the time required for half of the hormone to be eliminated from the bloodstream. Hormones are secreted by endocrine glands and other specialized cells into the bloodstream to bind to specific _____ (7) on or in their _____ (8). In a _____ (9) mechanism, hormones will bind only to receptor molecules that fit them exactly.

The _____ (10) is the link between the body/mind and the nerve endocrine function. During stress, it translates nerve impulses into hormone secretions by endocrine glands. The _____ (11), or hypophysis, is located in the head at about eye level. It sits in a recessed area in the sphenoid bone. It secretes hormones that regulate growth, fluid balance, lactation, and childbirth.

The _____ (12) gland lies on the trachea below the thyroid cartilage. It consists of a right and left lobe connected by a bridge (isthmus), resulting in a butterfly shape. It regulates metabolism in the body by maintaining an adequate amount of oxygen consumption at the cellular level.

The _____ (13) glands are made up of four round, pea-sized bodies located on the posterior surface of the thyroid lobes. Their hormone, parathormone (PTH), when combined with vitamin D, decreases the amount of calcium excreted, causes the release of calcium from bone, and absorbs more calcium from the gastrointestinal tract, resulting in an increase in blood levels of calcium and phosphorus.

The _____ (14) is a long, slender gland located behind the stomach. It is both an exocrine and endocrine gland.

We have two _____ (15) glands, one on top of each of our kidneys. Each gland consists of an outer layer called the cortex and inner portion called the medulla.

The _____ (16) are the male and female gonads. They are located in the pelvic cavity and produce sex hormones identical to those of the adrenal cortex.

The _____ (17) is a tiny gland inside the brain within the diencephalon and is surrounded by pia mater. The complete functions of this gland have not been identified. Serotonin, norepinephrine, dopamine, histamine, and other neurotransmitters and hormones have been identified from this gland, but its major function seems to be to secrete melatonin. The gland is light sensitive and is involved with regulating the rhythmic patterns of the body.

The _____ (18) gland is located deep to the sternum and mediastinum of the thorax and between the lungs at the level of T4 to T5. Often considered part of the lymphatic system and identified as the master gland of the immune system, it does have endocrine secretions.

PROBLEM-SOLVING EXERCISE

Read the problem presented. There is no correct answer. Instead, the exercise assists the student in the development of analysis and decision-making skills necessary in a professional practice.
1. Identify the facts presented in the information.
2. Identify the possibilities ("what if" statements) presented or develop your own possibilities that relate to the facts.
3. Evaluate each possibility in terms of the logical cause and effect and pros and cons.
4. Consider the feelings of the people involved.
5. Write down each in the space provided.
6. Develop your solution by answering the question posed.

PROBLEM

In the subclinical or early onset stages of many endocrine dysfunctions the symptoms are vague and may be easily mistaken for stress-related disease. More than any area of pathology, people may seek soft tissue and movement therapists to deal with what seem to be simple stress-related symptoms. In reality, many forms of stress-induced disease are endocrine related and can actually be managed by stress management lifestyle changes. Who is to know that a heavy stress load is not causing a substantial amount of endocrine dysfunction? Could it be possible that some early-stage endocrine dysfunction resolves itself when the body is better able to handle the stress load? Would the client be best served if stress management and a healthy lifestyle were the first intervention?

Of concern is the need to refer those with endocrine symptoms for proper diagnosis and the willingness for the medical community to take a look at symptoms of early-onset endocrine dysfunction. Changes in lifestyle and more generalized health approaches that support homeostasis can be used successfully after a thorough medical workup.

On the other side of this issue, even if a referral for diagnosis is made, it sometimes feels like we have to be really sick before the condition can be identified by standard laboratory tests. What do low or high "normals" mean? Are these ends of the normal spectrum the beginning of dysfunction? What is normal anyway? Endocrine function is so variable, depending on so many physiologic factors, that the result of medical tests could be easily questioned. Maybe running the same test on different days would give a more reliable norm for a particular person. Soft tissue and movement therapists need to be observant of subtle symptoms that could indicate endocrine dysfunction and refer to other health care professionals.

QUESTION

What is the responsibility for referral by the bodywork therapist and what type of education is necessary to support educated decisions in these matters? Analyze the information to formulate your response to the question posed. An example is provided as a guide to get you started, then you fill in at least two more statements.

Facts:
1. In the subclinical or early onset stages of many endocrine dysfunctions, the symptoms are vague and may be easily mistaken for stress-related disease.

2. _____
_____

3. _____
_____

Possibilities:
1. Bodywork therapists may not be adequately trained to recognize these symptoms.

2. _____
_____

3. _____
_____

Logical cause and effect and pros and cons:
1. Because the symptoms are not recognized, the bodywork practitioner may not refer clients.

2. _____
_____

3. _____
_____

Effect on people:
1. People may be confused by the symptoms and not understand the referral.

2. _____
_____

3. _____
_____

What is the responsibility for referral of the bodywork therapist and what type of education is necessary to support educated decisions in these matters?

_____

_____

_____

_____

_____

_____

_____

_____

_____

FURTHER STUDY

Using a comprehensive anatomy and physiology text (see Works Consulted list at the back of this book), identify chapters pertaining to the information presented in this chapter. Locate the information presented in this text and then elaborate by writing a paragraph of additional information on each of the following:

Hypothalamus:

_____

_____

_____

_____

_____

_____

_____

Growth hormone:

_____

_____

_____

_____

_____

_____

_____

_____

Type II, or non–insulin-dependent, diabetes:

_____

_____

_____

_____

_____

_____

_____

_____

Aldosterone:

_____

_____

_____

_____

_____

_____

_____

Pineal gland:

_____

_____

_____

_____

_____

_____

Thymus:

_____

_____

_____

_____

_____

_____

_____

Prostaglandins:

_____

_____

_____

_____

_____

_____

_____

PROFESSIONAL APPLICATION

Refer to Chapter 2 of this text to review negative feedback loops. Remember, if a stimulus (stress) disrupts homeostasis in a controlled condition monitored by receptors, afferent receptors send input to a control center. The signal is interpreted and output responses to effectors are sent to bring about a change or response that alters the controlled condition, returning it to balance.

If the response reverses the original stimulus, it is a negative feedback system. **Negative feedback systems** stabilize physiologic function and are responsible for maintaining a constant internal environment. Most feedback systems are of this type.

Identify a hyposecretion and hypersecretion pathologic condition resulting from a failure of the negative feedback loop control. Then develop a plan for using soft tissue and movement therapies to support the care received by the primary physician. Justify each recommendation.

Complete the following:

1. Identify the hormone and gland.

2. Identify the pathologic condition.

3. List possible medical interventions.

4. Develop the support care plan.

5. Justify the plan.

Hypersecretion:

1. _____

2. _____

3. _____

4. _____

5. _____

Hyposecretion:

1. _____

2. _____

3. _____

4. _____

5. _____

Answer Key

1. Pituitary, thyroid, parathyroid, adrenal, pineal, and thymus. Also the pancreas, ovaries, testes, and hypothalamus.

2. They are separate tissues in the body that secrete hormones. They include the heart and intestinal mucous membranes.

3. They mobilize the body's defenses against stressors; maintain electrolyte, water, and nutrient balance in the blood; and regulate cellular metabolism and energy balance. They direct the creation of our form, especially during reproduction, growth, and development.

4. The main difference is location. When they are found in the bloodstream or in a tissue, they are called hormones. When found in the synapses, they are neurotransmitters.

5. Hypersecretion is the release of too much hormone. It is often caused by tumors, immune system dysfunction (autoimmunity), and failure of the feedback mechanisms to regulate secretion.

6. Many factors can cause a gland to reduce its hormonal output. Hyposecretion may be caused by tumors, tissue death, or abnormal operation of the regulatory feedback loops. Abnormal immune function can also reduce hormonal output, as well as insensitivity of the target cells to tropic hormones.

FILL IN THE BLANK

1. fast acting
2. short
3. slow acting
4. long
5. hormone
6. half-life
7. receptors
8. target cells
9. lock-and-key
10. hypothalamus
11. pituitary
12. thyroid
13. parathyroid
14. pancreas
15. adrenal
16. testes and ovaries
17. pineal
18. thymus

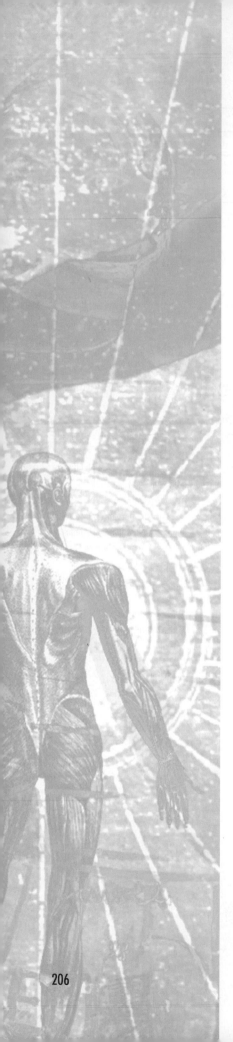

Section Three

The Body Moves

CHAPTER 7 THE SKELETAL SYSTEM
CHAPTER 8 THE JOINTS
CHAPTER 9 THE MUSCLES
CHAPTER 10 BIOMECHANICS BASICS

Soft tissue and movement professionals directly interact with the musculoskeletal system more than with any other body system. Because the musculoskeletal system and the rest of the body are interdependent, through the anatomy of this system we are able to influence the physiology of the entire body, supporting the maintenance of homeostasis.

A major portion of this text is devoted to the study of the anatomy of bones, joints, and muscles; the parts, we might say—and the body has lot of parts. Through an understanding of the design of movement, we can appreciate the physiology (function) of movement. This information will benefit the student in two ways:

- First, this knowledge is the foundation for the primary technical requirements of the soft tissue and movement discipline (e.g., therapeutic massage, shiatsu, polarity, yoga, and therapeutic exercise).
- Second, the student will be better able to work with other health care and service professionals as part of an interdisciplinary team, sharing information and treatments so as to best serve each client.

This unit begins with the study of the bones and ends with lessons in developing skills in assessment procedures, used to evaluate human movement, or biomechanics. The successive chapters build on each other, so that when the student reaches Chapter 10, Biomechanics Basics, she will be familiar with the terminology that describes biomechanics. With a solid foundation, the student will be able to predict the movement pattern of a particular bone, joint, or muscle unit.

Students should set themselves the following goals for this section:

1. Learn the names and landmarks of the bones and muscles.
2. Identify the attachment points of a muscle or group of muscles (the bones to which the ends of the muscle or muscles attach).
3. Identify the bones that move when the muscles contract and shorten. Usually one bone remains still while the other bone or bones are pulled toward or away from it. The point of motion is the joint.
4. Identify the types of action; for example, flexion, extension, and rotation.

Throughout the study of this section, the student will find it beneficial to refer to previous chapters to reinforce the knowledge and terminology needed to understand how we move.

Many references were consulted in the development of this section. Not all authorities agree on the specifics of the anatomy or the function of the musculoskeletal system. The most commonly accepted information has been adapted for use in this text.

Important clinicians, researchers, and teachers have been major influences in the development of this section; they include Dr. Janet Travell, Dr. David Simons, Dr. John Mennell, Dr. Philip Greenman, Dr. Leon Chaitow, Dr. David Gurvich, and Dr. John Warfel, to name a few.

The major resource for the activities in Chapter 10 was the classic text by Helen Hislop and Jacqueline Montgomery, *Daniels and Worthingham's Muscle Testing Techniques of Manual Examination*, first published in 1946 and now in its sixth edition (1995). The methods have been adapted and simplified for this text. Florence Kendall's "Muscle Testing Video Library" was a valuable tool in this simplification process. Another text used extensively in the development of Chapter 10 was *Therapeutic Exercise Foundations and Techniques* (third edition), by Carolyn Kisner and Lynn Allen Colby. These texts are listed in the Works Consulted section of this book.

All of these individuals, as well as countless others, supplied the base of information that has been organized for presentation in this section. It is important to remember and honor those who have gone before us.

Chapter 7

The Skeletal System

CHAPTER OUTLINE

Skeletal System Basics
Main functions of the skeletal system
Bones
Bone structure
Bone development
Articular cartilage
Ligaments
Classification of bones
Bone growth and repair
Skeletal changes caused by aging
Bony landmarks
Depressions and openings
Processes that form joints
Processes to which tendons and ligaments attach
Divisions of the skeleton

Individual Bony Framework by Region
Bones of the axial skeleton
Framework of the head
Framework of the trunk
Bones of the thorax
Bones of the appendicular skeleton
Bones of the upper division
Bones of the lower division

Pathology
Developmental problems
Spina bifida
Cleft palate
Osteogenesis imperfecta
Clubfoot (talipes)
Spinal curve abnormalities
Bone demineralization disorders
Osteoporosis
Paget's disease
Osteitis fibrosa cystica
Disorders caused by radiation therapy
Necrosis
Osteonecrosis or ischemic necrosis
Legg-Calvé-Perthes disease
Scheuermann's disease
Osteochondritis dissecans

CHAPTER OBJECTIVES

After completing this chapter, the student should be able to perform the following:

- List the seven main functions of the skeletal system.
- Describe the structure and development of bone.
- List and describe the six shapes of bone.
- Identify bony landmarks.
- Describe the two divisions of the skeleton and list the bones in each.
- List and describe the individual bones of the body by region.

KEY TERMS

Appendicular (ap-en-DIK-u-lar) *skeleton* The part of the skeleton composed of the limbs and their attachments.

Articulation (ar-tik-u-LAY-shun) Another word for joint, the structure created when bones connect to each other.

Axial (AK-see-al) *skeleton* The axis of the body; the axial skeleton consists of the head, vertebral column (the spine), and the ribs and sternum. It provides the body with form and protection.

Compact (dense) bone The hard portion of bone that protects spongy bone and provides the firm framework of the bone and the body. The osteocytes in this type of bone are located in concentric rings around a central haversian canal, through which nerves and blood vessels pass.

Endoskeleton The bony support structure found inside the human body; it accommodates growth.

Endosteum (en-DOSS-tee-um) A thin membrane of connective tissue that lines the marrow cavity of a bone.

Periosteum (PAIR-ee-OSS-tee-um) The thin membrane of connective tissue that covers bones except at articulations.

Piezoelectric (PIE-eh-zoh-EE-lek-trik) The quality of bones that allows them to deform slightly and vibrate when electrical currents pass through them and to produce minute electric current when deformed or compressed. Bone formation patterns follow lines of stress load directed by the piezoelectric currents.

Sesamoid (SES-ah-moyd) *bones* Round bones that often are embedded in tendons and joint capsules. The largest of these is the patella.

Spongy (cancellous) bone The lighter weight portion of bone, which is made up of trabeculae.

Trabeculae (tra-BEK-u-lee) An irregular meshing of small, bony plates that makes up spongy bone; its spaces are filled with red marrow.

What would we look like if we didn't have bones? Picture yourself as a mass of soft tissue with little form. Managing the forces of gravity would be almost impossible without the structure supplied by our skeletons. Getting from one place to another would be difficult. We would certainly be more susceptible to injury as we slithered around. Is it possible that we have taken our skeletons for granted? As we explore the most concrete aspect of our anatomy—the skeletal system—we will appreciate its functions even more, considering what life would be like without it (Activity 7-1).

Human beings have an **endoskeleton,** which means that our support structure is inside us and we grow around it. Some animals, such as lobsters, have an *exoskeleton,* a support structure that is on the outside of the body. Although an exoskeleton is appropriate for a lobster, it is not for a human being. Because an exoskeleton does not grow at the same rate as the rest of the body, it can become too small; also, it needs to be shed as a new one is grown. With an endoskeleton, growth is accommodated easily.

ACTIVITY 7-1

Draw a picture of a human being without bones.

In this section we will study the bones first. Because muscles attach to bones, learning the names, functions, and various landmarks of the bones helps in locating the muscles studied later in this section. Other chapters focus on the joints, on biomechanics, and on kinesiology (the action of muscles on joints in movement patterns).

Skeletal System Basics

The skeletal system comprises the bones, joints, and related connective tissues. The connective tissue component is extremely important to the functioning of the system. Because the bones do not have enough room for all the muscles to attach, the membranes between the bones and the ligaments at the joints function to expand the skeletal structure, allowing adequate space for muscle attachments. When the structures of the muscles and bones are combined, they form the functional unit known as the musculoskeletal system.

Bones connect at a joint, which is also known as an **articulation.** Bones are held together at joints by ligaments and other connective tissues. Muscles contract to produce the actions that move the joints. The actions of skeletal muscles are voluntary, coordinated by the nervous system.

MAIN FUNCTIONS OF THE SKELETAL SYSTEM

Besides the obvious functions of support and motion, bones have other extremely important roles, including the following:

- Supporting soft tissues and serving as a framework for the entire body
- Providing attachment points for muscles and ligaments
- Protecting delicate internal organs such as the brain, spinal cord, heart, and lungs
- Serving as levers to provide movement begun by the attached muscles
- Storing calcium, phosphorus, and other minerals for release to the body as needed
- Storing lipids for use as energy
- Producing blood cells in the red marrow

BONES

No matter their size, shape, or location, all bones are made of the same fundamental cells and matrix, are covered with the same sheets of connective tissue, and are nourished and stimulated by the same variety of vessels and nerves. Bones develop into different shapes, which serve specific functions.

The protective bones of the skull differ in shape from the supportive and lengthening bones of the limbs. Disease, injury, and aging affect both the structure and function of bones. The location and shape of a bone determine its function. The function of a bone can change its structure through a remodeling process, supporting once again the theme of interacting structure and function in a continuous, interdependent cycle.

Bones are hard, dense, and slightly elastic organs of the skeleton. They have their own system of blood, lymphatic vessels, and nerves. The body has 206 bones, with some individual variations; for example, some people have more or fewer **sesamoid bones,** a type of bone that develops within a tendon or joint capsule, and others may have an extra rib. Although all bones support the body, store calcium and other minerals, and house marrow for the production of red blood cells, some bones play more specific roles. The skull and the vertebral column protect the brain and spinal cord, and the bones of the limbs allow motion.

Bones are composed chiefly of bone tissue, called *osseous tissue.* Bones are not lifeless, but rather everchanging. The spaces between the cells of bone tissue are permeated with stony deposits of inorganic mineral salts of calcium and phosphorus, along with small amounts of magnesium, potassium, and sodium and carbonate ions. The cells dispersed among these mineral deposits are very much alive.

Two thirds of bone tissue is made up of inorganic minerals, which provide rigidity, and one third of bone tissue is composed of organic material, which provides elasticity. We all understand the need for bone to be rigid, but few of us realize that bone is also somewhat flexible. Without this elasticity, bone would break readily.

Bones are subject to mechanical strain. They must support the weight of the body, disperse the impact shock of activities such as walking, running, and jumping, and withstand the force of muscle contractions.

Bones have a **piezoelectric** quality. Piezoelectric substances such as the collagen in bones, deform slightly and vibrate when electric currents pass through them. In reverse, when stretched, twisted, or compressed, bone produces minute electric currents; the strength and direction of these currents change with the direction of the stress load. Bone formation patterns follow lines of stress load directed by these piezoelectric currents. Exactly how this happens is not yet fully understood.

Many cultural and healing traditions assert that certain kinds of stones and other crystalline substances, particular quartz, have healing qualities. Some spiritual places reputed to have healing qualities are located in areas of stony form, particularly granite, are structures constructed of stone (often granite), or contain statues made of stone. Quartz is considered a piezoelectric material, and granite, often used in building and sculpture, has a high concentration of quartz. We do know that very small electric currents can accelerate the healing of broken bones. Does this show a connection? In what way do the very small electric currents generated by bone affect homeostasis? Could a physiologic connection exist between the healing disciplines that use stones and these qualities of bone? These traditions are cross-cultural, suggesting the existence of some underlying, physiologically unified thread. The questions are interesting; the connection is plausible (Activity 7-2).

ACTIVITY 7-2

If you were to speculate about the piezoelectric quality of bones and other collagen connective tissues, what do you think would be the effects of the compressive, stretching, and twisting action of touch and movement therapies? List three. An example is provided to get you started.

Example The electric current produced by compression against bone during soft type methods may stimulate the so-called energetic mechanism of meridians, because these Oriental energy lines generally follow bones.

Your Turn

1. _____
   _____
   _____

2. _____
   _____
   _____

3. _____
   _____
   _____

Bone Structure

Bones share four features that allow them to work together as parts of the skeleton. Despite the different shapes of bones, they have these attributes in common:

1. Hard cells and a rigid matrix give bones strength and shape to sustain weight and movement.
2. Bones usually articulate with other bones, thereby transferring forces and movement through the skeleton.
3. A connective tissue structure, called the **periosteum,** covers every bone and provides vessels for nutrition, bone cells for growth, and attachments for tendons and ligaments.
4. Oppositional growth of new bone matrix and remodeling of existing bone matrix are responsible for shaping bones.

The structure and function of bones are intrinsically connected. Bones remodel themselves constantly, depending on the functional demand. Although it may seem static, the skeletal system is one of the body's more dynamic systems.

Bone Development

In the embryo, bone development begins near the end of the second month. The process that creates our skeleton is called *ossification.* Ossification is a two-part process: first, *chondroblasts,* or cartilage-forming cells, create the cartilage model of bones. Then, *osteoblasts,* or bone-building cells, develop the bone tissue from the cartilage model. This process does not create the hard bones with which we are familiar. Instead, these cells remain soft and pliable, allowing the fetus to remain flexible in order to exit the body more easily during birth.

Shortly after birth, *calcification* takes place. This hardening of the bones, called *osteogenesis,* occurs as calcium salts are deposited in the gel-like matrix of the forming bones. *Osteocytes* are mature bone cells, which maintain the bone during our lifetime.

The different areas of a bone contain one of two types of tissue, compact bone or spongy bone. **Compact (dense) bone** has very little space between its tissues. This hard portion of the bone makes up the main shaft of the long bones and the outer layer of other bones. It protects spongy bone and provides the firm framework of the bone and the body. The osteocytes in this type of bone are located in concentric rings around a central haversian canal, through which nerves and blood vessels pass.

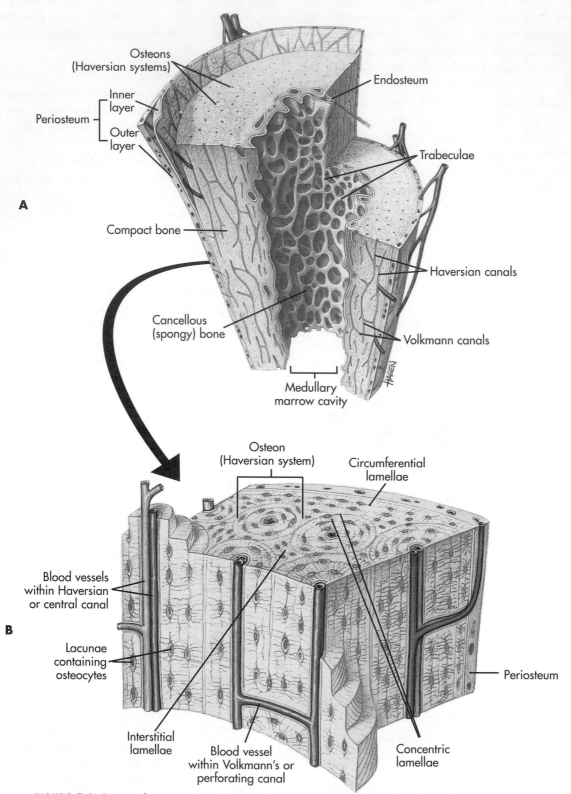

FIGURE 7-1   Structure of compact and cancellous bone. **A,** Longitudinal section of a long bone showing both cancellous and compact bone. **B,** Magnified view of compact bone.

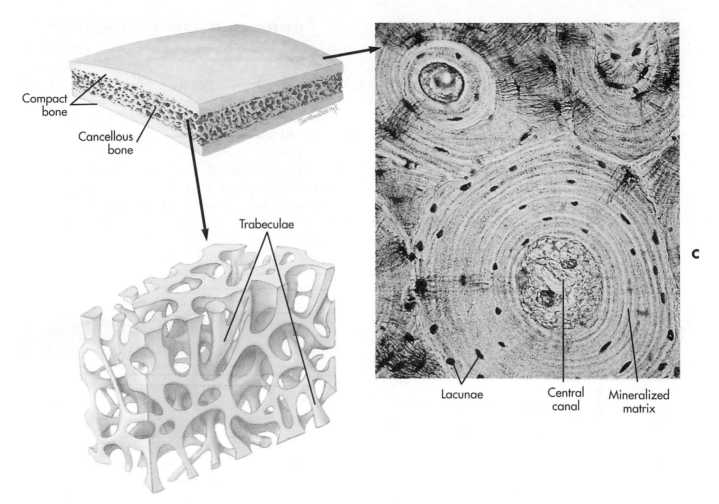

FIGURE 7-1, cont'd C, Section of a flat bone. Outer layers of compact bone surround cancellous bone. The fine structure of compact bone and cancellous bone is shown to the right. (From Thibodeau GA, Patton KT: *Anatomy and physiology,* ed 3, St Louis, 1996, Mosby.)

The second type, **spongy (cancellous) bone,** has larger spaces between cells than does compact bone, which makes the bones lighter in weight. Cancellous bone is made of an irregular meshing of small, bony plates, called **trabeculae,** and is found at the ends of the long bones or at the center of other bones. In some bones the trabecular spaces are filled with red marrow, which produces blood cells. Spongy bone tissue forms a supporting grid that can be altered mechanically by construction, destruction, or reorganization of the trabecular network. Piezoelectric current seems to be responsible for guiding these changes, which occur in response to postural change, muscle tension, and the stresses of weight.

Bones contain two kinds of marrow, red and yellow. *Red marrow,* which manufactures red blood cells, is found at the end of long bones and at the center of other bones of the thorax and pelvis. *Yellow marrow* of the "soup bone" type, which is largely fat, is found chiefly in the central cavities of the long bones.

Except for the ends that form joints, bones are covered with a thin membrane of connective tissue, which is called *periosteum.* On the inside of this membrane are osteoblasts, which are essential to bone formation during periods of growth and in the repair of bones. Blood and lymph vessels in the periosteum play an important role in the nourishment of bone tissue. Nerve fibers in the periosteum make their presence known when they are traumatized, such as when you get hit on the shin or fracture your arm.

A thinner membrane of connective tissue, called the **endosteum,** lines the marrow cavity of a bone; it, too, contains cells that aid in the growth and repair of bone tissue (Figure 7-1).

Articular Cartilage
Bones of synovial or movable joints make physical contact at their cartilaginous ends. The only remaining cartilage in bone is called *articular* (or *hyaline*) *cartilage;* articular cartilage is massaged by joint

movement, which aids the absorption of synovial fluid, oxygen, and nutrition. The degenerative process of arthritis involves the breakdown of articular cartilage. Cartilage is a form of connective tissue; it is smooth, slippery, porous, malleable, insensitive, and bloodless and is found wherever bones come together at synovial or freely movable joints. Because cartilage is an integral component of the synovial joint, it is discussed in more detail in Chapter 8.

Ligaments

Ligaments are dense bundles of parallel connective tissue fibers, primarily collagen. Ligaments connect bones and strengthen and stabilize the joints. They are not typically elastic nor do they have much stretch. Some joint positions place ligaments under tension, whereas other positions slacken them. Only a general mention of ligaments is made in this chapter. Because ligaments are specific to joint function, they also are discussed in more detail in Chapter 8.

CLASSIFICATION OF BONES

The bones of the skeleton are identified by their many different shapes. The customary classifications are as follows:

Flat bones: Generally more flat than round. Examples: the ribs and skull bones

Irregular bones: Have complex shapes that occur as two or more forms within the same bone structure. Examples: the vertebrae and scapula

Long bones: Longer in one axis than another. Bones of this type are characterized by a *medullary cavity,* a hollow *diaphysis,* or shaft of compact bone, and at least two *epiphyses,* which are active in the growth of long bones. Most of the bones of the arms and legs are long bones. The hollow structure of the diaphysis gives strength with light weight. Examples: the femur and ulna

Short bones: Shaped like long bones but much smaller. These bones make up the structures of the hands, fingers, feet, and toes. This shape of bone can also be classified as long bones. Example: the metacarpals

Cube-shaped bones (sometimes classified as short bones): Predominately cancellous bone with a thin cortex of compact bone and no cavity. Examples: the wrist bones (carpals) and ankle bones (tarsals)

Sesamoid bones: Round bones often embedded in tendons and joint capsules. Example: the patella.

BONE GROWTH AND REPAIR

In a long bone, the transformation of cartilage into bone begins at the center of the shaft. Later, secondary bone-forming centers develop across the ends of the bones at the epiphyses. The long bones continue to grow in length at these centers through childhood and into the late teens.

A growth spurt often is seen during puberty through the influence of the sex hormones estrogen and testosterone. Both hormones promote the growth of long bones; testosterone also increases bone density. At higher levels of estrogen, long bone growth stops; for this reason, women generally are shorter and have bones that are less dense than those of men (Activity 7-3).

ACTIVITY 7-3

Refer to Chapter 6, The Endocrine System, and explain the influence of the sex hormones on bone. Include the page number where you found the information.

An example is provided to get you started.

Example High estrogen levels slow the growth of girls, including the bones, at puberty (page 198).

Provide two more explanatory statements.

Your Turn

1.

2.

Identify two other hormones that affect bone formation. (*Hint:* see the sections in Chapter 6 on the thyroid and parathyroid glands.)

1.

2.

By the late teens or early twenties, again through the influence of the sex hormones, the epiphyses of the long bones close and the bones stop growing in length. Each bone-forming region hardens and can be seen in radiographic films as a thin line across the end of the bone. Physicians can judge the future growth of the bone by the appearance of these lines on the radiographic film.

As we grow, our bones widen and lengthen, and the central cavity follows this change in size. This all takes place because osteocytes are added in some areas of bone and reabsorbed in others.

As mentioned previously, children are more flexible because their bodies contain more cartilage and soft bone cells, since complete calcification has not yet taken place. In older adults, this is reversed; bone cells outnumber cartilage cells, and the bone is more brittle because it contains more minerals and fewer blood vessels. This makes the bones prone to fracture and slower to heal.

SKELETAL CHANGES CAUSED BY AGING

As we age, various changes occur in the skeleton. Loss of calcium begins earlier in women than in men. The bone matrix is not replaced as quickly because the

body produces less protein; this may lead to a problem with brittle bones. Also, bone fractures heal more slowly in elderly people. Beginning about age 40, the intervertebral disks begin to thin, and the average person loses ½ inch of height every 20 years. The vertebral bodies specifically lose height in our later years. The cartilage on the ribs calcifies, leading to a decrease in the diameter of the rib cage and a more barrel-shaped chest, caused by the lack of flexibility.

BONY LANDMARKS

The contour of bones varies and includes such configurations as flat areas, knobs, projections, spikes, dents, holes, and ridges. These landmarks often serve as regions for muscle attachment or provide passage or space for nerves and vessels. The student learns the bony landmarks, because this knowledge will assist her in learning muscle attachments later in this study (Activity 7-4).

Depressions and Openings
Canal: A tunnel or tube in bone. Example: the carotid canal in temporal bone
Fissure: A groove or slit between two bones. Example: the orbital fissure of the sphenoid bone
Foramen: An opening in a bone. Example: the verte-

ACTIVITY 7-4

For each of the landmarks listed, identify a metaphor that will help you remember what each represents. A few examples are provided to get you started.

Examples

Foramen: hula hoop

Groove: ditch

Sinus: cave

Now, make up some of your own.

Your Turn
Canal:

Fissure:

Foramen:

Fossa:

Groove:

Meatus:

Notch:

Sinus:

Sulcus:

Condyle:

Head:

Facet:

Process:

Trochlea:

Crest:

Epicondyle:

Spinous process, or spine:

Trochanter:

Tubercle:

Tuberosity:

bral foramen of the spinal column (through which the nerves pass)

Fossa: A depression in the surface or at the end of a bone. Example: the infraspinous and supraspinous fossae of the scapula

Groove: A depression in the bone that holds blood vessels, nerves, or tendons. Example: the radial groove of the humerus

Meatus: A tunnel or canal found in a bone. Example: the canal in the skull that extends from the external ear to the eardrum

Notch: An indentation or large groove. Example: the greater and lesser sciatic notches of the ilium

Sinus: An air cavity within a bone. Example: the frontal bones

Processes that Form Joints

Condyle: A rounded projection at the end of a bone that articulates with other bones to form a joint. Example: the medial condyle of the femur

Head: A rounded projection atop the neck of a bone. Example: the head of the femur

Facet: A smooth, flat surface. Example: the facet of a rib or vertebra

Process: Any prominent, bony growth that projects. Example: the olecranon process of the ulna

Trochlea: A pulley-shaped structure. Example: the trochlea of the humerus

Processes to Which Tendons and Ligaments Attach

Crest: A ridge on a bone. Example: the iliac crest

Epicondyle: A projection above a condyle. Example:

ACTIVITY 7-5

Match six similar sets of bones of the upper and lower appendicular skeleton. An example is provided.

Example Femur/humerus

Your Turn

1.

2.

3.

4.

5.

6.

the medial epicondyle of the femur

Line: A ridge that is smaller than a crest. Example: the linea aspera of the femur

Spinous process, spine, or spina: A sharp, bony or slender projection. Example: the spinous process of the vertebral column or scapula

Trochanter: One of two large, bony processes found only on the femur. Example: the greater or lesser trochanter

Tubercle: A small, rounded process. Example: the adductor tubercle of the femur

Tuberosity: A large, rounded protuberance. Example: the tibial tuberosity

DIVISIONS OF THE SKELETON

The skeleton is divided into two groups of bones: the axial skeleton and the appendicular skeleton.

The **axial skeleton,** which forms the axis of the body, consists of the head, vertebral column (spine), ribs, and sternum. It provides the body with form and protection. The **appendicular skeleton** is composed of the limbs of the body and their attachments (Activity 7-5). The shoulder and hip girdles, which have similar structures, are the connectors to the axial skeleton.

The long bones of the upper and lower limbs, in combination with the muscles, provide our fine and gross motor movements. Similar in design, these long bones are the humerus, radius, and ulna in the upper limbs and the femur, tibia, and fibula in the lower limbs. In the same manner, the short carpals of the wrist and the tarsals of the ankle allow for the flexibility needed in the hands and feet.

The six bones of the ear make up a third group of bones.

The more we study the basic construction of the skeletal system, the more we notice the elegant and simple pattern. Simplicity and repetition of form reflect this effective biomechanical design (Figure 7-2).

Individual Bony Framework by Region

BONES OF THE AXIAL SKELETON

Framework of the Head

The bony framework of the head, or skull, is made up of the cranial bones and the facial bones (Figure 7-3).

Eight cranial bones enclose and protect the brain:

- The *frontal bone* forms the forehead, the anterior portion of the roof of the skull, the top of the eye

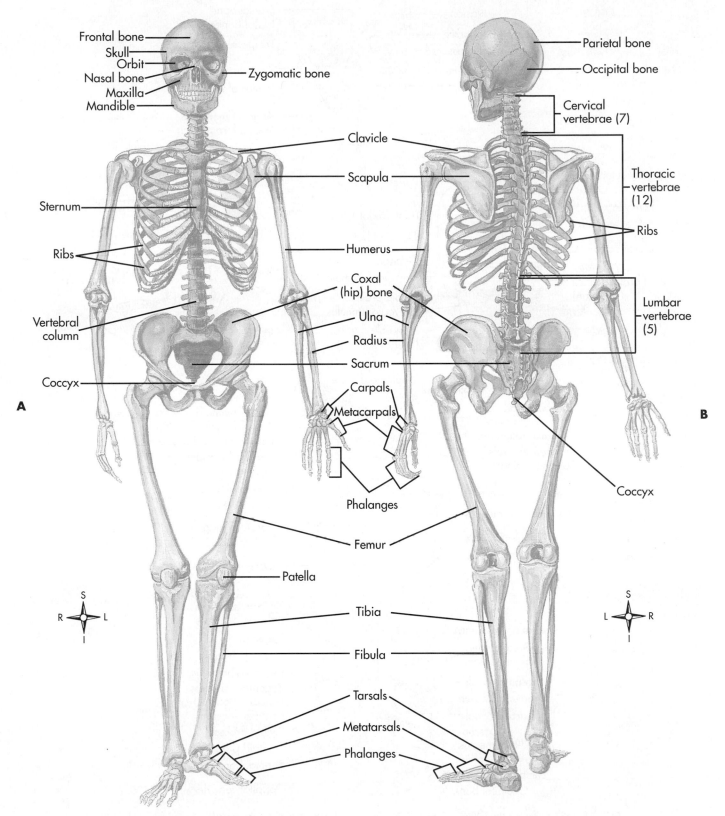

FIGURE 7-2 Skeleton. **A,** Anterior view. **B,** Posterior view. (From Thibodeau GA, Patton KT: *Anatomy and physiology,* ed 3, St Louis, 1996, Mosby.)

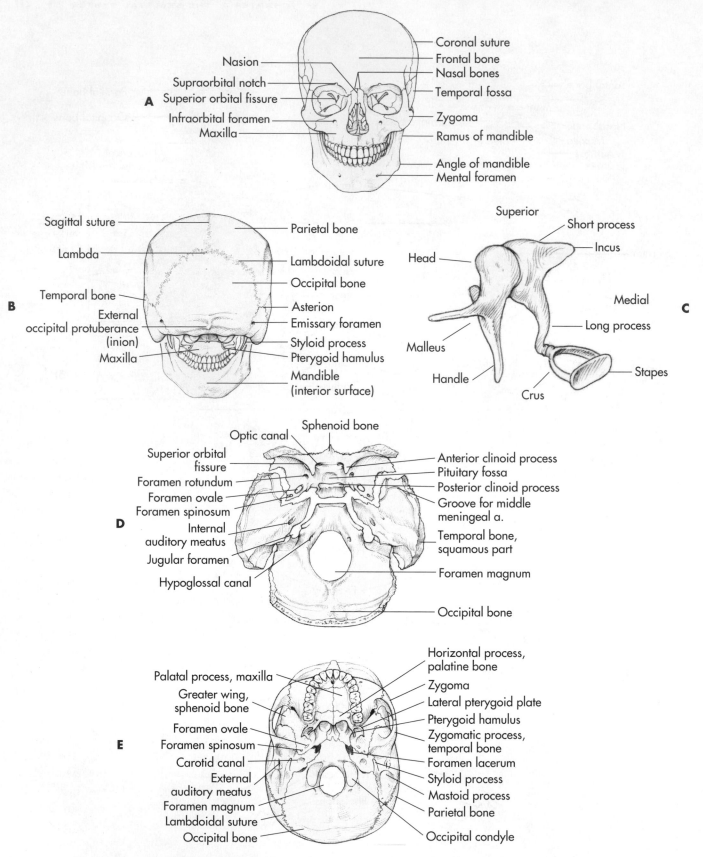

FIGURE 7-3 **A,** Anterior (frontal) view of the skull. **B,** Posterior view of the skull. **C,** The three ossicles. The malleus attaches to the inner surface of the tympanic membrane. The incus links the malleus to the stapes. The stapes is attached to the wall of the inner ear. **D,** Detailed view of the base of the skull. The sphenoid, occipital, and temporal bones are presented here as slightly separated to show that many of the important apertures traversing the floor of the skull are found within one of these bones or along their mutual borders. **E,** Basal view of the skull, showing several of the important foramina that convey nerves and vessels in and out of the cranial cavity. (From Mathers LH et al: *Clinical anatomy principles,* St Louis, 1996, Mosby.)

sockets, and part of the floor of the cranium. The frontal sinuses (air spaces) are within the frontal bone and open into the nasal cavities.

- Two *parietal bones* form most of the sides and top of the cranium.
- Two *temporal bones* form part of the side and part of the floor of the skull. Each temporal bone contains mastoid sinuses, an ear canal, an eardrum, and the middle and inner ears.
- The *ethmoid bone,* which is part of the anterior portion of the cranial floor, is a very light, spongy bone located between the eyes. It forms part of the medial wall of the eye sockets and most of the nasal roof. It contains some of the paranasal sinuses. An extension of the ethmoid bone forms most of the superior portion of the nasal septum. If this bone is fractured, its proximity to the brain means that cerebrospinal fluid (CSF) could leak into the nasal cavity. A runny nose that develops after a head injury could be the result of trauma to the sinuses or an indication of a serious condition.
- The *sphenoid bone* is in the middle of the base of the skull in front of the temporal bones. When viewed from above, it looks like a bat with its wings extended. The sphenoid sinuses are located within this bone. The *sella turcica,* or "Turkish saddle," is a cavity on the superior surface of the body of the sphenoid that supports the pituitary gland.
- The *occipital bone* forms the posterior portion and a large part of the base of the cranium. This large, curved bone provides attachments for muscles of the neck and trunk.

Fourteen facial bones form the front of the skull:

- The *mandible,* or lower jawbone, is the only voluntarily movable bone of the skull. The largest of the facial bones, it forms the chin, which is classified as a mental prominence. If the mandible is fractured, the upper and lower jaw may need to be immobilized by being wired together.
- Two *maxilla bones* unite to form the upper jawbone, part of the floor of the eye sockets, part of the roof of the mouth, including the front of the hard palate, and the outer walls and floor of the nasal cavity. Each maxilla contains the maxillary sinus, a large air space that empties into the nasal cavity.
- Two *zygomatic bones,* or cheekbones, form the prominences of the cheeks and a portion of the floor and outer wall of the eye sockets.
- Two small, oblong *nasal bones,* in the superior middle of the face, form the bridge of the nose.

- Two *lacrimal bones,* each about the size and shape of a fingernail, are posterior and lateral to the nasal bone. They form part of the medial wall of the eye sockets.
- The *vomer* is a triangular bone that forms the inferior and posterior nasal septum.
- Two L-shaped *palatine bones* form the posterior portion of the hard palate and part of the floor of the nasal cavity.
- Two *inferior nasal conchae* bones form a portion of the lateral wall of the nasal cavities. They work with the superior and middle conchae of the ethmoid bone to circulate and filter air that enters the nose.

In addition to the cranial and facial bones, other bones of the axial skeleton are found in the neck and head. The six *ossicles,* three in each middle ear, are discussed in Chapter 5. The *hyoid bone* is a U-shaped bone attached to the tongue. Although it is attached to the temporal bone by muscles and ligaments, it does not form an articulation with any other bones.

The structure of the skull is important to the function of other systems. Nerves and blood vessels enter and exit the skull through spaces, or foramina, in the base. Muscles attach to the various projections and prominences on the outside of the skull. The sinuses are air spaces that resonate the voice and remove some of the weight of the bones, making the head lighter (Figure 7-4).

Between the bones of the skull are specialized joints called *sutures.* The four most prominent sutures are the *sagittal suture,* between the parietal bones; the *lambdoid suture,* between the parietal bones and the occipital bone; the *coronal suture,* between the parietal bones and the frontal bones; and the *squamous suture,* between the temporal and parietal bones.

The infant skull

In the skull of an infant, bone formation is incomplete in some areas; these soft spots are called *fontanelles.* Found between the cranial bones, fontanels are formed from very dense connective tissue, which is replaced with bone as the infant grows. The fontanelles allow for compression of the skull as the infant travels through the birth canal and for expansion of the skull as the brain grows. They close when the child is 18 to 24 months old. The largest of the fontanelles is the *anterior fontanelle,* found near the front of the head at the junction between the two

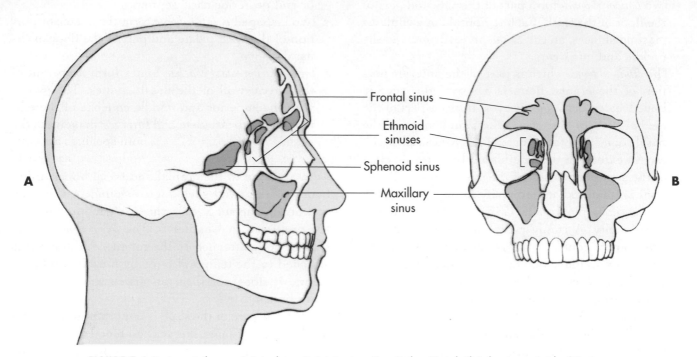

FIGURE 7-4 Air sinuses in the nose. **A,** Lateral view. **B,** Anterior view. (From Mathers LH et al: *Clinical anatomy principles,* St Louis, 1996, Mosby.)

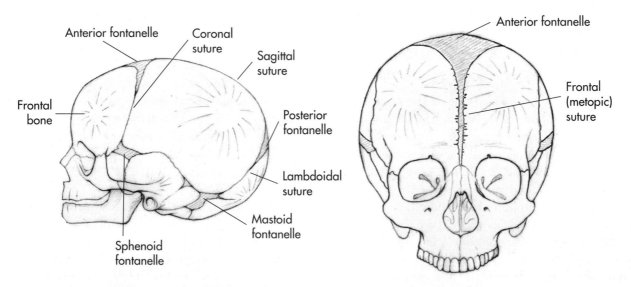

FIGURE 7-5 Infant skull. (From Mathers LH et al: *Clinical anatomy principles,* St Louis, 1996, Mosby.)

parietal bones and the frontal bone (Figure 7-5) (Activity 7-6).

Framework of the Trunk

The skeletal structure of the trunk is made up of the vertebral column and the bones of the chest. A child's vertebral column has 33 (or sometimes 34) irregularly shaped bones, which fuse in the lower portion to become 26 bones in the adult. Each of the vertebrae have two main sections, the anterior body and the posterior arch. All vertebrae, except the atlas and the axis, have the following characteristic features:

1. A drum-shaped *body*, or *centrum*, located toward the front (anterior), which serves as the weight-bearing portion of the bone

2. A *vertebral arch*, which is connected to the body by two *pedicles*—two *lamina* unite posteriorly to form the bony arch that encircles the spinal cord, called the *spinous process*. The spinous process usually can be felt just under the skin of the back. The thickened junctions between the pedicles and the laminae have superior and inferior cartilaginous articular facets and a laterally projecting *transverse process*.

3. Vertebrae that stack one on the other—each vertebra has a joint surface, called an *articular facet*, that provides the articulating surface for this stacking arrangement.

4. A large hole, or foramen, in the center of each vertebra—all the vertebrae are linked in a series by strong bands of connective tissue (ligaments), and these spaces form the spinal canal, a bony cylinder that protects the spinal cord. As the vertebrae stack, they form the *intervertebral foramina*, which allow passage of the spinal nerves.

Although not technically a part of the vertebrae, the *intervertebral disks* (or discs; both spellings are correct) between the vertebral bodies act as shock absorbers and spacers and provide flexibility. The disk consists of two components. The outer edge, or *annulus fibrosus*, is composed of concentric rings of fibrocartilage arranged like the layers of an onion. Internally, the center, or *nucleus pulposus*, is made of a gelatinous substance. If a disk ruptures, the fibrocartilage splits and the nucleus pulposus leaks. The disk becomes smaller and is less able to disperse pressure and maintain space between the vertebrae. In severe

ACTIVITY 7-6

The names of the eight cranial bones start with various letters. To help you remember them, make up a sentence that uses the first letter of each in whatever order works for you. Get creative!

Occipital

Parietal

Frontal

Temporal

Ethmoid

Sphenoid

Example Please Stop The Flying Ostrich Egg.

Your Turn

The facial bones are the following:

Nasal

Vomer

Lacrimal

Zygomatic

Palatine

Maxilla

Mandible

Inferior nasal concha

Make up a creative sentence that uses the first letter of each.

cases the vertebrae can impinge on nerves (Figures 7-6 and 7-7).

Ligaments

Three ligaments extend the length of the vertebral column. The *anterior longitudinal ligament* attaches to the front of the vertebral bodies and acts as a resis-

tance to extension. The *posterior longitudinal ligament* attaches to the back of the bodies and stabilizes flexion. The *supraspinous ligament* runs along the tips of the spinous processes and restrains flexion.

Other vertebral ligaments are placed between individual vertebra. The *ligamenta flava* connects the laminae of each adjacent vertebrae. The *interspinous*

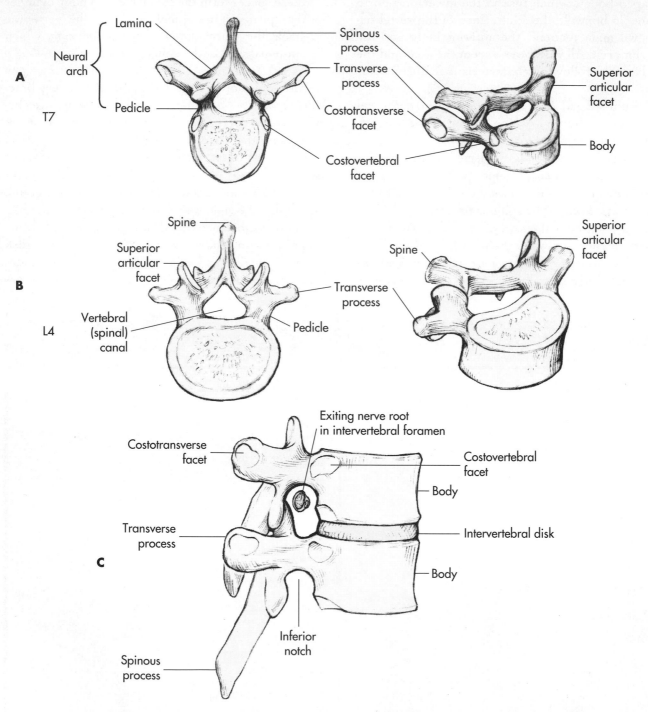

FIGURE 7-6   Common types of vertebrae (two views of T7 and L4 vertebrae). **A,** Superoinferior views. **B,** Right anterior oblique views. **C,** Intervertebral foramen. Vertebrae T5 and T6 have been articulated, and the resultant intervertebral foramen is shown with a segmental nerve in place. Blood vessels (not shown) enter and leave the interior of the vertebral canal through the intervertebral foramen. (From Mathers LH et al: *Clinical anatomy principles,* St Louis, 1996, Mosby.)

ligaments connect the spinous processes, and the *intertransverse ligaments* connect the transverse processes. Right-side bending stretches the left intertransverse ligaments and vice versa for left-side bending, which stretches the right intertransverse ligaments (Figure 7-8). Vertebral movement patterns are discussed in Chapter 8 (Activity 7-7).

The bones of the vertebral column are named and numbered on the basis of location, from the neck downward.

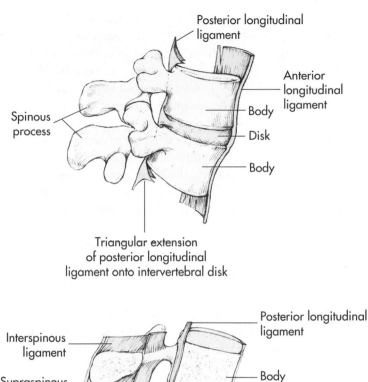

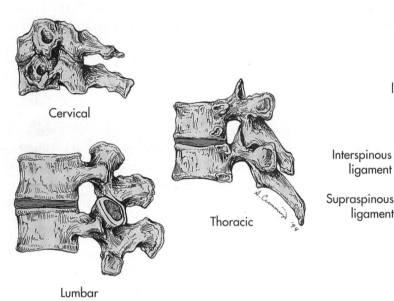

FIGURE 7-7 Three types of vertebrae. (Modified from Cramer GD, Darby SA: *Basic and clinical anatomy of the spine, spinal cord, and ANS,* St Louis, 1995, Mosby.)

FIGURE 7-8 Vertebral ligament. (From Mathers LH et al: *Clinical anatomy principles,* St Louis, 1996, Mosby.)

ACTIVITY 7-7

Draw either a thoracic or lumbar vertebra from the superior view and label the following areas. Be as accurate as you can without worrying about artistic ability. Looking at an anatomy picture or diagram will help.

Body (centrum)   Place drawing here.

Vertebral arch

Vertebral foramen

Pedicles

Lamina

Spinous process

Transverse process

Articular facet

Demifacets for ribs

Now draw two stack vertebrae and label the following:

Intervertebral disk   Place drawing here.

Intervertebral foramen

Anterior longitudinal ligament

Posterior longitudinal ligament

Supraspinous ligament

Ligamenta flava

Interspinous ligaments

Intertransverse ligaments

The seven *cervical vertebrae* (C1 to C7) are located in the neck. The first vertebra (C1), called the *atlas*, supports the head. When you nod your head "yes," the skull rocks on the atlas at the occipital condyles of the occipital bone. The atlas is greatly modified for articulation within the occipital region of the skull. It does not have a body or spinous process; rather, it essentially is a bony ring consisting of anterior and posterior arches and two lateral masses. The second cervical vertebra (C2), called the *axis*, serves as a pivot when the head is turned from side to side (as in the gesture "no"). It has a peglike *dens*, or *odontoid process*, projecting superiorly from its anterior side. The pivot joint of C1 to C2 consists of a ringlike structure that rotates around the dens. Considerable movement, especially as seen in rotation, is possible because of the design of this joint.

A strong, fibrous band called the *nuchal ligament*, runs along the notched spinous processes of C2 to C6 and helps support the weight of the head. The vertebral arteries heading toward the brainstem pass through the foramina of the transverse process of the upper six cervical vertebrae. These vessels are subject to stretching injuries with extreme cervical rotation of the hyperextended neck.

The 12 *thoracic vertebrae* (T1 to T12) are located in the thorax (the body area between the neck and diaphragm). The posterior ends of the 12 pairs of ribs are attached to these vertebrae at posterior demifacets (thought of as one half of a facet). T1 has a whole facet joint space for the first rib articulation and an inferior demifacet, which works with the corresponding superior demifacet of T2 for articulation with the second rib. T2 to T8 each has superior and inferior demifacets, which together form the vertebral portion of the articulation with the ribs. T9 has one superior demifacet, and T10 to T12 each has a whole facet to articulate with the ribs. The arrangement of the vertebrae in the thorax allows for a certain amount of flexion, extension, and side bending, but movements generally are limited, with most movement occurring at the thoracic-lumbar junction at T11, T12, and L1. The main functions of the thoracic vertebrae are to provide spaces on which to build the rib cage, which protects the heart and lungs, and to house the spinal cord.

The five *lumbar vertebrae* (L1 to L5) are located in the lower back. They are larger and heavier than the other vertebrae, which allows them to support more weight. The interlocking shape of the vertebrae makes rotation very difficult but facilitates flexion, extension, and side bending. L4 and L5 allow the most motion. Most disk injuries occur at L4 to L5 and S1, the area of the lumbar-sacral junction.

The *sacral vertebrae* are five separate bones in a child; however, they eventually fuse to form a single bone, the *sacrum*, in an adult. Wedged between the two hipbones, the sacrum completes the posterior part of the bony pelvis. Four transverse ridges are the remnants of intervertebral disks. At the ends of each ridge are paired sacral foramina, through which the branches of the sacral nerves pass.

The *coccyx*, or tailbone, consists of four or five tiny bones in a child. As we develop, they fuse to form a single bone in an adult.

Vertebral curves

When viewed from the side, the vertebral column can be seen to have curves that correspond to the groups of vertebrae. In a newborn, the entire column is a concave forward shape; this is the primary curve. When the infant begins to assume an erect posture, secondary curves, which are convex, form. For example, the cervical curve appears when the infant begins to hold up her head at about 3 months of age; the lumbar curve appears when she begins to walk. The curves of the vertebral column provide some of the resilience and spring so essential to walking and running.

The cervical region is concave, or has a *lordosis*. The thoracic region is convex, called a *kyphosis;* an abnormal lateral curvature of the thoracic region is called *scoliosis*. The lumbar region is concave again (lordosis can refer either to an exaggeration of the curvature or to the normal condition). The sacrum is convex toward the back..

Vertebral curvatures develop dysfunction generally from exaggerated posture, activity, obesity, pregnancy, trauma, and disease. These conditions have the same name as the normal curves but are considered abnormal if they are exaggerated enough to cause problems. For example, osteoporosis can lead to the development of a hump in the thoracic vertebrae, called *kyphosis* or *dowager's hump*. A swayback of the lower back is a lordosis. As mentioned earlier, abnormal lateral bending is called *scoliosis*. Any exaggerated curve puts a strain on the musculoskeletal posture mechanisms and may predispose a person to pain and impaired movement (Figure 7-9)(Activity 7-8).

BONES OF THE THORAX

The *thorax* is the body area between the base of the neck and the diaphragm muscle. The bones of the thorax form a cone-shaped cage. Twelve pairs of ribs form the bars of the cage, attaching to the sternum, or breastbone, anteriorly. The thorax protects the heart, the lungs, and other organs.

The *sternum* is fairly flat. It consists of three parts: the *manubrium* at the top, the *body* in the middle, and the *xiphoid process* at the lower end. The xiphoid process is used as a landmark in cardiopulmonary resuscitation (CPR) to locate the region for chest compression. Chest compressions are performed above the xiphoid process to avoid breaking it off the sternum (Figure 7-10)(Activity 7-9).

The *ribs* are elongated, flattened, and twisted bones. At the posterior end of each rib is a head, which has two facets for articulation with the bodies of the thoracic vertebrae. The neck of the rib is a constricted portion next to the head. The tubercle has an articular part, which is connected to the transverse process of a thoracic vertebra, and a nonarticular part for ligament attachment. The body, or shaft, is long and curved. The shaft also has a sharp bend, called the *costal angle*. The anterior end is joined to the costal cartilage. Most ribs articulate with two thoracic vertebrae at three points. As mentioned before, the two facets on the head of the rib contact the demifacets of the vertebral bodies, and the tubercle contacts the transverse process (Activity 7-10).

The 12 pairs of ribs are classified by their anterior attachments. The first seven pairs are the true ribs; they attach directly to the sternum via the costal cartilages. The next five pairs of ribs are known as the false ribs. The first three (or the eighth, ninth, and tenth ribs) attach to the cartilage of the rib above. The eleventh and twelfth pairs are referred to as floating ribs because they have no anterior attachment. Each of our ribs attaches to the posterior vertebrae. The intercostal spaces, between the ribs, contain muscles, blood vessels, and nerves.

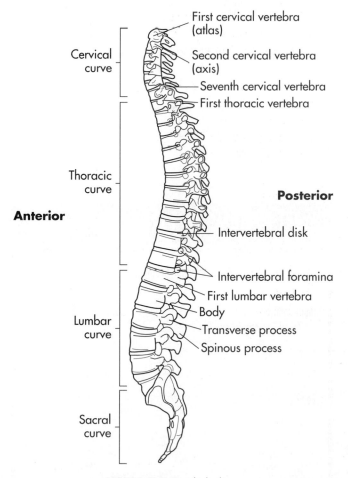

FIGURE 7-9 Vertebral column.

Cervical curve
First cervical vertebra (atlas)
Second cervical vertebra (axis)
Seventh cervical vertebra
First thoracic vertebra
Thoracic curve
Posterior
Anterior
Intervertebral disk
Intervertebral foramina
First lumbar vertebra
Body
Lumbar curve
Transverse process
Spinous process
Sacral curve

ACTIVITY 7-8

Draw the vertebral column and label the structures in the list below. Include the vertebral curve pattern and label the curves. Again, be accurate in your drawing but do not worry about artistic ability. Using diagrams or pictures from this text is helpful.

Atlas

Axis

Cervical vertebrae
(C1 to C7)

Nuchal ligament

Thoracic vertebrae
(T1 to T12)

Thoracic-lumbar junction
at T11, T12, and L1

Lumbar vertebrae
(L1 to L5)

Lumbar-sacral junction
at L4 to L5 and S1

Sacrum

Coccyx

Place drawing here.

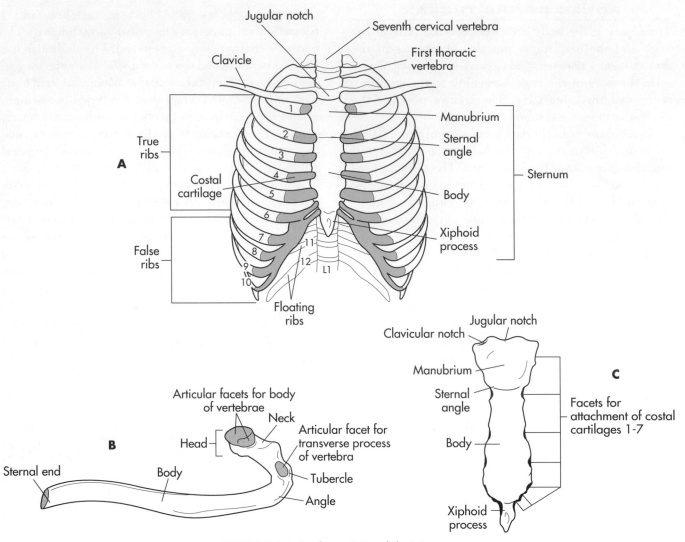

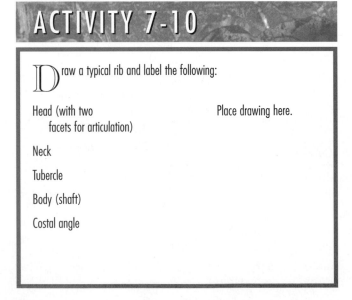

FIGURE 7-10   **A,** Rib cage. **B,** Typical rib. **C,** Sternum.

ACTIVITY 7-9

Draw the sternum and label the following:

Manubrium

Body

Xiphoid process

Place drawing here.

ACTIVITY 7-10

Draw a typical rib and label the following:

Head (with two
    facets for articulation)

Neck

Tubercle

Body (shaft)

Costal angle

Place drawing here.

BONES OF THE APPENDICULAR SKELETON

The appendicular skeleton may be considered as having two divisions, upper and lower.

The *upper division* includes the shoulders (or pectoral girdle); the arms between the shoulders and the elbows; the forearms between the elbows and the wrists; and the wrists, hands, and fingers. In everyday conversation we refer to the arm as the whole appendage from the shoulder to the wrist. In anatomic terms, the arm is the portion from shoulder to elbow. The only bony attachment of the pectoral girdle to the axial skeleton occurs at the sternoclavicular joint, the articulation of the clavicle and the manubrium.

The *lower division* includes the hips (or pelvic girdle); the thighs between the hips and knees; the legs between the knees and ankles; and the ankles, feet, and toes. Note that in anatomic terms, the leg is the portion from the knee to the ankle.

Bones of the Upper Division

The bones of the upper division can be divided into two groups. One group comprises the bones of the pectoral girdle, the *clavicle* and the *scapula* (some references include the manubrium, upper thoracic vertebrae, and first two ribs as functional units of the pectoral girdle). The other group includes the bones of the upper extremity.

Clavicle

The clavicle, or collarbone (Figure 7-11), is long and flat and has two bends, which gives it an S shape (Activity 7-11). The lateral clavicle articulates with the acromion, and together they form the upper portion of the shoulder. This structure functions as a strut by keeping the scapula posterior, which maintains the position of the glenoid fossa (the point of articulation of the humerus on the scapula). The clavicle articulates medially with the manubrium and the superior edges of the cartilage of the first rib to form the sternoclavicular joint. This fragile bone transmits force from the arms to the thorax. For this reason, when a person falls with arms outstretched, this bone often breaks or the joint separates when the clavicle hits the acromion.

Scapula

The scapula, or shoulder blade (Figure 7-12), is an irregular, triangular bone with a flat anterior surface. The posterior surface has a large spine and two major

processes, all easy to palpate. At the lateral end of the scapular spine is the *acromion process*, the highest point of the bony portion of the shoulder. The *coracoid process* is a fingerlike projection from the anterior portion of the superior border.

The three corners of this triangular-shaped bone are referred to as the inferior, superior, and lateral angles. The edges of the bone are also landmarks and attachment points for muscles; these are the medial, superior, and lateral borders. The medial border is also known as the vertebral border. The superior border is the hardest to palpate because it lies under the shoulder muscles. The lateral (or axillary) border is the thickest of the three. It contains the *glenoid cavity*, a shallow depression that articulates with the head of the humerus to form the shoulder joint. The supraspinous and infraspinous fossae and the fossa on the anterior portion of the scapula are attachment points for muscles that connect the shoulder to the thorax (Activity 7-12).

The second group of bones of the upper division comprises the bones of the upper extremity, which are the humerus, radius, ulna, and the bones of the wrist and hand.

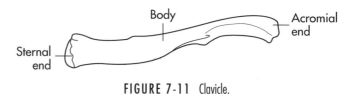

Body — Acromial end

Sternal end

FIGURE 7-11 Clavicle.

ACTIVITY 7-11

Draw the clavicle and label the following:

Articulation with the manubrium at the sternal end

Articulation with the acromion at the acromial end

Body

Place drawing here.

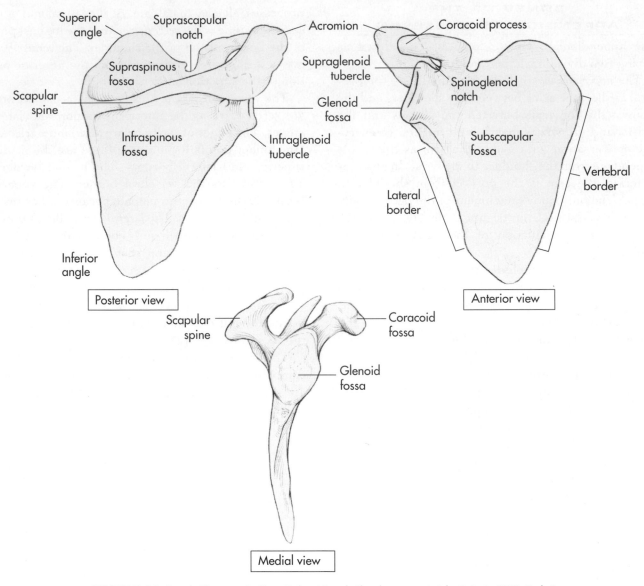

FIGURE 7-12 Scapula (three views). (From Mathers LH et al: *Clinical anatomy principles,* St Louis, 1996, Mosby.)

Humerus

The humerus, or arm bone (Figure 7-13), is a long bone. The head of the humerus, at the proximal end, forms the glenohumeral joint, which articulates with the glenoid fossa of the scapula.

The distal end of the humerus articulates with the radius and ulna to form the elbow joint. On the lateral edge of the distal end of the humerus is a rounded surface, called the *capitulum.* The medial edge of the distal end of the humerus forms a pulley-shaped surface, the trochlea.

Just above these projections on the anterior surface are the radial and coronoid (ulnar) fossae. The olecranon fossa is on the posterior surface. During flexion and extension, the radial head slides on the capitulum, and the trochlear notch of the ulna slides over the trochlea of the humerus.

In full flexion, the radial head and the ulnar coronoid process fit into the radial and coronoid fossae of the humerus. At full extension, the olecranon process of the ulna moves into the olecranon fossa of the humerus, which prevents extension beyond 180 degrees.

The medial and lateral epicondyles of the humerus are attachment points for muscles and are prone to problems from repetitive use (Activity 7-13).

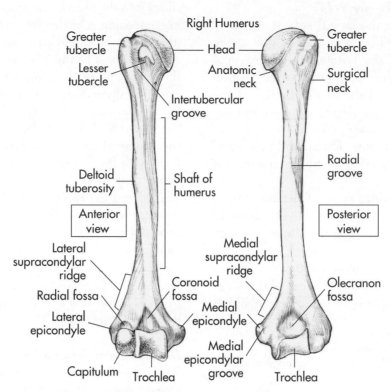

Right Humerus

Greater tubercle
Lesser tubercle
Head
Anatomic neck
Intertubercular groove
Greater tubercle
Surgical neck

Deltoid tuberosity
Shaft of humerus
Radial groove

Anterior view
Posterior view

Lateral supracondylar ridge
Medial supracondylar ridge
Radial fossa
Coronoid fossa
Olecranon fossa
Lateral epicondyle
Medial epicondyle
Capitulum
Trochlea
Medial epicondylar groove
Trochlea

FIGURE 7-13 Humerus (anterior and posterior views). (From Mathers LH et al: *Clinical anatomy principles,* St Louis, 1996, Mosby.)

ACTIVITY 7-12

Draw the posterior view of the scapula and label the following:

Acromion

Scapular spine

Inferior angle

Superior angle

Lateral border

Vertebral border

Glenoid fossa

Supraspinous fossa

Infraspinous fossa

Place drawing here.

ACTIVITY 7-13

Draw both the anterior and posterior views of the humerus and label the following:

Head

Greater tubercle

Lesser tubercle

Deltoid tuberosity

Capitulum

Trochlea

Radial fossa

Coronoid fossa

Olecranon fossa

Medial epicondyle

Lateral epicondyle

Diaphysis (shaft)

Place drawing here.

Bones of the forearm (Figure 7-14)

The radius, which is on the lateral side of the forearm, is narrow at the elbow and widens just above the wrist. The head of the radius, at the proximal end, articulates with the capitulum during flexion and extension. During full flexion, it slides into the radial fossa of the humerus. At the distal end of the radius, the articular surface combines with the carpals to form the wrist joint. The styloid process of the radius is a bony projection at the distal end, just above the thumb.

The ulna, which provides most of the stability of the forearm, lies on the medial side. Opposite in shape to the radius, it is wider at the elbow and narrower at the wrist. At its proximal end is the trochlear notch, which articulates with the trochlea of the humerus. The olecranon process is the large projection that most people refer to as their elbow. It slides into the olecranon process of the humerus during extension. On the anteroproximal surface of the ulna is the coronoid process, which moves into the coronoid fossa of the humerus during full flexion. At the distal end of the ulna is the head. The head of a bone usually is found at the proximal end, so do not become confused. The styloid process of the ulna is a bony landmark found above the wrist. Just beyond the proximal end is an articular disk, which articulates with the carpals to provide some of the movements of the wrist.

Between the radius and ulna lies the interosseous membrane, made of flexible connective tissue, which provides strength, support, and additional movement capabilities. The radius and ulna work together to produce many diverse, well-coordinated actions, both at the elbow and in the hand and wrist (Activity 7-14). The actions of the joint are discussed in more detail in Chapter 8.

Bones of the wrist and hand

The wrist contains the carpals, eight small, cube-shaped bones arranged in two rows of four. In the proximal row are the scaphoid, lunate, and triquetrum, which articulate with the radius to form the wrist joint. The pisiform is also in the first row but does not articulate with the radius. The distal row contains the trapezium, trapezoid, capitate, and hamate. Many skeletal injuries occur with falls on the hand, especially when it is forced into extreme hyper-

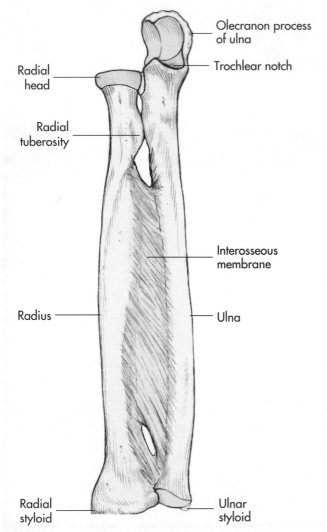

Olecranon process of ulna

Trochlear notch

Radial head

Radial tuberosity

Interosseous membrane

Radius

Ulna

Radial styloid

Ulnar styloid

FIGURE 7-14 Forearm bones. (From Mathers LH et al: *Clinical anatomy principles,* St Louis, 1996, Mosby.)

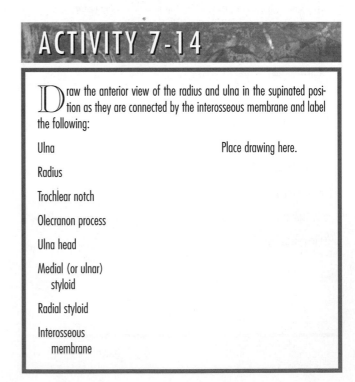

ACTIVITY 7-14

Draw the anterior view of the radius and ulna in the supinated position as they are connected by the interosseous membrane and label the following:

Ulna

Radius

Trochlear notch

Olecranon process

Ulna head

Medial (or ulnar) styloid

Radial styloid

Interosseous membrane

Place drawing here.

extension. Fractures of the scaphoid and radius are common because forces produced by a fall on the hand are transmitted through the scaphoid and lunate and absorbed by the radius.

The transverse arch of the wrist, formed by the carpals, is anteriorly concave. A wide, thick ligament, the *flexor retinaculum,* connects the pisiform and hamate to the scaphoid and trapezium. The dorsal side of the wrist has six tunnels for the extensor tendons, and the palmar side has two tunnels to carry nerves, arteries, and flexor tendons. The carpal tunnel, one of the palmar tunnels, is the most commonly traumatized. It contains the median nerve, which can become compressed, especially when repetitive movements of the fingers cause friction and inflammation.

In the palm of the hand are five metacarpal bones, short bones that form the framework of each hand. Knuckles are the rounded distal ends of the metacarpals.

Fourteen phalanges, or finger bones, are found in each hand, two for the thumb and three for each finger. Each of these short bones is called a phalanx. The first, or proximal phalanx, articulates with a metacarpal. The second and third, in the supine position, are referred to as the middle and distal phalanges. Note that the thumb has only a proximal phalanx and a distal phalanx (Figure 7-15) (Activities 7-15 and 7-16).

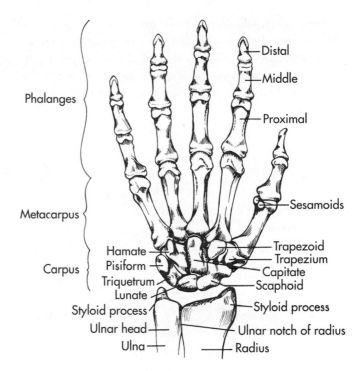

FIGURE 7-15 Volar view of the bones of the hand. (From Malone TR, McPoil T, Nitz AJ: *Orthopedic and sports physical therapy,* ed 3, St Louis, 1997, Mosby.)

ACTIVITY 7-15

Draw the wrist and hand and label the following:

Scaphoid

Lunate

Triquetrum

Pisiform

Trapezium

Trapezoid

Capitate

Hamate

Five metacarpal (metacarpus) bones

Fourteen phalanges

Place drawing here.

ACTIVITY 7-16

The following list names the bones of the upper limb:

Clavicle

Scapula

Humerus

Radius

Ulna

Carpals

Metacarpals

Phalanges

Make up a silly sentence to help you remember these bones by using the first letter of each name.

Bones of the Lower Division

The bones of the lower division are grouped together in a manner similar to that of the upper division. The two primary groups of the lower division are the bones of the pelvic girdle and the bones of the lower extremity.

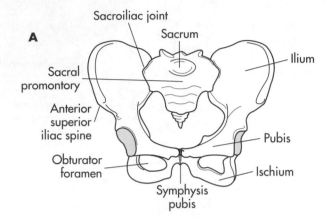

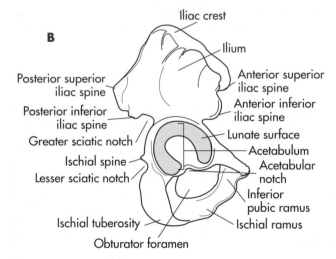

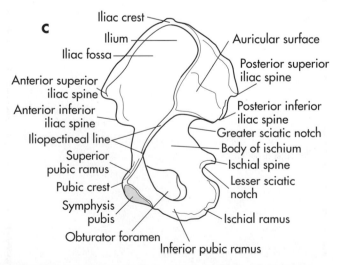

FIGURE 7-16 Pelvis. **A,** Anterior view. **B,** Lateral view. **C,** Medial view.

The bony pelvis (Figure 7-16) supports the trunk and the organs in the lower abdomen, or pelvic cavity. It also absorbs stress from the lower limbs when we are moving, whether walking or jumping. The female pelvis is adapted for pregnancy and childbirth and is wider and lighter than the male pelvis.

The pelvic girdle is a strong, bony ring composed of the *coxal bones* and the *sacrum.* Unlike the shoulder girdle, it is attached both anteriorly, at the symphysis pubis, and posteriorly, at the sacroiliac joint. Three bones fuse as we grow to create the coxae, or hipbones, which form the front and sides of the pelvic girdle. These three are the *ilium,* which forms the superior flared portion and is important for muscle attachments; the *ischium,* which is the inferior portion, and the strongest; and the *pubis,* which forms the anterior portion of the pelvis. In the middle of the pubis is the symphysis pubis, which is the anterior connection of the pelvis. The fibrocartilaginous disk

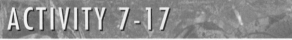

ACTIVITY 7-17

Draw anterior and lateral views of the pelvis and label the following:

Sacrum

Sacroiliac joint

Ilium

Ischium

Pubis

Symphysis pubis

Acetabulum

Iliac crest

Obturator foramen

Anterior superior
   iliac spine

Anterior inferior
   iliac spine

Posterior superior
   iliac spine

Posterior inferior
   iliac spine

Ischial tuberosity

Greater sciatic notch

Place drawing here.

at the symphysis pubis allows this joint to function as a shock absorber.

The posterior portion of the pelvic girdle is created from the sacrum, which is discussed in conjunction with the spine.

The lateral portion of the pelvis, where the ilium, ischium, and pubis fuse, creates a deep socket called the *acetabulum.* It articulates with the head of the femur to form the coxal (hip) joint.

At the superior portion is the iliac crest. On the anterior end of the crest is the anterior superior iliac spine (ASIS), which often is used as a bony landmark, especially in assessment and treatment. The posterior superior iliac spine (PSIS) is a bony prominence at the posterior end of the iliac crest. Just below the PSIS is the posterior joint of the pelvis, the sacroiliac (SI) joint. On the surface of the body is a small dimple or depression over the SI joint; the PSIS lies just above it (Activity 7-17).

The second group of bones of the lower division, that is, the bones of the lower extremity, are the femur and patella and the bones of the lower leg and foot.

Femur
The femur, or thigh bone (Figure 7-17), is the longest, strongest, and heaviest bone in the body. At the proximal end is the head, which has a smooth, spherical surface that fits into the acetabulum to form the hip joint. A depression in the center of the head, called the *fovea,* serves as an attachment for the ligamentum teres. All areas of the head except the fovea are covered with articular cartilage. The neck of the femur, distal to the head, is a common site of fracture in the elderly. The greater and lesser trochanters are projections that serve as muscle attachments. The shaft of the femur, as in most long bones, is triangular in cross section. On the posterior shaft is a prominent ridge, called the *linea aspera,* to which the adductor and vastus muscles attach. The lateral and medial condyles are smooth surfaces that articulate with the proximal tibia. Between the condyles is the anterior patellar surface. The lateral and medial epicondyles, which are above the condyles, are points of muscle attachment. The intercondylar fossa is a depression on the posterior surface between the condyles that articulates with the intercondylar eminence of the tibia. The menisci are cartilaginous cushions (lateral and medial) that lie between the femur and tibia (Activity 7-18).

Patella
The *patella,* or kneecap (Figure 7-18), is a sesamoid bone encased within the tendons of the quadriceps femoris, where it crosses the knee joint. The patella is

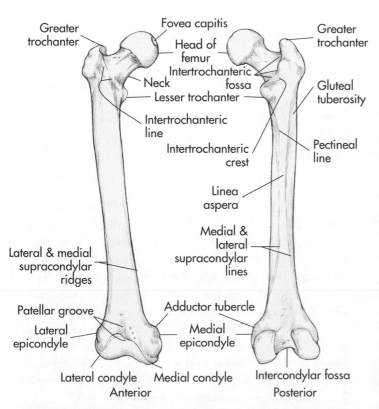

FIGURE 7-17 Femur (anterior and posterior views of the right femur). (From Mathers LH et al: *Clinical anatomy principles,* St Louis, 1996, Mosby.)

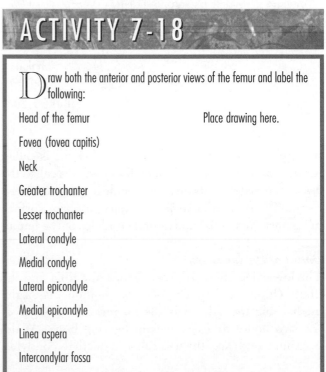

ACTIVITY 7-18

Draw both the anterior and posterior views of the femur and label the following:

Head of the femur

Fovea (fovea capitis)

Neck

Greater trochanter

Lesser trochanter

Lateral condyle

Medial condyle

Lateral epicondyle

Medial epicondyle

Linea aspera

Intercondylar fossa

Place drawing here.

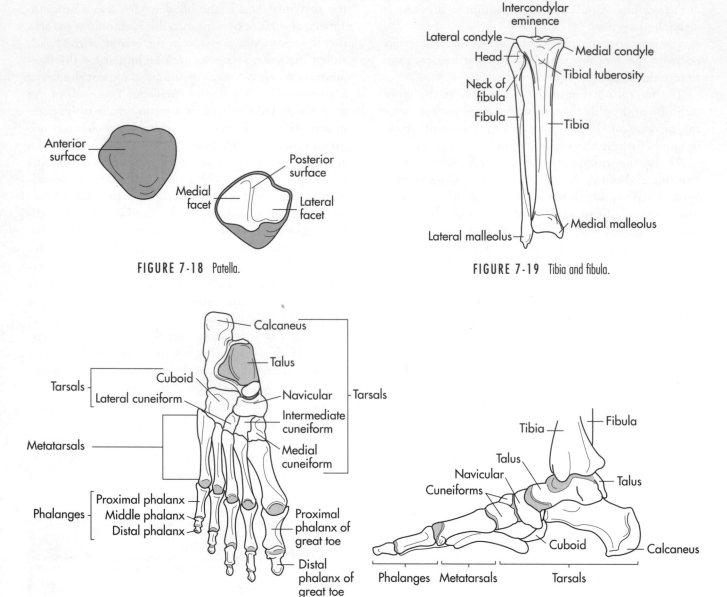

FIGURE 7-18 Patella.

FIGURE 7-19 Tibia and fibula.

FIGURE 7-20 Bones of the foot and ankle.

triangular in shape; the broad superior edge is called the *base,* and the more pointed inferior edge is called the *apex.* The patella sits in the trochlear groove of the femur. The two articular facets on its posterior surface fit against the medial and lateral condyles of the femur.

Bones of the lower leg

The lower leg comprises two bones, the tibia and the fibula (Figure 7-19). The *tibia,* or shinbone, is on the medial, big toe side. It is the longer and stronger of the two bones and is a weight-bearing bone. At the proximal end are the lateral and medial condyles, which fit against the identically named surface of the femur. The medial condyle is larger than the lateral condyle. The intercondylar eminence, a ridge that separates the two condyles, moves into the intercondylar fossa of the femur during knee flexion. The tibial tuberosity, at the proximal anterior superior tibia, is the attachment point for the patellar ligament. The distal end forms the medial malleolus, a bony landmark of the ankle. The tibia articulates with the fibula at the proximal end (the superior tibiofibular joint) and at the distal end (the distal tibiofibular joint). The tibia also articulates with the ankle bones.

The *fibula* is on the lateral side of the leg. This slender bone does not reach the knee joint and so does not bear weight. Its main function is to serve as an attachment for muscles and fascia. The head of the fibula articulates with the tibia. The distal end of the fibula, which forms the lateral malleolus, articulates with the talus. Despite its small size, the fibula can withstand more tensile pull and strain than any other bone in the body. As with the forearm, an interosseous membrane connects the tibia and fibula (Activity 7-19).

Bones of the foot

The structure of the foot (Figure 7-20) is similar to that of the hand. The difference lies in the fact that, because the foot supports the weight of the body, it must be stronger and does not have to be as mobile as the hand. The foot has 26 bones, 31 joints, and more than 20 intrinsic (inside the structure) muscles. Seven tarsal bones connect the foot to the leg. The largest is the calcaneus, or heel bone. The talus is the major weight-bearing bone of the foot during upright motions; it is next in size to the calcaneus.

The talus and calcaneus are the most posterior of the tarsal bones. They both articulate anteriorly with the other tarsals. The talus articulates with the tibia and fibula on its superior side and with the calcaneus inferiorly. Because no muscles insert on the talus, motion occurs by the movement of the bone and soft tissue structures around it. The other tarsals are cube shaped and lie between the talus, calcaneus, and the metatarsals; they are the anterior tarsals. The navicular articulates with the talus and cuneiforms. The cuboid articulates with the calcaneus. Together they form the transverse arch of the foot, also known as the instep. These gliding joints have less flexibility than the corresponding wrist bones.

Five short metatarsal bones form the instep, and the heads of these bones form the ball of the foot. They articulate proximally with the three cuneiforms and the cuboid and distally with the phalanges. Each of the metatarsals begins the actual formation of an individual toe. The phalanges are organized in the same way as in the hand. Each toe has three phalanges, except the great toe, which has two. The phalanges are identified in the same manner as in the hand (i.e., the first phalanx is known as the proximal phalanx) (Activities 7-20 and 7-21).

The plantar aponeurosis is a large band of connective tissue that begins at the inferior calcaneus and runs along the plantar surface of the foot, attaching at the toes. It adds stability to the arch of the foot but can shorten if the person commonly wears improperly fitting shoes. Plantar fasciitis is a painful condition caused by this shortening. Inflammation from repetitive use is common in track athletes. (For review of the bones, complete Activity 7-22.)

ACTIVITY 7-19

Draw the anterior view of the tibia and fibula and label the following:

Tibia

Fibula

Lateral condyle of the tibia

Medial condyle of the tibia

Intercondylar eminence

Tibial tuberosity

Head of the fibula

Neck of the fibula

Medial malleolus

Lateral malleolus

Place drawing here.

ACTIVITY 7-20

Draw the dorsal view of the bones of the foot and label the following:

Calcaneus

Talus

Cuboid

Navicular

Cuneiforms

Metatarsals

Phalanges

Place drawing here.

Pathologic Conditions

DEVELOPMENTAL PROBLEMS

Spina Bifida

If the vertebral arches in a growing fetus do not fuse into the spinous processes, the result is spina bifida. Instead of being protected by bone, the nerves of the dorsal spinal cord may be covered by a thin membrane, skin, muscle, or spinal meninges. This condition may range from a mild case, with the child showing no symptoms, to severe spinal cord damage and paraplegia. The most common site of the defect is the lumbosacral region.

Cleft Palate

Cleft palate is a congenital deformity involving a gap in the roof of the mouth from behind the teeth to the back of the mouth. Newborns with this defect may have difficulty nursing or swallowing because their mouths are open to the nasal cavities above. They suck in air rather than milk, or the milk may enter the nose instead of the esophagus. The condition usually is corrected surgically.

ACTIVITY 7-21

The list below names the bones of the lower limb:

Iilium

Ischium

Pubis

Femur

Patella

Tibia

Fibula

Tarsals

Metatarsals

Phalanges

Make up a silly sentence to help you remember these bones by using the first letter of each name.

Osteogenesis Imperfecta

Osteogenesis imperfecta is a group of hereditary disorders that appear in newborns or young children. The bones are deformed and extremely fragile as a result of demineralization and defective formation of connective tissue.

Clubfoot (Talipes)

Clubfoot is the most common of the lower extremity congenital deformities. In most cases one or both feet are bent downward and adducted; in other cases the feet are pointed upward and abducted. Mild cases respond to splinting and stretching, but severe cases require surgical correction. Clubfoot is more prominent in boys and may

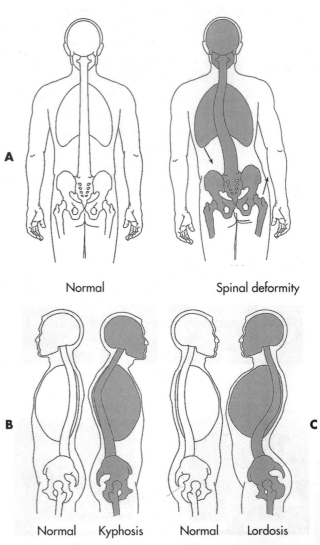

FIGURE 7-21 **A,** Deformity of the spine. Scoliosis is a lateral deviation of the spine. Arrows indicate the direction of the thoracic and pelvic tilt. **B,** Kyphosis, a flexion deformity of the spine. **C,** Lordosis and extension deformity of the spine. (Modified from Barkauskas VH et al: *Health and physical assessment,* ed 2, St Louis, 1998, Mosby.)

be the result of genetic predisposition or of the fetus' position in the womb.

Spinal Curve Abnormalities

Abnormal curvatures of the spine (Figure 7-21) may be congenital in origin; may result from paralysis or weakness or tension in spinal muscles; or may be the result of rapid growth of the body, especially after puberty. Bad posture habits, especially during periods of accelerated growth, can contribute to the problem. *Scoliosis*, a lateral curvature, is most often found in young girls, especially during or just after puberty, because of the rapid growth of the body. When discovered and treated early, good results are often seen. As was discussed previously, exaggeration of the thoracic curve is known as kyphosis (or hunchback), and excessive lumbar curvature is referred to as lordosis. One of the major problems caused by any extreme spinal curve is compression of the internal organs.

ACTIVITY 7-22

Locate each of the following bony landmarks on yourself. You may need to refer to the illustrations in this chapter.

Zygomatic bone (cheekbone)

Seventh cervical vertebra (the most pronounced of the cervical vertebrae, especially with the neck flexed)

Mastoid process of the temporal bones

Clavicle (collarbone)

Coracoid process of the scapula

Sternum (breastbone) between the ribs

Sternal notch of the manubrium

Xiphoid process (at the inferior end of the sternum; it has a pointed tip)

Scapula

    Acromion of the scapula (the highest point of the shoulder)

    Spine of the scapula

    Medial or vertebral border

    Lateral or axillary border

    Inferior angle

    Superior angle

    Lateral angle.

Humerus

    Greater and lesser tubercles

    Bicipital or intertubercular groove (runs between the two tubercles)

    Anatomic neck (just below the head of the humerus)

    Deltoid tuberosity (the insertion point for deltoid muscle)

    Lateral epicondyle (the bump at the distal end)

Medial epicondyle (the bump at the distal end)

Olecranon process (the point of the elbow)

Head of the radius (the bony knob just distal to the lateral epicondyle; you can feel it rolling during supination and pronation)

Pisiform bone (the lateral carpal bone on the anterior wrist)

Iliac crest (near the level of the waist)

Anterior superior iliac spine (ASIS)

Posterior superior iliac spine (PSIS)

Sacrum (the curved, triangular bone beneath the lumbar spine)

Coccyx (the caudal tip of the vertebral column, deep between the gluteal muscle masses)

Ischial tuberosity (the "sit bones" in the middle of the lower gluteals)

Pubic symphysis (the anterior midline joint of the pelvic girdle)

Femur

    Greater trochanter (large protuberance on the lateral side)

    Lesser trochanter (small elevation; on the medial side near top of inner thigh)

    Medial epicondyle

    Lateral epicondyle

Patella

Head of the fibula (the bump on the proximal anterior tibia, inferior to the patella)

Tibial tuberosity (the large bump just inferior to the patella)

Lateral malleolus

Medial malleolus

Calcaneus

INDICATIONS CONTRAINDICATIONS
For Soft Tissue and Movement Therapies

If skeletal problems create or are part of a permanent condition, supportive care is required. Soft tissue methods are helpful in managing compensatory muscle spasms and connective tissue changes. Any type of compressive force or joint movement methods are contraindicated for a fragile skeletal structure, regardless of the cause, unless carefully supervised by the appropriate medical professionals. Light, superficial methods, such as the gentle laying on of hands used in some forms of touch systems, might be indicated, again with supervision.

BONE DEMINERALIZATION DISORDERS

Osteoporosis

Osteoporosis is a disorder of the bone in which calcium and other minerals are lacking and bone protein is diminished. Under normal conditions, bone replaces itself with osteoblasts (bone-forming cells); with osteoporosis, this happens much more slowly, leaving the bones soft, fragile, and more likely to break. The condition is seen most often in postmenopausal women as a result of the decrease in hormone levels. It primarily affects the spine and pelvis. Other causes include deficiencies in the nutritional intake, absorption, or assimilation of protein and minerals, cigarette smoking, and inactivity. Treatments include hormone therapy (primarily estrogen, progesterone, and calcitonin), increasing exercise, and including more sources of calcium, magnesium, boron, and vitamin D in the daily diet.

Paget's Disease

Paget's disease, or osteitis deformans, occurs when the bones undergo normal periods of calcium loss followed by periods of excessive new cell growth. Bone cells are replaced with fibrous tissue and blood vessels. As a result, the bones harden, deform, and become susceptible to fracture. Currently, we know neither the cause nor a cure. The condition is most commonly found in men over 40 years of age.

Osteitis Fibrosa Cystica

In osteitis fibrosa cystica, bone tissue is replaced by fibrous tissue and cysts, making the bones weak and prone to fracture. This disorder is seen in long-standing hyperparathyroidism.

Disorders Caused by Radiation Therapy

When radiation is used to treat a bone disorder or is given as part of the treatment of a malignancy, bone may become brittle and fragile because of the changes in its structure. This happens if the bone is treated directly or if the treatment site involves bony structures.

INDICATIONS CONTRAINDICATIONS
For Soft Tissue and Movement Therapies

Caution is required before any soft tissue or movement therapy requiring any amount of compressive force is used on a client with a condition that causes demineralization of bone or that results in brittle, fragile bones. A fragile skeletal structure, regardless of the cause, is a contraindication for any type of compressive force or joint movement methods unless these are carefully supervised by the appropriate medical professionals. Light, superficial methods, such as the gentle laying on of hands used in some forms of touch systems, might be indicated with supervision. Bone involvement may be localized, such as with radiation treatment. In these cases, bodywork methods can be used on the unaffected areas and avoided over the involved area.

NECROSIS

Osteonecrosis (Ischemic Necrosis)

Various pathologic changes occur in the bone when its blood supply is diminished or cut off, or when infection, malignancy, or trauma occur. These conditions are among the common causes of hip pain and disability. The changes usually occur secondary to a primary disease such as lupus, especially when the disease is treated with glucocorticoids. Symptoms include pain during active motion and at night. Because of its slow, progressive deterioration, necrosis may go undiagnosed.

Legg-Calvé-Perthes Disease

More commonly known as Perthes disease, Legg-Calvé-Perthes disease involves degeneration and necrosis at the head of the femur, followed by recalcification. The disorder, most often seen in young boys, occurs when the vascular supply to the head of the femur is compromised, resulting in developmental deformity. The condition lasts about 3 years and may predispose the child to arthritis in the area as an adult. Symptoms include hip pain and gait abnormalities.

Scheuermann's Disease

Scheuermann's disease is most commonly caused by necrosis or inflammation in bone or in a disk of the thoracic vertebrae. It begins during puberty, is the result of genetic predisposition or trauma (or both), and leads to back pain and kyphosis. The excessive curvature is caused by the changes in the structure of the vertebrae, from columnar to wedge shaped.

Osteochondritis Dissecans

In osteochondritis dissecans, the cartilage and adjacent bone separate from the bone itself. This disorder is most common in adults and is caused by inflammation and necrosis of the particular area. At the affected joint, portions of dead tissue may break away and lodge in the joint capsule, restricting movement and causing pain. The condition is most often seen in the knee joint.

INDICATIONS CONTRAINDICATIONS

For Soft Tissue and Movement Therapies

Necrosis usually is a localized condition that requires regional avoidance of the involved bone area. Because soft tissue and movement therapies provide the generalized effect of enhanced circulation, indirect benefits might be realized with careful use of these methods. However, because these disorders are pathologic conditions, bodywork must be done with the permission and supervision of the primary health care provider.

GROWTH-RELATED DISEASE

Osgood-Schlatter Disease

Osgood-Schlatter disease, which affects the tibial tubercle, most often occurs in boys between 10 and 15 years of age. The tubercle becomes inflamed or separates from the tibia because of irritation caused when the patellar tendon pulls on the tubercle during periods of rapid growth or overuse of the quadriceps.

General Growing Pains

One of the many causes of growing pains occurs during growth spurts in children and adolescents when the bone grows faster than the attached muscles. The pain results when the muscle pulls on the pain-sensitive periosteum.

INDICATIONS CONTRAINDICATIONS

For Soft Tissue and Movement Therapies

Treatment of local areas may be contraindicated if inflammation or necrosis is present. General grow-

ing pains often are soothed by methods that do not introduce any sort of therapeutic inflammation, such as intense stretching and frictioning methods, which should be avoided. Methods that relax and lengthen the muscle and soften the connective tissue are appropriate.

INFECTIOUS DISEASE

Osteomyelitis

Osteomyelitis is an inflammation in the bone, bone marrow, or periosteum, usually caused by pyogenic (pus-producing) bacteria. The bacteria reach the bone through the bloodstream or by way of an injury in which the skin is broken. Osteomyelitis is most often seen in children, near the joints in the legs or arms. When promptly treated medically, the chance of a full recovery is excellent.

Tuberculosis

Tuberculosis is a systemic disease caused by the tubercular bacillus. Involvement in the skeletal system causes destruction of the bone tissue and necrosis. Tuberculosis of the spine, known as Pott's disease, affects mostly children. The onset of skeletal tuberculosis is insidious, usually marked by vague complaints of pain.

INDICATIONS CONTRAINDICATIONS

For Soft Tissue and Movement Therapies

Soft tissue and movement therapies are contraindicated in infectious disease unless carefully supervised by medical personnel. The therapist must always refer clients with vague pain symptoms for proper diagnosis.

TUMORS

Tumors in the skeletal system can be either primary or secondary. Primary tumors such as cysts or osteomas (bony knobs in or on a bone) are rare and usually benign. Some tumors are malignant such as osteosarcomas, which often arise in the femur or tibia of a young person. Some of the signs of malignancy are pain, unexplained swelling over a bone, a feeling of warmth on the skin, and prominent veins over the area.

Secondary tumors develop from primary sites, most often in the breast, lungs, or prostate. In older individuals, metastases from epithelial tumors or carcinomas of various organs can spread to the bones.

Tumors also can be found in cartilage. Osteochondroma is a benign tumor of the cartilage and bone tissue of long bones. Chondrosarcomas are malignant tumors of the cartilage.

INDICATIONS CONTRAINDICATIONS

For Soft Tissue and Movement Therapies

Prompt referral for diagnosis is a must for any sign that may indicate the growth of a tumor. Benign tumors are a local contraindication for soft tissue and movement therapies. These therapies are contraindicated for individuals with malignant tumors unless the therapist is supervised directly and carefully by the medical team.

NUTRITIONAL DISORDERS

Rickets

Rickets is a childhood disease that is extremely rare in the Western world, yet it still occurs with conditions of extreme nutritional deficiency. It is characterized by numerous bone deformities. Deficiency of the active form of vitamin D prevents the absorption of calcium and phosphorus through the intestine; these minerals, then, are not available for deposit in the bones, which remain soft and become distorted. The deformity patterns may be noticeable in older clients who had rickets as a child.

Osteoporosis

Osteoporosis, discussed in more detail on p. 238, also can be considered a nutritional disorder.

Scurvy

Scurvy is a vitamin C deficiency. Vitamin C is necessary for the production of collagen of the fibrous tissue and bone matrix. With scurvy, bone density is lost. Treatment involves increasing the vitamin intake, but some damage may be permanent. As with rickets, this disease is extremely rare in the Western world, but it can occur under conditions of inadequate nutrition, such as with eating disorders.

INDICATIONS CONTRAINDICATIONS

For Soft Tissue and Movement Therapies

Regardless of the cause, a fragile skeletal structure is a contraindication for any type of compressive force or joint movement methods unless these methods are carefully supervised by the appropriate medical professionals. Light, superficial methods such as the gentle laying on of hands used in some forms of touch systems, might be indicated, with supervision.

DISORDERS CAUSED BY TRAUMA

Whiplash

In whiplash, the anterior longitudinal ligament and cervical disks sometimes are injured.

Dislocation

A dislocation is the displacement of the bones of a joint; a subluxation is a partial dislocation.

Fractures

Severe force can fracture almost any bone. The term *fracture* means a break or rupture in a bone. Fractures may be classified as follows:

- *Compound (open) fracture*—The skin and other soft tissues are torn, and the bone protrudes through the skin.
- *Simple (closed) fracture*—The break in the bone does not break the skin or injure soft tissue.
- *Greenstick fracture*—The break in the bone is incomplete, producing a split such as might occur in a green piece of wood. This type is most common in children.
- *Impacted fracture*—The broken ends of the bones are jammed into each other.
- *Comminuted fracture*—The break involves more than one fracture line, with several fragments resulting, often with much soft tissue damage.
- *Complete fracture*—The break goes across the entire bone.
- *Incomplete fracture*—The break does not go across the entire bone.
- *Compression fracture*—The bone is squeezed or crushed (this type most often occurs in the spinal column).
- *Depressed fracture*—Bone in the skull is driven inward.
- *Stress fracture*—This type of fracture actually is a crack in the bone, often caused by repeated mechanical stress and strain.
- *Spiral fracture*—A break in which the bone is twisted apart. These fractures are relatively common in skiing accidents.

The signs and symptoms of fractures include local swelling, pain, loss of function or abnormal movement of the affected part, and deformities such as angulation, shortening, or rotation. Crepitation, a grating sound produced when bone fragments rub together, also may be heard. Pain may not occur immediately because of temporary loss of nerve function and shock.

The most important step in first aid for a fracture is to prevent movement of the affected parts. Expert help should be summoned immediately, and the area should be protected to prevent movement, leaving as much as possible "as is."

When a bone is fractured, blood vessels and periosteum rupture and blood seeps into the fracture site; this is called the *fracture hematoma,* which develops 48 to 72 hours after injury. The hematoma surrounding the fracture site provides a loose fibrin mesh in which fibroblasts and capillaries form granulation tissue that replaces the blood clot. Osteoblasts and chondroblasts become active in forming new bone and cartilage, and within approximately 7 days are dispersed throughout the soft tissue callus. This temporary bony union is called a *procallus.* Eventually the procallus is replaced by bone, and a rigid, bony callus is formed.

The healing process for a fractured bone usually takes 6 weeks, and it is essential that this process not be interrupted. Immobilization and casting often are required. Extensive soft tissue damage, including nerve damage and infection, can result secondary to the fracture. These conditions can continue to cause difficulties long after the bone itself has healed.

INDICATIONS CONTRAINDICATIONS

For Soft Tissue and Movement Therapies

Soft tissue and movement therapies are contraindicated locally over a trauma area until healing is complete. Very light, subtle methods of touch therapies (e.g., a gentle laying on of hands) may be beneficial in diminishing pain. The process usually is calming and soothing, which encourages healing through stress management. Bodywork methods are beneficial in supporting the rest of the body during the healing process, especially in managing compensation patterns caused by immobilization of an area, and in helping the client learn the use of crutches and canes.

Stress fractures may not be readily detected. Referral is indicated if the history would point toward a mechanical stress condition such as a participation in a recent athletic event (Activity 7-23).

ACTIVITY 7-23

List three benefits of soft tissue and movement therapies in dealing with pathologic conditions of the skeletal system.

Example Stress management promotes healing.

Your Turn

1. _____

2. _____

3. _____

List three contraindications for the use of soft tissue and movement therapies in dealing with pathologic conditions of the skeletal system.

Example Necrosis is locally contraindicated.

Your Turn

1. _____

2. _____

3. _____

Summary

This chapter has focused on the general structure of the skeletal system and the specific anatomy of the bones of the body. The various activities have reviewed and integrated the data so that the names, shapes, and functions of bones are familiar. This information is important to our study of the way the body moves as it continues in later chapters.

WORKBOOK SECTION

1. List the seven main functions of the skeletal system.

_____

_____

_____

_____

_____

_____

_____

_____

2. Describe the structure and development of bone.

_____

_____

_____

_____

_____

_____

_____

_____

_____

_____

_____

_____

_____

_____

_____

_____

_____

_____

3. List and describe the six shapes of bone.

_____

_____

_____

_____

_____

_____

_____

_____

_____

4. List and describe bony landmarks and give an example of each type.

_____

_____

_____

_____

_____

_____

_____

_____

_____

_____

_____

_____

_____

_____

_____

_____

_____

_____

5. Describe the two divisions of the skeleton and list the bones in each division.

_____

_____

_____

_____

_____

_____

_____

_____

_____

_____

FILL IN THE BLANK

The appendicular skeleton is composed of the _____ (1) of the body and their attachments. Another name for a joint is a (an) _____ (2).

The _____ (3) skeleton consists of the head, the vertebral column (spine), and the ribs and sternum. It provides the body with form and protection.

Compact bone is the_____ (4) portion of bone that protects spongy bone and provides the firm framework of the bone and the body. The osteocytes in this type of bone are located in concentric rings around a central _____ (5) canal, through which nerves and blood vessels pass.

The _____ (6) is a thin membrane of connective tissue that lines the marrow cavity of a bone.

An endoskeleton is found _____ (7) the human body; it accommodates growth.

The _____ (8) is a thin membrane of connective tissue that covers bones except at the articulations.

The_____ (9) quality of bones allows them to deform slightly and vibrate when electrical currents pass through them.

Sesamoid bones are round bones that often are embedded in tendons and joint capsules. The largest of these is the _____ (10).

Spongy bone is also known as _____ (11) bone.

_____ (12) are an irregular meshing of small, bony plates that make up spongy bone. Its spaces are filled with _____ (13) marrow.

EXERCISE

Identify each bone in the figure shown on p. 245 by filling in the blanks with the appropriate name.

A. _____

B. _____

C. _____

D. _____

E. _____

F. _____

G. _____

H. _____

I. _____

J. _____

K. _____

L. _____

M. _____

N. _____

O. _____

P. _____

Q. _____

R. _____

S. _____

T. _____

U. _____

V. _____

W. _____

X. _____

Y. _____

Z. _____

AA. _____

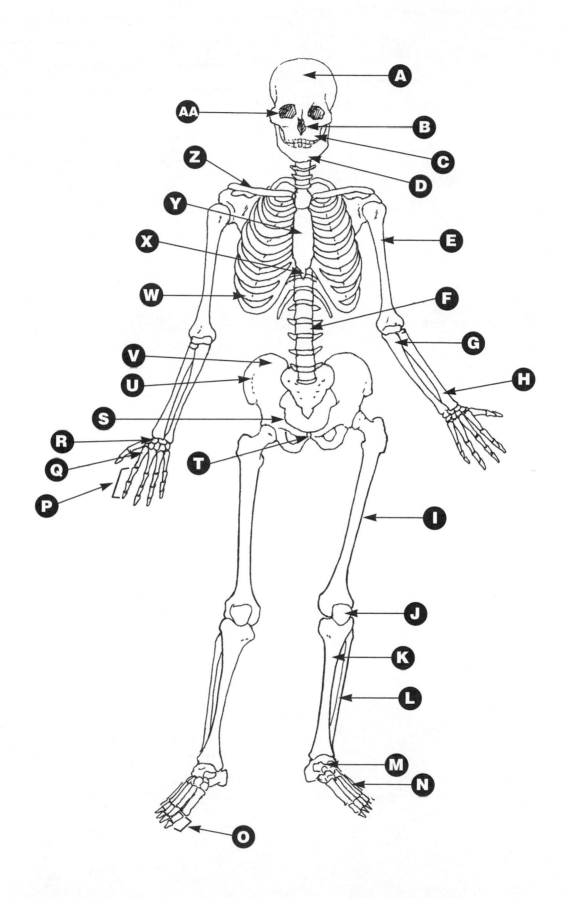

Now identify each part of the vertebral column, shown on p. 247, by filling in the blanks with the appropriate name.

A. _____

B. _____

C. _____

D. _____

E. _____

F. _____

G. _____

H. _____

I. _____

J. _____

K. _____

L. _____

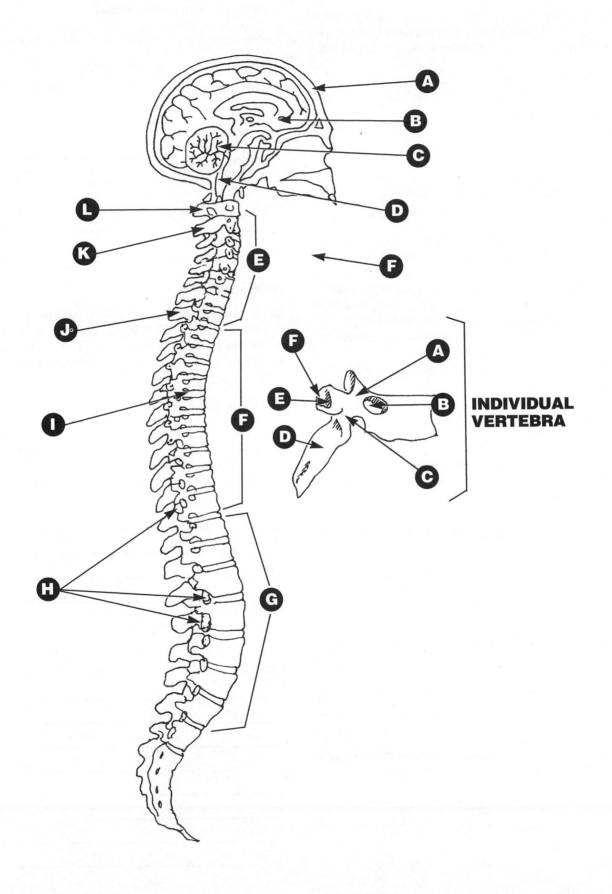

INDIVIDUAL VERTEBRA

PROBLEM SOLVING

Read the problem presented. There is no correct answer; rather, the exercise is intended to assist the student in developing the analytic and decision-making skills necessary in a professional practice. The following six steps can help you with this exercise:

1. Identify the facts presented in the information.
2. Identify the possibilities ("what if" statements) or develop your own possibilities from a careful reading of the facts.
3. Evaluate each possibility in terms of the logical cause and effect and the pros and cons.
4. Consider the effect on the people involved.
5. Write each down in the space provided.
6. Develop your solution by answering the question posed.

PROBLEM

The bones are not necessarily thought of as soft tissue. For this reason, direct work with the bones could be considered outside the scope of practice of the soft tissue or movement therapist. However, because muscles attach to bone and movement is related directly to bones, it seems logical that bones would be part of the anatomy and physiology affected by soft tissue and movement therapies. Any approach that promotes general well-being affects the entire body, including the bones.

In what way would you justify a scope of practice that included the bones as part of the body affected by soft tissue and movement therapies?

The first response is provided as a guide to get you started. Fill in at least two more statements

FACTS

1. Muscles attach to bones.

2. _____

3. _____

POSSIBILITIES

1. Direct work with bones could be considered outside the scope of practice for soft tissue and movement therapists.

2. _____

3. _____

LOGICAL CAUSE AND EFFECT

1. Logically, soft tissue and movement therapies will affect bone; therefore bones should be part of the scope of practice.

2. _____

3. _____

INFLUENCE ON PEOPLE

1. Clients may be uncertain as to who can address certain situations if the scope of practice lines is not clear.

2. _____

3. _____

How would you justify a scope of practice that includes the bones as part of the body affected by soft tissue and movement therapies?

_____

_____

_____

_____

_____

_____

_____

_____

_____

_____

FURTHER STUDY

Using a comprehensive anatomy and physiology text (see the Recommended Reading section of the list of Works Consulted), identify the chapters that pertain to the information presented in this chapter. Locate the information presented in this text and then elaborate by writing a paragraph of additional information on each of the following topics.

Piezoelectric quality of bones

_____

_____

_____

_____

_____

_____

_____

_____

_____

Remodeling process of bone

_____

_____

_____

_____

_____

_____

_____

Degenerative process of articular cartilage

_____

_____

_____

_____

_____

_____

_____

_____

Bone growth and repair

_____

_____

_____

_____

_____

_____

_____

_____

Skeletal changes caused by aging

_____

_____

_____

_____

_____

_____

_____

_____

Sinuses

_____

_____

_____

_____

_____

_____

_____

_____

The foot

_____

_____

_____

_____

_____

_____

_____

_____

Spinal curve abnormalities

_____

_____

_____

_____

_____

_____

_____

_____

Osteoporosis

_____

_____

_____

_____

_____

_____

_____

_____

_____

_____

Answer Key

1. (a) Supports soft tissues and serves as a framework for the entire body.
   (b) Provides attachment points for muscles and ligaments.
   (c) Protects delicate internal organs such as the brain, spinal cord, heart, and lungs.
   (d) Bones work as levers to provide movement begun by the attached muscles.
   (e) Stores calcium, phosphorus, and other minerals for release to the body as needed.
   (f) Stores lipids for use as energy.
   (g) Serves as production site for blood cells in the red marrow.

2. Bones are hard, dense, and slightly elastic organs of the skeleton. They have their own system of blood, lymphatic vessels, and nerves.

   The process that creates our skeleton is called *ossification*. Ossification is a two-part process: chondroblasts, or cartilage-forming cells, create the cartilage model of bones. Bone-building cells, called *osteoblasts,* develop the bone tissue from the cartilage model.

   Shortly after birth, calcification takes place. This hardening of the bones, called *osteogenesis,* occurs as calcium salts are deposited in the gel-like matrix of the forming bones.

   Osteocytes are mature bone cells, which maintain the bone during the lifetime. Bones are composed chiefly of bone tissue, called *osseous tissue.* Two thirds of bone tissue is composed of inorganic mineral, which gives rigidity, and one third is composed of organic components, which provide elasticity. Bones have a piezoelectric quality. The structure and function of bones are intrinsically connected. Bones remodel themselves constantly, depending on the functional demand.

   Compact (dense) bone has very little space between its tissues. This hard portion of the bone makes up the main shaft of the long bones and the outer layer of other bones. The osteocytes in this type of bone are located in concentric rings around a central haversian canal, through which nerves and blood vessels pass. Spongy (cancellous) bone has larger spaces between cells than compact bone, which makes cancellous bones lighter in weight. This type of bone is made of an irregular meshing of small, bony plates, called *trabeculae,* and is found at the ends of the long bones or at the center of other bones. In some bones the trabecular spaces are filled with red marrow, which produces blood cells. Bones contain red marrow and yellow marrow.

   Except for the ends that form joints, bones are covered with a thin membrane of connective tissue, called *periosteum*. A thinner membrane, the endosteum, lines the marrow cavity of a bone; it, too, contains cells that aid in the growth and repair of bone tissue. Bones of a synovial or movable joint make physical contact at their cartilaginous ends. The only remaining cartilage in bone is called *articular* (or *hyaline*) *cartilage.*

3. (a) Flat bones: Generally more flat than round. Examples: Ribs and skull bones.
   (b) Irregular bones: Have two or more complex shapes within the same bone structure. Examples: Vertebrae and scapula.
   (c) Long bones: Longer in one axis than another; characterized by a medullary cavity, a hollow diaphysis (shaft) of compact bone, and at least two epiphyses, which are active in the growth of long bones. Most of the bones of the arms and legs are long bones; the hollow structure of the diaphysis has the advantages of strength and light weight. Examples: Femur and ulna.
   (d) Short bones: Shaped like long bones but much smaller; these bones make up the structures of the hands and fingers and the feet and toes. This shape of bone also can be classified as long bone. Example: Metacarpals.
   (e) Cube-shaped bones (sometimes classified as short bones): Predominantly cancellous bone with a thin cortex of compact bone and no cavity. Examples: Wrist and ankle bones.
   (f) Sesamoid bones: Round bones that often are embedded in tendons and joint capsules. Example: Patella.

4. (a) Depressions and openings
   Canal: A tunnel or tube in bone. Example: Carotid canal in temporal bone.
   Fissure: A groove or slit between two bones. Example: Orbital fissure of sphenoid bone.
   Foramen: An opening in a bone. Example: Vertebral foramen of spinal column, through which the nerves pass.
   Fossa: A depression in the surface or at the end of a bone. Example: Infraspinous and supraspinous fossae of the scapula.
   Groove: A depression in the bone that holds blood vessels, nerves, or tendons. Example: Radial groove of the humerus.
   Meatus: A tunnel or canal found in a bone. Example: Canal in the skull from the external ear to the eardrum.
   Notch: An indentation or large groove. Example: Greater and lesser sciatic notches of the ilium.
   Sinus: Air cavity within a bone. Example: Frontal bones.
   (b) Processes that form joints
   Condyle: A rounded projection at the end of a bone that articulates with other bones to form a joint. Example: Medial condyle of the femur.
   Head: A rounded projection found on top of the neck of a bone. Example: Head of the femur.
   Facet: A smooth, flat surface. Example: Facet of a rib or vertebra.
   Process: Any prominent, bony growth that projects. Example: Olecranon process of the ulna.
   Trochlea: A pulley-shaped structure. Example: Trochlea of the humerus.
   (c) Processes to which tendons and ligaments attach
   Crest: A ridge on a bone. Example: Iliac crest.
   Epicondyle: A projection above a condyle. Example: Medial epicondyle of the femur.
   Line: A ridge that is smaller than a crest. Example: Linea aspera of the femur.

Spinous process, spine, or spina: A sharp, bony or slender projection. Example: Spinous process of the vertebral column or scapula.

Trochanter: One of two large, bony processes found only on the femur. Example: Greater or lesser trochanter.

Tubercle: A small, rounded process. Example: Adductor tubercle of the femur.

Tuberosity: A large, rounded protuberance. Example: Tibial tuberosity.

5. The two divisions of the skeleton are the axial skeleton and appendicular skeleton. The axial skeleton, which forms the axis of the body, consists of the head, vertebral column (spine), and the ribs and sternum. It provides the body with form and protection. The shoulder and hip girdles, which have similar structures, are the connectors to the axial skeleton.

The appendicular skeleton is composed of the limbs of the body and their attachments. The long bones of the upper and lower limbs, in combination with the muscles, provide fine and gross motor movements. Similar in design, these long bones are the humerus, radius, and ulna, and the femur, tibia, and fibula. In the same manner, the short carpals of the wrist and the tarsals of the ankle provide the flexibility needed in the hands and feet.

FILL IN THE BLANK

1. limbs
2. articulation
3. axial
4. hard
5. haversian
6. endosteum
7. inside
8. periosteum
9. piezoelectric
10. patella
11. cancellous
12. Trabeculae
13. red

EXERCISE

Answers for figure on p. 245.

A. Cranium
B. Nasal bone
C. Maxilla
D. Mandible
E. Humerus
F. Vertebral column
G. Ulna
H. Radius
I. Femur
J. Patella
K. Tibia
L. Fibula
M. Tarsals
N. Metatarsals
O. Phalanges
P. Phalanges
Q. Metacarpals
R. Carpals
S. Ischium
T. Pubis
U. Ilium
V. Innominate bone
W. Costal cartilage
X. Xiphoid process
Y. Sternum
Z. Clavicle
AA. Orbit

Answers for figure on p. 247.

A. Skull
B. Brain
C. Cerebellum
D. Brainstem
E. Cervical curve
F. Thoracic curve
G. Lumbar curve
H. Intervertebral foramina
I. Intervertebral disk
J. Seventh cervical vertebra
K. Second cervical vertebra (axis)
L. First cervical vertebra

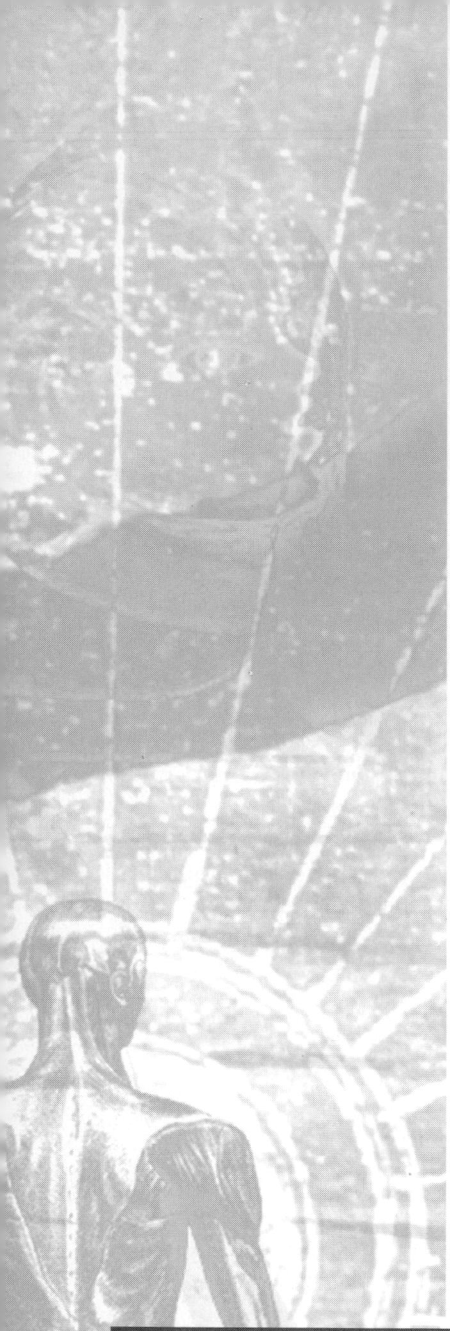

Chapter 8

The Joints

CHAPTER OUTLINE

Joint Overview
- Connective tissue and joint structure
  - *Collagen*
  - *Elastin*
  - *Bursae*
  - *Cartilage*
  - *Viscoelasticity of connective tissue*
- Joint categories
  - *Synarthrosis and diarthrosis*
- Forces and stress

Joint Motion
- Arthrokinematics
- Joint play
- Joint positions and stability
- Osteokinematics: range of motion (ROM)
  - *Hypomobility*
  - *Hypermobility*
- Movements of joints
  - *Terms used to describe general joint movements*
  - *Terms used to describe specific joint movements characteristic of the forearm, wrist, thumb, ankle, and foot*
  - *Terms used to describe specific joint movements characteristic of the shoulder girdle and shoulder joint*
  - *Terms used to describe specific joint movements characteristic of the spine*
  - *Classification of synovial joints by movements*
- Kinematic chains
  - *Closed kinematic chain*
  - *Open kinematic chain*

CHAPTER OBJECTIVES

After completing this chapter, the student should be able to perform the following:
- Describe the elementary principles of joint design.
- Define the two main types of joints.
- Define arthrokinematics and osteokinematics.
- Describe joint play.
- Describe the structures that contribute to joint stability.
- Identify pathologic conditions of joints and describe general treatment protocols used for intervention.
- Design a joint movement sequence for the body.

KEY TERMS

Anatomic range of motion (ROM) The amount of motion available to a joint based on the structure of the joint and determined by the shape of the joint surfaces, joint capsule, ligaments, muscle bulk, and surrounding musculo-tendinous and bony structures.

Articulation (ar-tik-yoo-LAY-shun) A joint where two or more bones meet to connect parts together and allow for movement in the body.

***Bursa* (Bursae pl.)** (BER-sah) A flat sac of synovial membrane in which the inner sides of the sac is separated by a fluid film. Bursae are located where moving structures are apt to rub.

Close-packed position The only position of a synovial joint in which the surfaces fit precisely together and maximal contact between the opposing surfaces occurs. The compression of joint surfaces permits no movement, and the joint possesses its greatest stability.

Closed kinematic chain The positioning of joints in such a way that motion at one of the joints is accompanied by motion at an adjacent joint.

Collagen (KOL-ah-jen) A fibrous tissue that provides stability to connective tissue structures of fascia, tendons, and ligaments. It makes up one fourth of the protein in the body.

Diarthrosis (dye-ar-THRO-sis) A freely movable synovial joint.

Elastin (e-LAS-tin) A fibrous tissue that has elastic properties and allows flexibility of connective tissue structures.

Fibrocartilage (fye-bro-KAR-ti-lij) A connective tissue that permits little motion in joints and structures. It is found in such places as the intervertebral disks and forms our ears.

Hyaline (HYE-ah-lin) ***cartilage*** The thin covering of articular connective tissue on the ends of the bones in freely movable joints in the adult skeleton. It forms a smooth, resilient, low-friction surface for the articulation of one bone with another, distributes forces, and helps absorb some of the pressure imposed on the joint surfaces.

Hypermobility A range of motion of a joint greater than would normally be permitted by the structure. It results in instability.

Hypomobility A range of motion of a joint less than what would normally be permitted by the structure. It results in restricted range of motion.

Joint capsule A connective tissue structure that indirectly connects the bony components of a joint.

Joint play The involuntary movement that occurs between articular surfaces that are separate from the range of motion of a joint produced by muscles. It is an essential component of joint motion and must occur for normal functioning of the joint.

Loose-packed position The position of a synovial joint in which the joint capsule is most lax. Joints tend to assume this position when inflammation occurs to accommodate the increased volume of synovial fluid.

Open kinematic chain A position in which the ends of the limbs or parts of the body are free to move without causing motion at another joint.

Pathologic range of motion The amount of motion at a joint that either fails to reach the normal physiologic range or exceeds normal anatomic limits of motion of that joint.

Physiologic range of motion The amount of motion available to a joint determined by the nervous system from information provided by joint sensory receptors. This information usually prevents a joint from being positioned where injury could occur.

Suture A synarthrotic joint in which two bony components are united by a thin layer of dense fibrous tissue.

Symphysis (SIM-fi-sis) A cartilaginous joint in which the two bony components are directly joined by fibrocartilage in the form of a disk or plate.

Synarthrosis (sin-ar-THRO-sis) A limited-movement, nonsynovial joint.

Synchondrosis (SIN-kond-ROE-sis) A joint in which the material used for connecting the two components is hyaline growth cartilage.

Syndesmosis (SIN-dez-mo-sis) A fibrous joint in which two bony components are joined directly by a ligament, cord, or aponeurotic membrane.

Synovial (si-NO-vee-al) *fluid* A thick, colorless, lubricating fluid that is secreted by the membrane of the joint cavity.

Synovial joint A freely moving joint allowing motion in one or more planes of action. Types of synovial joints include the following:

Ball-and-socket joint Allows movement in many directions around a central point. Ball-and-socket joints are formed when a ball-shaped convex surface is fitted into a concave socket. This type of joint gives the greatest freedom of movement, but it is also the most easily dislocated.

Condyloid (condylar) *joint* Allows movement in two directions, but one motion predominates.

Gliding joints Known also as synovial plane, gliding joints allow only a gliding motion in various planes.

Hinge joint Allows flexion and extension movement in one direction, changing the angle of the bones at the joint, like a door hinge.

Pivot joint Allows rotation around the length of the bone.

Saddle joint Is both convex in one plane and concave in the other with the surfaces fitting together like a rider on a saddle.

Viscoelasticity The combination of resistance offered by a fluid to a change of form and the ability of material to return to its original state after deformation. This term is used to describe connective tissue.

Joint Overview

Move. Wiggle. Put on some music and dance. Hug someone. Scratch your nose. Touch your toes. Joints are where we bend and twist. Body movement depends on joints. Many systemic body functions such as respiration and movement of blood and lymph depend on the mechanical pumping action of joint movement. For example, lymph nodes are often located at jointed areas so that with every movement the body massages the lymph system. The mechanical actions of breathing in and out depend on movement of the ribs. A firm understanding of the anatomy and physiology of jointed areas is necessary because soft tissue and movement therapists interact most directly with the somatic structures of the body wall (i.e., the muscles, connective tissue, joint structure, and bones) as the entry point to the entire body.

Metaphorically, joints are interdependent relationships. A joint cannot exist with only one bone; at least two must work together. Joints seldom operate independently of other joints, but instead an orchestrated, synchronized network of links develop similar to relationships within a family. Joints are passive and unable to function without the muscles. They can do nothing alone but depend on others to get the job done, just as do families, friends, and work teams. Joints and muscles need each other. Joints must move to be healthy and can only function best in the way they are designed to move.

So it is with us. People need to be active and do best when they work with their unique structure of personal gifts. A knee would not make a very good shoulder joint nor would the elbow be able to operate as a knee, but an elbow is designed to be a very good elbow and is essential and equal to the knee in the function of the body.

A joint or **articulation** is used to connect parts of a structure together. In the body the structures joined are the bones. Joints illustrate the strong relationship that exists between structure and function. The design of a joint depends on its function and vice versa. Joints that provide stability or static support are different from joints that provide mobility. In the body, structure such as bone shape and the way the bones attach at the joint determines joint function.

Each structure that is a part of a joint has one or more specific functions essential for the overall performance of the joint. Any disruption or change in any of the parts of a joint affect the total function of the joint.

Approximately 200 bones of various sizes and shapes in the human skeleton are connected by joints. Effective functioning of the total structure depends on the integrated action of many joints, some providing stability and some providing mobility. Generally, stability must be achieved before mobility. Joint capsules, ligaments, and tendons stabilize joints. Most joints serve a dual mobility/stability function.

Joint designs in the human body vary from simple to complex. The simplest human joints usually have stability as a primary function, whereas the more complex joints usually have mobility as a primary function. Joints that serve a single function are less complex than joints serving multiple functions. Complex joints are more likely to be affected by injury, disease, or aging than are simple joints because the complex joints have more parts and are subject to more wear and tear than stability joints (Activity 8-1).

CONNECTIVE TISSUE AND JOINT STRUCTURE

Connective tissue was first discussed in Chapter 1. More specific detail, as it relates to joint function, is provided in this chapter.

Connective tissue is used in the construction of human joints in the form of bones, ligaments, tendons, bursae, disks, plates, menisci, fat pads, membranes, and sesamoid bones.

As discussed in Chapter 1, the structure of the connective tissue is characterized by the presence of a large extracellular matrix and a wide dispersion of cells. The extracellular matrix has both a nonfibrous component, referred to as the ground substance, and a fibrous component.

The ground substance is composed of proteins responsible for attracting and binding water. The concentration of these proteins in the extracellular matrix of bone, cartilage, membranes, tendons, or ligaments affects the water content and therefore pliability of these structures. The nonfibrous component also plays an important role in protection of the connective tissue structure, strengthening it.

The fibrous component of the extracellular matrix contains two types of fibers: collagen and elastin.

Collagen

The primary fibrous component of the intercellular substance in dense fibrous tissue is **collagen** (white fibrous tissue). Collagen has a tensile strength similar to steel and is responsible for the functional stability of connective tissue structures.

Collagen fibers are nonelastic but still provide some limited mobility. In the relaxed position of some structures, collagen fibers assume a wavy configuration called *crimp*. The crimp or wave can be straightened out, allowing for some flexibility in the structure.

Collagen has piezoelectric properties that generate small electrical currents when deformed, and it oscillates or vibrates if electrical currents travel through it (Figure 8-1, *A*).

Elastin

Elastin or yellow fibrous tissue, has elastic properties that allow fibers to return to their original condition after a deforming force has been applied (Figure 8-1, *B*). The arrangement of the collagen fibers along with the collagen/elastin fiber ratio in various ligaments and tendons determines the ability of these structures to provide stability and mobility for a particular joint.

The fibrous component of the extracellular matrix in both ligaments and tendons contains a larger collagen content than elastin content. However, the ratio of collagen to elastin fibers and their arrangement varies considerably among different ligaments. Generally, the collagen fibers in tendons are arranged in a parallel configuration to handle pulling forces, whereas the collagen fibers in ligaments have a somewhat more varied arrangement, depending on the function of the ligament.

In addition to their usual connective tissue components, tendons and ligaments are surrounded by loose areolar connective tissue that forms either complete or partial sheaths around these structures. Double layers of connective tissue around the tendons at the wrist and hand form complete sheaths. These are sometimes called *sheathed tendons*. The sheath protects the tendon and produces synovial fluid, which helps reduce friction.

Bursae

Bursae are flat sacs of synovial membrane in which the inner sides of the sacs are separated by a fluid film. Bursae are located where moving structures are apt to rub. Subcutaneous bursae are located between the skin and bones. Subtendinous bursae are located between tendons and bones. Submuscular bursae are located between muscles and bones. Although most of us have bursa in the same places, bursae can form from demand if additional cushioning is needed.

ACTIVITY 8-1

Consider the following principles and characteristics of joint design. Write down a social interaction that is similar. Some examples are provided to get you started.

Example   Some joints provide stability.

Having my grandmother over to talk stabilizes my connection with my family and my past.

Some joints provide mobility.

Relationships with my teachers move my knowledge forward.

The structure of the joint determines the function of the joint.

The relationship I have with my dog is one of companionship, and the relationship I have with my chickens is one of a caretaker.

A breakdown or change of any joint structure will affect the entire joint function.

My son's divorce affected our entire immediate family, and the holidays were particularly difficult the first year.

Your Turn

Joints connect two or more bones together.

The design of a joint depends on its function.

Some joints provide stability.

Some joints provide mobility.

The structure of the joint determines the function of the joint.

Each part of the joint has a specific function that is essential to the whole function of the joint.

The breakdown of any joint structure will affect the entire joint function.

Complex joints are more likely to malfunction than simple joints.

Effective functioning of the whole body depends on the integrated action of many joints working together.

Generally, stability must be achieved before mobility.

Most joints serve a dual function of mobility and stability.

Simple joints provide more stability.

Complex joints provide more mobility.

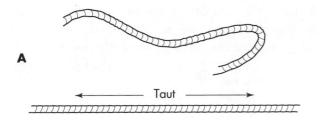

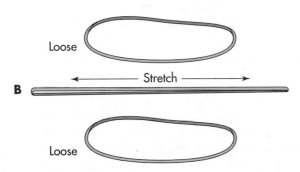

FIGURE 8-1 **A,** Collagen—like a rope. **B,** Elastin —like a rubber band.

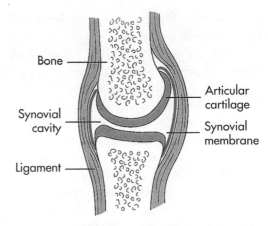

FIGURE 8-2 Articular cartilage in the joint capsule. (From Barkauskas VH et al: *Health and physical assessment,* ed 2, St Louis, 1998, Mosby.)

Cartilage

Cartilage is usually divided into two types: fibrocartilage and hyaline cartilage.

Fibrocartilage

Fibrocartilage is subdivided into white and yellow types.

White **fibrocartilage** consists primarily of collagen fibers and forms the cement in joints that permit little motion. This type of cartilage also forms the intervertebral disks and the menisci in the knees.

Yellow cartilage is found in the ears and epiglottis and differs from white fibrocartilage in that it has a higher ratio of elastin to collagen fibers.

Hyaline cartilage

Hyaline cartilage forms a thin covering of articular cartilage on the ends of the bones in freely movable joints in the adult skeleton. It forms a smooth, resilient, low-friction surface for the articulation of one bone with another. It also disperses joint pressure over a wider area. Any additional stresses applied to a joint distribute forces and help absorb some of the pressure imposed on the joint surfaces. These cartilaginous surfaces are capable of bearing and distributing weight over the lifetime of a person. Water is the most abundant component of hyaline cartilage

and, when combined with protein substances in the ground substance, forms a stiff gel (Figure 8-2).

Synovial fluid is distributed during joint motion or when the cartilage is compressed. The fluid flows back into the cartilage after motion or compression stops. Because hyaline cartilage is devoid of blood vessels and nerves in the adult, its nourishment is derived solely from this back-and-forth flow of fluid. The free flow of fluid is essential for the survival of cartilage as an aid to reducing friction. The effects of immobilization, in which compression of joint surfaces is absent or diminished, can cause hyaline cartilage to degenerate.

Bone is the hardest of all connective tissue found in the body. As with other forms of connective tissue, it consists of a cellular component, a ground substance, and a fibrous component.

☝ PRACTICAL APPLICATION

The availability of adequate water in the body is important to the function of connective tissue and cartilage. Studies have shown that certain types of disk and joint pain can be reduced with an increase in water intake. The connective tissues rehydrate whenever possible, and as they do, intervertebral disks expand somewhat, increasing the space between the vertebrae and reducing pressure on the nerves. In synovial joints a similar process takes place with a rehydration of the articular cartilage, as well as all of the connective tissue structures.

The benefit of most connective tissue modalities results from an increase in the pliability of the connective tissue. Because this pliability also depends on the water content of the tissue, unless adequate fluid is available for the protein to bind with, the connective tissue is unable to readily change structure. Therefore an increase in water intake, in combination with connective tissue modalities, seems a logical approach to take when working with joints. Drinking adequate amounts of water seems a simple thing to do, and the benefits are certainly demonstrable.

Movement is also essential to joint health. Soft tissue and movement therapies can support joint function and in some instances replace movement to encourage the production and distribution of synovial fluid in the joint. Methods that use both passive and active forms of movement are the modalities of choice in these instances.

Viscoelasticity of Connective Tissue

Although connective tissue appears in many forms throughout the body, all connective tissue exhibits the common property of **viscoelasticity.** The behavior of viscoelastic materials is a combination of the properties of elasticity and viscosity.

Elasticity refers to a material's ability to return to its original state after deformation. *Viscosity* refers to the resistance to a change of form offered by a fluid. When a constant compressive or tensile force deforms connective tissue, the tissue moves in the direction of the force and then attempts to return to its original state. Under normal conditions, viscoelastic materials initially modify in the direction of the force applied and then slowly return to their original state (called *creep*). If a connective tissue structure is held in a deformed position for an extended period of time, over days or weeks, the viscous creep pattern may become permanent, thus altering the structure and therefore the function of a joint.

When connective tissue is subjected to sudden, prolonged, or excessive forces, the elastic limits of the tissue may be exceeded, and the tissue may enter the *plastic range*. In the plastic range the tissue is permanently deformed and is no longer able to return to its original state after the removal of the deforming force. This situation is similar to what happens when ligaments are overstretched and become lax. The ligaments are no longer capable of returning to their original length after being elongated and remain in a partial state of elongation. Ligament laxity places a joint at risk for injury because it compromises an important source of joint support and protection.

When the plastic range of connective tissue is exceeded, a failure (break or tear) of the tissue occurs. In the case of a ligament or tendon, the failure may occur in the middle of the structures, through tearing and disruption of the connective tissue fibers. This is called a *rupture*. If the failure occurs through a tearing off of the bony attachment of the ligament or tendon, it is called an *avulsion*. When failure occurs in bony tissue, it is called a *fracture*.

Each type of connective tissue is able to undergo a certain percentage of deformation before failure. This percentage varies not only among the types of connective tissue but also within the various types. Generally, tendons can deform more than ligaments, ligaments are able to deform more than cartilage, and cartilage is able to deform more than bone.

PRACTICAL APPLICATION

Two types of general pathologic conditions develop with changes in elasticity and viscosity of connective tissue. One is that connective tissue becomes lax, as previously described. This most often happens with prolonged overstretching of joint structures or with a sudden trauma. Gymnastics, dancing, figure skating, and excessive use of stretching systems such as yoga can produce this condition. Too much flexibility results in instability. Remember, stability is established before mobility. When connective tissue is unstable around a joint, the muscles of the jointed area increase contraction to provide joint stability. This action pulls the bones of a joint together, decreasing joint space, which may result in increased friction in the joint capsule. Although this is a good short-term strategy, other problems with joint function such as predisposition to osteoarthritis develop over the long term.

Bodywork approaches can be used to manage the muscle contractions around the joint and support the compensation pattern by keeping the muscle contractions appropriate to the need for stabilization and minimizing the excessive pulling together of the bones of the joint. The use of certain types of frictioning techniques on individual connective tissue structures such as ligaments can create a therapeutic inflammation process. Because inflammation triggers the formation of connective tissue, it is possible to encourage the development of additional ligament structure. This procedure is combined with moderate immobilization necessary to allow the connective tissues to form and rehabilitative exercise to prevent adhesions from developing during the restructuring process. Therefore a combination of purposeful therapeutic inflammation, external stability in the form of moderate immobilization such as wrapping the area with elastic bandages or soft supports, and appropriate rehabilitation exercise that includes range of motion without resistance creates a broadening of the muscles or connective tissue structures of the area. A series of pulsing activities that do not stretch the tissues but instead mobilize the area through a gentle range of motion also increase stability in lax ligaments. This form of intervention for lax ligaments is a very slow and deliberate process.

Connective tissue also tends to shorten and dehydrate, pulling structures together and stiffening the area, thus decreasing mobility. In this situation too much stability is present. This situation tends to develop as a compensation pattern as a result of form altering in response to a change in function. Should the body need to alter position for an extended period of time such as static positions from working at a computer daily for hours at a time, connective tissue slowly alters to support that position. Also, generalized healing results in the laying down of connective tissue, which can thicken and shorten if the inflammatory process does not resolve itself effectively. In these types of situations the plastic component of connective tissue needs to be elongated in the direction of the shortening, the pliability restored, and the creep pattern redirected.

When stretching a shortened connective tissue structure to elongate it, the tissue should be warm. An appropriately intense but slow pulling or pushing force is then applied to the connective tissue area and sustained to produce creep and increase pliability. The goal is to extend the elastic range of connective tissue structures by altering the plastic range of shortened connective tissue. Myofascial-approach bodywork methods incorporate these principles. Movement methods such as yoga and other forms of slow, sustained stretching are based on similar principles. To access the plastic range of connective tissue, the protective muscle contraction initiated by the stretch-reflex response must be avoided. It is important to lengthen all muscle components to their available resting length before increasing the force to stretch beyond the elastic range to elongate the plastic component of connective tissue. As already mentioned, an adequate intake of water is essential for the success of these methods.

Some restricted joint function develops from the tissues surrounding the joint instead of within the capsule itself. Because of this, the entire area must be assessed for shortening. For example, shortening in either the lumbodorsal fascia or pectoral fascia can limit the range of motion of the shoulder joint. Over time, the reduction in movement will cause pathologic immobilization in the joint. Therefore any soft tissue or movement methods affecting joint function need to address the entire body broadly. Working with connective tissue is a slow process. Allowing time for the form to change gently and integrate effectively into the entire function of the jointed area and surrounding tissue is essential (Activities 8-2 and 8-3).

JOINT CATEGORIES

Synarthrosis and Diarthrosis

The joints of the human body are divided into two categories on the basis of the type of motion allowed at the joint and the methods and type of materials used to connect the bones at the articulating surfaces. The two categories of joints, or arthroses, are **synarthroses,**

ACTIVITY 8-2

Return to Chapter 1 and review the information about connective tissue. Summarize the information below.

ACTIVITY 8-3

Develop a therapeutic intervention process for a hypothetical connective tissue dysfunction. First, define and describe the assessment procedures you would use. Then develop a therapeutic goal for the area. Finally, develop treatments on the basis of the principles listed below. Do plans for both a hypermobile and hypomobile situation. Use therapy modalities you are presently studying in your technique classes. Remember that the actual implementation of such a plan would often be supervised by the appropriate health care professional, who would approve the plan before it is implemented. The principles are listed below, followed by an example.

PRINCIPLES

Assessment Principles

Hypermobility—connective tissue becomes lax.
- Too much flexibility results in instability.
- Muscle splinting develops to stabilize the area.

Hypomobility
- The entire area must be assessed for shortening.
- Over time, the reduction in movement will cause pathologic immobilization in the joint itself.
- Any soft tissue or movement methods affecting joint function need to address the body broadly.

Therapeutic Goals

Hypermobility
- Restore stability to connective tissue structures.
- Reduce muscle spasms surrounding the jointed area.

Hypomobility
- Extend the elastic range of connective tissue structures by altering the plastic range.
- Elongate the plastic component of connective tissue in the direction of the shortening.
- Restore pliability.
- Redirect the creep pattern.

Treatment Principles

Hypermobility
- Manage the muscle contraction around the joint to support the compensation pattern by keeping the muscle contraction appropriate to the need for stabilization and minimizing the excessive pulling of the joint cavity together.
- Apply frictioning techniques to individual connective tissue structures such as ligaments to create a therapeutic inflammation process.
- Combine this procedure with moderate immobilization.
- Use rehabilitative exercise to prevent adhesions from developing.

Hypomobility
- Avoid the protective muscle contraction initiated by the stretch reflex response to access the plastic range of connective tissue.
- Lengthen all muscle components to their available resting length before increasing the force to stretch beyond the elastic range to elongate the plastic component of shortened connective tissue.

To stretch out (elongate) a connective tissue structure:
1. Warm the tissue.
2. Use appropriately intense but slow pulling or pushing force.
3. Sustain the force for a period of time to produce creep and increase pliability.
4. Work toward the goal of extending the elastic range of connective tissue by altering the plastic range.
5. Make sure the person has an adequate intake of water.

Example

Situation: Hypermobile ankle from a bad sprain 3 years ago.

Assessment:
- Assess ankle for laxity in ligaments and other connective tissue structures by studying range of motion.
- Assess for muscle splinting and spasm with palpation.

Therapeutic goal:
- Increase stability of the ankle to prevent future ankle strains and sprains.

Treatment principles:
- Manage the muscle contraction around the joint with soft tissue methods.
- Create a therapeutic inflammation process by use of frictioning on the appropriate lax ligament.
- Suggest the client wrap the ankle for moderate immobilization.
- Teach client ways to move the frictioned area through a series of pulsing activities that do not stretch the tissues but instead mobilize the area through a gentle range of motion to prevent adhesions from developing.

Your Turn

Hypermobility

Situation:

Assessment:

Therapeutic goal:

which are nonsynovial limited-movement joints, and **diarthroses,** which are synovial, freely moveable joints.

Synarthroses

The material used to connect the bony components in synarthrodial joints is interosseus fibrous and cartilaginous connective tissue. The connective tissue directly unites one bone to another in a bone-solid connective tissue-bone configuration. Synarthroses are grouped into two divisions according to the type of connective tissue used in the union of bone to bone: fibrous joints and cartilaginous joints.

Fibrous joints

In fibrous joints the fibrous tissue directly connects bone to bone (Figure 8-3). Three different types of fibrous joints are found in the human body. They are sutures, gomphoses, and syndesmoses.

A **suture** is a joint in which two articulating bones are held together by a thin layer of dense fibrous tissue that is continuous with the periosteum. The ends of the bony components are grooved so that the edges interlock or overlap one another. This type of joint is found only in the skull. Early in life these sutures allow a small amount of movement. In adulthood the bones slowly grow together to form a synostosis in which little or no motion is possible. The sagittal suture is an example of a suture.

A gomphosis is a joint in which the bony components fit together similar to a peg in a hole. The only gomphosis joint that exists in the human body is found between a tooth and either the mandible or maxilla. In most adults the loss of teeth mainly results from disease processes that affect the connective tissue cementing or holding the teeth. Under normal conditions in the adult, these joints do not permit motion.

A **syndesmosis** is a fibrous joint in a ligament, cord, or aponeurotic membrane that joins the articulating bones. For example, the shaft of the tibia is joined directly to the shaft of the fibula by a membrane. A slight amount of motion at this joint accompanies movement at the knee and ankle joints.

PRACTICAL APPLICATION

One particular method of soft tissue work deals with the slight movements of the cranial sutures. It works to normalize the gentle cranial/sacral rhythm, of which the movement of the cranial

ACTIVITY 8-3—cont'd

Treatment principles:	Therapeutic goal:
	Treatment principles:
Hypomobility	
Situation:	
Assessment:	

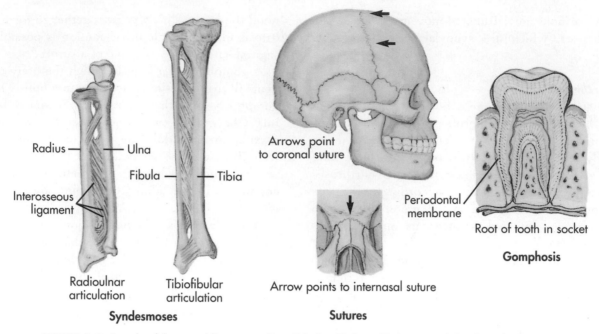

FIGURE 8-3 Examples of the types of fibrous joints. (From Thibodeau GA, Patton KT: *Anatomy and physiology*, ed 3, St Louis, 1996, Mosby.)

sutures is a part. Experts disagree about the mechanisms involved in the cranial rhythm and whether the cranial sutures do indeed move in the adult skull. Many theories exist, none of which has solid validation. The methods that work with the cranial sutures seem to have clinical validity, even if not agreed on scientific justification. Gentle pressure is used and more of an intent or thought of movement is experienced.

Cartilaginous joints

This type of joint is slightly movable and is also called *amphiarthrosis* (Figure 8-4). Either fibrocartilage or hyaline growth cartilage is used to hold one bony surface to another in a bone-cartilage-bone configuration. The two types of cartilaginous joints are symphyses and synchondroses.

A **symphysis** is a joint in which thin layers of hyaline cartilage over each bone are separated from each other by fibrocartilage in the form of disks or plates. The symphysis pubis is the articulation of the two pubic bones. Its structure allows for good stability, with the thick fibrocartilage providing a stable union between the two bones.

A **synchondrosis** is a joint in which a thin layer of hyaline growth cartilage connects the two bones. The cartilage forms a bond between the two ossifying centers of bone. This type of joint permits bone growth while providing stability and allowing a small amount of movement. When bone growth is complete, these joints ossify and convert to bony unions (synostoses). The first sternocostal joint is a synchondrosis. The adjacent surfaces of the first rib and sternum are directly connected by articular cartilage.

Diarthrosis or synovial joints

Most of our joints are synovial joints, which are freely moveable (Figure 8-5). All synovial joints are constructed in a similar fashion with the following features:

- A joint capsule formed of fibrous tissue surrounds the joint.
- A joint cavity is enclosed by the joint capsule.
- Synovial fluid forms a lubricating film over the joint surfaces.
- A synovial membrane lines the inner surface of the capsule.
- Hyaline cartilage covers the joint surfaces.

In **synovial joints** the ends of the bony components are free to move in relation to one another because no cartilaginous tissue directly connects the bones as in fibrous and cartilaginous joints. Instead, the bony components are indirectly connected to one another by means of a joint capsule, ligaments, and tendons.

The **joint capsule** is composed of two layers, an outer layer called the *stratum fibrosum* and an inner layer called the *stratum synovium*.

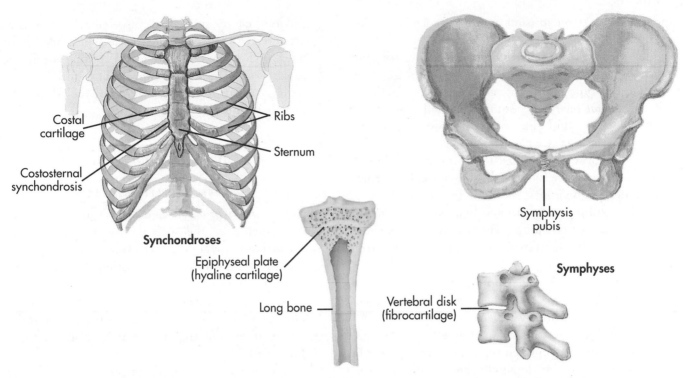

Synchondroses

Costal cartilage

Ribs

Costosternal synchondrosis

Sternum

Epiphyseal plate (hyaline cartilage)

Long bone

Symphysis pubis

Symphyses

Vertebral disk (fibrocartilage)

FIGURE 8-4 Examples of the types of cartilaginous joints. The epiphyseal plate between the epiphysis and diaphyses of a long bone is a temporary synchondrosis that does not move. The plate of hyaline cartilage is totally replaced by bone at skeletal maturity. (Most cartilaginous joints are amphiarthroses, or slightly moveable joints.) (From Thibodeau GA, Patton KT: *Anatomy and physiology,* ed 3, St Louis, 1996, Mosby.)

The stratum fibrosum, composed of dense fibrous tissue, completely surrounds the ends of the bones and is continuous with the periosteum of the adjoining bones. The outer layer is poorly vascularized but richly innervated by joint receptors. The receptors that are located in and around the joint capsule are able to detect the rate and direction of motion, compression, tension, vibration, and pain. *Hilton's law* states that a nerve trunk that supplies a joint also supplies the muscles of the joint and the skin over the insertion of the muscles. Therefore the stratum fibrosum is the source for extensive sensory data that affect the joint, muscles, and skin in the area.

The inner layer or stratum synovium of the joint capsule is highly vascularized but poorly innervated. It is insensitive to pain but undergoes vasodilatation in response to heat and vasoconstriction in response to cold. The stratum synovium produces matrix collagen and serves as an entry point for nutrients and an exit point for waste materials.

Ligaments and tendons play an important role in keeping joint surfaces together and often assist in guiding motion. Separation of joint surfaces is limited by passive tension in ligaments, the joint capsule,

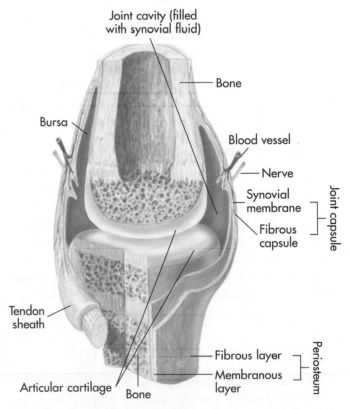

Joint cavity (filled with synovial fluid)

Bone

Bursa

Blood vessel

Nerve

Synovial membrane

Fibrous capsule

Joint capsule

Tendon sheath

Fibrous layer

Membranous layer

Periosteum

Articular cartilage

Bone

FIGURE 8-5 Structures of a synovial joint (the knee). (From Mourad LA: *Orthopedic disorders,* St Louis, 1991, Mosby.)

and tendons. Active tension in muscles also limits the separation of joint surfaces.

The bone surfaces in freely movable joints are protected by a smooth layer of articular cartilage. The bones in this type of joint have a space between them called the *joint cavity*. It contains a small amount of thick colorless fluid that resembles uncooked egg white. This lubricant, called *synovial fluid*, is secreted by the membrane that lines the joint cavity. Small sacs called *bursae* are filled with synovial fluid and are located near some joints. As discussed earlier, bursae lie in areas subject to stress and help ease movement over and around the joints. Such a design not only helps to provide stability for the joint but also permits motion.

The same structures that hold joints together also serve to maintain joint space or hold joints apart. When these structures weaken and become worn, the joint cavity is not maintained as effectively, and the ends of bone begin to contact each other and rub together. Friction develops; the end result is most often called *arthritis* but is more accurately called *degenerative joint disease*. In response to the pain, protective muscle spasms develop. Instead of increasing the joint space, which would alleviate the problem, the contraction of the muscles that surround the joint actually pull the ends of the bone, which together further decreases the space between the bones.

In addition, synovial joints often have accessory structures such as fibrocartilaginous disks and plates or menisci. Menisci, disks, and the synovial fluid help prevent excessive compression of opposing joint surfaces.

FORCES AND STRESS

Every time we take a step, push against an object with our arms, or bend and twist, our bones and joints have to dissipate the forces of stress imposed on them. Stress forces travel in straight lines. When they meet an obstacle such as a bend or curve in a bone, some forces are absorbed and others are reflected. Those absorbed will be transmitted to the soft tissues outside the bone, which helps dissipate excessive stress forces on joint surfaces.

🖐 PRACTICAL APPLICATION

Soft tissue and movement therapies can decrease the protective muscle spasm, which, in turn, allows some separation of bony structures in the joint and, as a result, provides a small increase in the joint cavity space. Because the muscle spasms are often protective in nature, decisions need to be made on how much reduction in spasm is desirable to increase space in the joint without totally eliminating the protective stability provided by the muscle splinting.

Joint Motion

ARTHROKINEMATICS

The term *arthrokinematics* is used to refer to accessory movements of the articulating surfaces of the bones at joint surfaces. Most often, one of the joint surfaces is more stable than the other and serves as a base for the motion, while the other surface moves on this relatively fixed base.

The terms *roll*, *slide*, and *spin* are used to describe the type of motion that the moving part performs (Figure 8-6).

A roll refers to the rolling of one joint surface on another, similar to a bowling ball rolling down an alley. In the knee the femoral condyles roll on the fixed tibial surface.

Sliding refers to the gliding of one component over another, as when you slide on ice. In the hand the

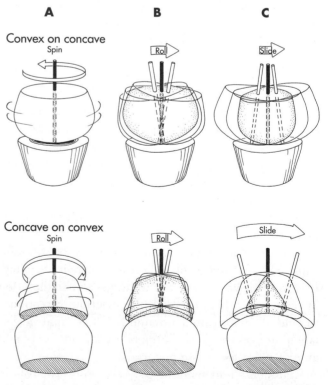

FIGURE 8-6 Accessory movements: **A,** spin; **B,** roll; **C,** slide. (From Malone TR, McPoil T, Nitz AJ: *Orthopedic and sports physical therapy*, ed 3, St Louis, 1997, Mosby.)

proximal phalanx slides over the fixed end of the metacarpal.

The term *spin* refers to a rotation of the movable component, as when a top spins. The head of the radius spins on the capitulum of the humerus during supination and pronation of the forearm.

Combinations of rolling, sliding, and spinning occur during the process of joint motion. A relatively large amount of motion can occur in a confined space by combining motions. When a moving component in a joint alternately rolls in one direction while sliding in the opposite direction, the range of motion available to the joint increases and opposing joint surfaces remain in contact with each other. Another method of increasing the range of available motion is by permitting both components to move at the same time. The humerus and the scapula move together during flexion/extension and during abduction/adduction at the glenohumeral joint.

JOINT PLAY

The involuntary movements that occur between articular surfaces, which have nothing to do with the range of motion of a joint produced by muscles, are an essential component of joint motion and must occur for the joint to function normally. Called **joint play,** these small movements are essential for proper joint function.

The rolling and sliding movements of the articular surfaces are not usually visible or under voluntary control. An externally applied force, such as that applied by a therapist or physician, can produce movement of one articular surface on another, and the amount of joint play present can be assessed. A door hinge is an excellent example. If you examine a door hinge, you will find that there are two plates, one attached to the door frame and one attached to the door. Between the two plates is a cylinder and inside the cylinder is a pin. The pin fits inside the cylinder and there is just enough space around it so that the pin is free to rotate in the cylinder, allowing the door to swing. The distance the door swings is comparable to the range of motion of a joint, whereas the amount of space in the cylinder that allows the pin to roll is comparable to joint play.

In an optimal situation a joint has a sufficient amount of play to allow normal motion of the joint. For the human body, the amount of joint play is almost always approximately ⅛ inch no matter which synovial joint is examined or the amount of range of motion of that joint. If the supporting joint structures are lax, the joint may have too much play and become unstable. If the joint structures are tight or inflammation or degeneration is present, the joint will have too little movement between the articular surfaces, the amount of joint play will be reduced, and range of motion may be restricted.

JOINT POSITIONS AND STABILITY

In most of our synovial joints the ends of the articulating surfaces of the bones are opposite in shape to each other, usually convex and concave. All synovial joints have only one position where the surfaces fit together and in which maximal contact between the opposing surfaces occurs. This is called the **close-packed position,** or locked position, and it allows no movement. The close-packed position is usually at the extreme end of the range of motion where the joint surfaces are compressed and the joint exhibits its greatest stability. The position of extension is the close-packed position for the elbow, knee, and interphalangeal joints. When not in this position, the joint is said to be in the **loose-packed position,** or unlocked, where the amount of contact is reduced and movements of spin, roll, and glide may occur (Figure 8-7, *A* and *B*). Each joint also has a least-packed position in which the capsule is at its most lax. Joints tend to assume this position when inflammation occurs to accommodate the increased volume of synovial fluid. In an injured joint that has swelling, the close-packed position is a position of discomfort. In the least-packed position the joint cavity has a greater volume; therefore it is a position of comfort.

Movement in and out of the close-packed position is likely to have a beneficial effect on joint nutrition because the movement squeezes out the synovial fluid during each compression against the cartilage, and the fluid is reabsorbed when the compression is removed.

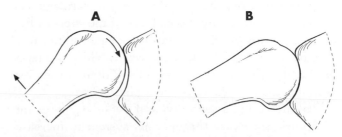

FIGURE 8-7 The congruence of articular surfaces: **A,** loose-packed position; **B,** close-packed position. (From Malone TR, McPoil T, Nitz AJ: *Orthopedic and sports physical therapy,* ed 3, St Louis, 1997, Mosby.)

OSTEOKINEMATICS:
RANGE OF MOTION (ROM)

Osteokinematics refers to the movement of the bones rather than the movement of the articular surfaces. There are three categories of range of motion (ROM): anatomic, physiologic, and pathologic.

The **anatomic range of motion** refers to the amount of motion available to a joint within its structural limits. The extent of the anatomic range is determined by a number of factors, including the shape of the joint surfaces, the joint capsule, ligaments, muscle bulk, and surrounding musculotendinous and bony structures. In some joints there are no bony joint limitations to motion, and the ROM is limited only by soft tissue structures. For example, the knee joint has no bony limitations to motion. Flexion is limited by soft tissues, often muscles, whereas extension stops with ligament stretch. Other joints have definite bony restrictions to motion in addition to soft tissue limitations. The elbow joint is limited in extension (close-packed position) by bony contact of the ulna with the olecranon fossa of the humerus.

The anatomic ROM may extend the limits of available movement to a point where joint injury can occur. Therefore many joints have established a **physiologic range of motion** set by the nervous system from information provided by joint sensory receptors. Usually this physiologic ROM is somewhat less than the anatomic ROM, preventing a joint from being positioned where injury could occur.

Pathologic range of motion occurs when motion at a joint either fails to reach the normal physiologic range or exceeds normal anatomic limits of motion. It may be either a structural or functional limit. Two main pathologic conditions exist: hypomobility and hypermobility.

Hypomobility

When the ROM is less than what would normally be permitted by the structure, the joint is hypomobile. **Hypomobility** may be caused by bony or cartilaginous blocks to motion or by the inability of the capsule, ligaments, or surrounding tissues to elongate sufficiently to allow a normal ROM. A *contracture*, which is a term used to describe the shortening of soft tissue structures around a joint, is one cause of hypomobility.

An increased sensitivity and reactivity of joint receptors can cause the nervous system to increase muscle tension patterns, which in turn would limit ROM because muscles would not relax to their normal resting length. The result would be hypomobility of joint movement even though nothing is dysfunctional in the joint itself. If this limited range is maintained, the joint capsule often alters and extends the dysfunction into the joint capsule itself by altering tissue structure. These conditions are much more difficult to manage because of the complexities of dysfunctional patterns and body-wide compensation.

Hypermobility

Hypermobility may be caused by a failure to limit motion by either the bony or soft tissues and results in instability. Weak or flaccid muscles can contribute to hypermobility because the muscles provide a stabilizing force to the joints. The joint may be subject to more trauma or damage because of excessive ROM, instability of the surrounding structures, or inability to withstand stresses.

✋ PRACTICAL APPLICATION

Both hypermobility and hypomobility of a joint may have undesirable effects, not only at the affected joint but also at adjacent joint structures because the body needs to develop compensation patterns to deal with the dysfunction.

Bodywork methods can be used to increase or decrease the ROM of a joint by helping to return a pathologic condition to a more normal ROM. By providing sensory stimulation to the joint nerve receptors, abnormal tension patterns of surrounding muscles can be disrupted and the restoration of homeostasis can restore ROM. Through the use of methods that elongate connective tissue structures, some forms of hypomobility can be reversed. Methods that create therapeutic inflammation, combined with appropriate rehabilitation, can sometimes increase stability in lax joint structures. Methods that strengthen surrounding muscles can provide alternative stabilizing forces when the joint is lax. Soft tissue work can manage the splinting action of the muscle so that spasm does not cause pain and pull the joint capsule together.

Finding the right combination of therapeutic care is not a precise protocol but more often an experimental decision-making process. Remember, any disruption of a part of the joint structure affects the entire joint function. When one joint is affected, the whole body must use compensation patterns to adjust. Over time, other joint movement patterns can become involved in dysfunction.

MOVEMENTS OF JOINTS

Joint design permits many different types of movement. Some joints only permit flexion and extension. Others permit a wide range of movements, depending largely on the joint structure. Some movement terms may be used to describe motion at several joints throughout the body, whereas other terms are relatively specific to a joint or group of joints (See Figure 3-9 A-EE).

Terms Used to Describe General Joint Movements

Flexion—Bending movement that results in a decrease of the angle in a joint by bringing bones together. An example is the elbow joint when the hand is drawn to the shoulder.

Extension—Straightening movement that results in an increase of the angle in a joint by moving bones apart. An example occurs when the hand is on the shoulder and moves away from the shoulder.

Abduction—Lateral movement away from the midline of the trunk. An example is moving the arms or legs to the side.

Adduction—Movement medially toward the midline of the trunk. An example is moving the arms to the side or the legs back to the anatomic position.

Diagonal abduction—Movement by a limb through a diagonal plane directly across and away from the midline of the body. An example is moving the right arm from in front of the left hip to in front of the right shoulder.

Diagonal adduction—Movement by a limb through a diagonal plane toward and across the midline of the body. An example is the return of the right arm from a flexed position to in front of the left hip.

Horizontal abduction—Movement of the humerus in the horizontal plane away from the midline of the body. It is also known as the horizontal extension or transverse abduction.

Horizontal adduction—Movement of the humerus in the horizontal plane toward the midline of the body. It is also known as horizontal flexion or transverse adduction.

Circumduction—Circular movement of a limb, combining the movement of flexion, extension, abduction, and adduction, to create a cone shape. An example is the shoulder joint moving in a circular fashion around a fixed point, as in doing arm circles.

Rotation—Twisting or turning of a bone on its own axis. An example is turning the head from side to side to indicate "no."

Internal rotation—Rotary movement around the longitudinal axis of a bone toward the midline of the body. It is also known as rotation medially, inward rotation, and medial rotation. An example is turning the palms of the hands from the anatomic position to facing backwards.

External rotation—Rotary movement around the longitudinal axis of a bone away from the midline of the body. It is also known as rotation laterally, outward rotation, and lateral rotation. An example is returning the palms from facing backward to the anatomic position, so they face forward.

Terms Used to Describe Specific Joint Movements Characteristic of the Forearm, Wrist, Thumb, Ankle, and Foot

Pronation—Internal rotation of the radius where it lies diagonally across the ulna, resulting in the palm-down position of the forearm.

Supination—External rotation of the radius where it lies parallel to the ulna, resulting in the palm-up position of the forearm.

Radial flexion, or wrist abduction—Abduction movement at the wrist of the thumb side of the hand toward the forearm.

Ulnar flexion, or wrist adduction—Adduction movement at the wrist of the little finger side of the hand toward the forearm.

Opposition of the thumb—Diagonal movement of the thumb across the palmar surface of the hand to make contact with the fingers.

Eversion—Turning of the sole of the foot outward or laterally. An example is moving our body weight to the inner edge of the foot.

Inversion—Turning of the sole of the foot inward or medially. An example is moving our body weight to the outer edge of the foot.

Dorsal flexion, or dorsiflexion—Flexion movement of the ankle that results in the top of the foot moving toward the anterior tibia.

Plantar flexion—Extension movement of the ankle that results in the foot and/or toes moving away from the body.

Terms Used to Describe Specific Joint Movements Characteristic of the Shoulder Girdle and Shoulder Joint

Elevation—Movement of the shoulder girdle to become closer to the ears. It occurs in shrugging of the shoulders.

Depression—Inferior movement of the shoulder girdle. An example is returning to the normal position from a shoulder shrug.

Protraction—Forward movement of the shoulder girdle away from the spine. It occurs in abduction of the scapula.

Retraction—Backward movement of the shoulder girdle toward the spine. Adduction of the scapula.

Rotation downward—Rotary movement of the scapula with the inferior angle of the scapula moving medially and downward. It occurs when the acromion process moves down.

Rotation upward—Rotary movement of the scapula with the inferior angle of the scapula moving laterally and upward. It occurs when the acromion process moves up.

Terms Used to Describe Specific Joint Movements Characteristic of the Spine

Lateral flexion (side bending)—Movement of the head and/or trunk laterally away from the midline. It occurs in abduction of the spine.

Reduction—Return of the spinal column to the anatomic position from lateral flexion. It occurs in adduction of the spine (Activity 8-4).

ACTIVITY 8-4

Find the definitions of the joint movements in Chapter 3 of this text and compare them to the ones you just studied in this chapter. Then, using both definitions, design a joint movement sequence that moves all the synovial joints in your body. An example is provided to get you started.

Example

Flexion

Drop chin to chest, make a fist, bend elbows so that hands touch the shoulders, bring a knee to chest and then repeat with other knee, bring the heel to buttocks and then repeat with other heel, curl toes toward the sole of the feet.

Your Turn

Abduction:

Adduction:

Diagonal abduction:

Diagonal adduction:

Extension:

Horizontal abduction:

Horizontal adduction:

Circumduction:

Rotation:

Pronation:

Supination:

Elevation:

Depression:

Protraction:

Retraction:

Rotation downward:

Rotation upward:

Radial flexion:

Ulnar flexion:

Opposition of the thumb:

Eversion:

Inversion:

Dorsal flexion:

Plantar flexion:

Lateral flexion (side bending):

Reduction:

Classification of Synovial Joints by Movements

Traditionally, synovial joints have been divided into three main categories on the basis of the number of axes at which motion occurs. A further subdivision of the joints is made on the basis of the shape and configuration of the ends of the bony components. The three main categories are uniaxial, biaxial, and triaxial (Figure 8-8).

A uniaxial joint is constructed so that visible motion of the bony components is allowed in only one of the planes of the body around a single axis. The two types of joints in this category are hinge joints and pivot joints.

A **hinge joint** allows flexion and extension in one direction, changing the angle of the bones at the joint, as in a door hinge. Examples include the elbow and interphalangeal joints.

A **pivot joint** allows rotation around the length of the bone. A pivot (trochoid) joint is a type of joint constructed so that one component is shaped like a ring and the other component is shaped so that it can rotate within the ring. Examples include the joint between the first and second cervical vertebrae and the joint at the proximal ends of the radius and the ulna.

Biaxial joints allow movement in two planes around two axes. The two types of joints in this category are condyloid joints and saddle joints.

A **condyloid joint**, also called a *synovial ellipsoid joint*, allows movement in two directions, but one motion dominates. The joint surfaces in a condyloid joint are shaped so that the concave surface of one bone is allowed to slide over the convex surface of another bone in two directions. Movements allowed are flexion, extension, abduction, and adduction. Examples include the wrist joint, metacarpophalangeal joints, metatarsophalangeal joints, and atlantooccipital joint.

Some condyloid joints allow flexion, extension, and rotation. Examples include the knee and temporomandibular joint. (Note that the knee is often classified as a hinge joint, but it is more accurately a condyloid joint.)

In a **saddle joint** each joint surface is both convex in one plane and concave in the other, and these surfaces fit together similar to a rider on a saddle. Movements allowed are flexion, extension, abduction, adduction, and a small degree of axial rotation.

Examples include the joint between the wrist and the metacarpal bone of the thumb (carpometacarpal joint), sternoclavicular joint, and ankle joint.

Triaxial or *multiaxial joints* are joints in which the bony components are free to move in three planes around the axes. Motion at these joints may also occur in oblique planes. The two types of joints in

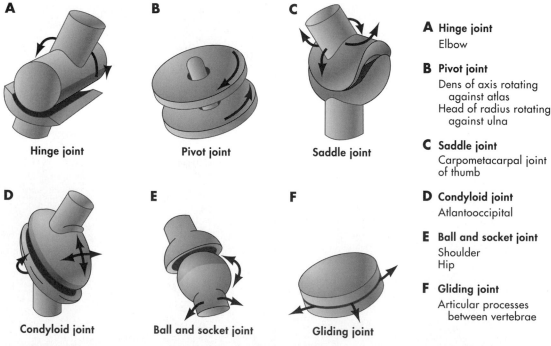

A Hinge joint
  Elbow

B Pivot joint
  Dens of axis rotating against atlas
  Head of radius rotating against ulna

C Saddle joint
  Carpometacarpal joint of thumb

D Condyloid joint
  Atlantooccipital

E Ball and socket joint
  Shoulder
  Hip

F Gliding joint
  Articular processes between vertebrae

Hinge joint   Pivot joint   Saddle joint

Condyloid joint   Ball and socket joint   Gliding joint

FIGURE 8-8   Synovial joint types. Uniaxial: **A,** hinge; **B,** pivot. Biaxial: **C,** saddle; **D,** condyloid. Triaxial (multiaxial): **E,** ball and socket; **F,** gliding. (From Thibodeau GA, Patton KT: *Anatomy and physiology,* ed 3, St Louis, 1996, Mosby.)

this category are ball-and-socket joints and plane or gliding joints.

A **ball-and-socket joint** allows movement in many directions around a central point. Ball-and-socket joints are formed when a ball-shaped convex surface is fitted into a concave socket. Movements allowed are flexion, extension, abduction, adduction, rotation, and circumduction. This type of joint gives the greatest freedom of movement, but it is also the most easily dislocated. Examples are the hip and shoulder joints.

Synovial plane joints, most often referred to as **gliding joints,** permit gliding between two or more bones. These joints allow only a gliding motion in various planes. The adjacent surfaces may glide on one another or rotate with respect to one another in any plane. Examples include the sacroiliac joint, superior tibiofibular joint, acromioclavicular joint, costovertebral joints, and joints between the vertebral arches.

KINEMATIC CHAINS

Kinematic chains describe the association between joints as they operate in relation to each other. The concept of kinematic chains is useful for analyzing human motion and the effects of injury and disease on the joints of the body. There are two types: closed kinematic chains and open kinematic chains.

Closed Kinematic Chain

Some joints of the human body are linked together into a series in which motion at one of the joints is accompanied by motion at an adjacent joint. This is called a **closed kinematic chain.** For instance, when a person is standing erect and bends both knees, simultaneous motion must occur at the ankle and hip joints. If the hand is used to apply a compressive force to a fixed object, a closed kinematic chain is created. The interaction between joints in the chain is predictable in terms of linked movement because the joints are interdependent. A change in the structure or function of one joint in the chain will usually cause a change in the function of a joint either immediately adjacent to the affected joint or at a distal joint. For example, if the ROM at the knee were limited, the hip and ankle joints would have to compensate so that the foot could clear the floor when a person is walking to avoid stumbling.

Open Kinematic Chain

When the ends of the limbs or parts of the body are free to move without causing motion at another joint, the system is referred to as an **open kinematic chain.**

The ends of our limbs are often not fixed but are free to move without necessarily causing motion at another joint. When the leg is lifted from the ground, the knee is free to bend without causing or changing motion at either the hip or ankle. The motion of waving the hand may occur at the wrist without causing motion of the elbow or shoulder. In an open kinematic chain, motion does not occur in a predictable fashion because joints may function either independently or in unison. For example, you can wave your whole upper limb by moving your arm at the shoulder or by moving only at the wrist.

PRACTICAL APPLICATION

An understanding of joint movement is fundamental to any soft tissue or movement therapy system. Many systems, particularly movement modalities, are based on body movement patterns provided by joints. A comparison of these systems, such as yoga, tai chi, or Feldenkrais, will reveal the intricate and interactive interplay of the joint moved either alone or in a dynamic combination of movement.

All types of athletes depend on proper functioning of their joints, as do dancers and others who purposefully move their bodies. These people often seek out soft tissue and movement therapies both to enhance their performance and maintain or restore optimal functioning. Especially when working with closed kinematic chains, all joints in the pattern need to be addressed for proper function to be restored in any particular area.

Identification and Palpation of Specific Joints

JOINTS OF THE SKULL

The joints of the skull are the cranial sutures and temporomandibular joint.

Cranial Sutures
- The coronal suture is the articulation of the frontal and the parietal bones.
- The sagittal suture is the articulation of the two parietal bones.
- The squamous suture is the articulation of the parietal and temporal bones.
- The lambdoidal suture is the articulation of the occipital and parietal bones.

Palpation

Place your fingertips on your eyebrows and slide them firmly up your forehead to the top of your skull, where you'll feel the first indentation. This is the coronal suture. Pressing your finger firmly into the suture, follow the indentation down on either side to where the suture ends, about midway between the top of the ear and the eye. Move posteriorly along the next indentation that arcs over your ear; this is the squamous suture. Behind the ear, just above the mastoid process, palpate the indentation that moves in an arc superiorly and posteriorly. This is the lambdoidal suture. At the midway point of the lambdoidal suture find the indentation that travels superiorly and anteriorly along the middle of the skull to join with the coronal suture. This is the sagittal suture (Figure 8-9, *A, B*).

Temporomandibular Joint

Articulating bones—Temporal bone and mandible
Joint type—Synovial condylar joint

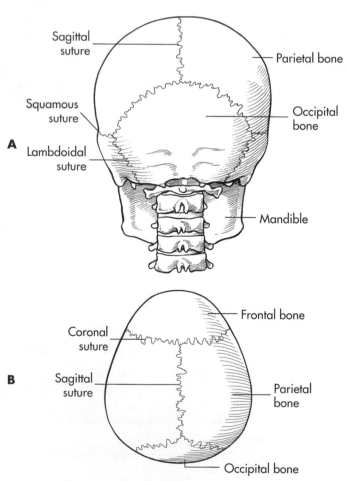

A

B

FIGURE 8-9 **A,** Posterior skull. **B,** Top view of skull. (Modified from D'Ambrogio KJ, Roth GB: *Positional release therapy: assessment and treatment of musculoskeletal dysfunction,* St Louis, 1997, Mosby.)

Ligaments—Lateral temporomandibular ligament from the zygomatic arch to the mandible; sphenomandibular ligament from the sphenoid to mandible (not pictured in Figure 8-10); stylomandibular ligament from the styloid process to the mandible
Movements—Depression, elevation, protrusion, retraction, lateral movements

The temporomandibular joint (TMJ) is one of the strongest joints in the body. It is the only biarticular joint in the body. This means that it has two separate articulating surfaces on one bone joining with two separate bones. This construction requires a balanced action in the joint so that both jointed areas work freely. When this is not the case, it results in temporomandibular joint dysfunction, or TMJD.

Palpation

Palpate the joint just in front of each ear as you open and close your jaw (Figure 8-10)(Activity 8-5).

SHOULDER JOINTS

The shoulder joints include the glenohumeral, sternoclavicular, and acromioclavicular joints and the scapulothoracic junction.

Glenohumeral Joint

Articulating bones—Humerus and scapula
Joint type—Synovial ball and socket
Ligaments—Glenohumeral: inferior, middle, and superior, from the glenoid cavity of the scapulae to head of humerus; coracohumeral ligament from coracoid process to greater and lesser tuberosity of humerus (not pictured in Figure 8-10)
Movements—Flexion, extension, abduction, adduction, medial (internal) rotation, lateral (external) rotation, circumduction

The glenohumeral joint is the main joint of the shoulder and the most mobile joint in the body. It is shallow, which allows for its high degree of mobility, but also accounts for its decreased stability. Most of the support for this joint is provided by the muscles,

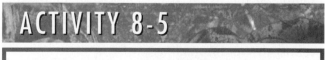

ACTIVITY 8-5

Move your TMJ through each of the movement patterns.

ligaments, and a loose joint capsule with very little support by the bony structures themselves. The tendons of the rotator cuff muscles provide additional stability (Figure 8-11).

Sternoclavicular Joint
Articulating bones—Clavicle and manubrium
Joint type—Synovial gliding joint
Ligaments—Anterior and posterior sternoclavicular from clavicle to sternum; interclavicular ligament joining both clavicles; costoclavicular ligament from clavicle to first rib; a fibrocartilaginous (articular) disk is located within the joint
Movements—elevation, depression, anterior and posterior movement, and rotation.

The movements of the sternoclavicular joint follow the movements of the scapula because no muscle

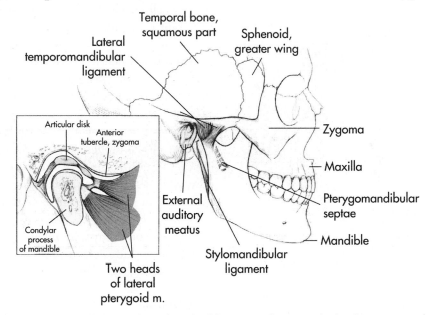

FIGURE 8-10 Temporomandibular joint/inset of articular disk. (From Mathers LH et al: *Clinical anatomy principles,* St Louis, 1996, Mosby.)

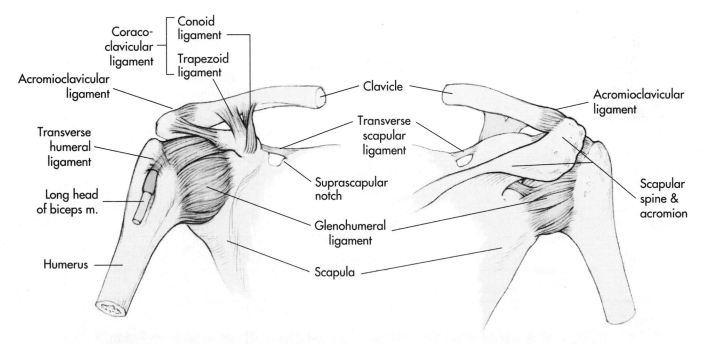

FIGURE 8-11 Ligaments of the shoulder. Anterior and posterior views. (From Mathers LH et al: *Clinical anatomy principles,* St Louis, 1996, Mosby.)

works directly on this joint. If mobility is decreased or lost in this joint, shoulder movement is directly affected. This joint is the only direct connection between the axial skeleton and the shoulder girdle and arm (Figure 8-12).

Acromioclavicular Joint (A/C Joint)

Articulating bones—Clavicle and scapula
Joint type—Synovial gliding joint

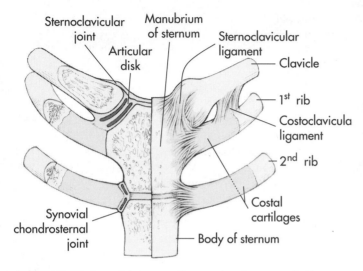

FIGURE 8-12 Joints of the sternum. The sternoclavicular joint is a double synovial joint, with an articular disk dividing the synovial cavity into two distinct compartments. (From Mathers LH et al: *Clinical anatomy principles,* St Louis, 1996, Mosby.)

Ligaments—Acromioclavicular from the acromion process to the clavicle; coracoclavicular ligament from the coracoid process to the clavicle
The acromioclavicular (A/C) joint may contain a fibrocartilaginous disk; NOTE: some people do not have an A/C joint
Movement—Anterior and posterior gliding, upward and downward rotation, and elevation and depression; movements that separate the joint are also possible; although a very small joint, it is important in shoulder action (Figure 8-13, *A, B*)

Scapulothoracic Junction

Although not a true joint because it does not involve bone-to-bone contact, the scapula moves across the thorax as the subscapularis and serratus anterior muscles glide over a subscapular bursa and fat pad. Most of the movement is a result of sternoclavicular action, with the rest of the action provided by movement in the acromioclavicular joint. If the scapula is limited in its movement, all shoulder movement will be directly restricted, although restrictions in adduction can be compensated for most easily. Its movements include elevation, depression, protraction, retraction, and upward and downward rotation.

Palpation

The position of three major points—the tip of the acromion, the greater tubercle of the humerus, and

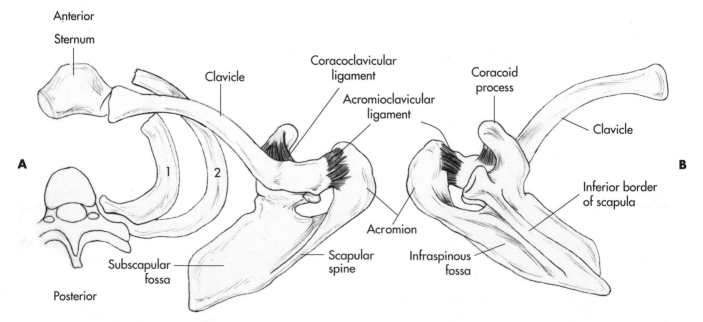

FIGURE 8-13 Acromial clavicular joint of the shoulder girdle. Superior **(A)** and inferior **(B)** views. The superior view illustrates the attachments of the lateral end of the clavicle, especially to the acromion and coracoid process. (From Mathers LH et al: *Clinical anatomy principles,* St Louis, 1996, Mosby.)

the coracoid process—will provide a clue as to the exact position of the shoulder. Beginning at the suprasternal notch, move slightly laterally to locate the sternoclavicular joint. To confirm the location of the joint, hold lightly while moving the same side arm into flexion and extension. Compare this joint movement with the direction of the scapular movements. Continue along the clavicle, following the convex curve of the medial two thirds and the concave curve of the lateral one third. Reach back to the spine of the scapula and follow it laterally; at its end move superiorly and anteriorly, where it becomes the acromion (the high point of the shoulder). This will be a large flat area, with a slight concavity. Find the anterior tip of the acromion and move slightly medially; the elevated ridge marks the start of the acromioclavicular joint. Move back to the top of the acromion, then laterally and inferiorly to the outer edge of the greater tubercle of the humerus. Moving anteriorly and medially, locate the lesser tubercle. Continuing medially on to the soft tissues of the anterior chest, press in to locate the coracoid process of the scapula just below the concave portion of the clavicle.

The glenohumeral joint, where the arm connects to the body, is easiest to palpate when the arm is either in passive extension or actively moving through circumduction. The fibrous capsule of the rotator cuff (muscles and tendons that surround the joint) often makes it hard to feel the bony structures. Of the four muscles of the rotator cuff, three—the supraspinatus, infraspinatus, and teres minor—insert together on the greater tubercle of the humerus, and their attachments are easiest to palpate. The fourth, the subscapularis, inserts on the lesser tubercle and is not easily palpated (Activity 8-6).

ELBOW JOINTS

The joints of the elbow are the ulnarhumeral, radiohumeral, and radioulnar joints.

Ulnarhumeral and Radiohumeral Joints
Articulating bones—Humerus with ulna, humerus with radius

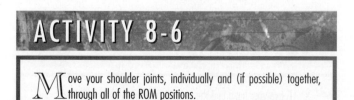

ACTIVITY 8-6

Move your shoulder joints, individually and (if possible) together, through all of the ROM positions.

Joint type—Synovial hinge

Ligaments—Ulnar collateral: anterior, posterior, transverse from the medial epicondyle of the humerus and olecranon processes of the ulna to the coronoid process; radial collateral from lateral epicondyle of the humerus to the annular ligament; annular ligament from anterior portion of radial notch around to the posterior margin of radial notch

Movements—Flexion, extension

Because of the bony structure and the support of muscles and ligaments, the elbow is a very stable joint. Most elbow action involves the ulnar and humeral portion of the joint, although the radius interacts with the humerus. The radius is on the thumb side of the forearm, and the ulna is on the little finger side. In anatomic position the radius is referred to as *lateral* and the ulna as *medial*. During flexion, the trochlear notch of the ulna slides on the humeral trochlea while the head of the radius slides on the capitulum. In extension the movements are reversed and stop when the olecranon process reaches its anatomic barrier at the olecranon fossa. This is one of the few areas in the body where a hard end feel and anatomic barrier occurs. Hyperextension is possible in those individuals who have a small olecranon process or a large olecranon fossa.

Radioulnar Joint
Articulating bones—Radius, ulna
Joint type—Synovial pivot
Ligaments—Annular ligament (see previous joint)
Movements—Pronation and supination

The radioulnar joint articulates at both the proximal and distal ends. It is listed as part of the elbow complex because it has the same soft tissue support as the elbow joint, and most of the actions occur in this area. The head of the radius moves both clockwise and counterclockwise around the ulna at the proximal end. During pronation, the radius crosses the ulna and ends diagonal to the ulna, providing for the palm to face down. Supination returns the radius and ulna to parallel positions, with the palm facing up, as in holding a bowl of soup (soup = supination, or up as in sUPination—a clue to remembering the position).

The interosseous membrane connects the ulna and radius. Its fibers run in a diagonal pattern perpendicular to one another. This membrane is taut during supination and relaxed in pronation. It is sometimes referred to as an articulation, just like the scapulothoracic junction (Figure 8-14).

Palpation

Locate the medial and lateral epicondyles of the humerus and the olecranon process of the ulna. A bursa lies between the olecranon process and the skin. If it can be palpated, it will feel like a small bubble. The synovial membrane is most accessible to examination between the olecranon and the epicondyles. The ulna can be traced by following the bony ridge toward the wrist from the olecranon. The area between the medial epicondyle and olecranon may be sensitive because of the proximity of the ulnar nerve.

Supinate and pronate your forearm and feel the radius rotate on the ulna (Activity 8-7).

JOINTS OF THE WRIST AND HAND

The joints of the wrist and hand include the radiocarpal and carpometacarpal joints.

Radiocarpal Wrist Joint

Articulating bones—Radius, scaphoid and lunate; some triquetrum involvement

Joint type—Synovial condyloid

Ligaments—Palmar radiocarpal ligament from the radius to the scaphoid, lunate, and triquetral; palmar ulnocarpal ligament from the ulna to the scaphoid, lunate, and triquetral; dorsal radiocarpal ligament from the radius to the scaphoid, lunate, and triquetral (See Figure 8-15, which shows the bones that these ligaments connect [ligaments not pictured])

Movements—Flexion, extension, radial and ulnar flexion

The wrist is called the *radiocarpal joint* because the radius alone articulates with the carpal bones. The ulna joins the wrist indirectly by a disk that articulates with the carpal bones. This allows pronation and supination to take place without affecting any wrist movements.

Hand Joints

This intricate pattern of joints is where all the movements involving the hand take place. The metacarpals and phalanges, which make up the palm of the hand and the fingers, form hinge joints permitting flexion and extension.

First carpometacarpal joint (the thumb)

Articulating bones—First metacarpal with trapezium

Joint type—Synovial saddle

Ligaments—Flexor retinaculum from the trapezium to the pisiform, with assistance from the articular capsule

Palmar aponeurosis

Movements—Flexion, extension, abduction, adduction, circumduction, and opposition

The hand is capable of a variety of functions that vary from the precise handling of objects to acts of great strength. The opposable thumb is unique to the human hand and allows us to grasp and manipulate objects. Because the thumb is rotated from the rest of the fingers in the resting position, the thumb faces the rest of the fingers. The joint capsule of the wrist is loose in the superior and inferior directions, allowing easy flexion and extension, but tight laterally and medially, allowing for minimal adduction and abduction. No circumduction occurs at the wrist. Instead, what appears to be a rotation is actually pronation and supination of the forearm combined with wrist flexion.

Palpation

At the wrist, locate the bony tips of the radius (laterally) and the ulna (medially). On the dorsum of the wrist, palpate the groove of the radiocarpal or wrist joint.

Each individual carpal bone within the hand cannot be readily identified, so instead palpate the carpal structure while moving the wrist. Palpate each of the five metacarpals and the proximal, middle, and distal phalanges. Remember the thumb lacks a middle phalanx. Partially flex your fingers, and find the groove marking the metacarpophalangeal joint of each finger. It is distal to the knuckle and can be felt best on either side of the extensor tendon (Activity 8-8).

ACTIVITY 8-7

Move your elbow through the ROM positions.

ACTIVITY 8-8

Move your hand and the wrist through each of the ROM positions.

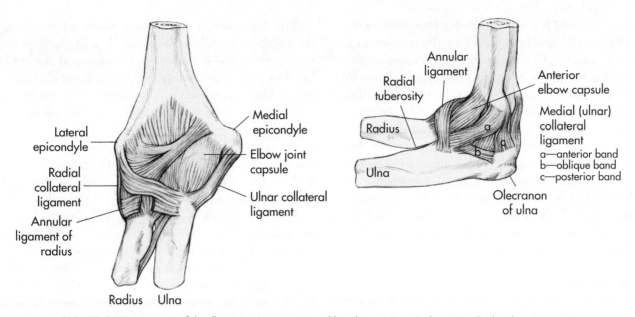

FIGURE 8-14 Ligaments of the elbow joint. Anteroposterior and lateral views. (From Mathers LH et al: *Clinical anatomy principles,* St Louis, 1996, Mosby.)

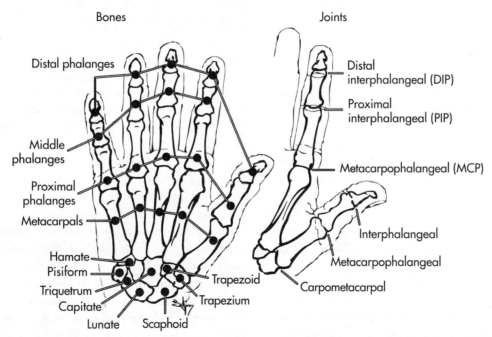

FIGURE 8-15 Joints of the hand and wrist. (From Brister SJ: *Mosbys' comprehensive physical therapist assistant board review,* St Louis, 1996, Mosby.)

JOINTS OF THE PELVIS AND HIP

The sacroiliac joint is a synovial gliding joint. The symphysis pubis is a cartilaginous symphysis, and the hip is a synovial ball-and-socket joint.

Sacroiliac Joint

Articulating bones—Sacrum and the two ilia
Ligaments—Sacroiliac ligament; ventral sacroiliac ligament covers the anterior and inferior aspects of

the joint; interosseous sacroiliac ligament links the sacrum and the iliac tuberosity; dorsal sacroiliac ligament (on the posterior aspect of the joint to the anterior surface of the sacrum) interfaces with the sacrotuberous ligament

This joint connects the pelvis to the trunk. It transfers the weight of the body to the hip and works as a shock absorber during walking and running. The movement allowed is a small but very important anterior and posterior and lateral and medial rotation in a side-lying figure-eight pattern. This rotary movement of the hips at the pelvis allows the vertebral column to remain relatively still as we walk. When the sacroiliac joint does not move, the lack of rotation is compensated for at the sacral lumbar junction, putting strain on the joint. No direct muscle action occurs on this joint. Instead, it moves as a result of other joint movements in the area, following the sacral movement.

Ligaments provide much support. They are more relaxed in the female. This laxity increases with hormones released during monthly cycles and especially during pregnancy (Figure 8-16).

Symphysis Pubis

Articulating bones—Between the two pubic bones

Ligaments—Superior pubic ligament supports the anterior, posterior, and superior aspect; arcuate pubic ligament supports the inferior aspect (these ligaments are not shown in Figure 8-16)

Movement—Slight separation, especially during pregnancy and delivery

The main function of this joint is to provide stability. It connects the left and right coxal (hip) bones anteriorly. Should this joint become misaligned, which can happen during childbirth or trauma such as a fall, the stability of the pelvis is compromised and many postural and soft tissue problems can result (see Figure 8-16).

Hip Joint

Articulating bones—Ilium, pubis, and ischium form the concave surface called the acetabulum; the femur

Ligaments—Iliofemoral ligament from the anterior superior iliac spine to the intertrochanteric line of the femur; ischiofemoral ligament from the ischium to the femur on the posterior side; pubofemoral ligament from the pubis to the intertrochanteric line of the femur on the anterior side; the ligamentum teres, also known as the ligament of the head of the femur, from the fovea to the acetabulum

A fibrocartilaginous ring called the labrum is attached around the edge of the acetabulum and is reinforced by the transverse acetabular ligament. This ring helps hold the femoral head in place by increasing the depth of the acetabulum.

Movements—Flexion, extension, abduction, adduction, medial rotation, lateral rotation, and circumduction

The hip joint is the most massive of the joints. Although a mobile ball-and-socket joint, it is less mobile than the shoulder joint because of the round head of the femur fitting into the deep socket of the acetabulum of the pelvis. This structure provides stability. In the anatomic position the femoral head is not fully in the hip socket. A better fit is when the femur is flexed to 90 degrees, slightly abducted, and laterally rotated. The most relaxed position is flexion, abduction, and lateral rotation such as found in relaxed sitting with the leg falling to the side.

The joint capsule is quite large. All ligaments become tight in lateral rotation and looser in medial rotation. The capsule is more loose in flexion than extension.

Usually the leg moves on the pelvis, but the pelvis can move on the leg if the leg is fixed. With the femur fixed, the pelvis can move forward, which tends to increase the lordosis of the lumbar spine. This is anteversion. Retroversion is the opposite movement that decreases lumbar lordosis. The pelvis can laterally flex and medially flex in connection with flexion of the lumbar spine (Figure 8-17).

Palpation

The hip joint lies deep within the body and is not directly palpable. The posterior edge of the greater trochanter of the femur is easiest to locate. It can be felt about a palm's width below the iliac crest. The superficial trochanteric bursa lies on the posterolateral surface of the greater trochanter. At the same level as the greater trochanter, locate the pubic tubercles. The symphysis pubis can be palpated at the anterior midline of the body. The sacroiliac joint can be palpated just inferior to the posterior superior iliac spine near the "dimples" of the gluteal area. The sacroiliac joint is not directly palpable because it is covered with ligaments, but movements there can be felt. A small rotary movement can be felt if the finger or thumb is held in this area while a person is walking, marching in place, or flexing or extending the trunk (Activity 8-9).

ACTIVITY 8-9

Move your hip through each of the ROM positions.

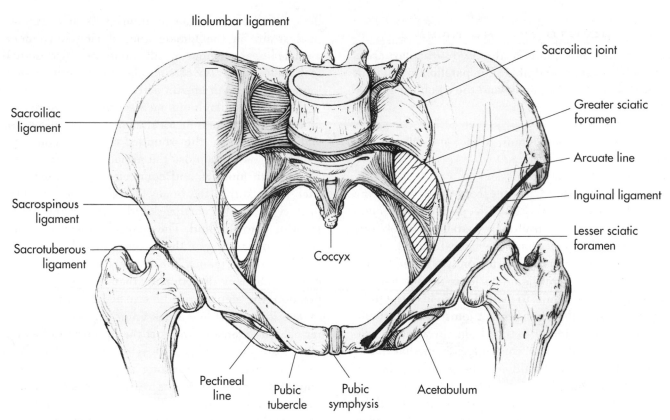

FIGURE 8-16 Pelvic ligaments, superoanterior view. These important ligaments give the pelvis its strength. (From Mathers LH et al: *Clinical anatomy principles,* St Louis, 1996, Mosby.)

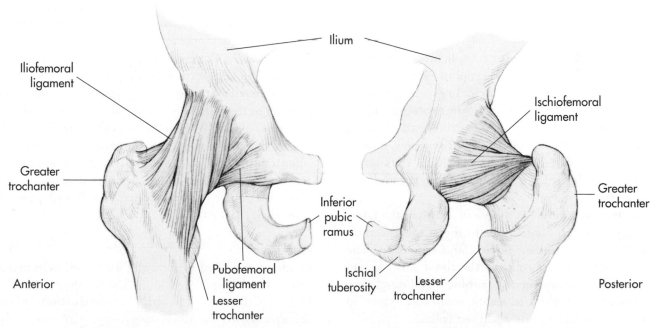

FIGURE 8-17 Ligaments of the hip joint. The three principal hip joint ligaments are arranged in a continuum that surrounds the joint. The iliofemoral ligament is especially important in limiting the extension of the hip. (From Mathers LH et al: *Clinical anatomy principles,* St Louis, 1996, Mosby.)

JOINTS OF THE KNEE

The tibiofemoral joint is the two articular areas between the femur and tibia. The patellofemoral joint is found between the patella and the trochlear groove of femur.

Articulating bones—Femur, tibia, and patella (or kneecap)

Joint type—Synovial condylar

Ligaments—Patellar ligament from the patella to the tibial tuberosity (the quadriceps femoris tendon also provides stability to the patella); the oblique popliteal ligament joins the lateral aspect of the fibrous capsule to the lateral condyle of the femur; the tibial collateral ligament joins the medial epicondyle of the femur to medial condyle of the tibia; the fibular collateral ligament joins the lateral epicondyle of the femur to the fibula; the anterior cruciate ligament joins the anterior medial intercondylar area of the tibia to the medial surface of the lateral condyle of the femur; the posterior cruciate ligament joins the posterior intercondylar area of the tibia to the medial condyle of the femur; the coronary ligament joins the menisci to the tibia; the transverse ligament joins the medial meniscus to the lateral meniscus

Medial and lateral meniscus

Movements—Flexion, extension, medial rotation, and lateral rotation

The knee joint is the most complicated joint in the body. It is not as stable as other joints, yet it is one of the most often used. The principal movements at the knee are flexion and extension. Some rotation is possible during flexion of the joint. Prolonged standing while the knee is in a slightly flexed position, instead of the normal locked extension position, puts stress on the articular surfaces of the condyles and can damage the cartilage.

The medial condyle is more curved than the lateral condyle, which contributes to the automatic rotation of the knee during flexion and extension. The femoral condyle first rolls off the tibial condyle and then glides, producing a combined rolling-gliding movement. The opposite action occurs in extension of the knee—first a glide and then rolling.

In the male the acetabulum is located almost directly above the knee. This allows for even distribution of weight-bearing forces during movement. In contrast, the wider female pelvis results in the knee being medial to the acetabulum. This arrangement puts strain on the female knee during movement. Female knees are not typically anatomically designed to handle the strain of running and repetitive flexion/extension with impact activities.

The fibrocartilaginous menisci provide more surface contact on the tibia for the femur. This allows for stability between the rounded femoral condyles, which sit on an almost flat tibia. The menisci are attached to muscles and connected by ligaments to each other and to the bones. These shock absorbers protect bone and cartilage and increase the movement of synovial fluid. The menisci move in the joint capsule, depending on the forces imposed on them. If the movement against the menisci is too abrupt or quickly changes direction so that they cannot shift position, the menisci can be crushed or torn.

The joint capsule is slack anteriorly and taut posteriorly in extension and just the opposite in flexion. The posterior knee capsule is thick and consists of two strong bands connecting the femoral and tibial condyles. These ligaments resist hyperextension of the joint and provide stability in the standing position in normal extension. In normal extension all the ligaments are taut and the joint can be passively stabilized without any muscular action. This is the most stable position for the knee.

The patella protects the knee joint from external impact such as falling forward onto the knees. The patella moves in a groove between the femoral condyles by the contraction of the quadriceps muscle. The more flexion, the greater the pull on the patella. The contraction of the quadriceps tends to pull the patella laterally during active extension. The position of the patella becomes somewhat unstable in this position. The patella provides an increased mechanical advantage for the quadriceps muscles when contracting to move the knee into extension. The knee is prone to injury because it relies on soft tissue for much of its support in a flexed position (Figure 8-18).

Palpation

Landmarks in and around the knee will help orient you to this complicated joint. Locate the flat medial surface of the tibia—the shin. Follow its anterior border upward to the tibial tuberosity. Move medially and follow the medial border of the tibia upward until it merges into a bony prominence—the medial tibial condyle. This is somewhat higher than the tibial tuberosity. In a comparable location on the other

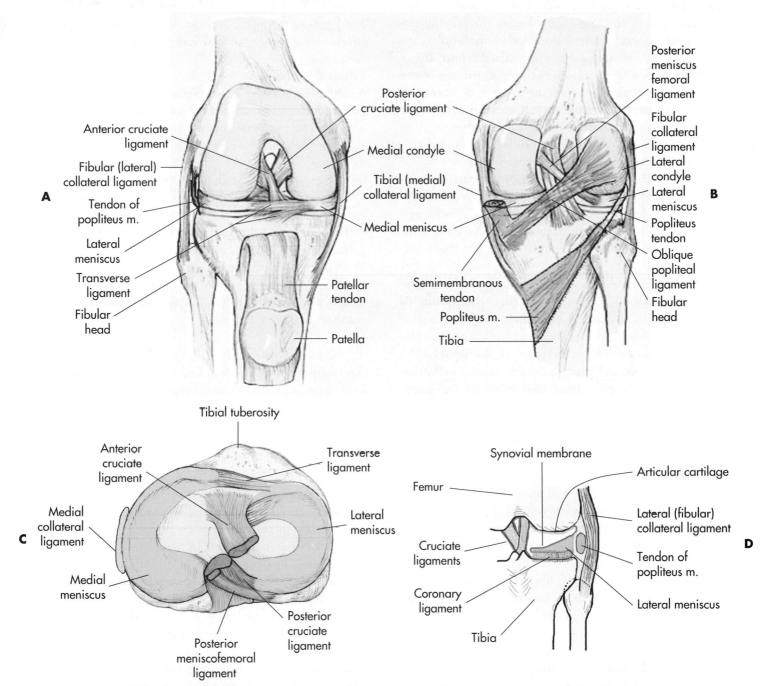

FIGURE 8-18 Knee joint opened, anterior and posterior view. **A,** Anterior view of the knee joint, opened by folding the patella and patellar ligament inferiorly. On the *lateral side* is the fibular collateral ligament, separated by the popliteal tendon from the lateral meniscus. On the *medial side*, the tibial collateral ligament is attached to the medial meniscus. The anterior and posterior cruciate ligaments are seen between the femoral condyles. **B,** Posterior view of the opened knee joint, with a more complete view of the posterior cruciate ligament. Also shown is the posterior meniscofemoral ligament. **C,** The femur is removed, showing the superior (articular) end of the right tibia. On the medial side is the gently curved medial meniscus and, on the lateral side, the more tightly curved lateral meniscus. The anterior end of the medial meniscus is anchored to the surface of the tibia by the transverse ligament. The cut ends of both the anterior and posterior cruciate ligaments are shown, as well as the meniscofemoral ligaments. **D,** This view of the lateral side of the knee illustrates the way the lateral meniscus is attached to the tibial plateau by the coronary ligaments. It is enclosed by synovial membrane, continuous with the general synovial lining of the joint space. (From Mathers LH et al: *Clinical anatomy principles,* St Louis, 1996, Mosby.)

side of the knee, find a similar prominence—the lateral condyle of the knee. Just below the level of the lateral tibial condyle, find the head of the fibula.

Now identify three parts of the distal femur. Bring your fingertips firmly down the medial surface of the thigh along a line where the inner seam of your pant leg would be. Your fingers will run up against an abrupt bony prominence, the adductor tubercle. Just below this is the medial epicondyle. The lateral epicondyle is found in a similar area on the other side.

The patella rests on the anterior articulating surface of the femur, roughly midway between the epicondyles. It lies within the tendon of the quadriceps muscles. This tendon continues below the knee joint, as the patellar tendon, and inserts on the tibial tuberosity.

Two collateral ligaments, one on each side of the knee, give medial and lateral stability to the joint. To feel the lateral collateral ligament, cross one leg so that your ankle rests on the opposite knee. Find the firm cord that runs from the lateral epicondyle of the femur to the head of the fibula. The medial collateral ligament is not palpable. Two cruciate ligaments cross obliquely within the knee and give it anteroposterior stability.

With the knee flexed to about 90 degrees, you can press your thumbs—one on each side of the patellar tendon—into the groove of the tibiofemoral joint. Note that the patella lies just above this joint line. As you press your thumbs downward, you can feel the edge of the upper surface of the tibia. Follow it medially, then laterally until you are stopped by the converging femur and tibia.

The medial and lateral menisci, crescent-shaped fibrocartilaginous pads that lie on the tibial plateaus, form cushions between the tibia and femur. By moving your thumbs up and toward the midline to the top of the patella, you can follow the articulating surface of the femur and identify the margins of the joint. The soft tissue in front of the joint space, on either side of the patellar tendon, is the infrapatellar fat pad.

Several bursae lie near the knee. The prepatellar bursa lies between the patella and the overlying skin, whereas the superficial infrapatellar bursa lies anterior to the patellar tendon.

Observe the concavities that are usually evident at each side and above the patella. In these areas is the synovial cavity of the knee joint. Although the synovium is not normally detectable, these areas may become swollen and tender when the joint is inflamed (Activity 8-10).

JOINTS OF THE ANKLE AND FOOT

The joints of the ankle and foot include the tibiotalar, inferior tibiofibular, and talocalcaneal joints.

Tibiotalar Joint

Articulating bones—Tibia, fibula and talus

Joint type—Synovial saddle joint (many resources classify as synovial hinge); saddle joint classification is due to the accessory movements in plantar flexion

Ligaments—Medial collateral or deltoid from the medial malleolus to the navicular, calcaneus, and talus; lateral collateral from the lateral malleolus to the talus and calcaneus; calcaneofibular from the fibula to the lateral calcaneus

Movements—Dorsiflexion (flexion) and plantar flexion (extension) with slight abduction, adduction, and rotation in plantar flexion caused by the other joints

The metatarsals and phalanges that make up the anterior portion of the foot and the toes form a hinge joint permitting flexion and extension (Figure 8-19).

Inferior Tibiofibular Joint and Talocalcaneal Joint

The inferior tibiofibular joint, a mortise joint, is a fibrous syndesmosis joint that holds the tibia and fibula together as one bone, forming the ankle joint. Immediately distal to the ankle joint is the talocalcaneal joint, or the articulation of the talus with the calcaneus. It is reinforced by the joint capsule and interosseous ligaments, which essentially make the talus and calcaneus one bone, just as the tibiofibular joint function make the tibia and fibula one bone. No muscles insert on the talus. It is moved indirectly by the structures surrounding it. Full dorsiflexion is the more stable position. Most sprained ankles occur in plantar flexion, where less stability is evident. This joint is more stable than mobile because of the structural support, but if these structures are injured, the joint can become very unstable.

Motions of the ankle joint itself are limited to dorsiflexion and plantar flexion, as previously stated.

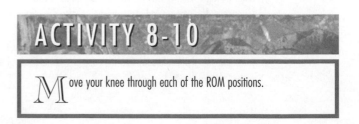

ACTIVITY 8-10

Move your knee through each of the ROM positions.

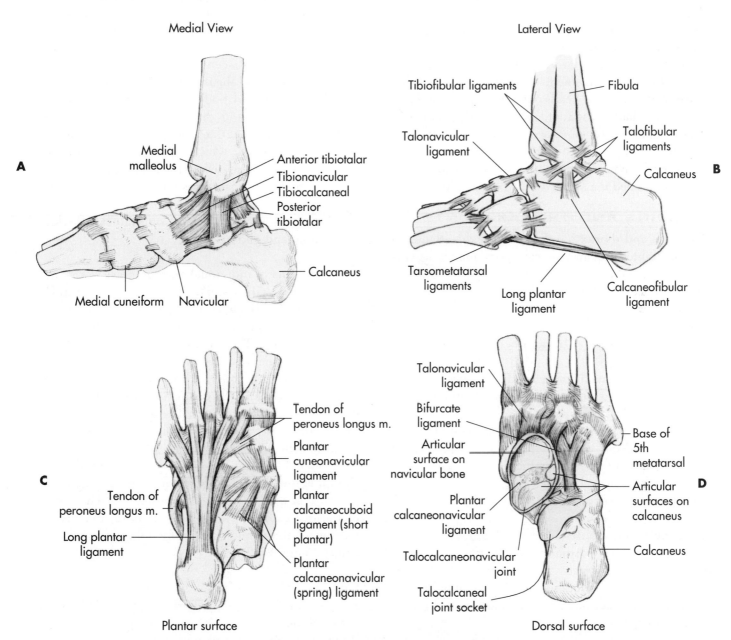

Medial View

Lateral View

Medial malleolus

Anterior tibiotalar
Tibionavicular
Tibiocalcaneal
Posterior tibiotalar

Calcaneus

Medial cuneiform   Navicular

A

Tibiofibular ligaments   Fibula

Talonavicular ligament   Talofibular ligaments

Calcaneus

B

Tarsometatarsal ligaments   Long plantar ligament   Calcaneofibular ligament

Tendon of peroneus longus m.

Plantar cuneonavicular ligament

Plantar calcaneocuboid ligament (short plantar)

Plantar calcaneonavicular (spring) ligament

Tendon of peroneus longus m.

Long plantar ligament

C

Plantar surface

Talonavicular ligament

Bifurcate ligament

Articular surface on navicular bone

Plantar calcaneonavicular ligament

Talocalcaneonavicular joint

Talocalcaneal joint socket

Base of 5th metatarsal

Articular surfaces on calcaneus

Calcaneus

D

Dorsal surface

FIGURE 8-19 A, Deltoid ligament. The deltoid ligament attaches the medial malleolus of the tibia to several underlying bones. It consists of anterior tibiotalar, tibionavicular, tibiocalcaneal, and posterotalar or tibiotalar portions. **B,** Ligaments of the ankle. **C,** Plantar ligaments of the foot, including the long plantar, short plantar, and spring ligaments. **D,** Carpal bones with the talus removed, showing the rounded socket in which it articulates (the talocalcaneonavicular joint). The bifurcate and talonavicular ligaments help stabilize the bones forming this articulation. (From Mathers LH et al: *Clinical anatomy principles,* St Louis, 1996, Mosby.)

Inversion and eversion of the foot are functions of the talocalcaneal and transverse tarsal joints (see Figure 8-19).

Palpation

The principal landmarks of the ankle are the medial malleolus, the bony prominence at the distal end of the tibia, and the lateral malleolus, at the distal end of the fibula. Ligaments extend from each malleolus into the foot. The heads of the metatarsals are palpable in the ball of the foot. These and the associated metatarsophalangeal joints are proximal to the webs of the toes. An imaginary line along the foot bones extending from the heads of the metatarsals to the calcaneous is called the *longitudinal arch* (Activity 8-11).

SPINE AND THORAX JOINTS

The spine and thorax joints consist of the atlantooccipital, atlantoaxial, and intervertebral joints, the vertebral arch, and the costovertebral, costochondral, and chondrosternal joints.

Atlantooccipital Joint

Articulating bones—Atlas and occipital bone at the occipital condyles
Joint type—Synovial condyloid (ellipsoid) joint
Movements—Flexion, extension, and lateral flexion

Atlantoaxial Joint (Atlantoepistropheal Joint) (Figure 8-20)

Articulating bones—Atlas and axis
Joint type—Synovial pivot
Movement—Rotation

Intervertebral Joints (Figure 8-21)

Articulating bones—Adjacent vertebrae
Joint type—Cartilaginous symphysis
Movements—Individual joints allow minimal movement; movement of entire spine as a whole unit is much larger

Vertebral Arch

Articulating bones—Superior and inferior articulating facets of adjacent vertebra.

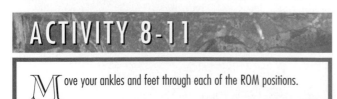

ACTIVITY 8-11

Move your ankles and feet through each of the ROM positions.

Joint type—Synovial gliding joints
Ligaments—Supraspinous ligament and interspinous ligaments between the spinous process of each vertebrae; this supraspinous ligament enlarges in the cervical region and becomes the ligamentum nuchae in the cervical area; intertransverse ligaments connect the transverse processes; ligamenti flavae connect adjacent laminae in the trunk; anterior longitudinal ligament, which connects the anterior vertebral body and disk to the anterior vertebral body and disk located directly above, runs the entire length of the spine; posterior longitudinal ligament, which connects the posterior vertebral body and disk to the above posterior vertebral body and disk, runs the entire length of the spine
Movements—Flexion, extension, lateral flexion, rotation, and gliding

Movements of individual vertebrae are slight, but the cumulative effect of main movements occur at C7 to T1, the cervical thoracic junction; T12 to L1, the thoracolumbar junction; and L5 to S1, the sacral lumbar junction. These areas, where one curve ends and another begins, are more flexible and more prone to injury. In flexion the body of the vertebrae moves forward, and the disk is compressed anteriorly and expanded posteriorly. The fluid nucleus moves toward the back. The posterior ligaments stabilize. In extension the opposite occurs.

A similar pattern is created in lateral flexion. Compression on the side of the flexion increases pressure in the disk on the opposite side. The action of the disks and the ligaments is more involved in movement than the actual bony components of the spine (Figure 8-22).

Costovertebral Joints

Articulating bones—Rib with facets on adjoining vertebrae
Joint Type—Synovial plane joints
Ligaments—Intraarticular ligament from the disk to the head of the rib, and radiate ligaments from the head of the rib to the vertebral body
Movement—Gliding (Figure 8-23)

Costochondral and Chondrosternal Joints

Articulating bones—Costochondral joints: first through the seventh ribs articulate with the costal cartilage; Chondrosternal joints: cartilage articulates with the sternum

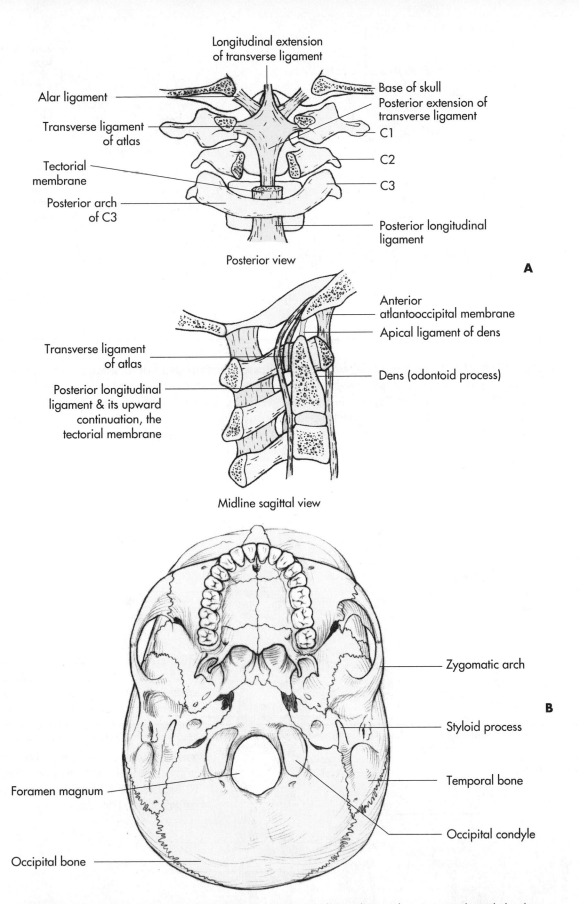

Longitudinal extension of transverse ligament

Alar ligament

Transverse ligament of atlas

Tectorial membrane

Posterior arch of C3

Base of skull

Posterior extension of transverse ligament

C1

C2

C3

Posterior longitudinal ligament

Posterior view

A

Transverse ligament of atlas

Posterior longitudinal ligament & its upward continuation, the tectorial membrane

Anterior atlantooccipital membrane

Apical ligament of dens

Dens (odontoid process)

Midline sagittal view

Zygomatic arch

B

Styloid process

Temporal bone

Foramen magnum

Occipital condyle

Occipital bone

FIGURE 8-20   A, Ligaments connecting the skull and vertebral column. Both C1 and C2 vertebrae are separately attached to the base of the skull to ensure maximal stability. The transverse ligament of the atlas prevents the dens from moving posteriorly and crushing the spinal cord as it passes through the lumen of the C1 vertebra. With its upward and downward extensions, the transverse ligament forms the cruciform ligament. **B,** Base of the skull. On this view, the large occipital condyles are shown. These are the surfaces at which the skull articulates with the C1 vertebra, the atlas. (From Mathers LH et al: *Clinical anatomy principles,* St Louis, 1996, Mosby.)

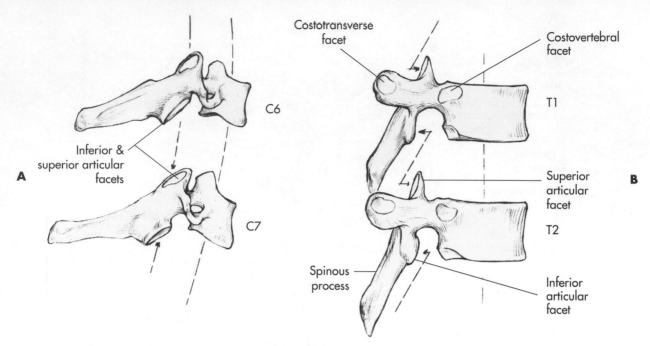

FIGURE 8-21 Vertebral articulations. In these two examples, pairs of articulated cervical and thoracic vertebrae are separated to show their points of attachment. In cervical vertebrae **(A)** the superior and inferior articular facets are nearly in the horizontal plane, whereas for thoracic vertebrae **(B)**, they are in the frontal plane. (In lumbar vertebrae [not shown] the articular facets are in the sagittal plane.) In **A**, the *dashed lines* indicate the position of the anterior and posterior borders of the spinal cord. In **B**, the *vertical dashed line* indicates the articulation of adjacent vertebral bodies. The *jagged dashed lines* indicate the way articular facets align with one another. (From Mathers LH et al: *Clinical anatomy principles,* St Louis, 1996, Mosby.)

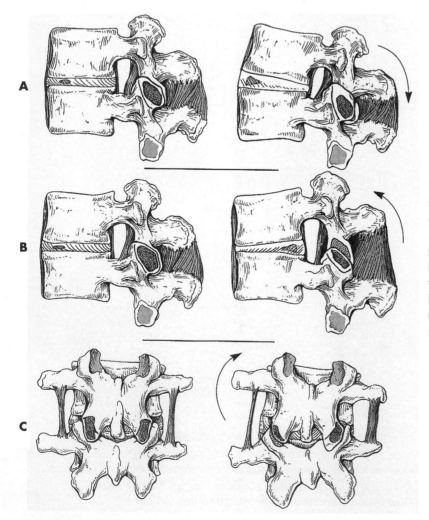

FIGURE 8-22 Motion between adjacent vertebrae. **A** through **C,** *Left,* Vertebrae in their neutral positions. **A,** *Right,* Vertebra in extension. The anterior longitudinal ligament is becoming taut. **B,** *Right,* Vertebra in flexion. Notice that the interspinous and supraspinous ligaments, as well as the ligamentum flavum, are being stretched. **C,** *Right,* Vertebra in lateral flexion. The left intertransverse ligament is becoming taut, and the right superior articular process is making contact with the right lamina. (From Cramer GD, Darby SA: *Basic and clinical anatomy of the spine, spinal cord and ANS,* St Louis, 1995, Mosby.)

Ligaments—Costochondral joints are synchondroses and have no ligaments for support; chondrosternal joints are synovial and are supported by an intraarticular ligament and a thin capsule

Movement—Similar to the movement of a handle on a bucket; movement of the thoracic cage occurs during respiration; small movement of the ribs at the costovertebral joints produces large movements anteriorly of the sternum and laterally of the rib shafts; the result is a change in diameter of the thoracic cage that shifts intrathoracic pressure and enables inspiration to occur (Figure 8-24)

Palpation

Beginning just below the skull, palpate the spinous processes of the cervical vertebrae. The spinous processes of C7 and often T1 are larger and more prominent. Continue along the thoracic spine, noticing the bony prominences of each vertebra. A line drawn between the iliac crest crosses the spinous process of L4 and L5. This is most often used as a reference point to locate the other vertebrae.

Viewed laterally, the spine has cervical and lumbar concavities and a thoracic convexity. The sacral curve forms a second convexity.

The most mobile portion of the spine is the neck. Flexion and extension occur chiefly between the head and the first cervical vertebrae, rotation occurs primarily between the first and second vertebrae, and lateral bending involves the cervical spine from the second to the seventh vertebrae.

Movements of the rest of the spine (i.e., from the sacrum to the base of the neck) are more difficult to measure than those in the neck and are subject to considerable individual variation. The most mobile areas

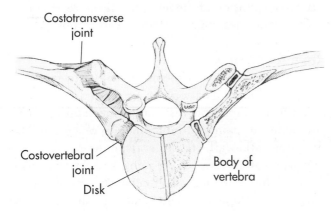

FIGURE 8-23 Joints between the ribs and vertebrae. On the left are shown the intact costovertebral and costotransverse joints, reinforced by ligaments. On the right the joints have been opened, revealing the synovial spaces within. (From Mathers LH et al :*Clinical anatomy principles*, St Louis, 1996, Mosby.)

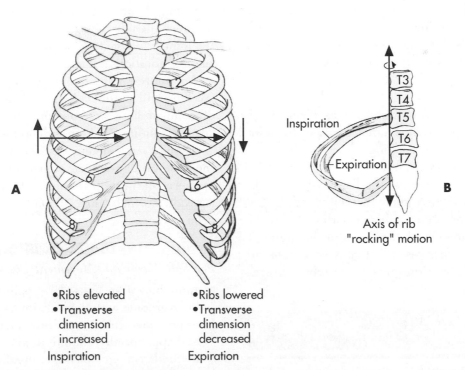

FIGURE 8-24 Rib cage and respirations. **A,** The rib cage in inspiration and expiration, illustrating the upward and lateral excursion that takes place at inspiration. This results in an increase in intrathoracic volume and the movement of air into the tracheobronchial tree. **B,** The "bucket handle" motion of a sample single rib during inspiration and expiration. (From Mathers LH et al: *Clinical anatomy principles*, St Louis, 1996, Mosby.)

are at the thoracolumbar junction of T11 to T12, L1, L4 to L5, and the lumbosacral joint. The angle at the lumbosacral joint is tipped anteriorly so that when the lumbar vertebra wants to slide forward, it is stopped by the contact between the articular facets of S1 and the inferior articular process of L5.

In the thoracic region, follow each rib from its costovertebral joint to the costal cartilage. Feel for the bucket handle motion of the ribs during breathing. Palpate each of the vertebrae, locating each spinous process. Then palpate again during rotation of the spine and identify the thoracolumbar junction of T11 to T12, L1, L4 to L5, and the lumbosacral joint.

What looks like spinal flexion takes place partly at the hips. For this reason, and because people differ in the length of their limbs, flexion cannot be estimated accurately by noting the distance of our fingertips from the floor when we bend over. On forward flexion, watch the lumbar area. Its normal concavity should flatten out (Activity 8-12).

Pathology of the Joints

GENERALIZED JOINT DISORDERS

Any process or event that disturbs the normal function of a specific joint structure will usually set up a chain of events that eventually affects every part of a joint and its surrounding structures. Most pathologic joint conditions fall into the following categories: injury, immobilization, and repetitive overuse.

Injury

Joint injuries are usually classified as dislocations and sprains. A dislocation is a dislodging of the joint parts. A sprain is the wrenching of a joint with rupture or tearing of the ligaments.

Injury such as the tearing of a ligament results in a lack of support for the joint. Instability causes the separation of the articulating bones with wobbling or deviation from the normal alignment of the bones of the joint. These changes in alignment create an abnormal joint distraction on the side where a liga-

ment is torn. As a result the other ligaments, tendons, and the joint capsule may become excessively stretched in the area of the injury.

The uninjured side of the joint can also be affected by being subjected to abnormal compression during weight bearing or movement. Compensation in movement patterns, from both instability and pain, can result in uneven pressure on the joint. Protective muscle spasms develop, limiting movement. In the short-term acute phase of injury, this action provides effective splinting of the area, but if the restriction in ROM continues, immobilization can result.

Immobilization

Immobilization is detrimental to joint structure and function. Immobilization can be caused by a cast or other form of external restraining mechanism such as a reaction to pain and inflammation or by paralysis. Immobilization affects the surrounding soft tissues, the articular surfaces of the joint, and the underlying bone. The detrimental effects of immobilization include development of fibrofatty connective tissue within the joint space, adhesions between the folds of the synovium, atrophy of cartilage, regional osteoporosis, weakening of ligaments at insertion sites, and a decrease in the water content of articular cartilage, tendons, ligaments, and the joint capsule. Swelling or immobilization of a joint also inhibits and weakens the muscles surrounding the joint; therefore the joint is unable to function normally and is at high risk for additional injury.

An injured joint subjected to inflammation and swelling will assume a loose or least- packed position of comfort in which the pressure within the joint space is minimized. Pain is decreased in this position. If the joint movement is restricted for a few weeks in the position of comfort, contractures can develop in the surrounding soft tissues and the joint capsule. As a result, normal range of joint motion will be compromised.

INDICATIONS CONTRAINDICATIONS

For Soft Tissue and Movement Therapies

Immobilization caused by pain and swelling can be overcome with the judicious and short-term use of pain medication, antiinflammatory medications, and appropriate rehabilitation exercise. Soft tissue methods such as massage, myofascial release, and trigger point work are often effective. The application of ice along with rehabilitation exercise is beneficial. Attention needs to be given to the scope

ACTIVITY 8-12

Move your spine and thorax through each of the ROM positions.

of practice and appropriate training to deal with rehabilitation programs. Management and rehabilitation of joint problems is a long-term process often requiring a multidisciplinary approach. Ice, soft tissue applications, and rehabilitation exercise are often methods of choice because they are drugless therapies. Ice is contraindicated in some conditions and thus should be used with caution. All three require active participation by the client, and the methods are not always pleasant. Compliance can be a problem, and the client needs to be motivated toward healing for the best results.

Immobilization from casts, splints, and so on is more difficult to handle. Physicians recognize that prolonged immobilization is undesirable and have developed forms of external stabilization that allow mobility. Dynamic moveable splinting devices such as air casts and continuous passive motion devices that are capable of moving joints passively and repeatedly through a specified position of the physiologic ROM have been beneficial in reducing immobilization in joints. Soft tissue modalities can be used to maintain pliability in accessible connective tissue structures. Soft tissue methods and movement approaches are beneficial in assisting a return to normal function after the splinting is removed.

Soft tissue and movement therapies also help manage compensatory patterns that develop because of casting and other forms of immobilization. Although direct work over an area that is actively healing is contraindicated, massage and other forms of soft tissue work, coupled with movement therapies, can manage the tension and possible pain that the rest of the body may develop from the changes in movement, sleeping positions, and so forth caused from the casting or immobilization process.

In paralysis conditions, soft tissue approaches and movement therapies can help to maintain and in some instances restore pliability of connective tissues. Movement therapies can passively replace joint movement and mimic compressive forces into the bones and jointed areas, helping to prevent contracture and any other detrimental effects of immobilization. Soft tissue and movement therapy intervention for those with paralysis needs to be supervised as part of a total treatment program. Care must be taken with pressure and intensity level because normal feedback mechanisms are disrupted.

Repetitive Overuse

Constant static stress on the joints such as occurs in prolonged standing, sitting, or squatting can damage joint structures. Ligaments subjected to constant tensile loads will creep and can undergo excessive lengthening.

Cartilage subjected to constant compressive loading also can creep and may undergo excessive deformation. Joints and their supporting structures subjected to repetitive loading can be injured and fail because they do not have time to recover their original dimensions before they are subjected to another loading cycle. These types of injuries are common in athletes, dancers, musicians, and factory and office workers.

INDICATIONS CONTRAINDICATIONS

For Soft Tissue and Movement Therapies

Rest, rehabilitative exercise, ergonomically correct equipment, education, and other similar methods are often used to treat and manage overuse syndromes. Soft tissue therapies can both restore and manage some types of connective tissue dysfunctions. Movement modalities can be used to balance movement function and reduce tension patterns.

SPECIFIC DISORDERS

Arthritis

The most common type of joint disorder is termed *arthritis*, which means "inflammation of the joint." Several different kinds of arthritis occur.

Degenerative Joint Disease

Osteoarthritis, or degenerative joint disease (DJD), usually first occurs in middle age and progresses with the aging process as a result of normal wear and tear. Although it appears to be a natural result of aging, such factors as obesity and repeated trauma can help bring it about earlier and more intensely. Osteoarthritis may be a genetic disorder. Although some inflammation may be present, it is a result of the degenerative process. The disease process involves the growth of new bone (called *spurs*) at the edges of the articular surfaces, thickening of the synovial membrane, atrophy of the cartilage, and calcification of the ligaments. Friction is increased between the joint surfaces, further increasing the degenerative process. Osteoarthritis occurs mostly in joints used in weight bearing, such as the hips, knees, and spinal column, but it can occur in most joints. It is not uncommon for joints that have been previously injured to later develop some arthritis. Pain is usually less intense in the morning and steadily worsens throughout the day.

In the hands, nodules on the dorsal lateral aspects of the distal interphalangeal joints, called *Heberden's nodes*, result from the bony overgrowth of osteoarthritis. Flexion and deviation deformities may develop. Usually hard and painless, they affect the middle-aged or elderly and are often associated with arthritic changes in other joints.

Methods of treatment include the use of nonsteroidal antiinflammatory and pain medications. Nonpharmaceutical interventions include moderate exercise that does not cause pain, the use of ice, and topical counterirritant ointments such as capsicum-based preparations. Soft tissue methods can manage excessive protective muscle spasms that may develop. Gentle traction or distraction methods can provide temporary relief. General systemic changes in the neurotransmitters and hormones that accompany exercise and many forms of bodywork can elevate mood and thus reduce pain perception.

Inflammatory Joint Disease

The three types of inflammatory joint disease are immune related, crystal-induced, and infectious.

Immune-related disease

Rheumatoid arthritis is the most common immune-related form of inflammatory joint disease. Lupus erythematosus can be the cause of immune-related arthritis. Rheumatoid arthritis has many characteristics similar to other autoimmune disorders in which antibodies attack normal body tissues. It is a crippling condition characterized by swelling of the joints in the hands, feet, and other parts of the body as a result of inflammation and overgrowth of the synovial membranes and other joint tissues. The disease process changes the composition and quantity of the synovial fluid, altering the lubrication of the joint. The articular cartilage is gradually destroyed, and the joint cavity develops adhesions: the surfaces become stuck together. The joints stiffen and may eventually become useless. The cause of rheumatoid arthritis is uncertain, and the interaction of multiple agents is probable. Genetic factors may influence susceptibility.

Treatment includes the use of various nonsteroidal antiinflammatory drugs. The administration of steroids and gold salts may provide some relief in severe conditions. Localized injection of steroids can reduce severe acute localized symptoms. The use of steroids is controversial, and benefits do not always outweigh the risks of long-term use.

INDICATIONS CONTRAINDICATIONS

For Soft Tissue and Movement Therapies

Because the progression and flare-ups of the disease are often stress related, the generalized gentle stress reduction methods provided by soft tissue and movement therapies may be beneficial in long-term management of the condition, if supervised as part of a total care program. Frictioning techniques or any other forms of bodywork that cause inflammation are to be avoided. General systemic changes in the neurotransmitters and hormones that accompany exercise and many forms of bodywork can elevate mood and thus reduce pain perception.

Crystal-induced disease

Gout is a form of arthritis caused by a disturbance of metabolism. One of the by-products of metabolism is uric acid, which normally is excreted in the urine. If an overproduction of uric acid occurs or for some reason not enough is excreted, the accumulated uric acid forms crystals, which are deposited as masses around the joints and other parts of the body. Gout is characterized by a very painful and tender, hot, dusky red swelling that extends beyond the margin of the joint. It is easily mistaken for cellulitis. Any joint can be involved, but the one most commonly affected is the metatarsophalangeal joint of the great toe. Most victims of gout are men past middle age. Treatment includes dietary modifications.

INDICATIONS CONTRAINDICATIONS

For Soft Tissue and Movement Therapies

Soft tissue and movement modalities are regionally contraindicated.

Infectious arthritis

Infectious arthritis can be brought on by such infections as rheumatic fever, gonorrhea, and tuberculosis. Gonorrheal arthritis is becoming widespread as a result of the tremendous increase in the number of cases of gonorrhea.

The joints and bones themselves are subject to attack by the tuberculosis organism, and the result may be gradual destruction of parts of the bone near the joint. The organism is carried by the bloodstream, usually from the lungs or lymph nodes, and may cause considerable damage before it is discovered. Several vertebrae sometimes are affected, or one hip or other single joint may be diseased. The client may complain only of difficulty in walking, and diagnosis is difficult unless an accompanying lung tuberculosis has been found. This disorder is most common in children. Referral for proper diagnosis is important.

INDICATIONS CONTRAINDICATIONS

For Soft Tissue and Movement Therapies

> Infectious disease is a contraindication for bodywork unless directly supervised by appropriate heath care professionals.

Ganglion

Ganglia are cystic, round, usually nontender swellings located along tendon sheaths or joint capsules. The dorsum of the hand and wrist is a frequent site of involvement. Flexion of the wrist makes ganglia more prominent, whereas extension tends to obscure them. Ganglia may also develop elsewhere on the hands, wrists, ankles, and feet.

INDICATIONS CONTRAINDICATIONS

For Soft Tissue and Movement Therapies

> Bodywork methods are regionally contraindicated.

Bursitis

Bursitis is one of the most common causes of joint pain. Inflammation of the bursae, especially those located between the bony prominences and a muscle or tendon such as in the shoulder, elbow, hip, or knee, usually results from trauma. Repetitive overuse, or rheumatoid or gouty arthritis, may also cause bursitis. A common treatment includes the use of rest during the acute phase but only for a short time to avoid pathologic immobilization. Analgesics and local injections of antiinflammatory medications can also be helpful. Ice, soft tissue methods that reduce any muscle tension contributing to the development of inflammation, and a readjustment of activities to reduce strain on the bursa are beneficial. Often a postural deviation changes the angle of function at a joint, resulting in irritation at an area of a bursae. Restoring normal postural alignment elevates the irritation and the bursitis may resolve itself.

Lateral Epicondylitis

Lateral epicondylitis (tennis elbow) follows repetitive extension of the wrist or pronation-supination of the forearm. Pain and tenderness develop at the lateral epicondyle and possibly in the proximal extensor

muscles. When the wrist is extended against resistance, pain increases. Treatment is similar to bursitis mentioned previously.

Medial Epicondylitis

Medial epicondylitis (golfer's or pitcher's elbow) follows repetitive wrist flexion, as in throwing. Tenderness is maximal at the medial epicondyle. Wrist flexion against resistance increases the pain. Again, treatment is similar to that of bursitis.

Adhesive Capsulitis (Frozen Shoulder)

Adhesive capsulitis refers to a mysterious fibrosis of the glenohumeral joint capsule, manifested by diffuse, dull, aching pain in the shoulder and progressive restriction of motion, but usually no localized tenderness. The condition is usually unilateral and most often occurs in persons 50 to 70 years of age. Onset is often preceded by some sort of pathologic condition, resulting in the joint being immobilized. Pathologic immobilization sets in. The course is chronic, lasting months to years, but the disorder often resolves itself spontaneously, at least partially. Treatment is with physical therapy, including ROM exercises.

INDICATIONS CONTRAINDICATIONS

For Soft Tissue and Movement Therapies

> Soft tissue and movement therapies can be a beneficial adjunctive treatment, especially with the symptomatic management of pain.

Backache

Backache is a common complaint. Although most often people complain of lower back pain, neck or cervical pain is also common. The usual cause is muscular and will be discussed later. Some joint causes are listed below.

Disorders of the intervertebral disks, especially those in the lower lumbar region, can cause back pain. Pain may be very severe, with muscle spasms and the resulting nerve impingement extending symptoms along the course of the nerve to the legs and groin. The condition can degenerate to a ruptured disk, which is a posterior or posterolateral protrusion of the nucleus pulposus through a tear in the annulus fibroses, placing pressure on nerves.

Abnormalities of the vertebrae or ligaments and other supporting structures include the following:

- Strains on the lumbosacral joint (where the lumbar region joins the sacrum) or strains on the sacroiliac joint (where the sacrum joins the ilium)

- Spondylolisthesis, or the moving forward of part of one vertebra on another; usually occurs at L5/S1
- Spondylitis, or inflammation of more than one vertebra
- Ankylosing spondylitis, or rheumatoid inflammatory disorder, in which the articular hyaline cartilage is destroyed, the bones fuse, and the spinal ligaments ossify; tends to begin in the sacroiliac joints and progress up the spine
- Spondylosis, or the formation of bony spurs at the disk margin of the vertebral bodies; causes degenerative changes in the intervertebral disks

Abnormal Spinal Curvatures

Abnormal spine curvatures result from postural deviation, especially the forward head position. Several types occur.

Flattening of the lumbar curve results in muscle spasm in the lumbar area and decreased spinal mobility. This combination of signs suggests the possibility of a herniated lumbar disk or, especially in men, ankylosing spondylitis.

Lordosis is an accentuation of the normal lumbar curve that develops to compensate for the protuberant abdomen of pregnancy or marked obesity. It may also compensate for kyphosis and flexion deformities of the hips.

Kyphosis—a rounded thoracic convexity—is common in aging. It occurs especially in women.

Gibbus is an angular deformity of a collapsed vertebra. Causes include metastatic cancer and tuberculosis of the spine.

List is a lateral tilt of the spine. When a plumb line dropped from the spinous process of T1 falls to one side of the gluteal cleft, a list is present. Causes include a herniated disk and painful spasms of the paravertebral muscles.

Scoliosis is a lateral curvature of the spine. It may be structural or functional. Structural scoliosis is typically associated with rotation of the vertebrae on one another, and the rib cage is accordingly deformed. This deformity is seen best when the client bends forward. On the side of the thoracic convexity, the ribs bulge posteriorly and are widely separated. On the opposite side, they are displaced anteriorly and are close together.

Functional scoliosis compensates for other abnormalities such as unequal leg lengths. It involves neither vertebral rotation nor thoracic deformity. The scoliosis disappears with forward flexion.

INDICATIONS CONTRAINDICATIONS

For Soft Tissue and Movement Therapies

Most backache can be prevented. The back muscles should not be used for lifting. Weight should be brought close to the body, above the hips if possible, and the legs allowed to do the actual lifting. An adequate exercise program is also important.

Soft tissue and movement modalities are effective in the management of backache. The benefits derived are from reduction in protective muscle spasm and generalized pain-modulating effects. Be aware that protective spasm provides stabilization. The goal is not to eliminate protective spasm but to support the body in management of dysfunctional patterns. Complex backache involving the joint structures requires that soft tissue methods be incorporated into a total treatment program with supervision by the appropriate health care professional.

Summary

A comprehensive understanding of joint structure and function is necessary for the effective practice of soft tissue and movement therapies. Bodywork methods can be used to support joint health and provide benefits in the management of joint dysfunction.

The health and strength of joint structures depend on a certain amount of stress and strain. Cartilage and bone nutrition and growth depend on joint movement and muscle contraction. Cartilage nutrition depends on joint movement through a full ROM to ensure that all of the articular cartilage receives the nutrients necessary for health. Ligaments and tendons depend on a normal amount of stress and strain to maintain and increase strength. Bone density and strength increase after the stress and strain created by muscle and joint activity. In contrast, bone density and strength decrease when stress and strain are absent.

Without stress and strain the joints do not function well, but with too much stress and strain a pathologic condition may develop. People are similar. We need to be exposed to challenges in life, but attempting to deal with too much can be overwhelming. The concept of balance is illustrated again—both in joint health and personal well-being.

WORKBOOK SECTION

1. Describe the elementary principles of joint design.

_____

_____

_____

_____

_____

_____

_____

_____

_____

_____

_____

_____

2. Define the two main types of joints.

_____

_____

_____

_____

_____

_____

_____

_____

3. Define arthrokinematics and osteokinematics and the three categories of ROM.

_____

_____

_____

_____

_____

_____

_____

_____

_____

_____

_____

_____

_____

_____

4. Describe joint play.

_____

_____

_____

_____

_____

5. List the structures that contribute to joint stability.

_____

_____

_____

_____

6. Identify the generalized joint disorders and describe a treatment protocol used for each.

_____

_____

_____

_____

_____

_____

_____

_____

FILL IN THE BLANK

_____ (1) refers to the amount of motion available to a joint within the anatomic limits of the joint structure. An articulation, or _____ (2) is where two or more bones meet to connect parts together and allow for movement in the body.

_____ (3) are flat sacs of synovial membrane in which the inner sides of the sacs are separated by a fluid film. Bursae are located where moving structures are apt to _____ (4).

A _____ (5) occurs when joints of the human body are linked together into a series in such a way that motion at one of the joints is accompanied by motion at an adjacent joint.

The _____ (6) is the only position in a synovial joint where the surfaces fit precisely together and maximal contact occurs between the opposing surfaces. Because the joint surfaces are _____ (7), they permit no movement, and the joint possesses its greatest stability.

Collagen is a fibrous tissue that provides stability to _____ (8) tissue structures. _____ (9) is a fibrous tissue that has elastic properties and allows flexibility of connective tissue structures.

Diarthrosis is a freely movable _____ (10) joint.

_____ (11) is a connective tissue that permits little motion in joints and structures. It is found in such places as the intervertebral disks and forms our ears.

Hyaline cartilage is the thin covering of _____ (12) connective tissue on the ends of the bones in freely movable joints in the adult skeleton.

Hypermobility occurs when the ROM of a joint is _____ (13) than would normally be permitted by the structure. It results in _____ _____ (14).

_____ (15) occurs when the ROM of a joint is less than what would normally be permitted by the structure. It results in _____ (16) ROM.

The joint _____ (17) is a connective tissue structure that indirectly connects the bony components of a joint.

Joint play is the _____ (18) movement that occurs between articular surfaces, which have nothing to do with the ROM of a joint produced by _____ (19). It is an essential component of joint motion and must occur for normal functioning of the joint.

The loose-packed position is the position of a synovial joint where the joint capsule is at its most _____ (20). Joints tend to assume this position when _____ (21) occurs to accommodate the increased volume of synovial fluid.

Open kinematic chain occurs when the ends of the limbs or parts of the body are free to move without causing _____ (22) at another joint.

_____ (23) ROM is the amount of motion at a joint that either fails to reach the normal physiologic range or exceeds normal anatomic limits of motion of that joint.

Physiologic ROM is the amount of motion available to a joint determined by the nervous system from information provided by joint _____ _____ (24) receptors. This information usually prevents a joint from being positioned where _____ _____ (25) could occur.

_____ (26) is a limited movement, nonsynovial joint.

A suture is a _____ (27) joint in which two bony components are united by a thin layer of dense fibrous tissue.

A symphysis is a _____ (28) joint in which the two bony components are directly joined by fibrocartilage in the form of a disk or plate.

Synchondrosis is a joint in which the material used for connecting the two components is _____ (29) growth cartilage.

Syndesmosis is a _____ (30) joint in which two bony components are joined directly by a ligament, cord, or aponeurotic membrane.

_____ (31) fluid is a thick, colorless, lubricating fluid that is secreted by the membrane of the joint cavity.

Types of _____ (32) joints include the following:

Hinge joint: allows flexion and extension movement in _____ (33) direction, changing the angle of the bones at the joint, similar to a door hinge.

_____ (34) joint: allows rotation around the length of the bone.

Condyloid (condylar) joints allow movement in _____ (35) directions, but one motion predominates.

A saddle joint is both _____ (36) in one plane and concave in the other, and these surfaces fit together like a rider on a saddle.

A _____ (37) joint allows movement in many directions around a central point.

Gliding joints, also known as synovial _____ (38) joints allow only a gliding motion in various planes.

_____ (39) is the combination of resistance offered by a fluid to a change of form and the ability of material to return to its original state after deformation. This term is used to describe _____ (40) tissue.

PROBLEM SOLVING

Read the problem presented. There is no correct answer. Instead the exercise assists the student in the development of analysis and decision-making skills necessary in a professional practice.

1. Identify the facts presented in the information.
2. Identify the possibilities ("what if" statements) presented or develop your own possibilities that relate to the facts.
3. Evaluate each possibility in terms of the logical cause and effect and pros and cons.
4. Consider the feelings of the people involved.
5. Write each down in the space provided.
6. Develop your solution by answering the question posed.

PROBLEM

All movement involves joints. Individuals who move for a living such as professional athletes or dancers are particularly susceptible to joint dysfunction. Injury is more than an inconvenience; it can put an end to a career. Many of these people continue to work in pain. Proper healing time is not allowed and additional damage may result.

Young children who begin to train for competition before puberty modify a more pliable joint structure. Hypermobility may result. As these people age, joint structure is compromised by laxity in the joints, and pain and various degrees of disability can result.

QUESTION

In what ways can a soft tissue and movement therapist use the information present in this chapter to educate the vulnerable client about the need for support of the joints so that accumulating damage does not continue?

FACTS

1. People who move professionally are susceptible to joint injury.
2. _____
3. _____

POSSIBILITIES

1. People may work with joint injury.
2. _____
3. _____

LOGICAL CAUSE AND EFFECT AND PROS AND CONS

1. Performance would not be as good.
2. _____
3. _____

IMPACT ON PEOPLE

1. The bodywork professional may feel frustrated working with someone who will not or cannot take time off for appropriate healing.
2. _____
3. _____

In what ways can a soft tissue and movement therapist use the information present in this chapter to educate the vulnerable client about the need for support of the joints so that accumulating damage does not continue?

_____
_____
_____
_____
_____
_____
_____
_____

PROFESSIONAL APPLICATION

Connective tissue plays an important role in joint health. For the modalities you are studying, what are the specific applications to connective tissue function? What other knowledge would you require to work more effectively with connective tissues? What referral base would be necessary to best support a client with connective tissue dysfunction affecting the joints?

_____
_____
_____
_____
_____
_____
_____
_____
_____
_____
_____
_____

FURTHER STUDY

Using a comprehensive anatomy and physiology text (see the Works Consulted list at the back of this book), elaborate on the following topics:

Connective tissue

_____

_____

_____

_____

_____

_____

_____

_____

_____

_____

_____

Cartilage

_____

_____

_____

_____

_____

_____

_____

_____

_____

_____

_____

_____

Kinematic chains

_____

_____

_____

_____

_____

_____

_____

_____

_____

_____

_____

Immobilization pathology

_____

_____

_____

_____

_____

_____

_____

_____

_____

_____

_____

_____

_____

Repetitive overuse syndrome

_____

_____

_____

_____

_____

_____

function of mobility and stability. Simple joints provide more stability. Complex joints provide more mobility.

2. The two main types of joints are synarthroses, which are nonsynovial limited-movement joints and consist of fibrous joints, and cartilaginous joints. Diarthroses, which are synovial, freely moveable joints, consist of the following:

- A joint capsule formed of fibrous tissue
- Hyaline cartilage covering the joint surfaces
- A joint cavity enclosed by the joint capsule
- Synovial fluid forming a film over the joint surfaces
- A synovial membrane lining the inner surface of the capsule

3. *Arthrokinematics* is used to refer to movements of joint surfaces. A *roll* refers to the rolling of one joint surface on another. *Sliding* refers to the gliding of one component over another. *Spin* refers to a rotation of the movable component. *Osteokinematics* refers to the movement of the bones rather than the movement of the articular surfaces. Three categories of *range of motion* exist: anatomic, physiologic, and pathologic. The *anatomic range of motion* refers to the amount of motion available to a joint within the anatomic limits of the joint structure. The anatomic range of motion may extend the limits of available range of motion to where joint injury can occur. Therefore many joints have established a physiologic range of motion set by the nervous system from information provided by joint sensory receptors. Usually this physiologic range of motion is somewhat less than the anatomic range of motion, preventing a joint from being positioned where injury could occur. Pathologic range of motion occurs when motion at a joint either fails to reach the normal physiologic range or exceeds normal anatomic limits of motion. Two main pathologic conditions exist: hypomobility and hypermobility.

4. The involuntary movement that occurs between articular surfaces, which has nothing to do with the range of motion of a joint produced by muscles, is an essential component of joint motion and must occur for the joint to function normally. In an optimal situation a joint has a sufficient amount of play to allow normal motion of the joint. If the supporting joint structures are lax, the joint may have too much play and become unstable. If the joint structures are tight, the joint will have too little movement between the articular surfaces, and the amount of motion will be restricted.

5. Structures contributing to bone stability include bone shape, ligaments, joint capsule, fibrocartilaginous rings, tendons, fascia, and muscles.

6. Most joint disorders fall into the following categories: injury, immobilization, and repetitive overuse. Joint injuries are usually classified as dislocations and sprains. A dislocation is a dislodging of the joint parts. A sprain is the wrenching of a joint with rupture or tearing of the ligaments.

Immobilization can be caused by a cast or other form of external restraining mechanism, as a reaction to pain and inflammation, or from paralysis. The detrimental effects of immobilization include development of fibrofatty connective tissue within the joint space; adhesions between the folds of the synovium; atrophy of cartilage; regional osteoporosis; weakening of ligaments at insertion sites; and a decrease in the water content of articular cartilage, tendons, liga-

Ergonomics

Answer Key

1. Some joints provide stability. Some joints provide mobility. The structure of the joint determines the function of the joint. A breakdown or change of any joint structure will affect the entire joint function. Joints connect two or more bones. The design of a joint depends on its function. Each part of the joint has a specific function that is essential to the whole function of the joint. Complex joints are more likely to malfunction than simple joints. Effective functioning of the whole body depends on the integrated action of many joints working together. Generally, stability must be achieved before mobility. Most joints serve a dual

ments, and the joint capsule. Swelling or immobilization of a joint also inhibits and weakens the muscles surrounding the joint; therefore the joint is unable to function normally and is at high risk for additional injury.

Repetitive overuse results from constant static stress on the joints such as occurs in prolonged standing, sitting, or squatting; it can damage joint structures. Ligaments subjected to constant tensile loads will creep and can undergo excessive lengthening.

Cartilage subjected to constant compressive loading also can creep and may undergo excessive deformation. Joints and their supporting structures subjected to repetitive loading can be injured and fail because they do not have time to recover their original dimensions before they are subjected to another loading cycle.

Soft tissue and movement therapies also help manage compensatory patterns that develop because of casting and other forms of immobilization. Although direct work over an area that is in an active healing process is contraindicated, massage and other forms of soft tissue work, coupled with movement therapies, can manage the tension and possible pain that the rest of the body may develop from the changes in movement, sleeping positions, and so on.

Rest, rehabilitative exercise, ergonomically correct equipment, and education are used to treat and manage overuse syndromes. Soft tissue therapies can both restore and manage some types of connective tissue dysfunctions. Movement modalities can be used to balance movement function and reduce tension patterns.

FILL IN THE BLANK

1. Anatomic range of motion (ROM)
2. joint
3. Bursae
4. rub
5. closed kinematic chain
6. close-packed position
7. compressed
8. connective
9. elastin
10. synovial
11. Fibrocartilage
12. articular
13. more
14. instability
15. Hypomobility
16. restricted
17. capsule
18. involuntary
19. muscles
20. lax
21. inflammation
22. motion
23. Pathologic
24. sensory
25. injury
26. Synarthrosis
27. synarthrotic
28. cartilaginous
29. hyaline
30. fibrous
31. Synovial
32. synovial
33. one
34. Pivot
35. two
36. convex
37. ball and socket
38. plane
39. Viscoelasticity
40. connective

Chapter 9

The Muscles

CHAPTER OUTLINE

Muscle Structure and Function
  Muscle tissue and the whole body
  Anatomy and physiology of muscle
    Muscle tone
    Types of muscle fiber
    Heat
    Blood supply
    Connective tissue
    Repair of muscle
    Attachments
    Muscle shapes
  Myotatic units or functional muscle groups
  Proprioceptors and reflexes
    Stretch reflex
    Tendon reflex
    Flexor reflex and crossed-extensor reflex
  Function of cardiac and smooth muscle tissue
    Cardiac muscle
    Smooth muscle

Individual Muscles
  Muscles of the face and head
    Muscles of facial expression
    Auricular (ear) muscles
    Eye muscles
    Muscles that move the mouth
    Muscles of mastication (chewing)
  Muscles of the neck
    Anterior triangle of the neck
    Suprahyoid muscles
    Infrahyoid muscles
    Posterior triangle of the neck
    Scalene group
  Deep muscles of the back and posterior neck
    Deep posterior cervical muscles
    Vertical muscles, erector spinae group
    Oblique muscles, transversospinalis group
    Suboccipital muscles

CHAPTER OBJECTIVES

After completing this chapter, the student should be able to perform the following:

- Describe the functions of muscles.
- List the three types of muscles.
- Describe the types of skeletal muscle fiber.
- List the components of myotatic units.
- Identify the origin, insertion, function, synergist, antagonist, and common trigger points of individual muscles.

KEY TERMS

Agonist A muscle that causes or controls joint motion through a specified plane of motion; known as a primary or prime mover.

All-or-none response The property of muscle contraction by which, when contraction is initiated, all the muscle fibers either contract to their full ability or do not contract at all.

Antagonist (an-TAG-a-nist) A muscle usually located on the opposite side of a joint from the agonist and having the opposite action. The antagonist works with the agonist by relaxing and allowing movement.

Contractility (kon-trak-TIL-i-tee) The ability of a muscle to shorten forcibly with adequate stimulation. This property sets muscle apart from all other types of tissue.

Deep fascia A coarse sheet of fibrous connective tissue that binds muscles into functional groups and forms partitions, called *intermuscular septa,* between muscle groups.

Dynamic force Force applied to an object that produces movement in or of the object.

Elasticity The ability of a muscle to recoil and resume its original resting length after being stretched.

Excitability The ability of a muscle to receive and respond to a stimulus.

Extensibility (eks-tensi-BIL-i-tee) The ability of a muscle to be stretched or extended.

Fixator (fik-SAY-tor) One of the stabilizing muscles surrounding a joint or body part that contract to fixate, or stabilize, the area, enabling another limb or body segment to exert force and move.

Insertion The distal attachment of a muscle; the part of a muscle that attaches farthest from the midline, or center, of the body.

Maximal stimulus The point at which all motor units of a muscle have been recruited and the muscle is unable to increase in strength.

Motor unit All the muscle fibers innervated by a single motor neuron.

Origin The proximal attachment of a muscle; the part that attaches closest to the midline (center) of the body. The least movable part of a muscle.

Oxygen debt The extra amount of oxygen that must be taken in to convert lactic acid to glucose or glycogen.

Static force Force applied to an object in such a way that it does not produce movement.

Synergist (SIN-er-jist) A muscle that aids or assists the action of the agonist but is not primarily responsible for the action; also known as a *guiding muscle*.

Threshold stimulus The stimulus at which the first observable muscle contraction occurs.

Tone A state of slight contraction in all skeletal muscle that enables the muscle to respond to stimulation.

Trigger points "A myofascial trigger point is a hyperirritable locus within a taut band of skeletal muscle, located in the muscular tissue and/or its associated fascia. The spot is painful on compression and can evoke characteristic referred pain and autonomic phenomena." (Travell, 1983).

Muscle Structure and Function

Muscles and their associated connective tissue make up the soft tissues of our bodies. In artistic terms, you could say that muscles and connective tissue are the medium of soft tissue and movement practitioners. Just as a sculptor needs to understand clay, the soft tissue therapist needs to understand muscles. Because soft tissue accounts for about half the body's tissue mass and most pain patterns find themselves connected to soft tissue dysfunctions of various types, the careful study of this area of anatomy and physiology is obviously important.

Volumes of material have been written about the intricacies of soft tissue structure and function. This text, by necessity, limits itself to the most clinically practical information as it relates to the methods used by soft tissue and movement therapists. Also, because this chapter is by no means an exhaustive study, the student is encouraged to make use of the list of Works Consulted at the back of this text. The wise student also should commit herself to continual formal study and self-study of this material.

The body has three types of muscle tissue: skeletal muscle, cardiac muscle, and smooth muscle. This chapter focuses on skeletal muscle tissue and provides a brief overview of cardiac and smooth muscle.

The word *muscle* means "little mouse." Apparently someone thought that muscle contractions looked like mice scurrying beneath the skin. A prominent functional characteristic of muscle is its ability to transform chemical energy from adenosine triphosphate (ATP) into mechanical energy. When this happens, muscle can exert force.

Force is energy applied in such a way that it initiates motion, changes the speed or direction of a motion, or alters the size and shape of an object. **Dynamic force** is force on an object that produces movement; **static force** does not produce movement.

Energy is defined technically as the capacity to do work. Many cultures use the words *force* and *energy* in referring to esoteric concepts. We find it in Eastern philosophy as *qi* or *prana*, and in the *Star Wars* movie trilogy as "The Force"—all these words translate to energy, vital force, life force. One doesn't have to stretch the imagination too far to see the metaphor of muscles in these more expansive concepts.

Muscle tissue transforms one form of energy into another and is able to produce force. Dynamic force creates movement and change; static force produces no movement or noticeable change, yet still expends energy. If therapeutic interaction can help transform static force into dynamic force, the energy to achieve therapeutic goals can be released; this often is the objective that soft tissue and movement professionals are seeking to achieve with their clients.

MUSCLE TISSUE AND THE WHOLE BODY

The functions of the three muscle types are integral to the maintenance of homeostasis of the whole body. The four major functions of muscle follow:

1. To produce movement
2. To generate heat
3. To maintain posture
4. To stabilize joints

All three types of muscle tissue produce the movement necessary for survival. Skeletal muscle moves the skeleton so that we can seek shelter, gather food, and protect ourselves. Skeletal, cardiac, and smooth muscles all produce movement, such as that involved in breathing, the heartbeat, digestion, and elimination.

The relative constancy of the body's internal temperature could not be maintained in a cool external environment if not for the "waste" heat generated by muscle tissue during contraction.

Maintenance of a relatively stable body posture is primarily a function of the skeletal-muscular system. The dynamic tension of muscle contraction opposes the force of gravity.

Stabilization of the joint structures is an often overlooked function of muscle. Especially in the more mobile joints, which by nature have a loose structural design, the dynamic contraction of muscles surrounding the joint provides external stability, supporting the structures of the joint proper.

A number of systems support the function of muscle tissues. The nervous system directly controls the contraction of skeletal muscle and smooth muscle. It also influences the rate of rhythmic contraction in cardiac muscle and visceral smooth muscle. The endocrine system produces hormones that promote repair of muscle tissue and assist the nervous system in regulating muscle contraction throughout the body. The blood delivers nutrients and carries away waste products. Nutrients for the muscle are ultimately procured by the digestive system. Work done by the body requires ATP, and glucose is the fuel for the manufacture of ATP. Potassium and insulin are required for glucose to enter the muscle cell. The digestive, respiratory, and urinary systems eliminate the waste products of muscle metabolism. Lactic acid is the end product of muscle work and is transported by the bloodstream to the liver, to be converted back to glucose; this process uses oxygen. The immune system helps defend muscle tissue against infection and cancer, as it does for all body tissues. Because the systems of the body function interdependently, muscle tissue gives to and receives from the entire body.

Muscles have the following four functional characteristics:

1. **Excitability** — Excitability is the ability to receive and respond to a stimulus. A stimulus is a change in the internal or external environment. One of the major reasons soft tissue and movement therapies are beneficial is that they provide specific forms of stimulus to the muscles, which in turn stimulate maintenance of homeostasis.

2. **Contractility** — Contractility is the ability to shorten forcibly with adequate stimulation. This property sets muscle apart from all other types of tissue. As mentioned earlier, muscle tissue interacts with all body systems, but it makes a unique contribution: the ability to contract allows the entire organism to move.

3. **Extensibility** — Extensibility is the ability to be stretched or extended. In any movement pattern, one group of muscles contracts while another group extends, together achieving stability, balance, and the ability to return to the neutral position. This interaction is the foundation of homeostasis, the ability to respond and return to balance.

4. **Elasticity** — Elasticity is the ability to recoil and resume the original resting length after being stretched. Elasticity also includes the ability to remember where the process began and return to the previous position (Activity 9-1).

ACTIVITY 9-1

Using the functional characteristics of muscle as a metaphor, provide examples of the ways in which your learning thus far has functioned like a muscle. Examples are provided to get you started.

Example

Excitability—The ability to receive and respond to a stimulus: Learning the names of the muscles is a new stimulus.

Contractility—The ability to shorten forcibly and produce movement when adequately stimulated: Using the information about the endocrine system has helped me better understand mood so that I can move more deliberately from one mood to another.

Extensibility—The ability to be stretched or extended: Seeking to understand the Eastern concepts in this text has stretched my belief system.

Elasticity—The ability to recoil and resume the original resting length after being stretched: My self-awareness has been reinforced by acquiring knowledge about my body.

Your Turn

Excitability—The ability to receive and respond to a stimulus:

Contractility—The ability to shorten forcibly and produce movement when adequately stimulated:

Extensibility—The ability to be stretched or extended:

Elasticity—The ability to recoil and resume the original resting length after being stretched:

ANATOMY AND PHYSIOLOGY OF MUSCLE

Each skeletal muscle is an individual organ made of hundreds and sometimes thousands of muscle fibers (or cells), large amounts of connective tissue and nerve fibers, and many blood vessels.

Skeletal muscle fibers are long, cylindric, tapered cells that have cross-striations created by the contractile structure inside. The sarcolemma is the plasma membrane that covers muscle cells. Numerous nuclei lie beneath the sarcolemma. The sarcoplasm of a muscle fiber is similar to the cytoplasm of other cells, but it contains large amounts of stored glycogen and a unique oxygen-binding protein called *myoglobin*. Myoglobin is a red pigment similar to hemoglobin that stores oxygen within the muscle cells.

Sarcomeres are the structural units of contraction in skeletal muscle fibers. Myofibrils, which are chains of sarcomeres, are packed side by side within the sarcoplasm. Thus the functional units of skeletal muscles actually are very small portions of the myofibrils, and each myofibril can be visualized as a chain of sarcomere units laid end to end (Figure 9-1).

When a muscle cell contracts, its individual sarcomeres shorten. Within a neuromuscular unit, after a contraction has been initiated, it cannot be stopped, and the muscle fibers either contract to their full ability or do not contract at all. This is called the **all-or-none response.**

Muscle contraction involves two types of myofilaments. The thick filaments are myosin, and the thin filaments are actin. Together they form cross-bridges. The actin and myosin filaments slide over one another, and shortening (contraction) of the myofibrils takes place. Sliding of these filaments continues as long as the calcium signal and ATP are present.

When the nervous system activates muscle fibers, the cross-bridges from the myosin attach to active sites on the actin subunits of the filaments, and the sliding begins. Each cross-bridge attaches and detaches several times during a contraction, working like a tiny ratchet to generate tension and pull the thin actin filaments toward the center of the sarco-

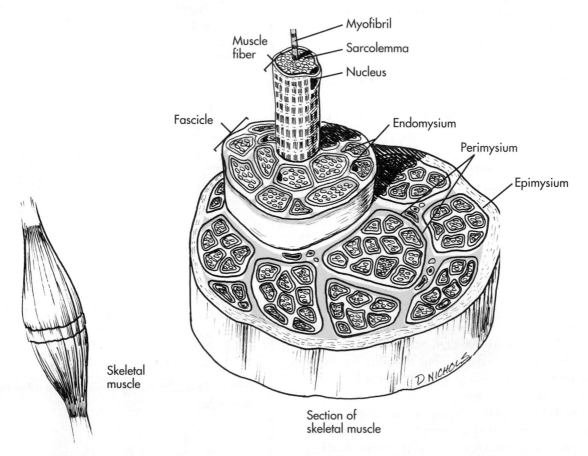

FIGURE 9-1 Section of skeletal muscle with contractile and noncontractile connective tissue. (From Shankman GA: *Fundamental orthopedic management for the physical therapist assistant,* St Louis, 1997, Mosby.)

mere. As this event occurs simultaneously in the sarcomeres throughout the cell, the muscle cell shortens. The attachment of myosin cross-bridges to actin requires calcium, and the nerve impulse leading to contraction causes an increase in calcium ions within the muscle cell (Figure 9-2).

Cardiac and smooth muscle are innervated by the autonomic division of the peripheral nervous system (PNS). Skeletal muscle is innervated by the somatic division of the PNS. Motor nerves stimulate the skeletal muscles to contract. The area of contact between the motor nerve and the muscle is the motor end plate, or myoneural (neuromuscular) junction. The motor end plate is a modified synapse consisting of a terminal bud of a nerve cell axon and a muscle fiber. When the nerve is stimulated, the terminal bud releases acetylcholine, and contraction follows (Figure 9-3).

A motor point is the location where the motor neuron enters the muscle and a visible contraction can be elicited with a minimal amount of stimulation. Motor points are most often located in the belly of the muscle. Muscles with a large belly may have more than one motor point. The motor point works in the same way a pilot light does in a gas furnace. Even though all the burners in the furnace are not on (much as with a muscle at rest), because of the pilot light, the furnace can respond quickly to the signal of the thermostat for more heat. The same holds true for the motor point area. Because it is always "on the alert," it can trigger the rest of the muscle to respond if needed. It would seem logical that the increased

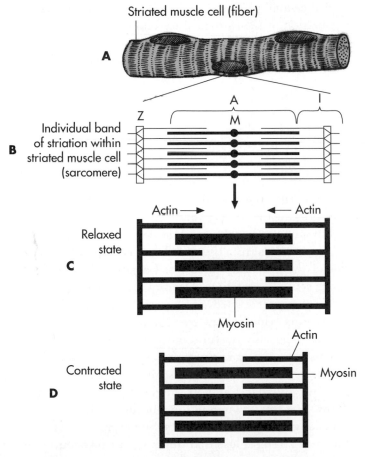

FIGURE 9-2 Striated muscle. **A,** Part of a single muscle cell, or fiber, with peripherally located nuclei. Vertical striations are evident within the cell. The repeating unit of this striation is the *sarcomere* **(B);** its major constituents are the proteins actin (*A*) and myosin (*M*), which slide in relation to each other to effect relaxation and elongation **(C)** or contraction **(D).** Neural signals stimulate the movement of calcium ions in the muscle fiber, and these ions stimulate the sliding movement of actin and myosin. (From Mathers LH et al: *Clinical anatomy principles,* St Louis, 1996, Mosby.)

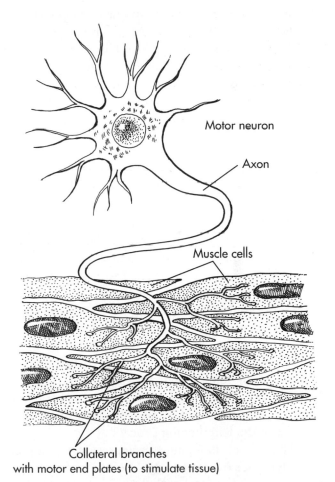

FIGURE 9-3 Motor unit. (From Scuderi GR, McCann PD, Bruno PJ: *Sports medicine: principles of primary care,* St Louis, 1997, Mosby.)

activity in these areas could lead to hyperstates in the muscle, called **trigger points.**

The classic definition of a trigger point, from the master of trigger point knowledge, Dr. Janet Travell, is this: "A myofascial trigger point is a hyperirritable locus within a taut band of skeletal muscle, located in the muscular tissue and/or its associated fascia. The spot is painful on compression and can evoke characteristic referred pain and autonomic phenomena."

A single motor neuron may innervate many muscle fibers, delivering stimuli to each one and making them all contract as a group; such a group is called a **motor unit.** The muscle fibers in a single motor unit are not clustered together but are spread throughout the muscle; thus the stimulation of a single motor unit causes a weak contraction of the entire muscle. The more strength that is needed, the more motor units are recruited. The size of the motor units determines whether a large muscle contracts forcefully or delicately. Large motor units with 700 fibers are found in the quadriceps femoris and other large, strong muscles that participate in running and walking. At the other extreme, three or four fibers per motor unit provide the muscles of the eyeball with the ability to produce delicate eye motions.

PRACTICAL APPLICATION

Trigger points are managed effectively with most soft tissue therapies. First, some sort of sensory stimulation is introduced to the trigger point area that interrupts the existing neurologic signal, and then the muscle is lengthened to restore the normal resting length. The most common approach involves compressing the trigger point, either with direct pressure or by pinching the point. The pressure is held for up to 30 seconds. After the application of pressure, the area of the trigger point in a muscle is lengthened. Muscle energy methods that use various types of muscle contraction, directed either to the muscle or its antagonist, assist in the lengthening process.

This theme has many variations; for example, applying ice over the trigger point instead of compression, followed by lengthening, often is successful. Methods that position the muscle fiber, holding the trigger point in an eased position and then gently lengthening, are effective for very tender trigger points. If fibrotic tissue changes have occurred around the trigger point, connective tissue stretching is necessary to elongate the connective tissue structures in the area.

A strong correlation exists between the locations of motor points, acupuncture points, and trigger points. However, assuming that these are all the same anatomic structure is simplistic. Researchers disagree about the differences and similarities of these areas. Acupuncture points correspond both to motor point locations and the locations of the Golgi tendon organs; this explains why trigger and acupuncture points can be found in both the belly and near the attachment ends of a muscle. Some agreement has been reached that these points correspond to neurovascular bundles in the muscles; this supports the idea of both a neurologic and vascular component of pathologic conditions of these points and the benefits of acupuncture and trigger point methods. Acupuncture points may be the nervous system aspect of the point phenomenon, and the trigger point may be the myofascial aspect of the same phenomenon. In this chicken-and-egg situation, it seems logical to follow the teaching of an old, wise, and experienced Russian physician, who says, "Where is pain, I rub" (Activity 9-2).

Muscle Tone

When the synapses in normal muscles stop firing, the muscles relax. Even so, they maintain a certain amount of contraction that keeps them ready to respond; this minimal amount of tautness is known as **tone.** Tone maintains the natural firmness of our muscles and their state of ready responsiveness. Appropriate amounts of tone help stabilize our joints and maintain our posture. Muscle tone is controlled by small signals from the spinal cord, brain, and spindles of the individual muscles. Because the stimulation is sent alternately to different sets of motor units within the muscle itself, some parts of the muscle are contracting while others are relaxing. This keeps the muscle, especially postural muscle, from tiring out.

This changeover in the signaling, which maintains muscle tone, can be demonstrated. Hold a heavy book in your hand as you slowly start to flex your elbow. The small twitch in the muscle occurs as there is a change-over in motor units. Sometimes it feels as if a small strength loss that quickly returns occurs.

Threshold stimulus

The stimulus at which the first noticeable muscle contraction occurs is called the **threshold stimulus.** Beyond this point the muscle contracts more vigorously as the intensity of the stimulus increases. The stimulus intensity beyond which the muscle fails to increase in strength is called the **maximal stimulus,**

ACTIVITY 9-2

Do you think the statement, "Where is pain, I rub" is a valid therapeutic approach? Use the clinical reasoning model to formulate your position.

What are the facts?
What is considered normal or balanced function?
What has happened?
What caused the imbalance?
What was done or is being done?
What has worked or not worked ?

What are the possibilities?
What does my intuition suggest?
What are the possible patterns of dysfunction?
What are the possible contributing factors?
What are possible interventions?
What might work?
What are other ways to look at the situation?
What do the data suggest?

What is the logical progression of the symptom pattern, contributing factors, and current behaviors?
What are the logical consequences of each intervention identified as a possibility?
What are the pros and cons of each intervention suggested?

What are the consequences of not acting?
What are the consequences of acting?

In terms of each intervention considered, what would be the impact on the people involved: client, practitioner and other professionals working with the client?
How does each person involved feel about the possible interventions?
Does the practitioner feel qualified to work with such situations?
Does a feeling of cooperation and agreement exist among all parties involved?

Summarize your reasons for determining the validity or invalidity of the statement, "Where is pain, I rub."

or the point at which all the muscle's motor units have been recruited. Thus the same muscle can apply both a gentle stroke and a firm slap.

Treppe

The first contraction of a muscle unit may be as little as one half the strength of those that occur in succession after it; this is called *treppe*. This stairstep effect is caused by many factors; for example, as the muscle begins work and produces heat, the muscle enzyme systems become more efficient, releasing more calcium ions. This produces a stronger contraction with each successive twitch during the beginning phase of muscle activity. Treppe is one reason why warming up before exercise is important.

Types of Muscle Fiber

Muscles contain fast, slow, and intermediate twitch fibers, which contract at different rates and with different characteristics, allowing muscles a wide range of action.

Fast-twitch (white) fibers contract more rapidly and forcefully, are larger than red fibers, and belong to larger motor units that fire when the nervous system demands rapid, powerful motion. They fatigue quickly and are considered anaerobic because they do not require much oxygen to contract.

Slow-twitch (red) fibers are smaller, contract more slowly and with less intensity, and belong to smaller motor units that respond during slower, more delicate movements. Red fibers do not fatigue quickly and can hold a contraction for a relatively long period. They contain much larger quantities of myoglobin and are classified as aerobic because they require oxygen for contraction. Some texts divide red twitch fibers into both fast and slow types.

Intermediate fibers combine the qualities of both red and white fibers to provide a rapid, moderately forceful contraction with moderate fatigue resistance.

Although the fiber composition varies from muscle to muscle, on the average, 50% of the fibers in a muscle are red, 35% are intermediate, and 15% are white. Up to 90% of the fibers in postural muscles are red fibers, whereas leg muscles contain a higher proportion of white and intermediate fibers.

The fiber configuration is greatly determined by genetics, but it can change as a result of demands made on the muscles. For example, the most successful sprinters are born with more white fibers in their leg muscles. To a certain extent, some others can be trained to be sprinters because the fiber configuration will adjust somewhat to demand.

White fibers, which are anaerobic, obtain ATP by converting glucose to lactic acid in the absence of oxygen. As a result, they fatigue more easily because the lactic acid accumulates and interferes with contraction. The liver needs oxygen to convert the lactic acid to glucose or glycogen. **Oxygen debt** is defined as the extra amount of oxygen that must be taken in to convert the lactic acid. Heavy breathing is primarily triggered by a high level of lactic acid in the blood, which stimulates the respiratory center of the brain. When the oxygen debt has been paid and lactic acid has been converted, breathing returns to normal.

Because of their aerobic quality, red fibers do not produce lactic acid. For this reason, postural muscles, which are composed mainly of red fibers, can sustain a contraction longer without fatiguing.

✋ PRACTICAL APPLICATION

The primary type of fiber in a muscle can affect the length of application of pressure methods (e.g., compression, direct pressure, acupressure) and tension methods (e.g., tensing and relaxing), which are used in progressive relaxation and muscle energy approaches. Red fibers often take longer to respond to these methods than white fibers.

Heat

Heat is a byproduct of muscle activity. Several homeostatic mechanisms such as radiation of heat from the skin's surface and sweating, prevent heat buildup from reaching dangerous levels. Shivering causes muscle contraction, which produces more heat.

Blood Supply

Contracting muscle fibers use tremendous amounts of oxygen and nutrients while giving off large amounts of metabolic waste. The blood delivers oxygen and nutrients and takes away waste products. Muscle tissue is highly vascularized, and the structure of capillaries in muscle has been modified so that they are long and winding. Thus when a muscle stretches, the capillaries can easily accommodate the change in shape.

Connective Tissue

Connective tissue is an essential part of the soft tissue or myofascial structure. A muscle cannot be separated from its extensive connective tissue network. The entire connective tissue network is one structure. Muscles do not just stick on bones; the connective tissue structure of the muscle and the bone blend into one tissue. Nerve and blood vessels do not just pass though holes in the connective tissue, rather, they are contained and supported in wrappings of connective tissue that intertwine. So when you pull on your little toe, you really do affect the inside of your head and every other structure in your body. No dysfunction is isolated; everything is connected.

Each individual muscle fiber is wrapped by several different layers of connective tissue. Each muscle fiber is surrounded by a fine sheath of connective tissue, called the *endomysium*. Several muscle fibers are wrapped together in side-by-side bundles, called *fascicles*, which in turn are wrapped in a collagenic sheath, the *perimysium*. The fascicles are bound together with more dense, fibrous connective tissue, called the *epimysium*, which surrounds the entire muscle. External to the epimysium is the **deep fascia,** an even coarser sheet of fibrous connective tissue that binds muscles into functional groups. The deep fascia forms partitions between muscle groups called *intermuscular septa*. All these connective tissue sheaths are continuous with one another. Near the ends of muscles the actual muscle fiber ends, but the connective tissue continues and converges to become the tendons and aponeuroses that join muscles to bones. The point where the muscle fiber ends and the tendon begins is called the *musculotendinous junction*. When muscle fibers contract, they pull on the connective tissue sheaths, which transmit the force to the bone to be moved. Because the individual skeletal muscle fibers are fragile, the connective tissue supports each cell, reinforces the muscle as a whole, and gives muscle tissue its natural elasticity. These sheaths also provide both entry and exit routes for the blood vessels and nerve fibers that serve the muscles, as well as a vast surface area for muscular attachment (Figure 9-4).

PRACTICAL APPLICATION

Soft tissue and movement therapies are most directly applied to the myofascial structure, the muscle fiber in the connective tissue network. The muscle fiber is most affected by the nervous system and responds to approaches that introduce stimulation to restore or support homeostasis.

The connective tissue network is more influenced by a mechanical approach that affects the viscous (colloid), elastic, and plastic components of this tissue. As described in Chapter 8, sustained, slow elongation of connective tissue, at an intensity sufficient to cause a change in the plastic and elastic properties, is necessary to affect these structures therapeutically. If too much resistance is applied to the tissue, the colloid gel responds with increased resistance. If not enough resistance is applied, the intensity will not be sufficient to effect change. As the fascia is stretched, manipulative mechanical energy is applied and the viscous component becomes softer and more pliable.

Most researchers agree that connective tissue changes are part of a degenerative process. Restoration of function helps reverse degenerative processes, supporting a return to homeostasis and an increase in well-being.

Repair of Muscle

Most of an adult's muscle cells are already in place at birth. Existing muscle fibers enlarge (hypertrophy) by as much as 30% of their original size. When a muscle is injured, it often is repaired with connective tissue. The body has a specific repair process for replacing muscle cells. Within hours of an injury, enzymes in the body begin to digest the damaged cell portion. Satellite cells, which are inactive during normal muscle activity, begin to form the new fibers by creating myotubes, which combine to form myofibrils. These new cells take on the characteristics of muscle fibers. Exercise influences the growth of satellite cells and aids in maintaining plasticity. Cardiac muscle has no satellite cells, and its damaged cells are replaced with fibrous tissue. Smooth muscle is well able to regenerate itself throughout life.

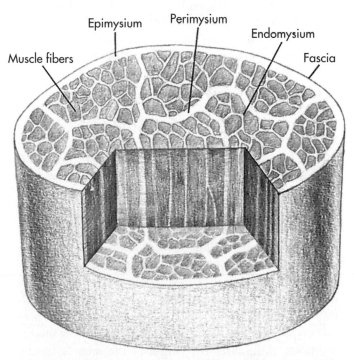

FIGURE 9-4 Structure of muscle fibers and their coverings. (From Thompson JM et al: *Mosby's clinical nursing*, ed 4, St Louis, 1997, Mosby.)

✋ PRACTICAL APPLICATION

The goals of healing for skeletal muscle tissue work are to promote satellite cell repair processes and manage the development of scar tissue. This allows the connective tissue structures that develop to be as normal as possible and stay pliable, so that they do not interfere with the function of the muscles. Stimulation of muscle function seems to encourage the satellite cells and support regeneration. Movement therapies can support these functions. Soft tissue methods can encourage appropriate mobile connective tissue development so that adhesions do not develop. Because connective tissue originates along the direction of tension, scar tissue can be encouraged to form along lines of external pressure provided by methods that orient, stroke, and pull the tissue in the direction of the desired connective tissue formation.

Areas of muscle healing that formed primarily with connective tissue by adhesion and random directional formation can be encouraged to re-heal through the use of soft tissue methods that introduce therapeutic inflammation. These methods need to be followed with appropriate rehabilitation processes that include broadening contractions to encourage mobility in the scar and decrease adhesion formation. The techniques are applied to small areas. Friction, which is a soft tissue method that moves muscle tissue against the muscle fiber configuration pattern, is the method most commonly used. Stretching methods that exceed the elastic range of connective tissue to alter the plastic range can pull apart adhesions and can be used to create the controlled area of inflammation.

Attachments

Most of our skeletal muscles span joints and are attached to bones or other structures in at least two places. In most cases a muscle starts on one bone and ends on another.

The terms most commonly used to describe these attachments are *origin* and *insertion*. The **origin** of a muscle is considered the least movable part, or the part that attaches closest to the midline or center of the body. The origin is known as the proximal attachment. The **insertion** is considered the most movable part, or the part that attaches farthest from the midline or center of the body. The insertion is known as the distal attachment. This text, as with most anatomy texts, designates the origin of the muscle by the most proximal location and the insertion by the most distal location. Some references avoid the confusion by simply referring to attachment sites. In some circumstances (e.g., when the psoas muscle flexes the trunk to the thigh with the legs fixed), the origin becomes the most movable attachment and the insertion the more fixed attachment. In most normal activities, however, the psoas muscle flexes the thigh to the trunk with the trunk fixed, therefore the insertion is the more movable attachment.

Muscles have two types of attachments, direct and indirect. In direct attachments, which are uncommon, the epimysium of the muscle blends into the periosteum of the bone or the perichondrium of cartilage. The more common form of muscle attachments is the indirect attachment, in which the muscle fascia extends beyond the muscles in a ropelike tendon or flat, broad aponeurosis. The tendon or aponeurosis blends into the connective tissue coverings and structures, including ligaments and other tendons, or into a seam of fibrous connective tissue, called a *raphe,* at the attachment site. The middle of the muscle or the area with the largest and broadest concentration of muscle fibers is the **belly** of the muscle.

Muscle Shapes

The bundles of muscle fibers, known as fascicles, form different patterns in muscles that result in the different shapes of muscles (Figure 9-5). These fascicle forms affect function, primarily the strength and direction of movement. The following are the more common patterns of fascicle arrangement:

Parallel—The fascicles are long and oriented parallel with the longitudinal axis of the muscle. Some of these muscles are straplike (e.g., the sartorius), and others are fusiform with an expanded belly (e.g., the biceps brachii).

Pennate—The fascicles are short, lie at an angle to the muscle, and attach to one or more tendons running the length of the muscles. A unipennate muscle (e.g., the extensor digitorum longus) has fascicles that insert on only one side of the tendon. A bipennate muscle (e.g., the rectus femoris) has fascicles that insert into the tendon from both sides; the result looks like a feather. A muscle resembling many feathers, all inserted into one large tendon, is called a *multipennate muscle.*

Circular—The fascicles are arranged in concentric rings around external body openings. These muscles, which contract to close the openings, are called *sphincters.*

A   **B**   **C**   **D**

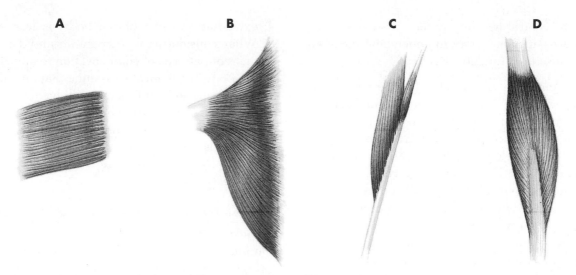

FIGURE 9-5 Muscle shape and fiber arrangement. **A,** Parallel. **B,** Convergent. **C,** Pennate. **D,** Bipennate. (From Thibodeau GA, Patton KT: *Anatomy and physiology,* ed 3, St Louis, 1996, Mosby.)

Convergent—The fascicle pattern begins with a broad origin and converges to blend with a much smaller tendon. The result is a triangular-shaped muscle (e.g., the pectoralis major).

The various patterns of fascicle arrangement determine the strength and amount of movement a muscle provides. Skeletal muscles can shorten to about 70% of their resting length when contracted. The longer and more parallel the muscle fibers to the muscle's long axis, the greater the muscle shortening. Parallel muscles shorten as a direct result of the shortening of their fibers; these muscles produce the greatest amount of shortening. They do this at the expense of strength; parallel muscles are not very powerful. The fibers of pennate muscles rotate around their tendon attachments. Pennate muscles can pack more fibers into the same amount of space as parallel fibers and so can produce the stronger contraction (Activity 9-3).

MYOTATIC UNITS
(FUNCTIONAL MUSCLE GROUPS)

Only rarely does any muscle act independently. Most muscles play a part in a movement pattern, just as actors do in a play. Roles can change, depending on the response required. A muscle can be the star, or prime mover, and in the next instant become one of the supporting cast. A moment later the very same muscle can assume the opposite role. The terms *agonist, prime mover, antagonist, synergist,* and *fixator* all describe the function of muscles in a complete movement pattern.

ACTIVITY 9-3

Draw the following muscle shapes:

Parallel

Pennate

Convergent

Because the central nervous system processes movement patterns, it is important to understand the interaction of muscles in functional units:

Agonist—A muscle or muscles that are the main force causing or controlling joint motion through a specified plane of motion; known as primary or prime movers, or muscles most involved

Synergist—A muscle that aids or assists the action of the agonists but is not primarily responsible for the action; known also as guiding muscles, they help refine movement and control any actions produced by other muscles

Antagonist—A muscle that has the opposite action to the agonist and usually is located on the opposite side of the joint; work in cooperation with agonist muscles by relaxing and allowing movement

Fixator (stabilizer)—A muscle that surrounds the joint or body segment and contracts to support or stabilize the area; enable another limb or body segment to work effectively; essential for establishing a firm base for the more distal joints to carry out movements

The agonist/prime mover interaction is relatively easy to visualize in muscles such as the biceps/triceps unit, but it becomes more complex when we consider that the deltoid and quadriceps, adductors and hamstrings form a functional unit because of our gait, or walking pattern. The various functional units that require muscles to cooperate in producing body-wide movements (e.g., walking or maintaining balance) need sophisticated reflex control by the nervous system. Reviewing the section on reflex arcs in Chapter 4 would be beneficial. When the role of stabilization is factored into a movement pattern, the functional (or myotatic) muscle group interaction becomes quite complex. Whenever maintaining posture is part of the pattern, a body-wide process truly is involved. Chapter 10 presents more on biomechanics.

✋ PRACTICAL APPLICATION

Often, effective application of soft tissue and movement therapies depends on the unraveling of these complex, functional group patterns of muscles. In many cases, addressing the entire body during each session in what is called a *general constitutional approach* is just as effective. Interventions that bring more general demand on the body to respond naturally address these complex patterns. Spot work, or addressing an isolated area and excluding the rest of the body, is less effective. When considering myotatic units and the development of patterns of compensation to any change in the body, it is logical to assume that any alteration in musculoskeletal function will have a body-wide effect. Because the components of the body are interdependent, everything affects everything else. Methods and treatment plans developed around generalized whole-body responses honor the innate body wisdom.

PROPRIOCEPTORS AND REFLEXES

If the central nervous system (CNS) is to coordinate motion, it must constantly be aware of any muscle action. Proprioceptors are sensory receptors that provide the CNS with information about position, movement, muscle tension, joint activity, and equilibrium. Methods that move, stretch, and apply tension to the muscles and joints stimulate the following receptors:

1. Muscles spindles—Respond both to sudden and to prolonged stretch
2. Tendon organs—Respond to tension in the muscle as it is relayed to the tendon; ligaments contain receptors that respond to strain at the joint to feedback information adjusting the tension patterns of associated muscles
3. Joint kinesthetic receptors in the joint capsule—Respond to pressure, acceleration, and deceleration of joint movement. The two main types of joint kinesthetic receptors are type II cutaneous mechanoreceptors and pacinian (lamellated) corpuscles.

Stimulation of nervous system receptors is interpreted and processed through the somatic reflex arcs. Reflexes are automatic responses triggered by changes in the environment that quickly and predictably restore homeostasis (Figure 9-6). The reflexes most often stimulated are the stretch reflex, tendon reflex, flexor reflex, and crossed-extensor reflex.

Stretch Reflex

The sensitivity of muscle spindles to stretching sets the level of muscle tone throughout the body. The stretch reflex is activated by the muscle spindles when a muscle is subjected to sudden or prolonged stretching. This activation causes a reflexive contraction of the same muscle. As was explained in Chapter 5, a muscle spindle produces nerve impulses, which are sent via a sensory neuron to the dorsal root of the spinal cord, where an impulse synapses with a motor neuron. The motor neuron carries the impulse to the stretched muscle, where a muscle action potential is generated, causing the muscle and its synergists to contract. Muscle contraction stops spindle cell discharge unless the muscle is held in an excessive stretch; a small amount of stretch reflex continues to be generated. The effect of the muscle stretch stimulates the stretch reflex, resulting in shortening of the muscle.

The principle of reciprocal inhibition comes into play during the stretch reflex. At the same time the original muscle is stimulated to contract, sensory signals are synapsing with association neurons to its antagonist or antagonists, inhibiting any signal through the motor neurons to the antagonists; this results in relaxation of the antagonist. To simplify, when one muscle contracts, its antagonist or opposing muscle group must relax. The pathway of this

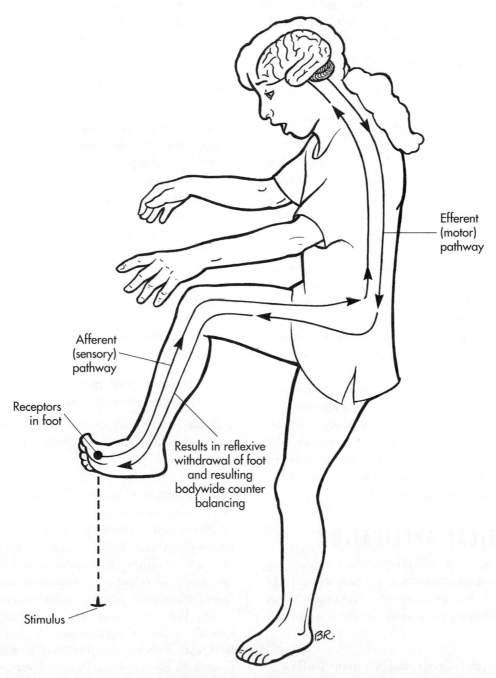

Efferent (motor) pathway

Afferent (sensory) pathway

Receptors in foot

Results in reflexive withdrawal of foot and resulting bodywide counter balancing

Stimulus

FIGURE 9-6 Reflex response. Local stimulation of a few specific receptors leads to a large number of outgoing impulses, which affect many muscles. (From Fritz S: *Mosby's fundamentals of therapeutic massage,* St Louis, 1995, Mosby.)

inhibition circuitry is called *reciprocal innervation* and can be initiated therapeutically to assist in muscle relaxation.

✋ PRACTICAL APPLICATION

Therapeutic methods can activate or strengthen weakened muscle patterns by stretching the muscles and initiating the stretch reflex. An awareness of this reflex response is important in all stretches intended to lengthen and relax the muscles. In these instances, the stretch reflex must be avoided. This system of reflexes frequently becomes hyperactive, resulting in an increase of muscle tension. Techniques using isometric and isotonic muscle contractions to relax and stretch muscles are helpful in resetting muscle tension patterns.

Tendon Reflex

The stretch reflex operates as a feedback mechanism that monitors and changes muscle length by initiating a muscle contraction; the tendon reflex, on the other hand, operates as a feedback mechanism that monitors and controls muscle tension by inducing muscle relaxation. This reflex is mediated by the tendon organs that detect and respond to changes in muscle tension caused by a sudden or intense muscle contraction. When the tendon organ is stimulated, it sends a signal along a sensory neuron to the spinal cord, where it synapses with an inhibitory association neuron, which inhibits the motor neurons that innervate the original muscle. This inhibition causes the muscle to relax.

At the same time the original muscle is inhibited from acting, a small increase occurs in the signal sent to the antagonist. The opposite of reciprocal inhibition, this signal causes a small contraction to take place in the antagonist. This signal can be initiated therapeutically to assist both in relaxing a tense muscle and in stimulating its antagonist.

✋ PRACTICAL APPLICATION

The most common technique used to stimulate the tendon reflex is an isometric (or isotonic) contraction, followed by postisometric relaxation. This technique increases tension at the tendon to elicit relaxation.

Flexor Reflex and Crossed-Extensor Reflex

The flexor (withdrawal) and crossed-extensor reflexes are polysynaptic reflex arcs. A single sensory neuron, most likely located in the skin, can activate several motor neurons. When these reflexes are stimulated, both sides of the body are affected through intersegmental reflex arcs. The flexor reflex withdraws the limb from an unpleasant or painful stimulus while the crossed-extensor reflex extends the limb on the opposite side of the spinal cord to maintain balance. Synchronized control over both the muscles contracting and those inhibited is handled through the circuitry of contralateral reflex arcs. These reflexes also explain why tension patterns are seldom found on one side of the body only.

As with the stretch reflex, the principle of reciprocal inhibition is active in flexor and extensor reflexes.

✋ PRACTICAL APPLICATION

The withdrawal response can stimulate opposite side patterns of tension or weakness. This is a powerful response because flexor or withdrawal reflexes take priority over all other reflex activity taking place simultaneously. Soft tissue and movement therapies can reset reflex patterns that are unproductive or that lead to discomfort and postural distortion from uneven contraction and relaxation muscle patterns. The effectiveness of the techniques depends on how efficiently the receptors for these reflexes are stimulated. The targeted receptor must be reached with the appropriate technique and intensity so that the reflex stimulated is allowed to function in the appropriate manner.

FUNCTION OF CARDIAC AND SMOOTH MUSCLE TISSUE

Cardiac and smooth muscle tissues operate by mechanisms similar to those in skeletal muscle tissues.

Cardiac Muscle

Cardiac muscle (Figure 9-7), also known as striated involuntary muscle, is found in only one organ of the body, the heart. Forming the bulk of the wall of each heart chamber, cardiac muscle contracts rhythmically and continuously to provide the pumping action necessary to maintain a relatively consistent blood flow through our internal environment.

The functional anatomy of cardiac muscle tissue resembles that of skeletal muscle, but it has specialized features related to its role of pumping blood continuously. Each cardiac muscle fiber contains parallel myofibrils composed of sarcomeres that give the whole fiber a striated appearance. However, the cardiac muscle fiber does not taper like a skeletal mus-

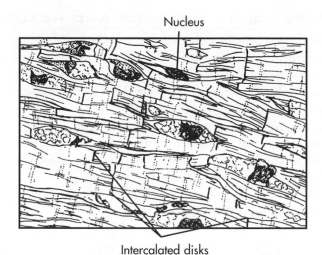

FIGURE 9-7   Cardiac muscle. The dark bands, called *intercalated disks,* which are characteristic of cardiac muscle, can be seen clearly in this tissue section. (From Thibodeau GA, Patton KT: *Anatomy and physiology,* ed 3, St Louis, 1996, Mosby.)

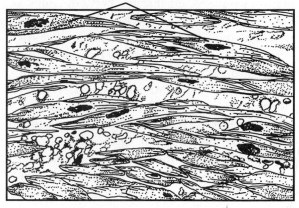

FIGURE 9-8   Smooth muscle. Note the central placement of nuclei in the spindle-shaped smooth muscle fibers. (From Thibodeau GA, Patton KT: *Anatomy and physiology,* ed 3, St Louis, 1996, Mosby.)

cle fiber; rather, it forms strong, electrically coupled junctions (intercalated disks) with other fibers. Cardiac muscle forms a continuous contractile band around the heart that conducts a single impulse across a continuous sarcolemma, allowing for an efficient, coordinated pumping action. This means that even though many adjacent cardiac muscle cells contract simultaneously, they have a prolonged contraction rather than a rapid twitch. Cardiac muscle does not normally run low on ATP and thus does not experience fatigue. Obviously, this characteristic of cardiac muscle is vital for keeping the heart pumping continuously.

Unlike skeletal muscle, in which a nervous impulse excites the sarcolemma to produce its own impulse, cardiac muscle is self-exciting. Cardiac muscle cells have a continuing rhythm of excitation and contraction on their own, although the rate of self-induced impulses can be altered by nervous or hormonal input.

Smooth Muscle

Smooth muscle (Figure 9-8) comprises small, tapered cells with single nuclei. The lack of striations in smooth muscle fibers is because thick and thin myofilaments are arranged quite differently than in skeletal or cardiac muscle fibers. These arrangements of myofilaments crisscross the cell and attach at their ends to the cell's plasma membrane.

When cross-bridges pull the thin filaments together, the muscle "balls up" and thus contracts the cell. Because the myofilaments are not organized into sarcomeres, they have more freedom of movement and

can contract a smooth muscle fiber to shorter lengths than in skeletal and cardiac muscle.

The two types of smooth muscle tissue are visceral muscle and multiunit muscle. In visceral, or single-unit, muscles, gap junctions join individual smooth muscles into large, continuous sheets, much like the fibers observed in cardiac muscle. This is the most common type of smooth muscle. It forms the muscular layer in the walls of many hollow structures such as the digestive, urinary, and reproductive tracts.

Similar to cardiac muscle, this type of smooth muscle commonly has a rhythmic self-excitation, or autorhythmicity (meaning "self-rhythm"), that spreads across the entire tissue. When these rhythmic, spreading waves of contraction become strong enough, they can push the contents of a hollow organ progressively along its lumen (the interior of a tubular structure). This type of contraction, called *peristalsis,* moves food along the digestive tract, assists the flow of urine to the bladder, and pushes a baby out of the womb during labor. Such contractions also can be coordinated to produce mixing movements in the stomach and other organs.

Multiunit smooth muscle tissue does not act as a single unit, as does visceral muscle; instead, it comprises many independent, single-cell units. Each independent fiber does not generate its own impulse, but rather responds only to nervous input. Although this type of smooth muscle can form thin sheets, as in the walls of large blood vessels, it more often is found in bundles (e.g., the erector pili muscles of the skin) or as single fibers, such as those surrounding small blood vessels.

Individual Muscles *

Although we understand that the body operates as a unit, the student must know the pieces making up that unit. The following section discusses the individual muscles most often encountered by soft tissue and movement professionals. Their primary function or functions, origin, insertion, innervation, synergists, antagonists and, if applicable, common trigger point areas and referred pain patterns are discussed. Activities such as palpation, movement, coloring, drawing and labeling the attachment points, and locating common trigger points reinforce the student's knowledge of the structure and function of individual muscles or groups of muscles.

Ideally, we would remember every single detail of each muscle, but most of us are not able to do so. A more realistic expectation in this study would be to get to know the muscles as you would a new friend. It helps to know where to find them, what they do, who their friends are, and what bothers them. To appreciate them as individuals, you do not need to know every single detail of the friend's life. If you need to know more about a muscle, you can always ask questions and look up additional material in reference texts as needed. Not all references agree about specific details, and different books list slightly different origins, insertions, functions, and so forth. Do not let this confuse you; as with most differing opinions, the answer is not black or white but somewhere in between in a range of gray.

The term *attachment* currently is used more than *origin* and *insertion* to describe muscle insertion points. The proximal attachment is usually the origin, and the distal attachment is usually the insertion. Most textbooks and reference books still use the terms *origin* and *insertion,* and to allow easy comparison, this text also uses that terminology.

NOTE: An illustration of each muscle is provided in this section. (Additional illustrations are found in the Color Plates.) If the Activity requires more than one muscle to be drawn, color each muscle a different color. Label the origin and the insertion with different colors, and use those colors consistently throughout all the Activities. Mark the trigger point or points in yet a third color, again being consistent throughout the Activities. Fine-point colored pencils will work best for these activities.

*Much of the material in this section is modified from Edwards D: *Mosby's anatomy flashcards: musculature, bones, and joints,* St Louis, 1998, Mosby.

MUSCLES OF THE FACE AND HEAD

The superficial muscles of the head, including those of the scalp and face, produce movement for facial expressions. The muscles vary in both shape and strength. Many adjacent muscles tend to be fused together. Unlike other muscles, they insert into skin or other muscles. Muscles of the head and face lift our eyebrows, flare our nostrils, and open and close our eyes and mouth. These muscles create our facial expressions, which are vital to nonverbal communication.

Muscles of Facial Expression

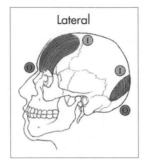

Lateral

Occipitofrontalis
(ok-SIP-ih-toe-fron-TAL-iss)
Meaning back of the head
    and related to the forehead
Sometimes described as separate muscles, the occipitalis and the frontalis
Function: Moves scalp forward and backward; assists in raising the eyebrows and wrinkling the forehead
Origin:
    Occipital belly—Lateral two thirds of the superior nuchal line of the occipital bone and the mastoid process of the temporal bone
    Frontal belly—Epicranial aponeurosis near the coronal suture

ACTIVITY 9-4

- Draw and color the occipitofrontalis in the space provided.
- Label the origin and insertion points: *O,* for the origin, *I,* for the insertion.
- Place an **X** on the trigger points.
- Palpate this muscle; identify the attachment points and the belly of the muscle.
- Move this muscle on yourself.

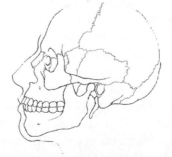

Insertion:
  Occipital belly—Galea aponeurotica
  Frontal belly—Galea aponeurotica in front of the coronal suture, the skin over the eyebrow, and the orbicularis oculi muscle
Innervation:
  Occipital—Posterior auricular branch of the facial nerve
  Frontal—Temporal branches of the facial nerve
Synergist: Frontalis and occipitalis bellies act as synergist together.
Antagonist: Procerus
Trigger points:
  Occipital—Near attachment at the galea aponeurotica
  Frontalis—Belly of the muscle over the eyebrow
Referred pain patterns: Eye, ear, and the scalp above the ear

See Activity 9-4

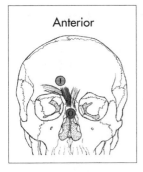

Anterior

Procerus (pro-SEHR-us)
Meaning tall
Function: Draws medial angles of the eyebrows downward; produces transverse wrinkles over the bridge of the nose
Origin: Fascia covering the lower part of the nasal bone and the upper part of the lateral nasal cartilage
Insertion: Skin over the lower forehead between the eyebrows
Innervation: Superior buccal branch of the facial nerve
Synergist: Corrugator supercilii procerus
Antagonist: Occipitofrontalis
Trigger point: No common trigger point identified

See Activity 9-5

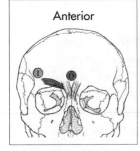

Anterior

Corrugator supercilii
Function: Draws the eyebrow downward and medially
Origin: Medial end of the superciliary arch
Insertion: Skin above the middle of the supraorbital margin
Innervation: Temporal branch of the facial nerve
Synergist: Procerus
Antagonist: Occipitofrontalis
Trigger point: No common trigger point identified

See Activity 9-6

ACTIVITY 9-5

- Draw and color the procerus in the space provided.
- Label the origin and insertion points: *O*, for the origin, *I*, for the insertion.
- Palpate this muscle; identify the attachment points and the belly of the muscle.
- Move this muscle on yourself.

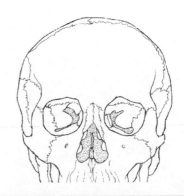

ACTIVITY 9-6

- Draw and color the corrugator supercilii in the space provided.
- Label the origin and insertion points: *O*, for the origin, *I*, for the insertion.
- Palpate this muscle; identify the attachment points and the belly of the muscle.
- Move this muscle on yourself.

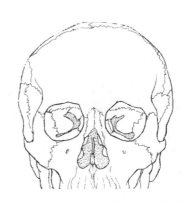

All subsequent figures in this chapter are taken from or modified from Edwards D: *Mosby's anatomy flashcards: musculature, bones, and joints,* St Louis, 1998, Mosby.

ACTIVITY 9-7

- Draw and color the transverse and alar nasalis in the space provided.
- Label the origin and insertion points: *O*, for the origin, *I*, for the insertion.
- Palpate this muscle; identify the attachment points and the belly of the muscle.
- Move this muscle on yourself.

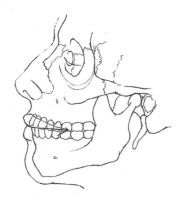

ACTIVITY 9-8

- Draw and color the anterior, posterior, and superior auricular muscles in the space provided.
- Label the origin and insertion points: *O*, for the origin, *I*, for the insertion.
- Palpate these muscles; identify the attachment points and the belly of the muscle.
- Move these muscles on yourself.

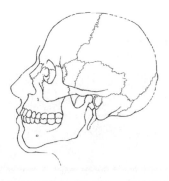

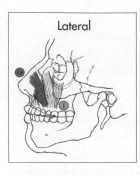

Lateral

Nasalis (transverse and alar) (nay-SAL-iss)
Meaning related to the nose
Function:
Transverse part (compressor naris)—Compresses the nasal aperture
Alar part (depressor naris)—Enlarges the nasal aperture
Origin:
Transverse—Maxilla, above and lateral to the incisive fossa
Alar—Nasal notch of the maxilla; lesser alar cartilage
Insertion: Aponeurosis of the procerus and the same muscle on the opposite side
Innervation: Superior buccal branch of the facial nerve (both)
Synergist: Levator labii superioris to the alar portions
Antagonist: Transverse and alar portions to one another
Trigger point: No common trigger point identified

See Activity 9-7

Auricular (Ear) Muscles (AW-ri-ku-lar)
Meaning belonging to the ear
As a group, these muscles move the ear

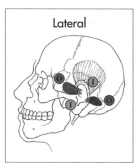

Lateral

Anterior auricular
Function: Draws the auricle forward and upward
Origin: Lateral edge of the epicranial aponeurosis
Insertion: Spine of the helix
Innervation: Temporal branches of the facial nerve

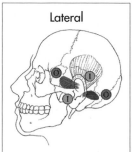

Lateral

Posterior auricular
Function: Draws auricle backward
Origin: Mastoid process of the temporal bone
Insertion: Inferior part of the cranial part of the conchae
Innervation: Posterior auricular branches of the facial nerve

Synergist: Not applicable
Antagonist: Portions to each other
Trigger point: No common trigger point identified

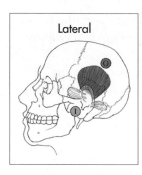

Lateral

Superior auricular

Function: Slightly raises auricle

Origin: Epicranial aponeurosis

Insertion: Upper part of the cranial surface of the auricle

Innervation: Temporal branches of the facial nerve

See Activity 9-8

Eye Muscles

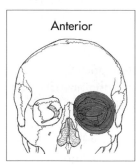

Anterior

Orbicularis oculi (or-BIK-you-LAR-iss OK-you-lee)
Meaning a small disk belonging to the eye

Function: Sphincter muscle of the eyelids; opens and closes the eyelids, can act voluntarily or reflexively; many of the upper orbital fibers of this muscle are inserted into the skin and subcutaneous tissue of the eyebrow; these constitute the depressor supercilii muscle

Origin:
   Orbital portion—Medial orbital margin
   Palpebral (eyelid) portion—Palpebral ligament
   Lacrimal portion—Lacrimal bone
Insertion:
   Orbital portion—Upper lid around the palpebral ligament
   Palpebral portion—Lateral palpebral raphe
   Lacrimal portion—Medial part of the upper and lower eyelids
Innervation: Temporal and zygomatic branches of the facial nerve
Synergist: Not applicable
Antagonists: Portions to itself
Trigger point: Superior orbital area above the eyelid
Referred pain pattern: To the nose

See Activity 9-9

Muscles That Move the Mouth

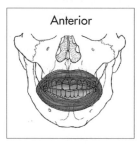

Anterior

Orbicularis oris (or-BIK-you-LAR-iss OR-iss)
Meaning a small disk belonging to the mouth

Function: Effects direct closure of the lips; brings the lips together and protrudes them forward

Origin and Insertion: Made up partly of fibers from other facial muscles and partly of fibers proper to the lips

Innervation: Lower buccal and mandibular branches of the facial nerve

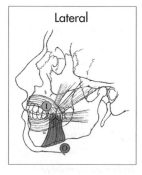

Lateral

Depressor anguli oris (de-PRESS-or ANG-you-lee OR-iss)
Meaning presses down the corner belonging to the mouth

Function: Draws the angle of the mouth downward and laterally in opening the mouth and in expressions of sadness

Origin: Oblique line of the mandible, below and lateral to the depressor labii inferioris

Insertion: Angle of the mouth with the orbicularis oris and the risorius

Innervation: Mandibular marginal branch of the facial nerve

ACTIVITY 9-9

- Draw and color the orbicularis oculi in the space provided.
- Label the origin and insertion points: *O*, for the origin, *I*, for the insertion.
- Place an **X** on the trigger point.
- Palpate this muscle and identify the attachment points and belly.
- Move this muscle on yourself.

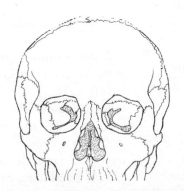

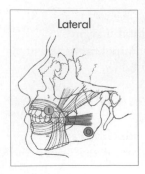

Risorius (rih-ZOR-ee-us)

Meaning causes one to laugh

Function: Retracts the angle of the mouth

Origin: Parotid fascia over the masseter muscle

Insertion: Skin at the angle of the mouth

Innervation: Buccal branches of the facial nerve

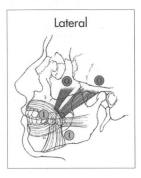

Zygomaticus major (ZYE-go-MAH-tih-kus)

Meaning connected to the yoke or connector; major meaning larger

Function: Draws the angle of the mouth upward and laterally, as in laughing

Origin: Zygomatic bone in front of the zygomatico-temporal suture

Insertion: Angle of the mouth, blending with the levator anguli oris, orbicularis oris, and depressor anguli oris

Innervation: Buccal branches of the facial nerve

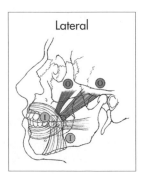

Zygomaticus minor (ZYE-go-MAH-tih-kus)

Meaning connected to the yoke or connector; minor meaning smaller

Function: Elevates the upper lip and produces nasolabial furrow

Origin: Lateral surface of the zygomatic bone, immediately behind zygomaticomaxillary suture

Insertion: Angle of the mouth, blending with the levator anguli oris, orbicularis oris, and depressor anguli oris

Innervation: Buccal branches of the facial nerve

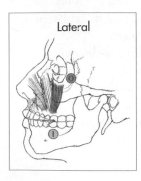

Levator labii superioris (le-VAY-tor LAY-bee-eye su-PEER-ee-OR-iss)

Meaning one that raises the lip; superioris meaning above or upper

Function: Raises and everts the upper lip

Origin: Maxilla and zygomatic bone, from the lower margin of the orbital opening immediately above the infraorbital foramen

Insertion: Muscular substance of the upper lip

Innervation: Buccal branches of the facial nerve

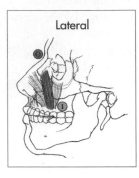

Levator labii superioris alaeque nasi (le-VAY-tor LAY-bee-eye su-PEER-ee-OR-iss AL-ek-wee NAY-see)

Meaning one that raises the lip and belonging to the wing of the nose; superioris meaning above or upper

Function:

Lateral slip—Raises and everts the upper lip

Medial slip—Acts as a dilator of the nostril

Origin: Upper part of the frontal process of the maxilla

Insertion: Divides into the lateral slip, which inserts into the lateral part of the upper lip, and the medial slip, which inserts into the greater alar cartilage and the skin of the nasal ala

Innervation: Buccal branches of the facial nerve

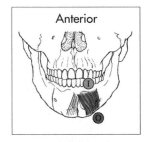

Depressor labii inferioris (de-PRESS-or LAY-bee-eye in-FEAR-ee-or-iss)

Meaning presses down the lip; inferioris meaning lower or beneath

Function: Draws the lower lip downward and slightly laterally during mastication

Origin: Oblique line of the mandible, between the symphysis menti and the mental foramen

Insertion: Skin of the lower lip, blending with the orbicularis oris

Innervation: Buccal branches of the facial nerve

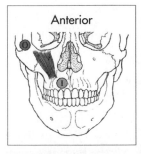

Levator anguli oris (le-VAY-tor ANG-you-ee OR-iss)

Meaning one that raises the corner of the mouth

Function: Elevates the angle of the mouth; instrumental in producing nasolabial furrow

Origin: Canine fossa, just below the infraorbital foramen

Insertion: Angle of the mouth, intermingling with the zygomaticus major, depressor anguli oris, and orbicularis oris

Innervation: Buccal branches of the facial nerve

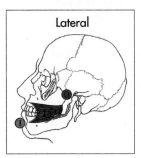
Lateral

Buccinator
(BUK-sin-ate-or) *trumpet*
Meaning trumpeter
Function: Aids in mastication; forces air out between the lips; compresses the cheek
Origin: Alveolar process of maxilla and mandible; pterygomandibular raphe

Insertion: Angle of the mouth, blending with fibers of the orbicularis oris

Innervation: Lower buccal branches of the facial nerve

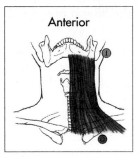
Anterior

Platysma (PLAH-tiz-ma)
Meaning a flat plate
Function: Draws down the lower lip and the angle of the mouth; draws the skin over the clavicle upward
Origin: Fascia covering the upper parts of the pectoralis major and deltoideus

Insertion: Anterior fibers; interlaced with fibers of the muscle of the other side

Innervation: Cervical branch of the facial nerve

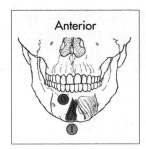
Anterior

Mentalis (men-TAL-iss)
Meaning related to the chin
Function: Raises and protrudes the lower lip, at the same time wrinkling the skin of the chin
Origin: Mandible
Insertion: Skin of the chin
Innervation: Mandibular marginal branch of the facial nerve

Elements common to the muscles that move the mouth

Synergists: Levators to levators and depressors to depressors

Antagonists: Levators to depressors

Trigger points: No common trigger points identified. Those that form are likely located in the belly of the muscle.

See Activity 9-10

Muscles of Mastication (Chewing)

Four main pairs of muscles are involved in mastication (chewing or biting) because they move the temporomandibular joint (TMJ). These are very powerful muscles. The masseter and temporalis muscles are the prime movers of jaw closure and biting. Grinding movements are provided by the medial and lateral pterygoid muscles. The buccinator muscles keep the cheeks close to the teeth to help us chew. The tongue is composed of specialized muscle fibers that curl, squeeze, and fold the tongue.

ACTIVITY 9-10

- Draw and color the following muscles in the space provided: orbicularis oris, depressor anguli oris, risorius, zygomaticus major and minor, levator labii superioris, levator labii superioris alaeque nasi, depressor labii inferioris, levator anguli oris, buccinator, platysma, and mentalis.
- Label the origin and insertion points: *O,* for the origin, *I,* for the insertion.

- Palpate these muscles; identify the attachment points and the belly of the muscle.
- Move these muscles on yourself.
NOTE: Levators help us smile.
Depressors help us frown.

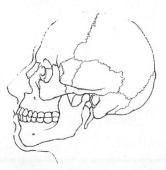

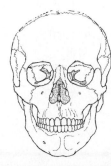

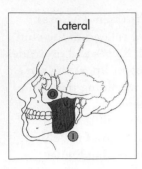

Lateral

Masseter (mah-SEAT-er)
Meaning one who chews
Function: Elevates the
   mandible to close the teeth
   when chewing
Origin:
   Superficial portion—
      Anterior two thirds of
      the lower border of the
      zygomatic arch
Deep portion—Medial surface of the zygomatic
   arch
Insertion: Ramus and angle of the mandible
Innervation: Mandibular division of the trigeminal
   nerve
Synergists: Temporalis, pterygoids
Antagonists: Geniohyoid, omohyoid, hypoglossus,
   and digastric
NOTE: Gravity, although not a muscle, plays a part
   in the antagonist pattern.
Trigger points: Superior at the tendinous junction
   near the zygomatic arch and in the belly of the
   muscle
Referred pain patterns: Upper and lower jaw, the ear,
   and the eyebrow

See Activity 9-11

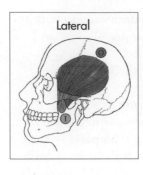

Lateral

Temporalis
(TEMP-or-AL-iss)
Meaning related to the temple of the head
Function: Elevates the
   mandible, closing the
   mouth and clenching the
   teeth; also contributes to
   side-to-side grinding
   movements
Origin: Temporal fossa, deep surface of the temporal
   fascia
Insertion: Ramus of the mandible; medial surface and
   anterior border of the coronoid process
Innervation: Anterior and posterior deep temporal
   nerve from the mandibular portion of the trigeminal nerve
Synergists: Masseter, superior and medial pterygoids
Antagonists: Inferior division of the lateral pterygoid,
   omohyoid, digastric
Trigger points: Anterior, medial, and posterior along
   the inferior aspect of the muscle near the tendinous junction at the coronoid process of the
   mandible
Referred pain patterns: Temporal region, eyebrow,
   upper teeth

See Activity 9-12

ACTIVITY 9-11

- Draw and color the masseter in the space provided.
- Label the origin and insertion points: *O,* for the origin, *I,* for the insertion.
- Place an **X** on the trigger points.
- Palpate this muscle; identify the attachment points and the belly of the muscle.
- Move this muscle on yourself.

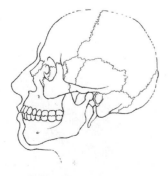

ACTIVITY 9-12

- Draw and color the temporalis in the space provided.
- Label the origin and insertion points: *O,* for the origin, *I,* for the insertion.
- Place an **X** on the trigger points.
- Palpate this muscle; identify the attachment points and the belly of the muscle.
- Move this muscle on yourself.

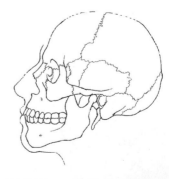

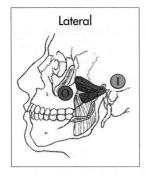

Lateral (external) pterygoid
(TEAR-ih-goyd)

Meaning wing shaped; lateral meaning to the side

Functions:
>Produces side-to-side movement of the jaw
>
>Superior division assists in opening the mouth by pulling forward the condylar process of the mandible and the articular disk
>
>Inferior division protrudes and depresses the mandible

Origin:
>Superior head—Greater wing of the sphenoid bone
>
>Inferior head—Lateral surface of the lateral pterygoid plate

Insertion: Front of the neck of the mandible; articular capsule and disk of the temporomandibular articulation

Innervation: Mandibular division of the trigeminal nerve

Synergists:
>Inferior division—Digastric, suprahyoid
>
>Superior division—Masseter, temporalis

Antagonists: Superior and inferior divisions are antagonistic to each other

Trigger points: Belly of both divisions of the muscle

Referred pain pattern: Cheek and TMJ

See Activity 9-13

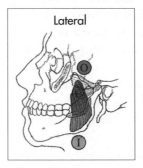

Medial pterygoid
(TEAR-ih-goyd)

Meaning wing shaped; medial meaning related to the middle

Function:
>Assists in elevating the mandible and laterally deviating to the opposite side

Acts with the inferior lateral pterygoids, helps protrude the mandible

Origin: Medial surface of the lateral pterygoid plate; pyramidal surface of the palatine bone

Insertion: Posteroinferior aspect of the medial surface of the ramus and the angle of the mandible

Innervation: Mandibular division of the trigeminal nerve

Synergists: Acting bilaterally—Masseter and temporalis

Antagonist: Acting unilaterally—Medial pterygoid on opposite side

Trigger points: Belly of the muscle, with best access inside the mouth

Referred pain pattern: Back of the throat, into the ear

See Activity 9-14

ACTIVITY 9-13

- Draw and color the lateral pterygoid in the space provided.
- Label the origin and insertion points: *O,* for the origin, *I,* for the insertion.
- Place an **X** on the trigger points.
- Palpate this muscle; identify the attachment points and the belly of the muscle.
- Move this muscle on yourself.

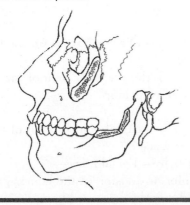

ACTIVITY 9-14

- Draw and color the medial pterygoid in the space provided.
- Label the origin and insertion points: *O,* for the origin, *I,* for the insertion.
- Place an **X** on the trigger points.
- Palpate this muscle; identify the attachment points and the belly of the muscle.
- Move this muscle on yourself.

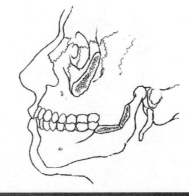

MUSCLES OF THE NECK

The sternocleidomastoid muscles divide the neck into the anterior and posterior triangles. Most of the muscles of the anterior neck assist in swallowing. Muscles that attach to the head and axial skeleton provide head movements. The sternocleidomastoid muscles are the major neck flexors. Lateral head movements are created by the sternocleidomastoid and the deeper neck muscles, including the scalenes, and by several straplike muscles of the vertebral column at the back of the neck. Head extension is accomplished by the splenius muscles, under the trapezius. The sternocleidomastoid assists in head extension if the neck is stabilized.

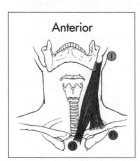

Sternocleidomastoid
(STER-no-CLY-do-mast-oyd) Meaning connecting to the sternum, clavicle, and mastoid process of the skull

Function:

Acting together—Assists longus colli in flexing the cervical portion of the vertebral column forward; resists forceful backward movement of the head; with head fixed, assists in elevating thorax during forced inspiration; assists in stabilizing the head in space when the mandible moves

Acting singly—Tilts head toward the shoulder on the same side; rotates the head to the opposite side

Origin:

Sternal head—Upper aspect of anterior surface of manubrium sterni

Clavicular head—Superior border of the anterior surface of the medial third of the clavicle

Insertion: Upper surface of the mastoid process and lateral half of the superior nuchal line

Innervation: Accessory nerve and ventral rami of second and third cervical spinal nerves

Synergists: Trapezius, scalenes, longus colli, and splenius on the opposite side

Antagonists: Acting unilaterally—Antagonistic to each other and to the trapezius on the opposite side during rotation; to splenius muscles on the same side

Trigger points: Several points the entire length of both divisions of the muscle

Referred pain pattern: Head and face, particularly the occipital region, ear, and forehead; autonomic nervous system phenomena and proprioceptive disturbances are common

See Activity 9-15

Anterior Triangle of the Neck

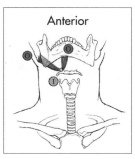

Digastric (dye-GAS-trik)
Meaning connecting bellies
NOTE: Considered part of the suprahyoid muscles

Function: Depresses the mandible to open the mouth and elevate the hyoid bone; the posterior belly is especially active in swallowing and chewing

Origin:

Posterior belly—Mastoid notch of the temporal bone

Anterior belly—Digastric fossa on the base of the mandible

Insertion: Body of the greater cornu of the hyoid bone via a fibrous loop

Innervation:

Anterior belly—Mylohyoid branch of the inferior alveolar nerve

Posterior belly—Facial nerve

Synergists: Inferior division of the lateral pterygoid, infrahyoid muscles

ACTIVITY 9-15

- Draw and color the sternocleidomastoid in the space provided.
- Label the origin and insertion points: *O*, for the origin, *I*, for the insertion.
- Place an **X** on the trigger points.
- Palpate this muscle; identify the attachment points and the belly of the muscle.
- Move this muscle on yourself.

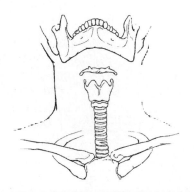

Antagonists: Elevators of the mandible, including the masseter, temporalis, medial pterygoid, and superior division of the lateral pterygoid

Trigger points: Belly of each division of the muscle

Referred pain pattern: Sternocleidomastoid area and bottom front teeth

See Activity 9-16

Suprahyoid Muscles

NOTE: As a group these muscles are located superior to the hyoid bone; they affect the movement of the tongue

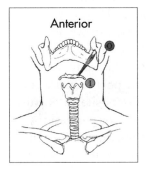
Anterior

Stylohyoid
(STY-low-HY-oyd)

Meaning pen and U-shaped

Function: Elevates and draws back the hyoid bone, elongating the floor of the mouth, and lifts the tongue

Origin: Posterior surface of the styloid process

Insertion: Body of the hyoid bone, at the junction with the greater cornu

Innervation: Facial nerve

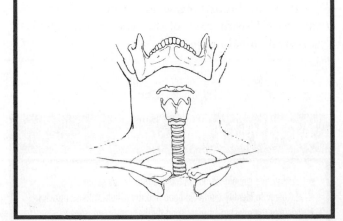

ACTIVITY 9-16

- Draw and color the digastric in the space provided.
- Label the origin and insertion points: *O,* for the origin *I,* for the insertion.
- Place an **X** on the trigger points.
- Palpate this muscle; identify the attachment points and the belly of the muscle.
- Move this muscle on yourself.

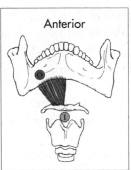
Anterior

Mylohyoid (MY-lo-HY-oyd)

Meaning molar and U-shaped

Function: Elevates the hyoid bone; elevates the floor of the mouth in the first stages of swallowing

Origin: Mylohyoid line of the mandible

Insertion:
Posterior fibers—Front of the body of the hyoid bone near the lower border
Middle and anterior fibers—Median fibrous raphe stretching from the symphysis menti to the hyoid bone

Innervation: Mylohyoid branch on the inferior alveolar nerve

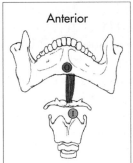
Anterior

Geniohyoid (JEEN-ee-oh-HY-oyd)

Meaning chin and U-shaped

Function: Elevates the hyoid bone and tongue and draws the tongue forward

Origin: Inferior mental spine on the back of the symphysis of the mandible

Insertion: Anterior surface of the body of the hyoid bone

Innervation: Mylohyoid branch of the inferior alveolar nerve

Infrahyoid Muscles

NOTE: These muscles are located inferior to the hyoid bone; as a group, they influence swallowing and the production of sound

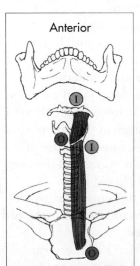
Anterior

Sternohyoid
(stern-oh-hy-OID)

Meaning chest and U-shaped

Function: Depresses the hyoid bone after it has been elevated in swallowing; most likely plays a part in speech and mastication

Origin: Posterior surface of the medial end of the clavicle; posterior sternoclavicular ligament; upper and posterior part of the manubrium

Insertion: Inferior border of the body of the hyoid bone

Innervation: Branches from the ansa cervicalis

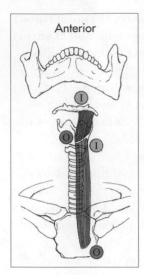

Anterior

Sternothyroid
(stern-o-thy-ROID)
Meaning chest and shaped like a shield
Function: Draws the larynx and thyroid cartilage downward after they have been elevated
Origin: Posterior surface of the manubrium and cartilage of the first rib
Insertion: Oblique line on the lamina of the thyroid cartilage
Innervation: Branches from the ansa cervicalis

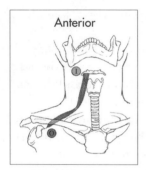

Anterior

Omohyoid
(OH-mo-HY-oyd)
Meaning shoulder and U-shaped
Function: Depresses the hyoid bone after it has been elevated; retracts the hyoid and larynx
Origin:
Inferior belly—Cranial border of the scapula near the scapular notch, suprascapular ligament; ends as a tendon under the sternocleidomastoid
Superior belly—From the tendon of the inferior belly near the sternocleidomastoid
Insertion: Lower border of the body of the hyoid bone
Innervation: Branches from the ansa cervicalis

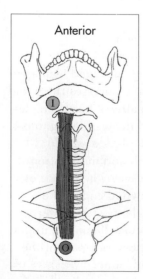

Anterior

Thyrohyoid
(thy-ro-hy-OID)
Meaning door and U-shaped
Function: Depresses the hyoid bone and the larynx; elevates the thyroid cartilage
Origin: Lamina of the thyroid cartilage at the oblique line
Insertion: Lower border of the greater cornu and the body of the hyoid bone

Elements common to the suprahyoid and infrahyoid muscles
Innervation: First cervical spinal nerve via the hypoglossal nerve

Synergists: Members of the suprahyoid group assists each other, as do members of the infrahyoid group
Antagonists: Generally, the suprahyoid group is antagonistic to the infrahyoid group
Trigger points: Likely to form in belly of muscles

See Activity 9-17

Posterior Triangle of the Neck

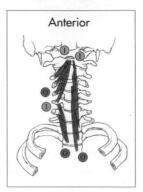

Anterior

Longus colli
(LON-gus KOAL-ee)
Meaning long and belonging to the neck
Function: Bends the neck forward; oblique portion bends it laterally; inferior oblique portion rotates it to the opposite side; pairs with the longus capitis, and the two can be compared with the psoas major and minor in the lumbar region
Origin:
Inferior oblique portion—Front of the bodies at the first two or three thoracic vertebrae
Superior oblique portion—Anterior tubercles of the transverse processes of the third, fourth, and fifth cervical vertebrae
Vertical portion—Front of the bodies of the lower three cervical vertebrae and the upper three thoracic vertebrae
Insertion:
Inferior—Anterior tubercles of the transverse processes of the fifth and sixth cervical vertebrae
Superior—Anterior tubercle of the atlas
Vertical—Front of the bodies of the second, third, and fourth cervical vertebrae
Innervation: Ventral rami of the second through sixth cervical spinal nerves

ACTIVITY 9-17

- Palpate the suprahyoid and infrahyoid muscles as groups.
- Swallow to identify the hyoid bone and the action of these muscles.
- Identify the attachment points and the belly of the muscles.

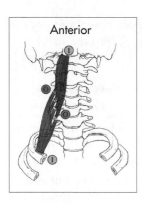

Anterior

Longus capitis
(LON-gus KAP-ih-tiss)
Meaning long and belonging to the head
Function: Flexes and rotates the cervical vertebrae and the head
Origin: Anterior tubercle of the transverse processes of the third through sixth cervical vertebrae

Insertion: Inferior surface of the basilar part of the occipital bone
Innervation: Muscular branches of the first through fourth cervical nerves

Elements common to the posterior triangle of the neck muscles
Synergists: Sternocleidomastoid, scalenes
Antagonists: Neck extensor group
Trigger points: Longus colli and longus capitis lie deep in the neck behind the larynx; although they may set up trigger points similar to any other muscle, they are very difficult to palpate and as such no specific trigger point locations have been identified
NOTE: The longus colli and capitis are important muscles to consider in any whiplash type of neck injury

See Activity 9-18

Scalene Group

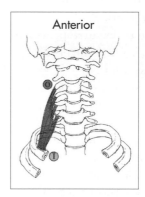

Anterior

Scalenus anterior
(SKAY-leen-us)
Meaning triangular with unequal sides; anterior meaning before or in front
Function: Bends the cervical portion of the vertebral column forward and laterally and rotates to the opposite side; assists in elevation of the first rib and thus functions as an accessory muscle of respiration
Origin: Anterior tubercle of the transverse processes of the third through sixth cervical vertebrae
Insertion: Scalene tubercle on the inner border of the first rib; upper surface of the first rib
Innervation: Ventral rami of the fourth through sixth cervical spinal nerves

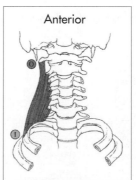

Anterior

Scalenus medius
(SKAY-leen-us)
Meaning triangular with unequal sides; medius meaning middle
Function: Acting from above, helps to raise the first rib and thus functions as an accessory muscle of respiration; acting from below, bends the cervical part of the vertebral column to the same side
Origin: Transverse process of the axis; front of the posterior tubercles of the transverse processes of the second through seventh cervical vertebrae

ACTIVITY 9-18

- Draw and color the longus colli and capitis in the space provided.
- Label the origin and insertion points: *O,* for the origin, *I,* for the insertion.
- Move these muscles on yourself.

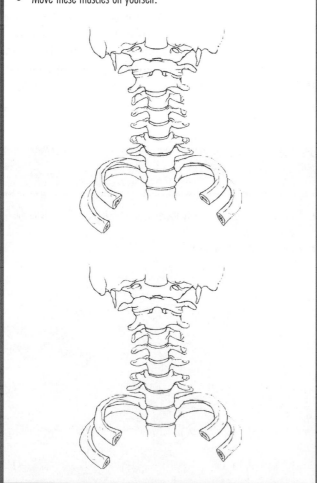

Insertion: Upper surface of the first rib

Innervation: Ventral rami of the third through eighth cervical spinal nerves

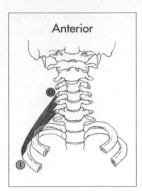

Anterior

Scalenus posterior
(SKAY-leen-us)

Meaning triangular with unequal sides; posterior meaning behind

Function: When the second rib is fixed, bends the lower end of the cervical portion of the vertebral column to the same side; when the upper attachment is fixed, helps to elevate the second rib and thus functions as an accessory muscle of respiration

Origin: Posterior tubercle of the transverse processes of the fourth through sixth cervical vertebrae

Insertion: Outer surface of the second rib

Innervation: Ventral rami of the sixth through eighth cervical spinal nerves

Elements common to the scalene group

Synergists: Scalene muscles on one side are synergistic with each other; sternocleidomastoid, upper trapezius, levator scapulae, omohyoid, pectoralis minor

Antagonists: Scalene muscles antagonize each other in lateral flexion

Trigger points: Belly of each muscle near the rib attachment points

Referred pain pattern: Pectoral region, rhomboid region, and the entire length of the arm, into the hand

See Activity 9-19

DEEP MUSCLES OF THE BACK AND POSTERIOR NECK

The splenius muscles are responsible for head extension. Trunk movements are effected by the deep or intrinsic back muscles associated with the vertebral column. These muscles also play an important role in maintaining the normal curvature of the spine. The deep muscles of the back form a complex column that extends from the sacrum to the skull. It helps to think of each of the individual deep back muscles as a string which, when pulled, causes one or more vertebrae to move on the vertebrae below. Because the attachments of the different muscle groups overlap extensively, entire regions of the vertebral column can be moved simultaneously and smoothly. Acting together, the deep back muscles can extend and hyperextend the spine. Contraction of muscles on only one side initiates lateral bending and rotation of the back, neck, or head.

The largest deep back muscle group is the erector spinae group. Assisting the long muscles of the back are a number of short muscles that extend from one vertebra to the next; these small intrinsic muscles act as stabilizers for the spine.

ACTIVITY 9-19

- Draw and color the scalenus anterior, medius, and posterior in the space provided.
- Label the origin and insertion points: *O,* for the origin, *I,* for the insertion.
- Place an **X** on the trigger points.

- Palpate these muscles; identify the attachment points and the belly of the muscle.
- Move these muscles on yourself.

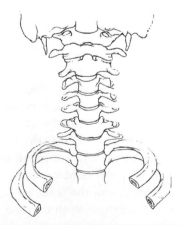

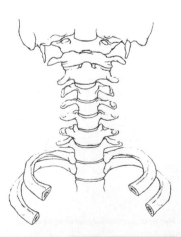

Deep Posterior Cervical Muscles

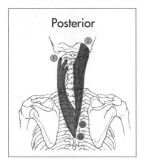

Posterior

Splenius capitis and cervicis
(SPLEEN-ee-us CAP-ih-tiss, SIR-vih-kiss)
Meaning bandage; capitis meaning head; cervicis meaning belonging to the neck

Function:
>   Together—To extend the head and neck

Separately—To draw the head dorsally and laterally and rotate to the same side

Origin:
  Capitis—Fascia and the spinous processes of the seventh cervical and first four thoracic vertebrae
  Cervicis—Spinous processes of the third through sixth thoracic vertebrae

Insertion:
  Capitis—Lateral one third of the superior nuchal line of the occipital bone underneath the attachment of the sternocleidomastoid and the mastoid process of the temporal bone
  Cervicis—Posterior tubercles of the transverse processes of the upper three cervical vertebrae

Innervation:
  Capitis—Dorsal rami of the middle cervical nerves
  Cervicis—Dorsal rami of the lower cervical nerves

Synergists: Posterior cervical extension group; for rotation—levator scapulae on the same side, and on the opposite side the upper trapezius, semispinalis capitis, deep paraspinals, and sternocleidomastoid

Antagonists: For extension—anterior flexor cervical group and sternocleidomastoid; for rotation—levator scapulae on the opposite side and on the same side the upper trapezius, semispinalis capitis, deep paraspinals, and sternocleidomastoid

Trigger points: Belly of the muscles closer to the head

Referred pain patterns: To the top of the skull (the pain often feels as if it is inside the head), to the eye, and into the shoulder

See Activity 9-20

Vertical Muscles, Erector Spinae Group (Sacrospinalis) (ee-REK-tor SPINE-eye)
The muscles in this group are the principal extensors of the vertebral motion segments.

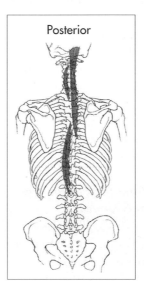

Posterior

Spinalis thoracis, cervicis, and capitis (spy-NAL-iss thor-AH-kiss, SIR-vih-kiss, CAP-ih-tiss)
Meaning related to the spine, chest, neck, and head

Function: Extends, rotates, and laterally flexes the vertebral column

Origin:
  Thoracis—Spinous processes of the first two lumbar and the last two thoracic vertebrae
  Cervicis—Spinous processes of the first and second thoracic and the seventh cervical vertebrae

Capitis—Transverse processes of the upper seven thoracic and the seventh cervical vertebrae; articular processes of the fourth through sixth cervical vertebrae

Insertion:
  Thoracis—Spinous processes of the fourth through eighth thoracic vertebrae
  Cervicis—Spinous processes of the second and third cervical vertebrae
  Capitis—Between the superior and inferior nuchal lines of the occipital bone

Innervation: Dorsal rami of the lower cervical, thoracic, and lumbar spinal nerve

ACTIVITY 9-20

- Draw and color the splenius capitis and cervicis in the space provided.
- Label the origin and insertion points: *O*, for the origin, *I*, for the insertion.
- Place an **X** on the trigger points.
- Palpate these muscles; identify the attachment points and the belly of the muscle.
- Move these muscles on yourself.

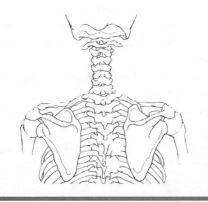

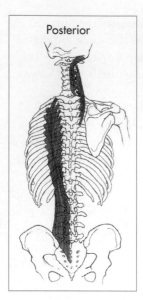

Posterior

Longissimus thoracis, cervicis, and capitis

(lon-GISS-ih-mus thor-AH-kiss, SIR-vih-kiss, CAP-ih-tiss)

Meaning the longest; related to the chest, neck, and head

Function: Extends, rotates, and laterally flexes the vertebral column

Origin:

Thoracis—Transverse processes of the lumbar vertebrae; lumbocostal aponeurosis

Cervicis—Transverse processes of the upper five thoracic vertebrae

Capitis—Transverse processes of the upper four or five thoracic vertebrae; articular processes of the lower three or four cervical vertebrae

Insertion:

Thoracis—Transverse processes of all thoracic vertebrae; lower nine or 10 ribs

Cervicis—Posterior tubercles of the transverse processes of the second through sixth cervical vertebrae

Capitis—Mastoid process of the temporal bone

Innervation: Dorsal rami of the lower cervical, thoracic, and lumbar spinal nerves

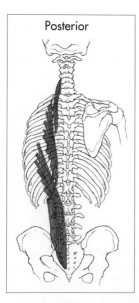

Posterior

Iliocostalis lumborum, thoracis, and cervicis

(ILL-ee-oh-kos-TAL-iss lum-BOR-um, thor-AH-kiss, SIR-vih-kiss)

Meaning connecting the ilium to the ribs and loins, chest and neck

Function: Extension, rotation, and lateral flexion of the vertebral column and lateral movement of the pelvis

Origin:

Lumborum—Body of the sacrospinalis

Thoracis—Lower six ribs medial to the tendons of the iliocostalis lumborum

Cervicis—Angles of the third through sixth ribs

Insertion:

Lumborum—Inferior border at the angles of the last six ribs

Thoracis—Superior border at the angles of the upper six ribs

Cervicis—Posterior tubercles of the transverse processes of the fourth through sixth cervical vertebrae

Innervation: Dorsal rami of the lower cervical, thoracic, and lumbar spinal nerves

Oblique Muscles, Transversospinalis Group

This group of muscles extends the motion segments of the back and rotates the thoracic and cervical vertebral joints.

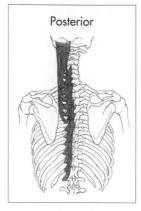

Posterior

Semispinalis thoracis, cervicis, and capitis

(sem-ee-spy-NAL-us thor-AH-kiss, SIR-vih-kiss, CAP-ih-tiss)

Meaning half and the spine, as related to the chest, neck, and head

Function: Extension and lateral flexion of the head and vertebral column; extension of the head and rotation to the opposite side; extension of the pelvis

Origin:

Thoracis—Transverse processes of the last six thoracic vertebrae

Cervicis—Transverse processes of the upper six thoracic and articular processes of the lower four cervical vertebrae

Capitis—Transverse processes of the upper six thoracic vertebrae and the seventh cervical vertebrae; articular processes of the fourth through sixth cervical vertebrae

Insertion:

Thoracis—Spinous processes of the first four thoracic and the last two cervical vertebrae

Cervicis—Spinous processes of the second through fifth cervical vertebrae

Capitis—Between the superior and inferior nuchal lines of the occipital bone

Innervation:

Thoracis—Dorsal rami of the upper six thoracic spinal nerves

Cervicis—Dorsal rami of the lower three cervical spinal nerves

Capitis—Dorsal rami of the first six cervical spinal nerves

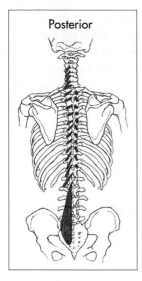

Posterior

Multifidi (mul-tih-FYE-eye)
Meaning many split parts
Function: Aids in extension and lateral flexion of the vertebral column
Origin: Articular processes of the last four cervical vertebrae; transverse processes of all thoracic vertebrae; mammillary processes of the lumbar vertebrae; posterosuperior iliac spine; posterior sacroiliac ligaments; back of the sacrum
Insertion: Spinous processes of the vertebra above the vertebra of origin
Innervation: Dorsal rami of the spinal nerves

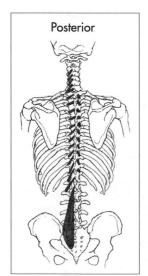

Posterior

Rotators (ro-TA-torz)
Meaning one that rotates
Function: Extend the vertebral column and rotate toward opposite side
Origin: Transverse process of one thoracic vertebra (11 pairs total)
Insertion: Base of the spinous process of the vertebra above
Innervation: Dorsal rami of spinal nerves

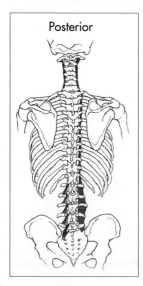

Posterior

Intertransversarii lumborum, thoracis, and cervicis
(inter-TRANS-ver-SAIR-ee-ee lum-BOR-um, thor-AH-kiss, SIR-vih-kiss)
Meaning between or among the transverse processes of the vertebrae and the loins, chest, and neck
Function: Aid in lateral flexion of the vertebral column
Origin and Insertion: Between spinous processes of the cervical, thoracic, and lumbar vertebrae (best developed in the cervical and lumbar regions)
Innervation: Ventral and dorsal rami of the spinal nerves

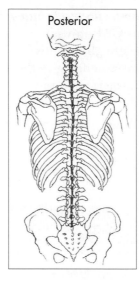

Posterior

Interspinalis
(inter-spy-NAL-eez)
Meaning between or among the parts of the spine
Function: Aid in extension of the vertebral column
Origin and Insertion: Between the spines of the vertebrae
Innervation: Posterior primary rami of the spinal nerves

Elements common to the erector spinae and transversospinalis group
Synergists: Extension is assisted by the serratus posterior inferior and the quadratus lumborum; rotation is assisted by the abdominal obliques
Antagonists: Extension—abdominal and psoas muscles; rotation—abdominal oblique muscles on the opposite side
Trigger points: The most common site for trigger points is the superficial long-fibered, longitudinal muscles in the erector spinae group; trigger points usually are found in the midscapular and lumbar regions
Referred pain patterns: Scapular, lumbar, abdominal, and gluteal areas

See Activity 9-21

Suboccipital Muscles
As a group these muscles extend and rotate the head.

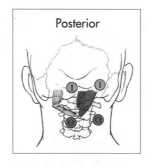

Posterior

Rectus capitis posterior major
(REK-tus CAP-ih-tiss)
Meaning straight; capitis meaning belonging to the head; posterior meaning behind; major meaning larger
Function: Extends the head and turns the face toward the same side
Origin: Spinous process of the axis
Insertion: Lateral aspect of the inferior nuchal line of the occipital bone lateral to the rectus capitis posterior minor
Innervation: Dorsal ramus of the first cervical spinal nerve

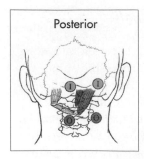

Posterior

Rectus capitis posterior minor
(REK-tus CAP-ih-tiss)
Meaning straight; capitis
   meaning belonging to the
   head; posterior meaning
   behind; minor meaning
   smaller
Function: Extends the head

NOTE: Recent myographic studies indicate that this muscle does not act in extension but rather functions as a restraint to flexion and forward movement of the head; its proximal attachment weaves into the dura through the foramen magnum (Greenman, 1996)
Origin: Posterior tubercle of the atlas
Insertion: Medial aspect of the inferior nuchal line of the occipital bone just above the foramen magnum
Innervation: Dorsal ramus of the first spinal nerve

ACTIVITY 9-21

- Draw and color the erector spinae and transversospinalis muscles in the space provided.
- Label the origin and insertion points: *O,* for the origin, *I,* for the insertion.
- Place an **X** on the trigger points.
- Palpate these muscles; identify the attachment points and the belly of the muscles.
- Move these muscles on yourself.

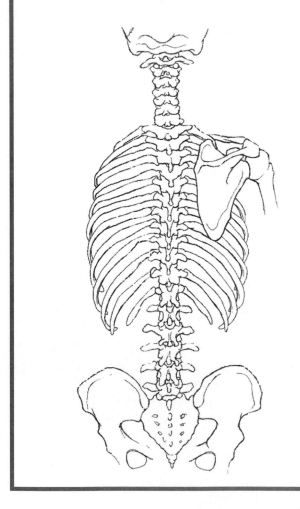

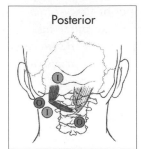

Posterior

Oblique capitis superior
(oh-BLEEK CAP-ih-tiss)
Meaning slanting; capitis
   meaning head; superior
   meaning above or higher
Function: Bends the head
   backward and to the same
   side
Origin: Superior surface of the transverse process of the atlas
Insertion: Between the superior and inferior nuchal lines of the occipital bone, lateral to the semi-spinalis capitis
Innervation: Dorsal ramus of the first cervical spinal nerve

ACTIVITY 9-22

- Draw and color the suboccipital muscles in the space provided.
- Label the origin and insertion points: *O,* for the origin, *I,* for the insertion.
- Place an **X** on the trigger points.
- Palpate these muscles; identify the attachment points and the belly of the muscle.
- Move these muscles on yourself.

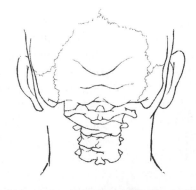

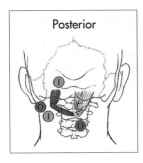

Posterior

Oblique capitis inferior
(oh-BLEEK CAP-ih-tiss)
Meaning slanting; capitis
meaning head; inferior
meaning lower or beneath
Function: Turns the face
toward the same side
Origin: Spinous process and
upper part of the lamina
of the axis
Insertion: Inferior and posterior aspect of the transverse process of the atlas
Innervation: Dorsal ramus of the first cervical spinal nerve

Elements common to the suboccipital muscles
Synergists:
Extension—Semispinalis capitis
Rotation—Splenius capitis on the same side and the sternocleidomastoid on the opposite side
Antagonists:
Extension—Longus capitis and rectus capitis anterior
Rotation—Splenius capitis on the opposite side and the sternocleidomastoid on the same side
Trigger points: Belly of the muscle, located with deep palpation at the base of the skull
Referred pain pattern: Around the ear on the same side
See Activity 9-22

MUSCLES OF THE TORSO

Muscles of the Thorax and Posterior Abdominal Wall
The primary function of the deep muscles of the thorax is to create movements necessary for breathing. Three layers of muscle form the anterolateral wall of the thorax, just as three layers of muscle forms the abdominal wall. Some anatomists have considered these muscle groups as one group. However, unlike the abdominal muscles, the thoracic muscles are very short, extending between the ribs. When they contract, they draw the somewhat flexible ribs closer together. The external intercostals lift the ribs for inspiration. The internal intercostals from the intermediate layer depress the ribs for forced expiration. Quiet expiration is largely a passive process and results from relaxation of the external intercostals and diaphragm and the elastic recoil of the lungs. The transversus thoracis is the deepest layer, and even in this age of scientific knowledge, we still do not know for sure what this muscle does.

The diaphragm is the most important muscle of inspiration. It forms a muscular partition between the thoracic and abdominopelvic cavities. When relaxed, the diaphragm is dome shaped, but when it contracts, it moves inferiorly and flattens, increasing the volume of the thoracic cavity. The alternating contraction and relaxation of the diaphragm cause pressure changes in the abdominopelvic cavity that assist the return of venous blood and lymph fluid to the heart. The diaphragm can be contracted to increase the intraabdominal pressure voluntarily to help evacuate urine or feces or to deliver a baby. An increase in intraabdominal pressure aids in lifting weight. When we take a deep breath to fixate our diaphragm, the abdominal pressure can be raised enough to support the spine while lifting a heavy weight. Fibers from both the quadratus lumborum and psoas muscles weave into the diaphragm. With this direct relationship, we can see how low back function and breathing function are interrelated.

Forced breathing involves a number of other muscles that insert into the ribs. During forced inspiration the scalenes and sternocleidomastoid muscles may assist in lifting the ribs. Contraction of the abdominal wall muscles assists respiration.

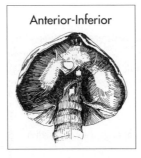

Anterior-Inferior

Diaphragm (DYE-ah-fram)
Meaning a fence or wall
Function: Respiration; during
inspiration (breathing in),
diaphragmatic contractions
increase the capacity of the
thoracic cavity; during
expiration (breathing out),
the diaphragm relaxes
Origin: First three lumbar vertebrae, the lower six costal cartilages, and the inner surface of the xiphoid process
Insertion: Muscle fibers arch upward and inward to end in tendinous fibers, which form the central tendon; the central tendon is a large aponeurosis
NOTE: The diaphragm is a broad, thin muscle that spans the thoracoabdominal cavity, separating the thorax from the abdomen; the origin is the edges of the bowl; the insertion is not attached to any solid structure; rather, the middle of the plastic wrap becomes a thickened fascial structure; when the muscle component of the diaphragm contracts, it pulls and flattens the central tendon

Innervation: Phrenic nerve

Synergists: Accessory respiratory muscles: intercostals, scalenes, sternocleidomastoids, scapular elevators, abdominals, pectoral muscles, serratus anterior, trapezius, quadratus lumborum

Antagonists: Difficult to discern; transversus thoracis reduces the thoracic cavity and therefore acts in opposition to the diaphragm; because this is an unpaired muscle, it is likely that no direct antagonist patterns exist; an antagonist pattern for any of the synergists could have an indirect influence on the function of the diaphragm

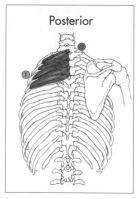

Serratus posterior superior
(suhr-Rate-us)

Meaning saw shaped; posterior meaning behind; superior meaning above

Function: Assists in lifting the ribs during inspiration

Origin: Lower portion of the ligamentum nuchae; spines of vertebrae C7 to T3

Insertion: Upper borders and external surfaces of the second through fifth ribs, just lateral to their angles

Innervation: Second through fifth intercostal nerves

ACTIVITY 9-23

- Draw and color the serratus posterior superior and inferior in the space provided.
- Label the origin and insertion points: *O,* for the origin, *I,* for the insertion.
- Place an **X** on the trigger points.
- Palpate these muscles; identify the attachment points and the belly of the muscle.
- Move these muscles on yourself.

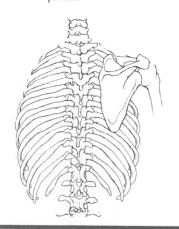

NOTE: This muscle lies under the rhomboids next to the ribs

Synergists: Intercostals and scalenes

Antagonists: Muscles of expiration

Trigger points: Under the scapula near the insertion of the muscle on the ribs

Referred pain pattern: Under the upper portion of the scapula

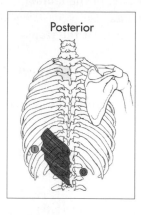

Serratus posterior inferior
(suhr-RATE-us)

Meaning saw shaped; posterior meaning behind; inferior meaning below

Function: Depresses last four ribs

NOTE: Some studies disagree that this is the function, finding no electromyographic activity of this muscle during respiration

Origin: Spines of T11, T12, and L1 to L3; supraspinous ligament; thoracolumbar fascia

Insertion: Inferior borders and outer surfaces of the lower four ribs, just lateral to the angles

Innervation: Thoracic spinal nerves T9 to T12

Synergist: Quadratus lumborum

Antagonists: Although questionable, antagonist patterns could be associated with the muscles of inspiration

Trigger points: Belly of the muscle near the eleventh rib

Referred pain pattern: Nagging ache in the area of the muscle

See Activity 9-23

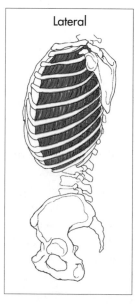

External intercostals
(inter-KOS-tals)

Meaning between or among the ribs; external meaning on the outside

Function: Draw adjacent ribs together; lift ribs, increasing the volume of the thoracic cavity

Origin: Eleven total, each arising from the caudal border of a rib

Insertion: Superior border of the rib below

Innervation: Adjacent intercostal nerves

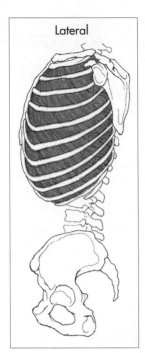

Lateral

Internal intercostals
(inter-KOS-tals)

Meaning between or among the ribs; internal meaning on the inside

Function: Draw adjacent ribs together; lower ribs, decreasing volume of thoracic cavity

Origin: Ridge of inner surface of a rib and corresponding costal cartilage

Insertion: Cranial border of the rib below

Innervation: Adjacent intercostal nerves

Innermost Intercostals (inter-KOS-tals)

Meaning between or among the ribs

The muscles of this small group attach to the internal aspects of two adjoining ribs. They are believed to act in conjunction with the internal intercostals.

ACTIVITY 9-24

- Draw and color the external and internal intercostals in the space provided.
- Label the origin and insertion points: *O*, for the origin, *I*, for the insertion.
- Place an **X** on the trigger points.
- Palpate these muscles; identify the attachment points and the belly of the muscle.
- Move these muscles on yourself.

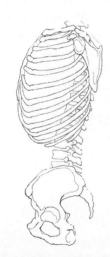
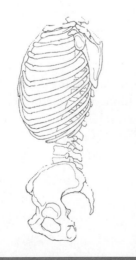

Transversus thoracis
(trans-VER-sus thor-AH-kiss)

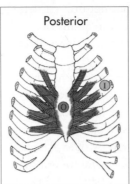

Posterior

Meaning lying crosswise and related to the chest

Function: Draws anterior portion of the ribs caudally (reduces thoracic cavity)

Origin: Inner surface of the body of the sternum (caudal one third); xiphoid process; sternal ends of the costal cartilages of the last three or four true ribs

Insertion: Costal cartilages of the second through sixth ribs

Innervation: Adjacent intercostal nerves

NOTE: This muscle is on the inside of the rib cage

Elements common to the innermost intercostals

Synergists: Intercostals, scalenes, sternocleidomastoids, scapular elevators, abdominals, pectoral muscles, serratus anterior, trapezius, quadratus lumborum

Antagonists: External and internal intercostals are antagonistic to each other

Trigger points: The intercostals can develop trigger points, which are located by palpating the muscles between the ribs

Referred pain pattern: Spans the intercostal segment

See Activity 9-24

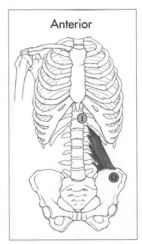

Anterior

Quadratus lumborum
(KWAD-rate-us-lum-BOR-um)

Meaning square shaped and of the loins

Function: Draws last rib downward; flexes lumbar vertebral column laterally to the same side; acting bilaterally, stabilizes and extends the lumbar spine and assists forced exhalation, as when coughing; assists normal inhalation by stabilizing the diaphragm and the twelfth rib

Origin: Iliolumbar ligament; posterior portion of the iliac crest

Insertion: Inferior border of the last rib; transverse processes of the first four lumbar vertebrae

Innervation: Ventral rami of the twelfth thoracic and upper three lumbar spinal nerves

NOTE: Quadratus lumborum fibers are oriented in three directions and operate as distinct units; the pectoralis and trapezius muscles are similar in form

Synergists: Abdominals, psoas, erector spinae, latissimus dorsi

Antagonist: Because of the fiber arrangement, the muscle is a self-antagonist; the primary antagonist of one quadratus lumborum is the corresponding muscle on the opposite side

Trigger points: Laterally near the rib or iliac attachment and medially near the iliac attachment at the transverse process of the lumbar vertebra

Referred pain pattern: Gluteal and groin area, sacroiliac joint and greater trochanter; these points are implicated in most low back pain; the duel function of lumbar stabilization and respiration can cause severe pain in the low back with a cough or sneeze if these trigger points are active

See Activity 9-25

ACTIVITY 9-25

- Draw and color the quadratus lumborum in the space provided.
- Label the origin and insertion points: *O,* for the origin, *I,* for the insertion.
- Place an **X** on the trigger points.
- Palpate this muscle; identify the attachment points and the belly of the muscle.
- Move this muscle on yourself.

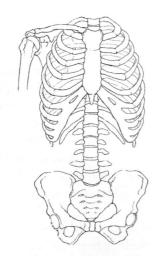

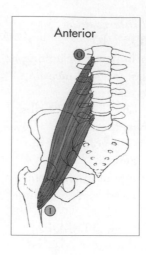

Anterior

Psoas major (SO-as)

Meaning muscle of the loins; major meaning larger

Function:

With origin fixed—Flexes the hip joint by flexing the femur on the trunk; may assist in lateral rotation of the hip joint; helps to maintain upright posture

With insertion fixed— Acting bilaterally, flexes the hip joint by flexing the trunk on the femur; can assist extension of the lumbar spine, increasing lumbar lordosis; acting unilaterally, assists in lateral flexion of the trunk toward the same side

Origin: Bodies and corresponding intervertebral disks of last thoracic and all lumbar vertebrae; anterior surface of transverse processes of all lumbar vertebrae; tendinous arches extending across the sides of the bodies of the lumbar vertebrae

Insertion: Lesser trochanter of the femur

Innervation: Ventral rami of lumbar nerves L2, L3, and L4

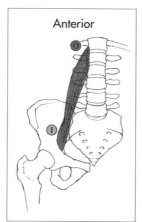

Anterior

Psoas minor (SO-as)

Meaning muscle of the loins; minor meaning smaller

Function: Flexes the pelvis on the lumbar spine and vice versa

NOTE: Absent in half of all people

Origin: Sides of the bodies of the twelfth thoracic and first lumbar vertebrae; from the intervertebral disk between them

Insertion: Pectineal line of the ilium, iliopectineal eminence, iliac fascia

Innervation: Branch from L1 and L2 nerves

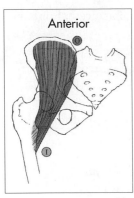

Anterior

Iliacus (ILL-ee-AK-us)
Meaning of the hip
Function:
    With origin fixed—Flexes
        the hip joint; may assist
        in lateral rotation and
        abduction of the hip
        joint
    With insertion fixed—
        Acting bilaterally, flexes
        the hip joint by flexing
        the trunk on the femur; tilts pelvis forward
        when legs are fixed
Origin: Internal lip of the iliac crest; anterior sacro-
    iliac, lumbosacral, and iliolumbar ligaments;
    superior two thirds of the iliac fossa; ala of the
    sacrum
Insertion: Femur, just distal to the lesser trochanter;
    lateral side of the tendon of the psoas major
Innervation: Muscular branches of the femoral nerve
    L2, L3, and L4

Elements common to the psoas major and minor and iliacus

Synergist: Rectus femoris, pectineus, sartorius, ten-
    sor fasciae latae, gracilis, adductors

Antagonists: Gluteus maximus, hamstrings
Trigger points: Psoas near both attachment points and
    the iliacus; inner border of the ilium behind the
    anterior superior iliac spine
Referred pain pattern: Entire lumbar area into the
    superior gluteal region, as well as the front of the
    thigh; may be associated with menstrual aching
    and can mimic appendicitis

See Activity 9-26

Muscles of the Anterior Abdominal Wall

The abdominal muscles and extensive fascia form the anterior abdominal wall. The muscle fiber arrangement produces a crisscross fiber pattern similar to plywood, with vertical support provided by the rectus abdominis and the pyramidalis. These muscles attach either directly or indirectly to a strong, fibrous cord in the midline of the abdomen called the *linea alba,* which is formed from the anterior abdominal aponeurosis and a fusion of three aponeuroses into a single tendinous band. It extends from the xiphoid process to the symphysis pubis and contains the umbilicus.

As a group these muscles act to compress the abdominal contents during expiration, urination, and defecation. They help maintain pressure on the curve of the low back, resisting excessive lumbar lordosis. In conjunction with the deep muscles of the back, the abdominals prevent hyperextension of the spine and splint the entire trunk of the body.

ACTIVITY 9-26

- Draw and color the psoas major and minor and the iliacus in the space provided.
- Label the origin and insertion points: *O,* for the origin, *I,* for the insertion.
- Place an **X** on the trigger points.
- Palpate these muscles; identify the attachment points and the belly of the muscle.
- Move these muscles on yourself.

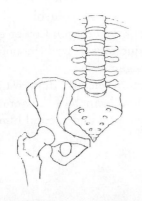

Transversus abdominis
(TRAN-ver-sus
ab-DAHM-in-is)
Meaning lying crosswise and
    of the abdomen
    NOTE: Innermost layer of
    the abdominal wall just ante-
    rior to the peritoneum
Function: Constricts the
    abdomen and supports the
    abdominal viscera
Origin: Inner surfaces of the
    cartilages of the last six
    ribs; anterior three
    fourths of the iliac crest;
    lateral one third of the
    inguinal ligament; thora-
    columbar fascia
Insertion: Linea alba, abdominal aponeurosis, pubis
Innervation: Ventral rami of the lower six thoracic
    and first lumbar spinal nerves

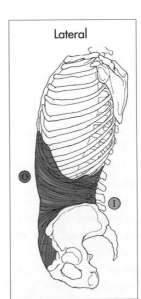

Lateral

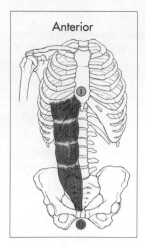

Rectus abdominis
(REK-tus ab-DAHM-in-is)

Meaning straight and of the abdomen

Function: Flexes the vertebral column, bringing the sternum toward the pelvis; compresses the abdominal cavity

Origin: Crest of the pubis and the pubic symphysis

Insertion: Cartilages of the fifth, sixth, and seventh ribs; xiphoid process of the sternum

Innervation: Anterior primary rami of the lower six intercostal nerves

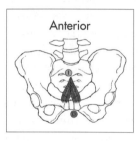

Pyramidalis
(peer-AM-id-al-iss)

Meaning pyramid shaped

Function: Tenses the linea alba to compress the abdomen and support the abdominal viscera; active in forced expiration

Origin: Ventral surface of the pubis and the pubic ligament

Insertion: Linea alba (between the pubis and the umbilicus)

Innervation: Muscular branches of the twelfth thoracic spinal nerve

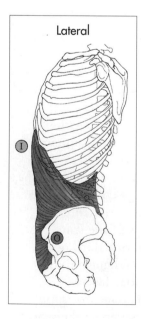

Internal oblique
(oh-BLEEK)

Meaning to the inside and slanting

Function:

Compresses the abdominal cavity

Both sides acting—Flexes the vertebral column, bringing the costal cartilage toward the pubis

One side acting—Laterally bends and rotates the vertebral column (brings the shoulder of the opposite side forward)

Origin: Inguinal ligament; iliac fascia; anterior two thirds of the middle lip of the iliac crest; lumbar fascia

Insertion: Upper fibers into cartilages of last three ribs; the remainder into the aponeurosis extending from the tenth costal cartilage to the pubic bone into the linea alba

Innervation: Ventral rami of the lower six thoracic and first lumbar spinal nerves

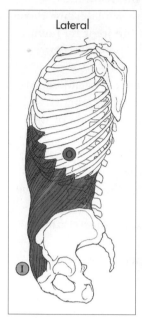

External oblique
(oh-BLEEK)

Meaning on the outside and slanting

Function:

Compresses the abdominal cavity

Both sides acting—Flexes the vertebral column, bringing the pubis toward the xiphoid process of sternum

One side acting— Laterally bends and rotates the vertebral column (brings the shoulder of the same side forward)

Origin: External surface of the lower eight ribs by interdigital slips

Insertion: Outer lip of the iliac crest, and the linea alba

Innervation: Ventral rami of the lower six thoracic spinal nerves

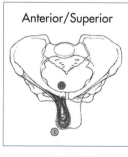

Cremaster (KREE-mast-er)

Meaning a suspender

Function: Pulls the testes up toward the superficial inguinal ring; although a striated muscle, it usually is not under voluntary control

Origin: Lower edge of the internal oblique muscle and the middle aspect of the inguinal ligament

Insertion: Pubic tubercle and the crest of the pubis

Innervation: Genital branch of the genitofemoral nerve from the first and second lumbar spinal nerves

Elements common to the anterior abdominal wall muscles

Synergists: Quadratus lumborum and diaphragm; rotation—lower serratus anterior and posterior, latissimus dorsi, iliocostalis

Antagonists: Flexion—paraspinal extensor group; rotation—contralateral muscles

Trigger points: Located throughout the area but concentrated more in the external circle of the abdominal wall rather than toward the middle near the umbilicus; the exceptions are points often found in the rectus abdominis just below the umbilicus on either side of the linea alba

Referred pain pattern: Pain likely to appear in the same quadrant and in the back; these trigger points are capable of causing somatovisceral responses (e.g., vomiting, nausea, intestinal problems, diarrhea, bladder symptoms, and pain).

See Activity 9-27

Pelvic and Perineal Muscles

The levator ani and the coccygeus muscles form the pelvic floor (also called the *pelvic diaphragm*). These muscles close the inferior outlet of the pelvis, support and elevate the pelvic floor, and counterbalance increased intraabdominal pressure, which would expel the contents of the bladder, rectum, and uterus.

The pelvic diaphragm has openings for the rectum, urethra, and vagina.

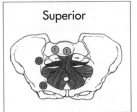

Superior

Levator ani
(le-VAY-tor AIN-eye)
Meaning one that raises; ani meaning belonging to the anus or rectum

Function: Forms the floor of the pelvic cavity; constricts the lower end of the rectum and vagina; supports and slightly raises the pelvic floor

Origin: Pelvic surfaces of the pubis; inner surface of the ischial spine; the obturator fascia

Insertion: Last two segments of the coccyx; anococcygeal raphe uniting with fibers from the opposite side; the sides of the rectum anterior into the perineal body

Innervation: Muscular branches of the perineal division of the pudendal nerve

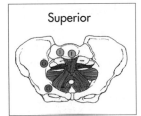

Superior

Coccygeus (kok-SIH-jee-us)
Meaning related to the coccyx or tailbone

Function: Pulls forward and supports the coccyx; exerts rotary tension on the

ACTIVITY 9-27

- Draw and color the anterior abdominal wall muscles in the space provided.
- Label the origin and insertion points: *O,* for the origin, *I,* for the insertion.
- Place an **X** on the trigger points.
- Palpate these muscles; identify the attachment points and the belly of the muscle.
- Move these muscles on yourself.

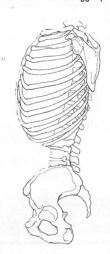 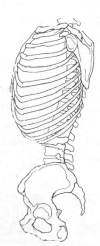 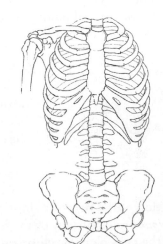

sacroiliac joint; with the levator ani and piriformis muscles, assists in closing the posterior part of the pelvic outlet and forms the supporting muscular diaphragm for the pelvic viscera

Origin: Pelvic surface of the spine of the ischium and the sacrospinous ligament

Insertion: Margin of the coccyx and the side of the fifth segment of the sacrum

Innervation: Branch of the fourth and fifth sacral nerves

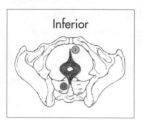

External sphincter ani
(SFINK-tur AIN-eye)
Meaning band and related to the anus or rectum; external meaning on the outside

Function: Closes the anal orifice

Origin: Superficial fibers from the anococcygeal raphe; deeper fibers surround the anal canal

Insertion: Superficial fibers surround the anus, meeting posteriorly at the coccyx and anteriorly at the central point of the perineum

Innervation: Perineal branch of the fourth sacral nerve and the inferior rectal branch of the pudendal nerve

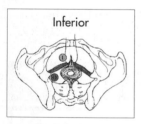

Superficial transverse perineals (pair-i-NEE-als)
Meaning crossing or around; to empty or defecate; superficial meaning on the top

Function: Simultaneous contraction of both muscles helps to fix the perineal body

Origin: Medial and anterior part of the ischial tuberosity

Insertion: Central tendinous point of the perineum

Innervation: Perineal branches of the pudendal nerve

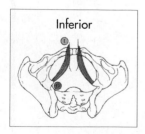

Ischiocavernosus
(ISS-she-oh-KAV-ern-oh-sus)
Meaning hip and cavernlike

Function: Compresses the crus penis, which obstructs venous return and therefore is believed to play a part in maintaining erection of the penis or clitoris

Origin: Inner surface of the ischial tuberosity behind the crus penis or clitoris; ramus of the ischium on both sides of the crus

Insertion: Aponeuroses on the sides and undersurface of the crus penis or clitoris

Innervation: Perineal branch of the pudendal nerve (S2 to S4)

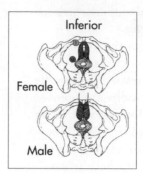

Bulbospongiosus
(BUL-bo-SPON-jee-oh-sus)
Meaning bulb and spongy

Function: Aids in emptying the urethra; it is relaxed during the greater part of micturition, coming into action only at the end of the process, and it can be used to arrest urination; it constricts the orifice of the vagina and contributes to erection of the penis and clitoris

Origin: Central tendinous point of the perineum, with fiber surrounding the vaginal orifice and vestibular bulbs (female)

Insertion: Lower surface of the perineal membrane; dorsal surface of the corpus spongiosum; deep fascia on the dorsum of the penis; corpora cavernosa clitoris (female)

Innervation: Perineal branch of the pudendal nerve (S2 to S4)

Elements common to the pelvic and perineal muscles

Synergist: All muscles are synergistic with each other; the gluteus maximus supports the closure of the anus

Antagonists: No direct antagonist pattern to the pelvic floor has been identified in the literature; however, because the gluteus maximus is powerfully synergistic with these muscles, it could be assumed that antagonist patterns to the gluteus maximus would have an antagonistic influence on the pelvic floor muscles

Trigger points: Trigger points do develop in these muscles; these trigger points usually can be palpated internally, either rectally or vaginally

Referred pain patterns: To the pelvic floor itself and to the coccyx region

See Activity 9-28

ACTIVITY 9-28

- Move your pelvic floor muscles.

MUSCLES OF SCAPULAR STABILIZATION

The muscles of scapular stabilization hold the scapula to the wall of the thorax and move the scapula. The arrangement of the muscle attachments to the scapula requires cooperative interaction to produce movement. Several muscles must act together to elevate or depress the scapula or to effect other scapular movements.

The prime movers of shoulder elevation are the trapezius and the levator scapulae, which work together to shrug the shoulder. The opposite rotational effects of the trapezius and levator scapulae counterbalance each other.

Scapular depression results largely from gravitational pull, but when the scapula is depressed against resistance, the trapezius and serratus anterior are active. Serratus anterior activity creates the forward (pushing) movements of abduction of the scapula on the chest wall. Retraction (adduction) of the scapula is effected by the trapezius and the rhomboids.

Although the serratus anterior and trapezius muscles are antagonists in the forward/backward movements of the scapula, they act together to coordinate the rotational scapular movements. The clavicles rotate around their own axes during scapular movements, giving these movements stability and precision.

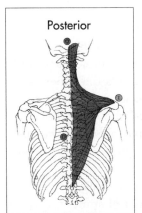

Posterior

Trapezius (TRAP-eez-ee-us)
Meaning a figure with four unequal sides
Function:

Upper trapezius elevates the shoulder and, with the shoulder fixed, can assist in drawing the head backward and laterally to tilt chin; the middle portion adducts the scapula, draws back the acromion process, and rotates the scapula; lower fibers depress the scapula; the entire muscle, acting bilaterally, assists extension of the cervical and thoracic spine

Levator scapula—Upper fibers elevate scapula and with it the point of the shoulder

Serratus anterior—Rotates scapula in forward direction so that the arm can be raised overhead

Rhomboids—Retracts the scapula

NOTE: This muscle consists of three distinct parts and can be considered as three separate muscles
Origin:

Upper trapezius—External occipital protuberance; nuchal line, ligamentum nuchae; spinous process of the seventh cervical vertebrae

Middle trapezius—Spinous processes of the first through fifth thoracic vertebrae

Lower trapezius—Spinous processes of the sixth through twelfth thoracic vertebrae

Insertion:

Upper trapezius—Lateral one third of the clavicle; acromion process of the scapula

Middle trapezius—Superior lip of the spine of the scapula

Lower trapezius—Apex of the spine of the scapula

Innervation: Accessory nerve and ventral rami of third and fourth cervical spinal nerves

Synergists:

Upper trapezius—Sternocleidomastoid, supraspinatus, deltoids

Middle trapezius—Rhomboids, deltoid, supraspinatus, and long head of the biceps brachii

ACTIVITY 9-29

- Draw and color the trapezius in the space provided.
- Label the origin and insertion points: *O,* for the origin, *I,* for the insertion.
- Place an **X** on the trigger points.
- Palpate this muscle; identify the attachment points and the belly of the muscle.
- Move this muscle on yourself.

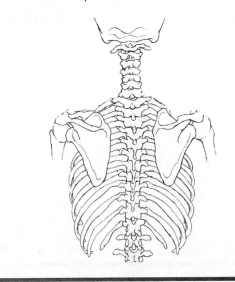

Lower trapezius—Anterior serratus, abductors of the arm supraspinatus and deltoids

Antagonists:

Upper trapezius—Serratus anterior and lower trapezius

Middle trapezius—Pectoralis major

Lower trapezius—Upper trapezius

Trigger points: Upper trapezius near the acromion and clavicular attachments; middle trapezius near the spine of the scapula; lower trapezius in the belly of the muscle

Referred pain patterns: Neck behind the ear and to the temple; subscapular area

See Activity 9-29

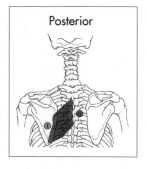

Rhomboid major
(rom-BOYD)

Meaning shaped like a rhombus, which is a parallelogram with oblique angles; major meaning larger

Function: Adducts and elevates the scapula and rotates it so that the glenoid cavity faces caudally

Origin: Spinous processes of the second through fifth thoracic vertebrae

ACTIVITY 9-30

- Draw and color the rhomboid major and minor in the space provided.
- Label the origin and insertion points: *O,* for the origin, *I,* for the insertion.
- Place an **X** on the trigger points.
- Palpate these muscles; identify the attachment points and the belly of the muscle.
- Move these muscles on yourself.

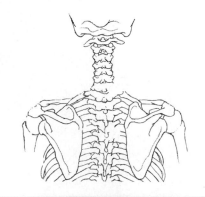

Insertion: Medial border of the scapula, between the spine and the inferior angle

Innervation: Dorsal scapular nerve (C4 to C5)

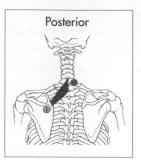

Rhomboid minor
(rom-BOYD)

Meaning shaped like a rhombus, which is a parallelogram with oblique angles; minor meaning smaller

Function: Adducts and elevates the scapula and rotates it so that the glenoid cavity faces caudally

Origin: Ligamentum nuchae; spine of the seventh cervical and first thoracic vertebrae

Insertion: Medial border at the root of the spine of the scapula

Innervation: Dorsal scapular nerve (C4 to C5)

Synergists: Trapezius, levator scapulae, latissimus dorsi

Antagonists: Pectorals

Trigger points: At the attachment point near the scapular border

Referred pain pattern: Scapular region

See Activity 9-30

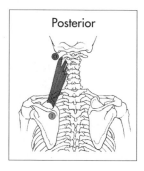

Levator scapula
(le-VAY-tor SKAP-you-la)

Meaning to raise up and of the shoulder

Function: Raises the scapula and draws it medially; with the scapula fixed, bends the neck laterally and rotates it to the same side

Origin: Transverse processes of the atlas and axis and the third and fourth cervical vertebrae

Insertion: Vertebral border of the scapula between the superior angle and the root of spine

NOTE: The levator scapula is a large muscle. It has a rotation, or twist, that occurs in its design so that the attachments at the atlas and axis are from muscle fibers that attach to the inferior portion of the vertebral border of the scapula and the attachment at C4 are from fibers at the superior portion of the vertebral border. This produces a combined rotation pattern whereby the head rotates so that the chin points to the acromion process and provides some extension while the scapula is pulled up and forward.

Innervation: Third and fourth cervical spinal nerves and dorsal scapular nerve

Synergists: Splenius cervicis and the scalenes

Antagonists: Serratus anterior and the latissimus dorsi

Trigger points: Belly of the muscle just as it begins the rotation and at the attachment near the scapula

Referred pain patterns: Angle of the neck at the trigger point and along the vertebral border of the scapula

See Activity 9-31

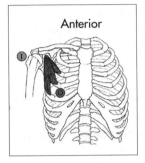

Anterior

Pectoralis minor
(PEK-tor-al-iss)

Meaning related to the chest; minor meaning smaller

Function: Assists in drawing the scapula forward around the chest wall; rotates the scapula so as to depress the point of the shoulder; assists in forced inspiration and therefore is an accessory respiratory muscle

Origin: Third, fourth, and fifth ribs near the cartilage and the aponeurosis covering the intercostals

Insertion: Coracoid process of the scapula

Innervation: Medial pectoral nerve (C7 to C8)

Synergists: Upper trapezius, levator scapulae, sternocleidomastoids, scalenes in forced respiration; pectoralis major, latissimus dorsi in depression of the scapula

Antagonists: Rhomboids, lower trapezius

Trigger points: Near the attachment at the coracoid process and at the belly of the muscle

Referred pain pattern: May mimic angina; front of the chest from the shoulder and down the ulnar side of the arm into the fingers

See Activity 9-32

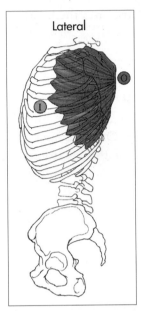

Lateral

Serratus anterior
(ser-RATE-us)

Meaning sawlike; anterior meaning toward the front

Function: Abducts or protracts the scapula; rotates the scapula so that the glenoid cavity faces cranially; holds the medial border of the scapula firmly against the thorax and prevents winging of the scapula; raises the ribs with the scapula fixed and therefore is an accessory muscle of respiration

Origin: Outer surfaces and superior borders of the upper eight or nine ribs

ACTIVITY 9-31

- Draw and color the levator scapula in the space provided.
- Label the origin and insertion points: *O,* for the origin, *I,* for the insertion.
- Place an **X** on the trigger points.
- Palpate this muscle; identify the attachment points and the belly of the muscle.
- Move this muscle on yourself.

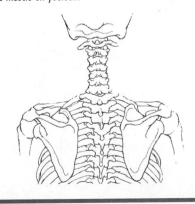

ACTIVITY 9-32

- Draw and color the pectoralis minor in the space provided.
- Label the origin and insertion points: *O,* for the origin, *I,* for the insertion.
- Place an **X** on the trigger points.
- Palpate this muscle; identify the attachment points and the belly of the muscle.
- Move this muscle on yourself.

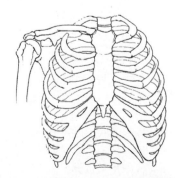

Insertion: Costal surface of the vertebral border of
the scapula
NOTE: This muscle lies along the ribs and is under
the scapula
Innervation: Long thoracic nerve (C5 to C7)
Synergists: Pectoralis minor and major
Antagonists: Latissimus dorsi, rhomboids, middle
trapezius
Trigger points: Along the midaxillary line near the ribs
Referred pain patterns: Side and back of the chest and
down the ulnar aspect of the arm into the hand

See Activity 9-33

MUSCLES OF THE
MUSCULOTENDINOUS
(ROTATOR) CUFF

Nine muscles cross over the ball-and-socket joint of
the shoulder to stabilize this joint. Of these nine, the
four SITS muscles are known as the rotator cuff
muscles; they are the *s*upraspinatus, *i*nfraspinatus,
*t*eres minor, and *s*ubscapularis. The SITS muscles
originate on the scapula, and their tendons blend
with the fibrous capsule of the shoulder joint. The
main functions of these muscles are to hold the head
of the humerus in the glenoid cavity and to reinforce
the joint capsule.

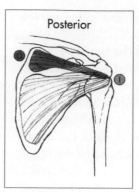
Posterior

Supraspinatus
(SOO-prah-spy-NAH-tus)
Meaning above the spine
Function: Abducts the arm;
acts to stabilize the
humeral head in the
glenoid cavity during
movements of the shoul-
der joint
Origin: Medial two thirds of
the supraspinous fossa of
the scapula; supraspinous fascia
Insertion: Superior facet of the greater tubercle of
the humerus and the capsule of the shoulder joint
Innervation: Suprascapular nerve C5 to C6
Synergists: Middle deltoid, upper trapezius for
abduction of the arm; the rotator cuff muscles
assist each other in stabilizing the humerus in the
glenoid fossa, and the anterior serratus stabilizes
the scapula
Antagonists: Latissimus dorsi, teres major, teres minor
Trigger points: In the belly of the muscle and near the
tendon at the humerus
Referred pain pattern: Shoulder, deltoid, and down the
arm to the elbow

See Activity 9-34

ACTIVITY 9-33

- Draw and color the serratus anterior in the space provided.
- Label the origin and insertion points: *O,* for the origin, *I,* for the insertion.
- Place an **X** on the trigger points.
- Palpate this muscle; identify the attachment points and the belly of the muscle.
- Move this muscle on yourself.

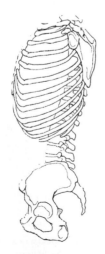

ACTIVITY 9-34

- Draw and color the supraspinatus in the space provided.
- Label the origin and insertion points: *O,* for the origin, *I,* for the insertion.
- Place an **X** on the trigger points.
- Palpate this muscle; identify the attachment points and the belly of the muscle.
- Move this muscle on yourself.

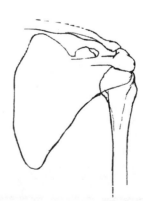

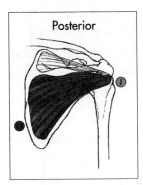

Posterior

Infraspinatus
(in-fra-spy-NAH-tus)
Meaning below the spine

Function: Lateral or external rotation of the arm at the shoulder; acts to stabilize the humeral head in the glenoid cavity during movements of the shoulder joint

Origin: Medial two thirds of the infraspinous fascia

Insertion: Middle facet of the greater tubercle of the humerus and the capsule of the shoulder joint

Innervation: Suprascapular nerve C5 to C6

Synergists: Teres minor, posterior deltoid, supraspinatus

Antagonists: Subscapularis, pectoralis major, anterior deltoid

Trigger points: Belly of the muscle below the spine of the scapula and near the medial border of the scapula

Referred pain patterns: Deep into the shoulder and deltoid area, down the arm, suboccipital area, medial border of the scapula

See Activity 9-35

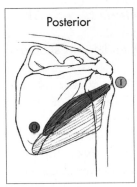

Posterior

Teres minor (TEAR-eze)
Meaning smooth and round; minor meaning smaller

Function: Adduction and lateral rotation of the arm; acts to establish the humeral head in the glenoid cavity during movements of the shoulder joint

Origin: Upper two thirds, dorsal surface of the lateral border of the scapula

Insertion: Lowest facet of the greater tuberosity of the humerus and the capsule of the shoulder joint

Innervation: Suprascapular nerve C5 to C6

Synergists: Infraspinatus, rotator cuff muscles, posterior fibers of the deltoid

Antagonists: Subscapularis, pectoralis major, anterior deltoid

Trigger points: Belly of the muscle nearer the attachment on the humerus

Referred pain pattern: Posterior deltoid region

See Activity 9-36

ACTIVITY 9-35

- Draw and color the infraspinatus in the space provided.
- Label the origin and insertion points: *O,* for the origin, *I,* for the insertion.
- Place an **X** on the trigger points.
- Palpate this muscle; identify the attachment points and the belly of the muscle.
- Move this muscle on yourself.

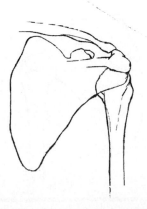

ACTIVITY 9-36

- Draw and color the teres minor in the space provided.
- Label the origin and insertion points: *O,* for the origin, *I,* for the insertion.
- Place an **X** on the trigger points.
- Palpate this muscle; identify the attachment points and the belly of the muscle.
- Move this muscle on yourself.

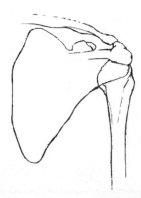

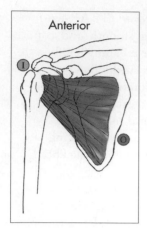

Anterior

Subscapularis (sub-SKAP-you-LAR-iss)

Meaning under the shoulder blade

NOTE: This muscle often is implicated in "frozen shoulder" syndromes

Function: Rotates humerus medially, draws it forward and down when the arm is raised

Origin: Subscapular fossa

Insertion: Lesser tuberosity of the humerus and the capsule of the shoulder joint

Innervation: Upper and lower subscapular nerves

Synergists: Rotator cuff muscles, teres major, latissimus dorsi, pectoralis major

Antagonists: Infraspinatus, teres minor

Trigger points: Access through the axilla near the attachment at the humerus and at the belly of the muscle

Referred pain pattern: Posterior deltoid, scapular region, triceps area and into the wrist

See Activity 9-37

MUSCLES OF THE SHOULDER JOINT

In general, any muscle that attaches anterior to the shoulder joint can flex the arm, and any muscle that attaches posterior to the shoulder joint can extend the arm. The deltoid is the prime mover of arm abduction. The main antagonists are the pectoralis major anteriorly and the latissimus dorsi posteriorly. Depending on the location and insertion points, the various muscles acting on the humerus also provide lateral and medial rotation of the shoulder joint. The interaction of these muscles is complex, and each muscle contributes to more than one movement.

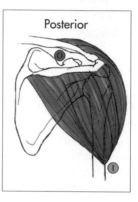

Posterior

Deltoid (del-TOYD)

Meaning triangular in shape

NOTE: This muscle functions in three distinct patterns and can be thought of as three different muscles

Function:

Anterior deltoid—Flexion and medial rotation of the arm

Middle deltoid—Abduction of the arm

Posterior deltoid—Extension and lateral rotation of the arm

ACTIVITY 9-37

- Draw and color the subscapularis in the space provided.
- Label the origin and insertion points: *O,* for the origin, *I,* for the insertion.
- Place an **X** on the trigger points.
- Palpate this muscle; identify the attachment points and the belly of the muscle.
- Move this muscle on yourself.

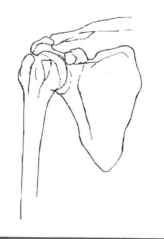

ACTIVITY 9-38

- Draw and color the deltoid in the space provided.
- Label the origin and insertion points: *O,* for the origin, *I,* for the insertion.
- Place an **X** on the trigger points.
- Palpate this muscle; identify the attachment points and the belly of the muscle.
- Move this muscle on yourself.

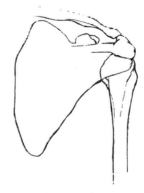

Origin:

Anterior deltoid—Superior surface, lateral third of the clavicle

Middle deltoid—Lateral margin and superior surface of the acromion

Posterior deltoid—Posterior border of the spine of the scapula

Insertion: Deltoid tuberosity of the humerus

Innervation: Axillary nerve C5 to C6

Synergists:

Anterior deltoid—Coracobrachialis, clavicular section of the pectoralis major, long head of the biceps brachii

Middle deltoid—Supraspinatus, biceps brachii

Posterior deltoid—Long head of the triceps brachii, latissimus dorsi, teres major

Antagonists: Anterior and posterior deltoid are antagonistic to each other; middle deltoid is opposed by the pectoralis major and latissimus dorsi

Trigger points:

Anterior deltoid—Near the clavicular attachment

Posterior and middle deltoid—In the belly of the muscles

Referred pain pattern: Deltoid region and down the lateral side of the arm

See Activity 9-38

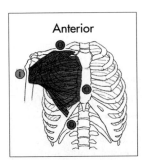

Pectoralis major

(PEK-tor-al-iss)

Meaning of the chest; major meaning larger

Function:

With origin fixed—Adducts and draws the humerus forward and medially rotates it

With insertion fixed and arm abducted—Assists in elevating the thorax (as in forced inspiration)

Origin: Ventral surface of the sternum down to the seventh rib; sternal half of the clavicle; cartilage of all true ribs; aponeurosis of the external oblique muscle

Insertion: Lateral lip of the bicipital groove of the humerus

NOTE: The attachment pattern for this muscle is complex; it consists of several overlapping sheets of muscles in a fan arrangement; the muscle is divided into clavicular, sternal, costal, and abdominal sections, each able to function independently

Innervation: Medial and lateral pectoral nerves

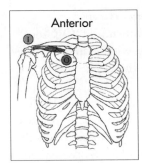

Subclavius

(sub-KLAVE-ee-us)

Meaning below and little key (referring to the clavicle)

NOTE: This muscle often is considered in conjunction with the clavicular portion of the pectoralis major

Function: Draws the shoulder forward and down and steadies the clavicle

Origin: Junction of the first rib and its costal cartilage

Insertion: Inferior surface of the clavicle

Innervation: Fifth and sixth cervical nerves C5 to C6

Elements common to the pectoralis major and subclavius muscles

Synergists: All sections contract together during strong adduction of the arm

Clavicular section—Anterior deltoid, coracobrachialis, subclavius, anterior scalene, sternocleidomastoid on the same side

Costal and abdominal sections—Latissimus dorsi, lower trapezius, lower serratus anterior

Antagonists: Rhomboids and trapezius for horizontal adduction, supraspinatus and deltoids for abduction

Trigger points: Belly of the muscle in each portion

Referred pain pattern: Chest and breast and down the ulnar aspect of the arm to the fourth and fifth fingers

See Activity 9-39

ACTIVITY 9-39

- Draw and color the pectoralis major and the subclavius in the space provided.
- Label the origin and insertion points: *O,* for the origin, *I,* for the insertion.
- Place an **X** on the trigger points.
- Palpate these muscles; identify the attachment points and the belly of the muscle.
- Move these muscles on yourself.

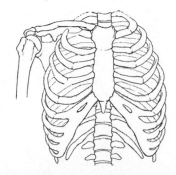

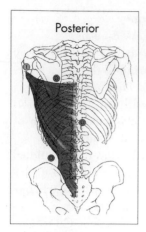

Posterior

Latissimus dorsi
(la-TISS-ih-mus DOR-see)
Meaning widest and belonging to the back

Function:

With origin fixed—Medially or internally rotates, adducts, and extends the shoulder; depresses the shoulder girdle and assists in lateral flexion of the trunk

With insertion fixed—Assists in tilting the pelvis anteriorly and laterally

Acting bilaterally—Assists in hyperextending the spine and tilting the pelvis anteriorly

Origin: Spinous processes of the last six vertebrae; posterior one third of the external lip of the iliac crest; posterior layer of the thoracolumbar fascia; last three or four ribs

Insertion: Intertubercular groove of the humerus with the teres major

NOTE: The latissimus dorsi is fan shaped and has a rotated or twisted insertion, which accounts for the rotation function; the latissimus fibers twist around the teres major muscle

Innervation: Thoracodorsal nerve C6 to C8

Synergists: Teres major, the long head of the triceps brachii, sternocostal portion of the pectoralis major, external obliques of the abdominal group

Antagonists: Scalenes, upper trapezius, clavicular portion of the pectoralis major

Trigger points: Posterior axillary area just as the muscle begins to twist around the teres major; belly of the muscle near the rib attachments

Referred pain pattern: Just below the scapula and into the ulnar side of the arm; anterior deltoid region and abdominal oblique area

See Activity 9-40

ACTIVITY 9-40

- Draw and color the latissimus dorsi in the space provided.
- Label the origin and insertion points: *O*, for the origin, *I*, for the insertion.
- Place an **X** on the trigger points.
- Palpate this muscle; identify the attachment points and the belly of the muscle.
- Move this muscle on yourself.

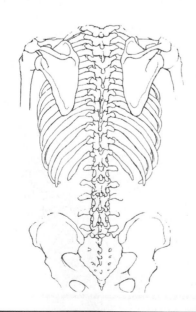

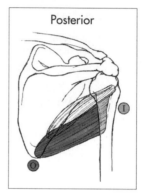

Posterior

Teres major (TEAR-eze)
Meaning smooth and round; major meaning larger

Function: Medial or internal rotation, adduction, and extension of the arm

Origin: Dorsal surfaces of inferior angle and lower third of lateral border of scapula

ACTIVITY 9-41

- Draw and color the teres major in the space provided.
- Label the origin and insertion points: *O*, for the origin, *I*, for the insertion.
- Place an **X** on the trigger points.
- Palpate this muscle; identify the attachment points and the belly of the muscle.
- Move this muscle on yourself.

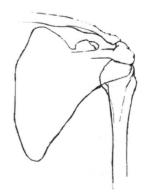

Insertion: Medial lip of bicipital groove of the humerus

Innervation: Lower subscapular nerve C5 to C6

Synergists: Latissimus dorsi, long head of the triceps brachii

Antagonists: Pectoralis major, teres minor

Trigger points: Near the musculotendinous junction at both attachments; points at the attachments at the humerus are best reached through the axilla

Referred pain pattern: Posterior deltoid region and down the dorsal portion of the arm

See Activity 9-41

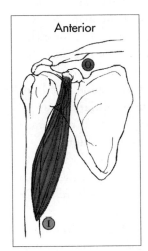

Coracobrachialis (KORE-koe-BRAY-kee-AL-iss)

Meaning crow's beak and of the arm

Function: Flexion and adduction of the humerus

Origin: Tip of the coracoid process of the scapula

Insertion: Anteromedial surface of the middle of the humeral shaft, opposite the deltoid tuberosity

Innervation: Musculocutaneous nerve C5 to C6

ACTIVITY 9-42

- Draw and color the coracobrachialis in the space provided.
- Label the origin and insertion points: *O,* for the origin, *I,* for the insertion.
- Place an **X** on the trigger points.
- Palpate this muscle; identify the attachment points and the belly of the muscle.
- Move this muscle on yourself.

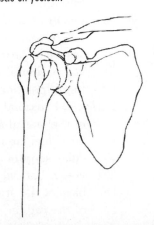

Synergists: Anterior deltoid, short head of the biceps brachii, pectoralis major, subscapularis, infraspinatus, teres major and minor, long head of the triceps brachii

Antagonists: Posterior deltoid, latissimus dorsi

Trigger points: Near musculotendinous junction and the coracoid attachment

Referred pain pattern: Posterior aspect of the arm down the triceps and dorsal forearm into the dorsal hand

See Activity 9-42

MUSCLES OF THE ELBOW AND RADIOULNAR JOINTS

The elbow is a hinge joint, and movements produced by these muscles are limited almost entirely to flexion and extension of the forearm. Posterior arm muscles are extensors; anterior arm muscles provide elbow flexion. The strongest elbow flexor is the brachialis. Pronation and supination take place at the radioulnar joint.

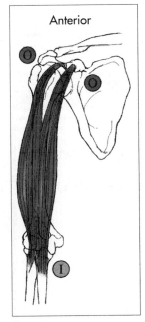

Biceps brachii

(BI-seps BRAY-kee-ee)

Meaning two heads and of the arm

Function:

Flexion of the arm; the long head may assist with abduction if the humerus is laterally rotated

With origin fixed—Flexes the forearm toward the humerus; supinates the forearm

With insertion fixed—Flexes the elbow joint, moving the humerus toward the forearm, as in a pull-up or chin-up

Origin:

Long head—Supraglenoid tubercle of the scapula

Short head—Tip of the coracoid process of the scapula

Insertion: Tuberosity of the radius; aponeurosis of the origin of the flexor muscles in the forearm

Innervation: Musculocutaneous nerve C5 to C6

Synergists: Brachialis, brachioradialis and supinator muscles to flex the forearm at the elbow; anterior deltoid and supraspinatus to abduct the arm at

ACTIVITY 9-43

- Draw and color the biceps brachii in the space provided.
- Label the origin and insertion points: *O,* for the origin, *I,* for the insertion.
- Place an **X** on the trigger points.
- Palpate this muscle; identify the attachment points and the belly of the muscle.
- Move this muscle on yourself.

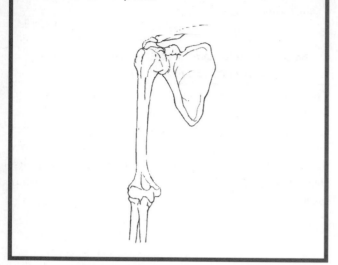

ACTIVITY 9-44

- Draw and color the brachialis in the space provided.
- Label the origin and insertion points: *O,* for the origin, *I,* for the insertion.
- Place an **X** on the trigger points.
- Palpate this muscle; identify the attachment points and the belly of the muscle.
- Move this muscle on yourself.

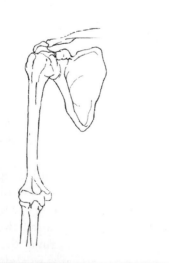

the shoulder; the coracobrachialis assists the short head in adduction at the shoulder

Antagonist: Triceps brachii

Trigger points: In the belly of the long and short heads, nearer the elbow

Referred pain pattern: Front of the shoulder at the anterior deltoid region and into the scapular region; also into the antecubital space or the front of the elbow

See Activity 9-43

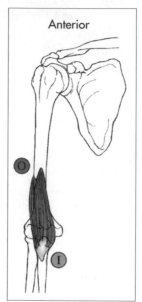

Anterior

Brachialis
(BRAY-kee-AL-iss)
Meaning of the arm

Function: Flexes the forearm

Origin: Distal one half of the anterior surface of the humerus; medial and lateral intermuscular septae

Insertion: Coronoid process, tuberosity of the ulna

Innervation: Musculocutaneous and radial nerves C5 to C6

Synergists: Biceps brachii, brachioradialis

Antagonist: Triceps brachii

Trigger points: Several locations in the belly of the muscle

Referred pain pattern: Primarily to the thumb, with some pain in the anterior deltoid area and at the elbow

See Activity 9-44

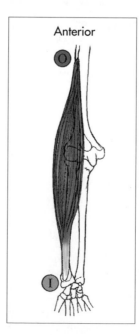

Anterior

Brachioradialis (BRAY-kee-oh-RAY-dee-AL-iss)
Meaning related to the arm and radius

Function: Flexes the elbow joint after movement has been initiated by the biceps and the brachialis; assists in pronation and supination of the forearm to midposition

Origin: Proximal two thirds of the lateral supracondylar ridge; lateral intermuscular septum

Insertion: Lateral side of the base of the styloid process of the radius

Innervation: Radial nerve C5 to C6
Synergists: Biceps brachii, brachialis
Antagonist: Triceps brachii
Trigger points: Belly of the muscle
Referred pain pattern: Wrist and base of the thumb in the web space between the thumb and index finger and to the lateral epicondyle at the elbow

See Activity 9-45

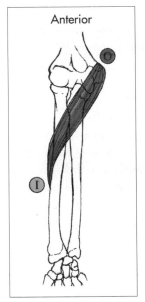
Anterior

Pronator teres
(PRO-nay-tor TEAR-eez)
Meaning one that causes pronation; round and smooth
Function: Pronates the forearm; assists in flexing the elbow joint
Origin:
Humeral head—Immediately above the medial epicondyle of the humerus; common flexor tendon; deep antebrachial fascia
Ulnar head—Medial side of the coronoid process of the ulna

Insertion: Middle of lateral surface of radius
Innervation Median nerve C6 to C7
Synergist: Pronator quadratus
Antagonists Supinator, biceps brachii
Trigger points: Belly of the muscle near the elbow attachment
Referred pain pattern: Radial side of the forearm into the wrist and thumb

See Activity 9-46

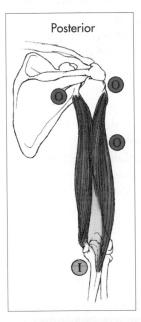
Posterior

Triceps brachii
(TRY-seps BRAY-kee-ee)
Meaning three heads and of the arm
Function: Extension of the forearm; in addition, the long head adducts and may assist in extension of the humerus
Origin:
Long head—Infraglenoid tubercle of the scapula
Short (or lateral) head—Lateral and posterior surfaces of the proximal

ACTIVITY 9-45

- Draw and color the brachioradialis in the space provided.
- Label the origin and insertion points: *O*, for the origin, *I*, for the insertion.
- Place an **X** on the trigger points.
- Palpate this muscle; identify the attachment points and the belly of the muscle.
- Move this muscle on yourself.

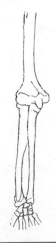

ACTIVITY 9-46

- Draw and color the pronator teres in the space provided.
- Label the origin and insertion points: *O*, for the origin, *I*, for the insertion.
- Place an **X** on the trigger points.
- Palpate this muscle; identify the attachment points and the belly of the muscle.
- Move this muscle on yourself.

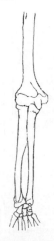

one half of the body of the humerus; lateral intermuscular septum

Medial head—Distal two thirds of the medial and posterior surfaces of the humerus below the radial groove; medial intermuscular septum

Insertion: Posterior surface of olecranon process of the ulna; antebrachial fascia

Innervation: Radial nerve C6 to C8

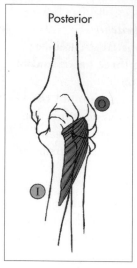

Posterior

Anconeus (an-koe-NEE-us)
Meaning elbow

Function: Assists the triceps in extension of the elbow joint and stabilizes the joint capsule

Origin: Posterior surface of the lateral epicondyle of the humerus

Insertion: Lateral side of the olecranon process; upper one fourth of the posterior surface of the body of the ulna

Innervation: Radial nerve C7 to C8

Elements common to the triceps brachii and anconeus muscles

Synergists: The triceps brachii and anconeus are synergistic to each other; the long head of the triceps brachii is synergistic to the latissimus dorsi, teres major, and teres minor

Antagonists: Biceps brachii, brachialis

Trigger points: Belly of each head of the triceps, and in the belly of the anconeus

Referred pain pattern:

Triceps brachii—Length of the posterior arm
Anconeus—Elbow at the lateral epicondyle

See Activity 9-47

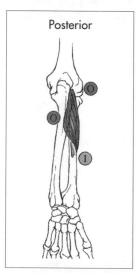

Posterior

Supinator
(SOOP-in-ATE-or)
Meaning to cause supination

Function: Supinates the forearm; assists with flexion of the forearm at the elbow when the hand is held half way between supination and pronation

Origin: Lateral epicondyle of the humerus; radial collateral ligament of the elbow joint; annular ligament of the radius; supinator crest of the ulna

ACTIVITY 9-47

- Draw and color the triceps brachii and the anconeus in the space provided.
- Label the origin and insertion points: *O,* for the origin, *I,* for the insertion.
- Place an **X** on the trigger points.
- Palpate these muscles; identify the attachment points and the belly of the muscle.
- Move these muscles on yourself.

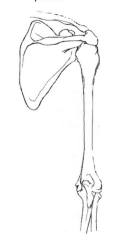

ACTIVITY 9-48

- Draw and color the supinator and the pronator quadratus in the space provided.
- Label the origin and insertion points: *O,* for the origin, *I,* for the insertion.
- Place an **X** on the trigger points of the supinator.
- Palpate these muscles; identify the attachment points and the belly of the muscle.
- Move these muscles on yourself.

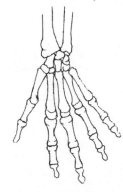 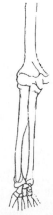

Insertion: Lateral surface of the upper one third of the body of the radius, covering part of the anterior and posterior surfaces

NOTE: The supinator is a large muscle that wraps around the bones of the forearm

Innervation: Deep branch of the radial nerve C5 to C6

Synergists: Biceps brachii, all forearm flexors

Antagonists: Pronator teres, pronator quadratus

Trigger points: Near the radius in the antecubital space

Referred pain pattern: Lateral epicondyle and dorsal web of the thumb; mimics tennis elbow

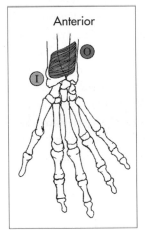

Pronator quadratus (PRO-nay-tor KWAD-rate-us)

Meaning to cause pronation; square shaped

Function: Pronation of the forearm

NOTE: The pronator quadratus is the primary pronator of the forearm

Origin: Medial side, anterior surface of the distal one fourth of the ulna

Insertion: Lateral side, anterior surface of the distal one fourth of the radius

Innervation: Anterior interosseous branch of the median nerve C8 to T1

Synergist: Pronator teres

Antagonists: Supinators

Trigger points: No common trigger points identified

See Activity 9-48

MUSCLES OF THE WRIST AND HAND JOINTS

If the muscles that move the hand actually were located in the hand, it would be too bulky to be functional. The bellies of these muscles are closer to the elbow, tapering to long insertion tendons in the wrist and hand. The long, tendinous insertions are secured by strong ligaments, called the *flexor* and *extensor retinacula* and are surrounded by synovial tendon sheaths that assist their movements and reduce friction. Many of the forearm muscles attach on the humerus and cross both the elbow and the wrist joints; however, their action on the elbow is insignificant. The forearm muscles are subdivided by fascial sheets into the anterior and posterior compartments, each having a superficial and a deep layer of muscles. Most muscles of the anterior compartment are wrist and finger flexors; the muscles of the posterior compartment are mainly wrist and finger extensors.

Anterior Flexor Group, Superficial Layer

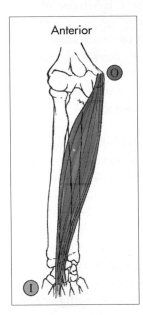

Flexor carpi radialis (FLEKS-or KAR-pee RAY-dee-al-iss)

Meaning to bend; of the wrist; related to the radius

Function: Flexes and abducts the wrist; may assist in pronation of the forearm and flexion of the elbow

Origin: Common flexor tendon from the medial epicondyle of the humerus; deep antebrachial fascia

Insertion: Base of the second and third metacarpal bones

Innervation: Median nerve C6 to C7

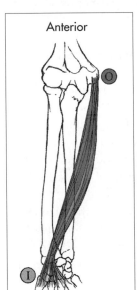

Palmaris longus (pal-MAR-iss LONG-us)

Meaning related to the palm; long

Function: Tenses the palmar fascia and flexes the wrist; may assist in flexion of the elbow and pronation of the forearm

Origin: Common flexor tendon from the medial epicondyle of the humerus; deep antebrachial fascia

Insertion: Flexor retinaculum; palmar aponeurosis

NOTE: The tendon of the palmaris longus is above the antebrachial fascia of the wrist and can be seen if one cups the hand and flexes the wrist; this muscle is absent in about one fourth of the population

Innervation: Median nerve C6 to C8

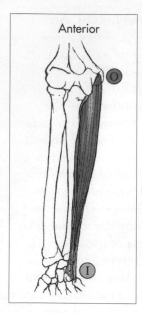

Anterior

Flexor carpi ulnaris (FLEKS-or KAR-pee ul-NAR-iss)

Meaning to bend; of the wrist; related to the ulna

Function: Flexes and adducts the wrist; may assist in elbow flexion

Origin:

Humeral head—Common flexor tendon from the medial epicondyle of the humerus

Ulnar head—Olecranon; proximal two thirds of the posterior border of the ulna; deep antebrachial fascia

Insertion: Pisiform bone and, indirectly, by ligaments to the hamate and fifth metacarpal bones

Innervation: Ulnar nerve C8 to T1

Anterior Flexor Group, Intermediate Layer

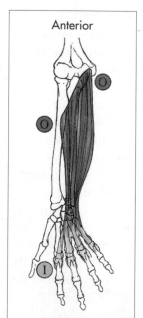

Anterior

Flexor digitorum superficialis (FLEKS-or DIH-jih-TOR-um soo-per-fish-ee-AL-us)

Meaning to bend; of the fingers or toes; related to the top or surface

Function: Flexes the proximal interphalangeal joints of the second through fifth digits; assists in flexion of the wrist

Origin:

Humeral head—Common flexor tendon from the medial epicondyle of the humerus; ulnar collateral ligament of the elbow joint; deep antebrachial fascia

Ulnar head—Medial side of the coronoid process of the ulna

Radial head—Oblique line of the radius

Insertion: Sides of the palmar surface of the middle phalanges of the second through fifth digits

Innervation: Median nerve C7 to C8 and T1

Anterior Flexor Group, Deep Layer

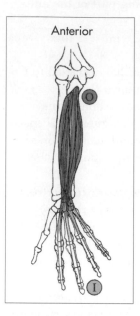

Anterior

Flexor digitorum profundus (FLEKS-or DIH-jih-TOR-um pro-FUND-us)

Meaning to bend; related to the fingers or toes; deep

Function: Flexes the distal interphalangeal joints of the second through fifth digits; assists in flexion of the proximal interphalangeal and metacarpophalangeal joints; assists in adduction of the index, ring, and little fingers and in flexion of the wrist

Origin: Medial and anterior surfaces of the proximal three fourths of the ulna; interosseous membrane; deep antebrachial fascia

Insertion: By four tendons into the distal phalanges of digits two through four on the anterior surface

Innervation:

Medial part—Ulnar nerve

Lateral part—Anterior interosseous branch of the median nerve C7 to C8 and T1

ACTIVITY 9-49

- Draw and color the anterior flexor group in the space provided.
- Label the origin and insertion points: *O*, for the origin, *I*, for the insertion.
- Place an **X** on the trigger points.
- Palpate these muscles; identify the attachment points and the belly of the muscle.
- Move these muscles on yourself.

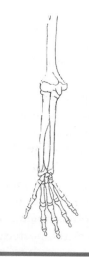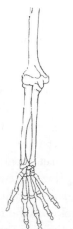

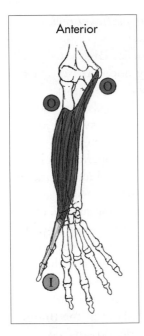

Flexor pollicis longus

(FLEKS-or POLL-ik-iss LONG-us)

Meaning to bend; of the thumb; long

Function: Flexes interphalangeal joint of the thumb; assists in flexion of the metacarpophalangeal and carpometacarpal joints

Origin: Anterior surface of the radius below the tuberosity; medial border of the coronoid process of the ulna; interosseous membrane

Insertion: Palmar surface of the base of the distal phalanx of the thumb

Innervation: Anterior interosseous branch of the median nerve C8 to T1

Elements common to the anterior flexor group muscles

Synergists: All flexors are synergistic with one another

Antagonists: Primary antagonist is the extensor carpi radialis, along with the entire extensor group

Trigger points: In the belly of each muscle

Referred pain pattern: Into the wrist and fingers

See Activity 9-49

Posterior Extensor Group, Superficial Layer

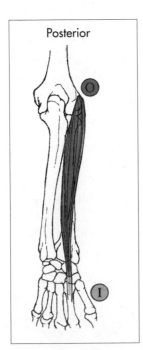

Extensor carpi radialis longus

(ex-STEN-sur KAR-pee RAY-dee-al-iss LONG-us)

Meaning one that stretches; related to the thumb; long

Function: Extends and abducts the wrist; may assist in flexion of the elbow

Origin: Distal one third of the lateral supracondylar ridge of the humerus; lateral intermuscular septum

Insertion: Dorsal surface of the base of the second metacarpal bone on the radial side

Innervation: Radial nerve C6 to C7

Extensor carpi radialis brevis

(ex-STEN-sur KAR-pee RAY-dee-al-iss BREV-us)

Meaning one that stretches; of the wrist; related to the radius; short

Function: Extends the wrist and assists in abduction of wrist

Origin: Common extensor tendon from the lateral epicondyle of the humerus; radial collateral ligament of the elbow joint; deep antebrachial fascia

Insertion: Dorsal surface of the base of the third metacarpal bone

Innervation: Posterior interosseous branch of the radial nerve C6 to C7

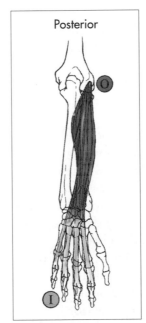

Extensor digitorum

(ex-STEN-sur DIH-jih-TOR-um)

Meaning one that stretches; of the fingers or toes

Function: Extends the metacarpophalangeal joints; extends the interphalangeal joint of the second through fifth digits (in conjunction with the lumbricales and interossei); assists in extension of the wrist

Origin: Common extensor tendon from the lateral epicondyle of the humerus; intermuscular septa

Insertion: By four tendons to the lateral and dorsal surface of the phalanges of the second through fifth digits

Innervation: Posterior interosseous branch of the radial nerve C6 to C8

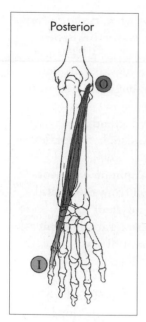

Posterior

Extensor digiti minimi

(ex-STEN-sur   DIH-jih-tee MIN-ih-mee)

Meaning one that stretches; of the fingers or toes; smallest

Function: Extends the metacarpophalangeal and (in conjunction with the interosseous and lumbrical muscles) the interphalangeal joints of the little finger; assists in abduction of the little finger

Origin: Common extensor tendon from the lateral epicondyle of the humerus; intermuscular septa

Insertion: Dorsum of the little finger with the extensor digitorum tendon

Innervation: Posterior interosseous branch of the radial nerve C6 to C8

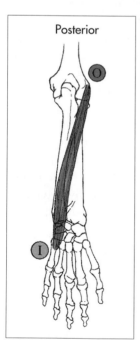

Posterior

Extensor carpi ulnaris

(ex-STEN-sur KAR-pee ul-NAR-iss)

Meaning one that stretches; of the wrist; related to the ulna

Function: Extends and abducts the wrist

Origin: Common extensor from the lateral epicondyle of the humerus; aponeurosis from the posterior border of the ulna

Insertion: Medial side of the base of the fifth metacarpal bone

Innervation: Posterior interosseous branch of the radial nerve C6 to C8

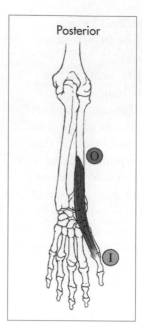

Posterior

Extensor pollicis brevis (ex-STEN-sur POLL-ik-iss BREV-us)

Meaning one that stretches; of the thumb; short

Function: Extends and abducts the carpometacarpal joint of the thumb; extends the metacarpophalangeal joint; assists in abduction (radially) of the wrist

Origin: Posterior surface of the body of the radius distal to the origin of the abductor pollicis longus and the interosseous membrane

Insertion: Base of the proximal phalanx of the thumb on the dorsal surface

Innervation: Posterior interosseous branch of the radial nerve C6 to C8

Posterior Extensor Group, Deep Layer

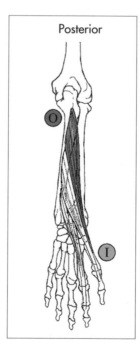

Posterior

Abductor pollicis longus

(ab-DUCK-tur   POLL-ik-iss LONG-us)

Meaning one that leads away; of the thumb; long

Function: Abducts and extends the carpometacarpal joint of the thumb; abducts (radially) and assists in wrist flexion

Origin: Posterior surface of the body of the ulna distal to the origin of the supinator; interosseous membrane; posterior surface of the middle one third of the body of the radius

Insertion: Base of the first metacarpal bone on the radial side

Innervation: Posterior interosseous branch of the radial nerve C6 to C8

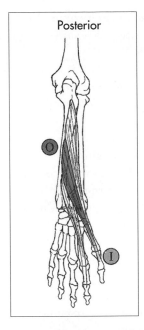

Posterior

Extensor pollicis longus (ex-STEN-sur POLL-ik-iss LONG-us)
Meaning one that stretches; of the thumb; long
Function: Extends the interphalangeal joint and assists in extension of the metacarpophalangeal and carpometacarpal joints of the thumb; assists in abduction and extension of the wrist
Origin: Middle one third of the posterior surface of the ulna distal to the origin of the abductor pollicis longus and the interosseous membrane
Insertion: Dorsal surface of the base of the distal phalanx of the thumb
Innervation: Posterior interosseous branch of the radial nerve C6 to C8

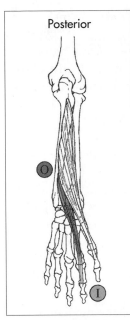

Posterior

Extensor indicis (ex-STEN-sur IN-dih-kiss)
Meaning one that stretches; of the index finger
Function: Extends the metacarpophalangeal joint and, in conjunction with the lumbrical and interosseous muscles, extends the interphalangeal joints of the index finger; may assist in adduction of the index finger
Origin: Posterior surface of the ulna and the interosseous membrane
Insertion: Into extensor expansion of index finger with extensor digitorum longus tendon
Innervation: Posterior interosseous branch of the radial nerve C6 to C8

Elements common to the posterior extensor group muscles

Synergists: For extension, all extensors are synergistic with each other; for radial deviation of the hand, the extensor carpi radialis muscles are synergistic with the flexor carpi radialis; for ulnar deviation, the extensor and flexor carpi ulnaris muscles are synergistic
Antagonists: The flexor group; the ulnar deviation and radial deviation groups are antagonistic to each other
Trigger points: Belly of each muscle, located nearer the elbow
Referred pain pattern: From the lateral epicondyle at the elbow down the dorsum of the forearm to various parts of the hand, especially to the web of the thumb

See Activity 9-50

INTRINSIC MUSCLES OF THE HAND

The small muscles found in the hand are called *intrinsic muscles*. The complex and intricate nature of these muscles allows for an almost limitless variety of fine hand movements. The delicacy of the muscles and the interactive pattern of their layout are unique to the human hand.

ACTIVITY 9-50

- Draw and color the muscles of the superficial layer and those of the deep layer of the posterior extensor group in the space provided.
- Label the origin and insertion points: *O,* for the origin, *I,* for the insertion.
- Place an **X** on the trigger points.
- Palpate these muscles; identify the attachment points and the belly of the muscle.
- Move these muscles on yourself.

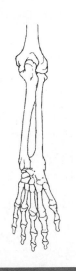
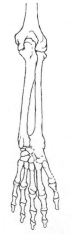

Thenar Eminence Muscles (THEE-nar)

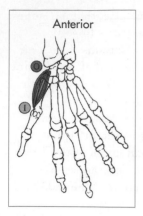

Anterior

Opponens pollicis
(oh-PONE-ens POLL-ik-iss)
Meaning opposing; of the thumb
Function: Adducts the carpometacarpal joint of the thumb; adducts and assists in flexion of the metacarpophalangeal joint; aids in opposition of the thumb to each of the other digits
Origin: Transverse carpal ligament; trapezium bone

Insertion: Anterior surface on the radial side of the first metacarpal bone
Innervation: Muscular branches of the median nerve

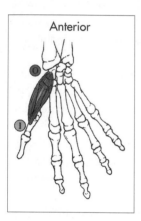

Anterior

Abductor pollicis brevis
(ab-DUCK-tur POLL-ik-iss BREV-us)
Meaning one that leads away; of the thumb; short
Function: Abducts and aids in opposition of the thumb
Origin: Flexor retinaculum; tubercle of the trapezium bone; tubercle of the scaphoid bone

Insertion: Radial side of the base of the proximal phalanx of the thumb; extensor expansion
Innervation: Median nerve C8 to T1

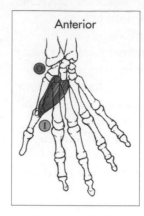

Anterior

Flexor pollicis brevis
(FLEKS-or POLL-ik-iss BREV-us)
Meaning one that bends; of the thumb; short
Function: Flexes the proximal phalanx of the thumb; assists in opposition of the thumb
Origin:
    Superficial head—Flexor retinaculum; trapezium bone
Deep head—Trapezoid and capitate bones
Insertion: Radial side of the base of the proximal phalanx of the thumb; extensor expansion
Innervation:
    Superficial head—Median nerve
    Deep head—Deep branch of the ulnar nerve C8 to T1

Elements common to the thenar eminence muscles

Synergists: The opponens pollicis, abductor pollicis brevis, and flexor pollicis brevis are synergistic
Antagonists: Abductors and extensors of the thumb
Trigger points: In the belly of the muscles
Referred pain pattern: Into the thumb and the wrist

See Activity 9-51

ACTIVITY 9-51

- Draw and color the thenar muscles (the opponens pollicis, the abductor pollicis brevis, and the flexor pollicis brevis) in the space provided.
- Label the origin and insertion points: *O,* for the origin, *I,* for the insertion.
- Place an **X** on the trigger points.

- Palpate these muscles; identify the attachment points and the belly of the muscle.
- Move these muscles on yourself.

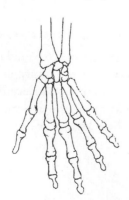

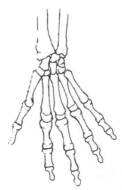

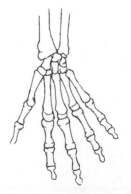

Hypothenar Muscles

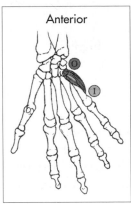

Anterior

Opponens digiti minimi
(oh-PONE-ens DIH-jih-tee MIN-ih-mee)

Meaning opposing; of the fingers or toes; smallest

Function: Flexion and slight rotation of the carpometacarpal joint of the little finger; helps to cup the palm of the hand

Origin: Transverse carpal ligament and the hamate bone

Insertion: Entire length of the fifth metacarpal bone on the ulnar side

Innervation: Deep volar branch of the ulnar nerve C8 to T1

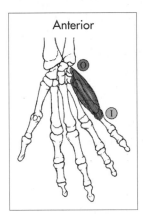

Anterior

Abductor digiti minimi
(ab-DUCK-tur DIH-jih-tee MIN-ih-mee)

Meaning one that leads away; of the fingers or toes; smallest

Function: Abducts and assists in flexion of the metacarpophalangeal joint of the little finger

Origin: Tendon of the flexor carpi ulnaris and the pisiform bone

Insertion: Base of the proximal phalanx of the little finger on the ulnar side; aponeurosis of the extensor digiti minimi

Innervation: Deep branch of the ulnar nerve C8 to T1

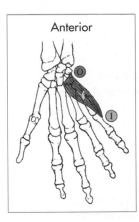

Anterior

Flexor digiti minimi (brevis) (FLEKS-or DIH-jih-tee MIN-ih-mee BREV-us)

Meaning one that bends; of the fingers or toes; short

Function: Flexes the metacarpophalangeal joint of the little finger; assists in opposition of the little finger to the thumb

Origin: Hook of the hamate bone; flexor retinaculum

Insertion: Base of the proximal phalanx of the little finger on the ulnar side

Innervation: Deep branch of the ulnar nerve C8 to T1

Elements common to the hypothenar muscles

Synergists: These muscles are synergistic

Antagonists: Finger extensors

Trigger points: In the belly of the muscles

Referred pain pattern: Into the little finger and wrist

See Activity 9-52

ACTIVITY 9-52

- Draw and color the hypothenar muscles (the opponens digiti minimi, the abductor digiti minimi, and the flexor digiti minimi [brevis]) in the space provided.
- Label the origin and insertion points: *O,* for the origin, *I,* for the insertion.
- Place an **X** on the trigger points.
- Palpate these muscles; identify the attachment points and the belly of the muscle.
- Move these muscles on yourself.

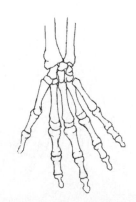

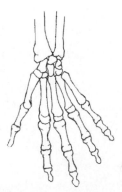

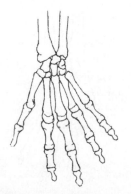

Deep Muscles of the Hand

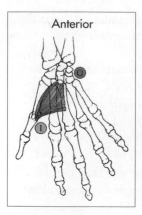

Anterior

Adductor pollicis (ab-
DUCK-tur POLL-ik-iss)
Meaning one that leads
away; of the thumb
Function: Adducts the thumb
and aids in opposition
Origin:
Oblique head—Trapezium,
trapezoid, and capitate
bones and the base of
the second and third
metacarpal bones
Transverse head—Palmar surface of the third
metacarpal
Insertion: Ulnar side of the base of the proximal phalanx of the thumb
Innervation: Deep branch of the ulnar nerve C8 to T1

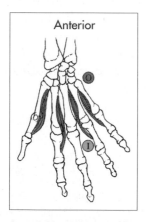

Anterior

Palmar interosseus (pol-
MARE INT-er-OSS-ee-us)
Meaning of the palm and
among the bones
Function: Adducts the index,
ring, and little fingers
toward the middle digit
Origin:
First—Ulnar side of the
first metacarpal bone
Second—Ulnar side of the
second metacarpal bone

Third—Radial side of the fourth metacarpal bone
Fourth—Radial side of the fifth metacarpal bone
Insertion:
First—Ulnar side of the thumb
Second—Ulnar side of the index finger
Third—Radial side of the ring finger
Fourth—Radial side of the little finger
Innervation: Deep branch of the ulnar nerve C8 to T1

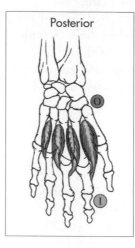

Posterior

Dorsal interosseus (dor-SAL
INT-er-OSS-ee-us)
Meaning related to the back
and between or among the
bones
Function: Abducts the index,
middle, and ring fingers
from the midline of the
hand
Origin:
First (lateral head)—
Proximal one half of the
ulnar border of the first
metacarpal bone
First (medial head)—Radial border of the second
metacarpal bone
Second, third, and fourth—Adjacent sides of the
metacarpal bones in each interspace
Insertion:
First—Radial side of the proximal phalanx of the
second digit
Second—Radial side of the proximal phalanx of
the third digit

ACTIVITY 9-53

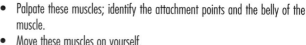

- Draw and color the deep muscles of the hand in the space provided.
- Label the origin and insertion points: *O,* for the origin, *I,* for the insertion.
- Place an **X** on the trigger points.

- Palpate these muscles; identify the attachment points and the belly of the muscle.
- Move these muscles on yourself.

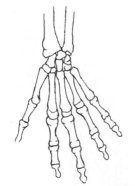
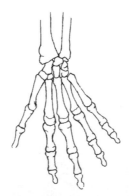
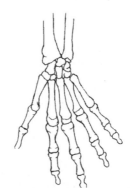
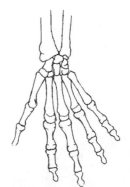

Third—Ulnar side of the proximal phalanx of the third digit

Fourth—Ulnar side of the proximal phalanx of the fourth digit

Innervation: Deep branch of the ulnar nerve C8 to T1

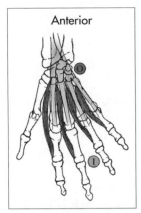

Lumbricales
(LUM-brih-kals)

Meaning earthworm

Function: Extend the interphalangeal joints and simultaneously flex the metacarpophalangeal joint of the second through fifth digits

Origin:

First and second—Radial surface of the flexor profundus tendons of the index and middle fingers, respectively

Third—Adjacent sides of the flexor profundus tendons of the middle and ring fingers

Fourth—Adjacent sides of the flexor profundus tendons of the ring and little fingers

Insertion: Into the radial border of the extensor expansion on the dorsal aspect of the digits

Innervation:

First and second—Median nerve

Third and fourth—Deep ulnar nerve C8 to T1

Elements common to the deep muscles of the hand

Synergists: Dorsal and palmar interossei are synergistic for flexion at the metacarpophalangeal joint and extension of the two most distal phalanges; the interossei and the lumbricales are synergistic

Antagonists: Dorsal and palmar interossei are antagonists for adduction, abduction, and rotation

Trigger points: In the belly of the muscles

Referred pain pattern: Into the associated finger; commonly associated with Heberden's nodes, which develop on the dorsolateral or dorsomedial aspect of the terminal phalanx at its joint

See Activity 9-53

MUSCLES OF THE GLUTEAL REGION

The muscles of the gluteal region are some of the most powerful muscles of the body. The more superficial muscles, especially the large gluteus maximus, extend the thigh during forceful extension. The gluteus medius and minimus abduct and rotate the thigh medially. The deep lateral rotators are six small, deep muscles of the gluteal region that oppose medial rotation.

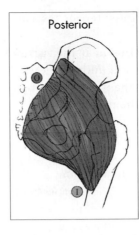

Gluteus maximus
(GLUE-tee-us MAX-uh-mus)

Meaning buttocks; greatest or largest

Function: Extends and laterally rotates the hip joint; lower fibers assist in adduction of the hip joint; with femur fixed, assists in extension of the trunk; these muscles are important postural muscles that help maintain the upright posture; the gluteus maximus is active primarily during strenuous activity, such as running, jumping, and climbing stairs

Origin: Posterior gluteal line of the ilium; dorsal surface of the lower aspect of the sacrum and the side of the coccyx; sacrotuberous ligament and gluteal aponeurosis; aponeurosis of the erector spinae

Insertion: Iliotibial tract of the fascia lata; gluteal tuberosity of the femur

Innervation: Inferior gluteal nerve L5 to S1 and S2

Synergists: Longissimus, iliocostalis, hamstrings as extensors of the trunk; piriformis in lateral rotation of the thigh; tensor fasciae latae for abduction

ACTIVITY 9-54

- Draw and color the gluteus maximus in the space provided.
- Label the origin and insertion points: *O,* for the origin, *I,* for the insertion.
- Place an **X** on the trigger points.
- Palpate this muscle; identify the attachment points and the belly of the muscle.
- Move this muscle on yourself.

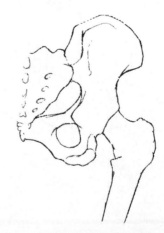

Antagonists: Iliopsoas; rectus femoris; tensor fasciae latae for lateral rotation

Trigger points: Three main areas: one near the sacrum at the musculotendinous junction midway down from the iliac crest; two near the ischial tuberosity; and three in the belly of the muscle nearer the lower fibers

Referred pain pattern: Regionally into the gluteal region, especially to the ischial tuberosity, the tip of the greater trochanter, and the sacrum

See Activity 9-54

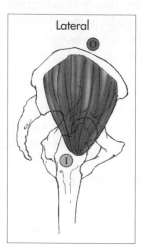

Lateral

Gluteus medius
(GLUE-tee-us MEED-ee-us)
Meaning buttocks; middle

Function: Abducts the hip joint; anterior fibers medially rotate and assist in flexion of the hip joint; posterior fibers laterally rotate and assist in extension of the hip joint; stabilizes the pelvis when a person is standing on one foot

Origin: Outer surface of the ilium between the iliac

ACTIVITY 9-55

- Draw and color the gluteus medius in the space provided.
- Label the origin and insertion points: *O*, for the origin, *I*, for the insertion.
- Place an **X** on the trigger points.
- Palpate this muscle; identify the attachment points and the belly of the muscle.
- Move this muscle on yourself.

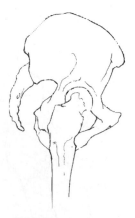

crest, the posterior gluteal line above and the anterior gluteal line below, and the gluteal aponeurosis

Insertion: Lateral surface of the greater trochanter of the femur

Innervation: Superior gluteal nerve L4 to L5 and S1

Synergists: For abduction—Gluteus minimus, tensor fasciae latae, sartorius, piriformis, upper fibers of the gluteus maximus, iliopsoas

Antagonists: The adductors

Trigger points: Along the musculotendinous junction at the iliac crest

Referred pain pattern: Low back, posterior crest of the ilium to the sacrum, and to the posterior and lateral areas of the buttock into the upper thigh

See Activity 9-55

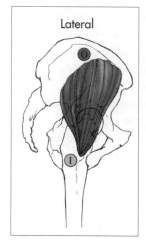

Lateral

Gluteus minimus
(GLUE-tee-us MIN-ih-mus)
Meaning buttocks; smallest

Function: Abducts the hip joint and medially rotates the thigh when the limb is extended; keeps the pelvis level when a person is standing on one foot

Origin: Outer surface of the ilium between the anterior and inferior gluteal lines; margin of the greater sciatic notch

Insertion: Anterior border of the greater trochanter

Innervation: Superior gluteal nerve L4 to L5 and S1

Synergists: Tensor fasciae latae; gluteus medius

Antagonists:

Medial rotation—Gluteus maximus, piriformis, deep lateral hip rotators

Abduction—Adductor muscles

Trigger points: Belly of the muscle

Referred pain pattern: Lower lateral buttock and down the lateral to posterior aspect of the thigh, knee, and leg to the ankle

See Activity 9-56

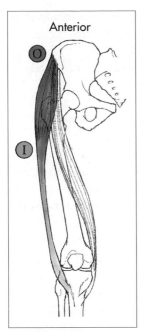

Anterior

Tensor fasciae latae
(TEN-sore FAH-she-eye
LAT-eye)
Meaning one that stretches;
bands or bandages; wide
Function: Flexes, medially
rotates, and may assist in
abduction of the hip joint;
assists in extension of the
knee; tenses the fascia
lata, counterbalancing the
backward pull of the glu-
teus maximus on the ilio-
tibial tract
Origin: Anterior aspect of the
outer lip of the iliac crest;
outer surface of the anteri-
or superior iliac spine
Insertion: Middle and proxi-
mal thirds of the thigh along the iliotibial tract
Innervation: Superior gluteal nerve L4 to L5 and S1
Synergists: Gluteus medius, gluteus minimus
Antagonists: Gluteus maximus, deep lateral hip rotators, adductors

Trigger points: In the belly of the muscle and near the
insertion
Referred pain pattern: Localized in the hip and down
the lateral side of the leg to the knee

See Activity 9-57

Deep Lateral Rotators

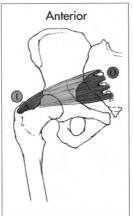

Anterior

Piriformis
(PEER-ih-FOR-miss)
Meaning pear shaped
Function: Lateral rotation and
abduction of the hip joint
when the limb is flexed
Origin: Pelvic surface (inner
surface) of the sacrum
between the first through
fourth sacral foramina;
margin of the greater sciatic
foramen; pelvic surface of
the sacrotuberous ligament
Insertion: Superior border of the greater trochanter
of the femur
Innervation: S1 to S2

ACTIVITY 9-56

- Draw and color the gluteus minimus in the space provided.
- Label the origin and insertion points: *O,* for the origin, *I,* for the insertion.
- Place an **X** on the trigger points.
- Palpate this muscle; identify the attachment points and the belly of the muscle.
- Move this muscle on yourself.

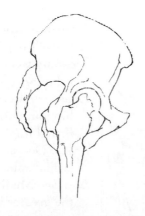

ACTIVITY 9-57

- Draw and color the tensor fasciae latae in the space provided.
- Label the origin and insertion points: *O,* for the origin, *I,* for the insertion.
- Place an **X** on the trigger points.
- Palpate this muscle; identify the attachment points and the belly of the muscle.
- Move this muscle on yourself.

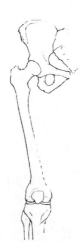

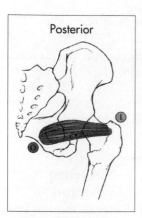

Posterior

Obturator internus
(OB-tur-ATE-or in-TER-nus)
Meaning one that covers an
    opening; interior
Function: Laterally rotates the
    hip joint; extends and
    abducts the hip when the
    limb is flexed
Origin: Pelvic surface of the
    obturator membrane and
    the margins of the obtura-
    tor foramen; internal sur-
face of the pubis; ramus of the ischium; obturator
fascia

ACTIVITY 9-58

- Draw and color the deep lateral rotators in the space provided.
- Label the origin and insertion points: *O,* for the origin, *I,* for the insertion.
- Place an **X** on the trigger points.
- Palpate these muscles; identify the attachment points and the belly of the muscle.
- Move these muscles on yourself.

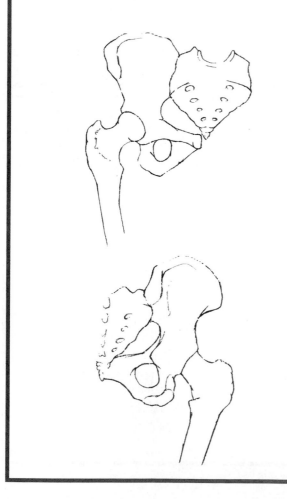

Insertion: Medial surface of the greater trochanter of
    the femur, anterior and superior to the
    trochanteric fossa
Innervation: Nerve to obturator internus L5 to S1
    and S2

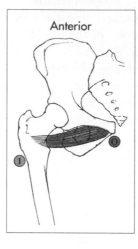

Anterior

Obturator externus
(OB-tur-ATE-or
ex-STIR-nus)
Meaning one that covers an
    opening; exterior
Function: Laterally rotates the
    hip joint
Origin: Medial side of the
    obturator foramen; rami of
    the pubis and ischium;
    external surface of the
    obturator membrane
Insertion: Trochanteric fossa
    of the femur
Innervation: Posterior branch of the obturator nerve
    L3 to L4

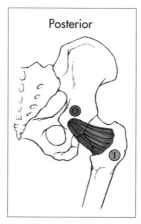

Posterior

Quadratus femoris
(kwad-RATE-us FEM-or-iss)
Meaning square shaped;
    related to the thigh
Function: Laterally rotates the
    hip joint and adducts the
    thigh
Origin: Upper part of the lat-
    eral border of the ischial
    tuberosity
Insertion: Small tubercle on the
    upper part of the trochan-
    teric crest of the femur
Innervation: Nerve to quadratus femoris L4 to L5
    and S1

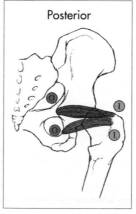

Posterior

Gemellus superior
(JEM-ell-us)
Meaning twin; superior
    meaning above
Function: Laterally rotates the
    hip joint; abducts the
    flexed thigh
Origin: Dorsal surface of the
    ischial spine
Insertion: Medial surface of
    the greater trochanter of

the femur, blending with the tendon of the obturator internus

Innervation: Nerve to obturator internus L4 to S1 and S2

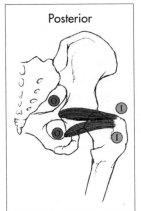

Posterior

Gemellus inferior
(JEM-ell-us)
Meaning twin; inferior meaning below

Function: Laterally rotates the hip joint; abducts the flexed thigh

Origin: Upper part of the ischial tuberosity

Insertion: Medial surface of the greater trochanter

Innervation: Nerve to the quadratus femoris and gemellus inferior

Elements common to the deep lateral rotator muscles

Synergists: All deep lateral hip rotators are synergistic with one another; other synergists are the gluteus maximus, long head of the biceps femoris, sartorius, posterior fibers of the gluteus medius and minimus

Antagonists: Semitendinosus, semimembranosus, tensor fasciae latae, posterior and anterior fibers of the gluteus medius and minimus

Trigger points: The main trigger points are in the piriformis muscle near the origin and the insertion; tension in this muscle may cause entrapment of the sciatic nerve, which normally passes under the piriformis but in some individuals passes through the muscles, predisposing the person to nerve entrapment

Referred pain pattern: Sacroiliac region, entire buttock and down the posterior thigh to just above the knee

See Activity 9-58

MUSCLES OF THE POSTERIOR THIGH

Hamstring Group
The hamstring muscle group crosses two joints, the hip and the knee. These muscles extend the thigh and flex the knee. The muscles of the massive hamstring group are the main extensors of the thigh.

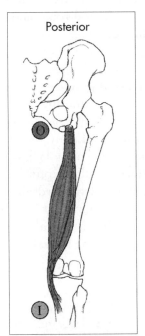

Posterior

Semimembranosus
(SEM-ee-MEM-bran-oh-sus)
Meaning half membrane

Function: Flexes the knee and medially rotates the knee joint when the knee is semiflexed; extends and assists in medial rotation of the hip joint

Origin: Upper lateral aspect of the ischial tuberosity

Insertion: Posteromedial aspect of the medial condyle of the tibia

Innervation: Tibial portion of the sciatic nerve L4 to L5, S1, and S2

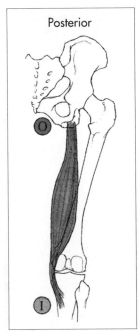

Posterior

Semitendinosus
(SEM-ee-TEN-din-oh-sus)
Meaning half tendon

Function: Flexes the knee and medially rotates the knee joint when the knee is semiflexed; extends and assists in medial rotation of the hip joint

Origin: Distal part of the medial aspect of the ischial tuberosity

Insertion: Proximal part of the medial surface of the body of the femur; deep fascia of the leg

Innervation: Tibial portion of the sciatic nerve L4 to L5, S1, and S2

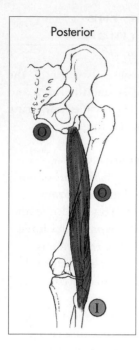

Posterior

Biceps femoris

(BI-seps FEM-or-iss)

Meaning two headed; related to the thigh

Function: Flexes and laterally rotates the knee joint when the knee is semiflexed; long head also extends and assists in lateral rotation of the hip joint

Origin:

Long head—Posterior part of the ischial tuberosity and the sacrotuberous ligament

Short head—Lateral lip of the linea aspera; lateral intermuscular septum; proximal two thirds of the supracondylar line

Insertion: Lateral side of the fibular head; lateral condyle of the tibia; deep fascia on the lateral aspect of the leg

Innervation:

Long head—Tibial division of the sciatic nerve

Short head—Peroneal division of the sciatic nerve L5 to S1 and S2

Elements common to the hamstring group of muscles

Synergists: Hip extension is assisted by the gluteus maximus, posterior adductor magnus, and posterior portions of the gluteus medius and minimus; knee flexion is assisted by the sartorius, gracilis, gastrocnemius, and plantaris; medial rotation is assisted by the popliteus, sartorius, and gracilis

Antagonists: Hip extension is opposed by the iliopsoas, tensor fasciae latae, rectus femoris, sartorius, and pectineus; knee flexion is opposed by the quadriceps femoris muscle group

Trigger points: Several areas in the belly of each of the muscles and at the musculotendinous junction nearer the knee

Referred pain pattern: Ischial tuberosity, back of the knee, and the entire posterior leg to midcalf

See Activity 9-59

ACTIVITY 9-59

- Draw and color the muscles of the hamstring group (the semimembranosus, the semitendinosus, and the biceps femoris) in the space provided.
- Label the origin and insertion points: *O*, for the origin, *I*, for the insertion.
- Place an X on the trigger points.
- Palpate these muscles; identify the attachment points and the belly of the muscle.
- Move these muscles on yourself.

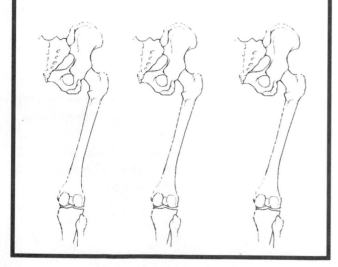

MUSCLES OF THE MEDIAL THIGH

The medial thigh muscles, called the *adductor group,* adduct the thigh. Abduction and adduction of the thighs keeps the body's weight balanced over the weight-bearing leg when a person is walking.

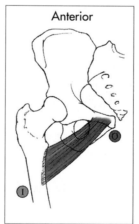

Anterior

Pectineus (PEK-tih-NEE-us)

Meaning related to the pubic bone

Function: Adducts, flexes, and assists in medial rotation of the hip joint

Origin: Surface of the superior ramus of the pubis among the iliopectineal eminence and pubic tubercle and the pectineal line

Insertion: Line extending from the lesser trochanter to the linea aspera

Innervation: Femoral nerve L2 to L3 and L4

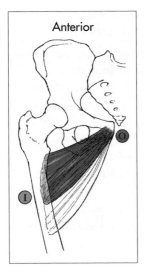

Adductor brevis
(ad-DUCK-tur BREV-us)
Meaning to lead toward; short

Function: Adducts and assists in flexing the hip joint

Origin: Outer surface of the inferior ramus of the pubis between the gracilis and the obturator externus

Insertion: Line extending from the lesser trochanter to the linea aspera

Innervation: Obturator nerve L2 to L3 and L4

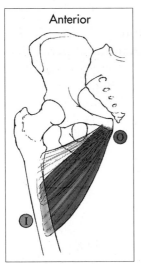

Adductor longus
(ad-DUCK-tur LONG-us)
Meaning to lead toward; long

Function: Adducts and assists in flexing the hip joint

Origin: Anterior pubis between crest and symphysis

Insertion: Middle one half of the medial lip of the linea aspera

Innervation: Obturator nerve L2 to L3 and L4

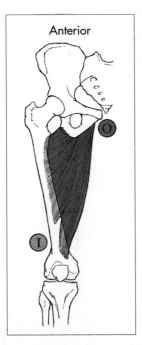

Adductor magnus
(ad-DUCK-tur MAG-nus)
Meaning to lead toward; great

Function: Adducts the hip joint; upper portion medially rotates and flexes while the lower portion laterally rotates and extends the hip joint

Origin: Inferior ramus of the pubis and the ramus of the ischium (anterior fibers); posterior fibers of the ischial tuberosity

Insertion: Line extending from the greater trochanter to the linea aspera; linea aspera; medial supracondylar line; adductor tubercle of the femur

Innervation: Obturator and tibial division of sciatic nerves L3 to L4 and L5

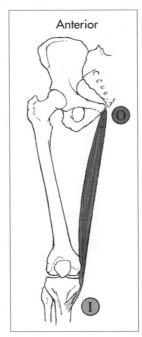

Gracilis (GRASS-ill-iss)
Meaning slender

Function: Adducts and flexes the hip joint; flexes and medially rotates the knee joint when the knee is semiflexed; assists in controlling the valgus angulation of the knee

Origin: Inferior one half of the symphysis pubis; inferior ramus of the pubic bone

Insertion: Upper surface of the medial body of the tibia distal to the condyle

Innervation: Obturator nerve L2 to L3

Elements common to the medial thigh muscles

Synergists: All muscles of the medial thigh are synergistic with one another for adduction

Antagonists: Gluteus medius and minimus; tensor fasciae latae

Trigger points: Various locations in the belly of each muscle and near the ischial tuberosity attachment

Referred pain pattern: Deep in the groin into the medial thigh and downward to the knee and shin

See Activity 9-60

ACTIVITY 9-60

- Draw and color the muscles of the medial thigh (the pectineus, the adductor brevis, the adductor longus, the adductor magnus, and the gracilis) in the space provided.
- Label the origin and insertion points: *O*, for the origin, *I*, for the insertion.
- Place an **X** on the trigger points.
- Palpate these muscles; identify the attachment points and the belly of the muscle.
- Move these muscles on yourself.

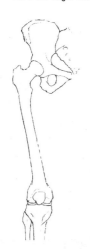

MUSCLES OF THE ANTERIOR THIGH

The main extensors of the knee joint are the quadriceps muscles. The quadriceps and hamstring muscle groups obviously are antagonistic to each other, yet together they ensure the stability of the knee joint. The sartorius and rectus femoris are also hip flexors.

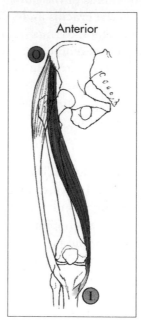

Sartorius (sar-TOR-ee-us) Meaning tailor, or to sit cross-legged

Function: Flexes, laterally rotates, and abducts the hip joint; also flexes the torso toward the thigh when the leg is fixed; flexes and assists in medial rotation of the knee joint

Origin: Anterior superior iliac spine and upper half of the iliac notch

Insertion: Proximal part of the medial aspect of the body of the tibia

Innervation: Femoral nerve L2 to L3

Quadriceps Femoris Group
(KWAD-rih-seps FEM-or-iss)
Meaning four headed; related to the thigh

ACTIVITY 9-61

- Draw and color the muscles of the anterior thigh (the sartorius, the rectus femoris, the vastus lateralis, the vastus medialis, and the vastus intermedius) in the space provided.
- Label the origin and insertion points: *O*, for the origin, *I*, for the insertion.

- Place an **X** on the trigger points.
- Palpate these muscles; identify the attachment points and the belly of the muscle.
- Move these muscles on yourself.

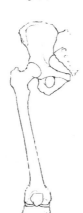
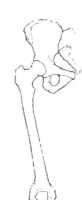
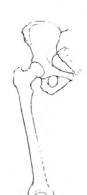

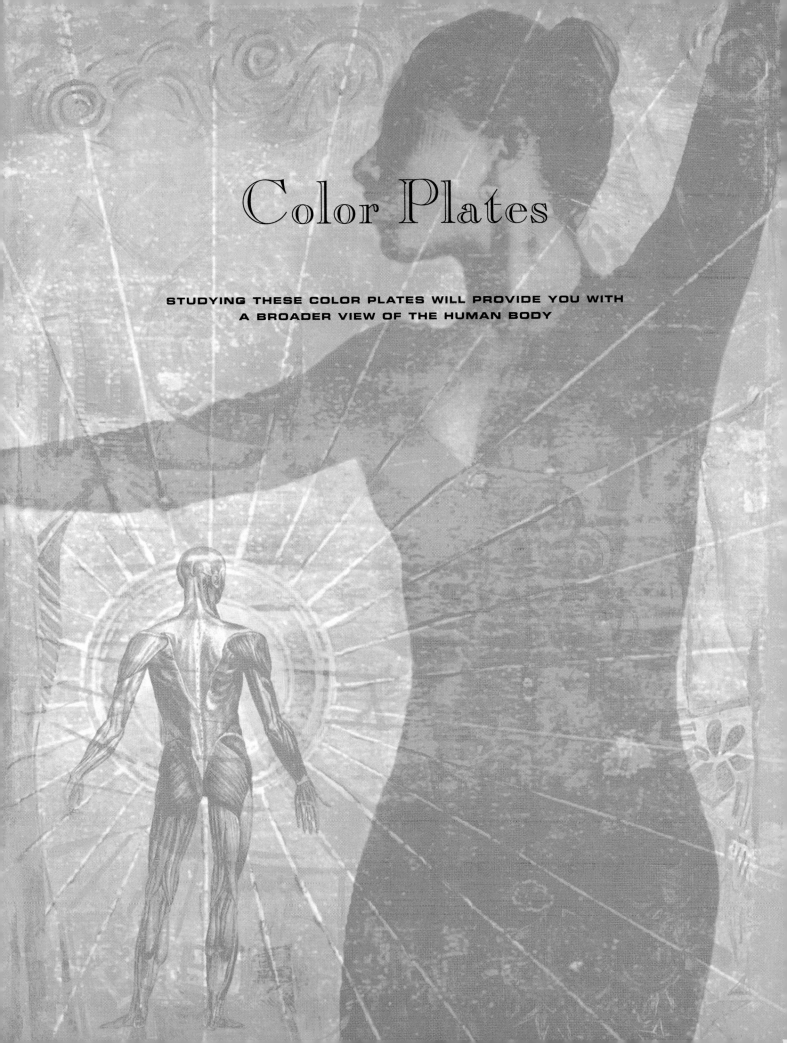

Color Plates

STUDYING THESE COLOR PLATES WILL PROVIDE YOU WITH
A BROADER VIEW OF THE HUMAN BODY

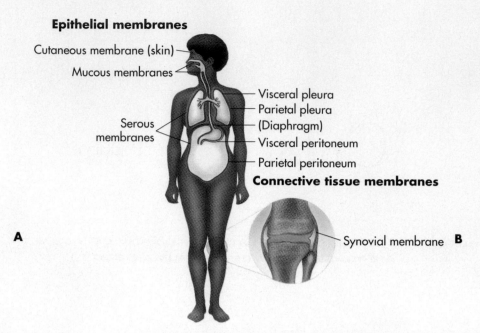

Epithelial membranes

Cutaneous membrane (skin)

Mucous membranes

Visceral pleura
Parietal pleura
(Diaphragm)
Visceral peritoneum
Parietal peritoneum

Serous membranes

Connective tissue membranes

Synovial membrane

A

B

PLATE 1 **Types of body membranes. A,** Epithelial membranes, including cutaneous membrane (skin), serious membranes (parietal and visceral pleura and peritoneum), and mucous membranes. **B,** Connective tissue membranes, including synovial membranes. (From Thibodeau GA, Patton KT: *The human body in health and disease,* ed 2, St Louis, 1997, Mosby.)

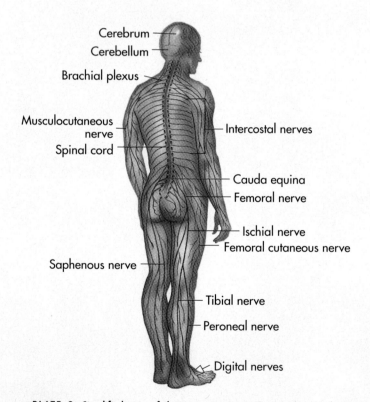

Cerebrum
Cerebellum
Brachial plexus

Musculocutaneous nerve
Spinal cord

Intercostal nerves

Cauda equina
Femoral nerve

Ischial nerve
Femoral cutaneous nerve

Saphenous nerve

Tibial nerve
Peroneal nerve

Digital nerves

PLATE 2 **Simplified view of the nervous system.** (From LaFleur Brooks M: *Exploring medical language: a student-directed approach,* ed 3, St Louis, 1994, Mosby.)

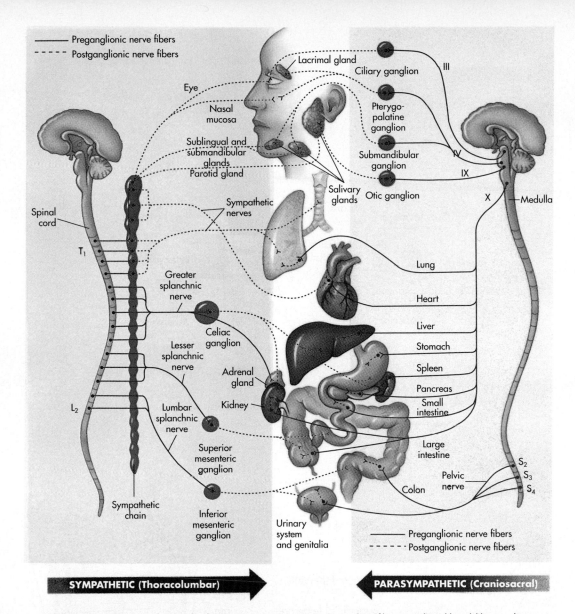

Preganglionic nerve fibers
Postganglionic nerve fibers

Lacrimal gland
Ciliary ganglion
III
Eye
Nasal mucosa
Pterygopalatine ganglion
Sublingual and submandibular glands
Parotid gland
Submandibular ganglion
IV
Salivary glands
Otic ganglion
IX
Sympathetic nerves
X
Medulla

Spinal cord
T₁

Greater splanchnic nerve
Celiac ganglion
Lesser splanchnic nerve
Adrenal gland
Kidney
Lumbar splanchnic nerve
L₂
Superior mesenteric ganglion
Sympathetic chain
Inferior mesenteric ganglion
Urinary system and genitalia

Lung
Heart
Liver
Stomach
Spleen
Pancreas
Small intestine
Large intestine
Colon
Pelvic nerve
S₂
S₃
S₄

Preganglionic nerve fibers
Postganglionic nerve fibers

SYMPATHETIC (Thoracolumbar)　　　**PARASYMPATHETIC (Craniosacral)**

PLATE 3 **Innervation of organs by the autonomic nervous system.** Preganglionic fibers are indicated by solid lines, and postganglionic fibers are indicated by broken lines. (From Seeley RR, Stephens TD, Tate P: *Anatomy and physiology*, St Louis, 1995, Mosby.)

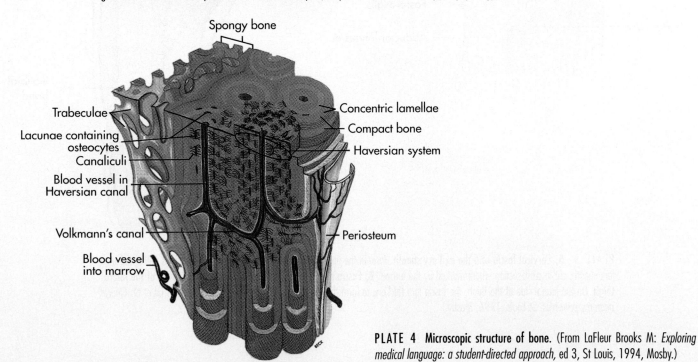

Spongy bone

Trabeculae
Lacunae containing osteocytes
Canaliculi
Blood vessel in Haversian canal
Volkmann's canal
Blood vessel into marrow

Concentric lamellae
Compact bone
Haversian system
Periosteum

PLATE 4 **Microscopic structure of bone.** (From LaFleur Brooks M: *Exploring medical language: a student-directed approach*, ed 3, St Louis, 1994, Mosby.)

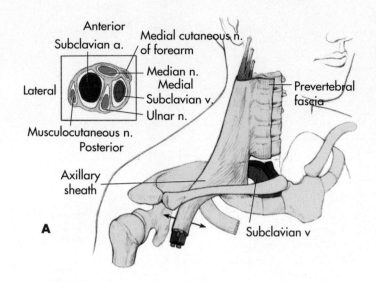

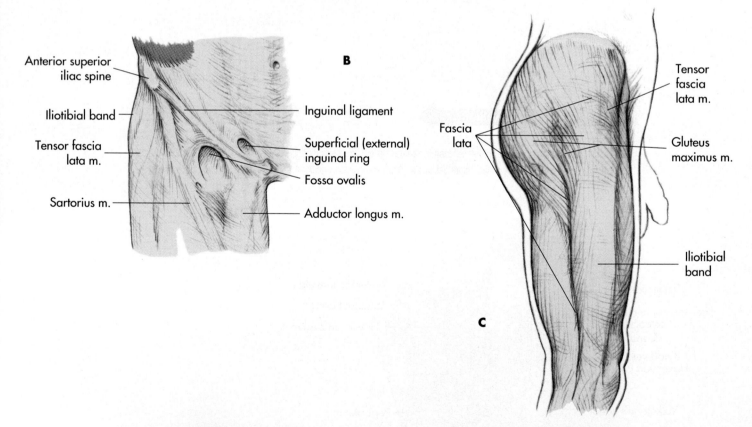

PLATE 5 **A, Cervical fascia and the axillary sheath.** *Inset* in the upper left shows the relationships of structures within the axillary sheath, cut in cross-section where marked by the arrows. **B, Fascia of the upper anterior thigh. C, Deep fascia of the lateral thigh.** On the lateral side of the thigh, the fascia lata thickens to form the elongated iliotibial band. (From Mathers LH et al: *Clinical anatomy principles,* St Louis, 1996, Mosby.)

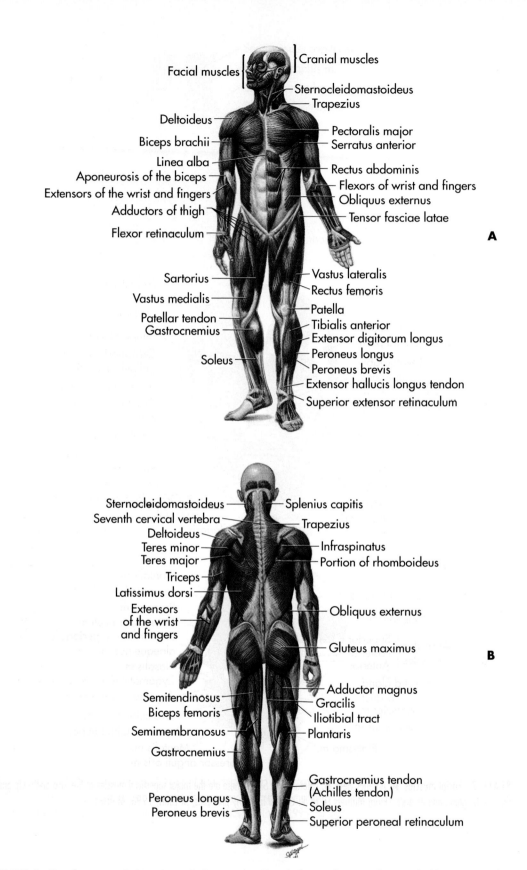

Facial muscles
Cranial muscles
Sternocleidomastoideus
Trapezius
Deltoideus
Biceps brachii
Pectoralis major
Serratus anterior
Linea alba
Aponeurosis of the biceps
Rectus abdominis
Extensors of the wrist and fingers
Flexors of wrist and fingers
Adductors of thigh
Obliquus externus
Flexor retinaculum
Tensor fasciae latae

Sartorius
Vastus lateralis
Rectus femoris
Vastus medialis
Patellar tendon
Patella
Gastrocnemius
Tibialis anterior
Extensor digitorum longus
Peroneus longus
Peroneus brevis
Soleus
Extensor hallucis longus tendon
Superior extensor retinaculum

A

Sternocleidomastoideus
Splenius capitis
Seventh cervical vertebra
Trapezius
Deltoideus
Teres minor
Infraspinatus
Teres major
Portion of rhomboideus
Triceps
Latissimus dorsi
Extensors of the wrist and fingers
Obliquus externus

Gluteus maximus

B

Semitendinosus
Adductor magnus
Biceps femoris
Gracilis
Iliotibial tract
Semimembranosus
Plantaris
Gastrocnemius

Gastrocnemius tendon (Achilles tendon)
Peroneus longus
Soleus
Peroneus brevis
Superior peroneal retinaculum

PLATE 6 Muscular system. A, Anterior view. **B,** Posterior view. (From LaFleur Brooks, M: *Exploring medical language: a student-directed approach,* ed 3, St Louis, 1994, Mosby.)

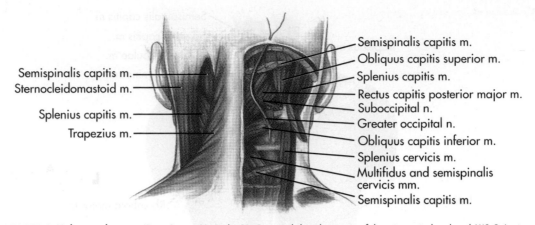

Semispinalis capitis m.
Sternocleidomastoid m.
Splenius capitis m.
Trapezius m.

Semispinalis capitis m.
Obliquus capitis superior m.
Splenius capitis m.
Rectus capitis posterior major m.
Suboccipital n.
Greater occipital n.
Obliquus capitis inferior m.
Splenius cervicis m.
Multifidus and semispinalis cervicis mm.
Semispinalis capitis m.

PLATE 9 **Suboccipital region.** (From Cramer GD, Darby SA: *Basic and clinical anatomy of the spine, spinal cord, and ANS,* St Louis, 1995, Mosby.)

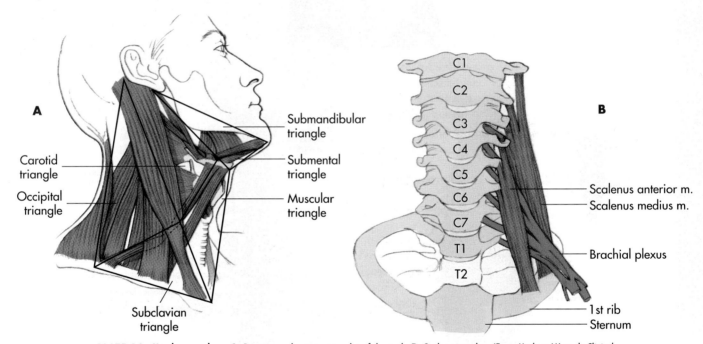

A

Carotid triangle
Occipital triangle
Subclavian triangle

Submandibular triangle
Submental triangle
Muscular triangle

B

C1
C2
C3
C4
C5
C6
C7
T1
T2

Scalenus anterior m.
Scalenus medius m.
Brachial plexus
1st rib
Sternum

PLATE 10 **Neck muscles. A,** Posterior and anterior triangles of the neck. **B,** Scalene muscles. (From Mathers LH et al: *Clinical anatomy principles,* St Louis, 1996, Mosby.)

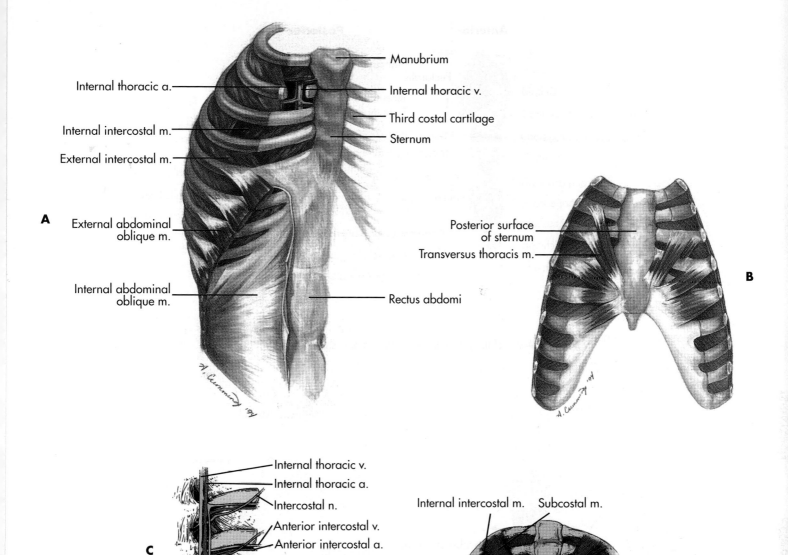

A

Manubrium

Internal thoracic a.

Internal thoracic v.

Third costal cartilage

Internal intercostal m.

Sternum

External intercostal m.

External abdominal oblique m.

Posterior surface of sternum

Transversus thoracis m.

B

Internal abdominal oblique m.

Rectus abdomi

Internal thoracic v.

Internal thoracic a.

Intercostal n.

Anterior intercostal v.

Anterior intercostal a.

Internal intercostal m.   Subcostal m.

C

D

PLATE 11 Thoracic structures. A, Anterolateral view of the thoracic and abdominal walls. *Upper aspect,* Cutaway view of the medial intercostal spaces demonstrating the internal thoracic artery and vein. The external intercostal muscle has been reflected between two ribs to show the internal intercostal muscle to best advantage. The external abdominal oblique muscle has also been reflected and cut away to reveal the internal abdominal oblique muscle. **B,** Internal view of the anterior thoracic wall showing the transversus thoracis muscle. **C,** Detail of *B* showing several intercostal spaces just lateral to the sternum. **D,** Internal view of the posterior thoracici wall showing several subcostal muscles. (From Cramer GD, SA: *Basic and clinical anatomy of the spine, spinal cord, and ANS,* St Louis, 1995, Mosby.)

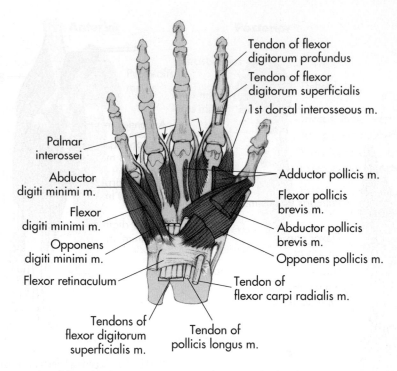

Tendon of flexor digitorum profundus

Tendon of flexor digitorum superficialis

1st dorsal interosseous m.

Palmar interossei

Abductor digiti minimi m.

Flexor digiti minimi m.

Opponens digiti minimi m.

Flexor retinaculum

Adductor pollicis m.

Flexor pollicis brevis m.

Abductor pollicis brevis m.

Opponens pollicis m.

Tendon of flexor carpi radialis m.

Tendons of flexor digitorum superficialis m.

Tendon of pollicis longus m.

PLATE 17 **Deeper muscles of the palm. Anterior view.** (From Mathers LH et al: *Clinical anatomy principles,* St Louis, 1996, Mosby.)

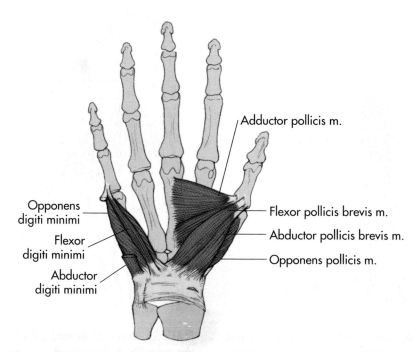

Adductor pollicis m.

Opponens digiti minimi

Flexor digiti minimi

Abductor digiti minimi

Flexor pollicis brevis m.

Abductor pollicis brevis m.

Opponens pollicis m.

PLATE 18 **Thenar and hypothenar muscles.** (From Mathers LH et al: *Clinical anatomy principles,* St Louis, 1996, Mosby.)

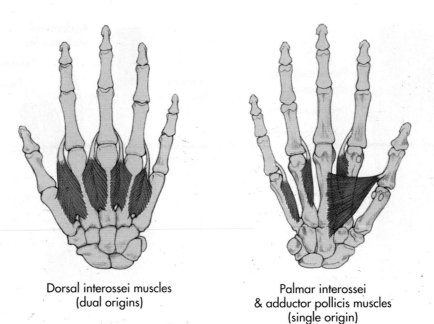

Dorsal interossei muscles
(dual origins)

Palmar interossei
& adductor pollicis muscles
(single origin)

PLATE 19 **Interosseous muscles and adductor pollicis.** (From Mathers LH et al: *Clinical anatomy principles,* St Louis, 1996, Mosby.)

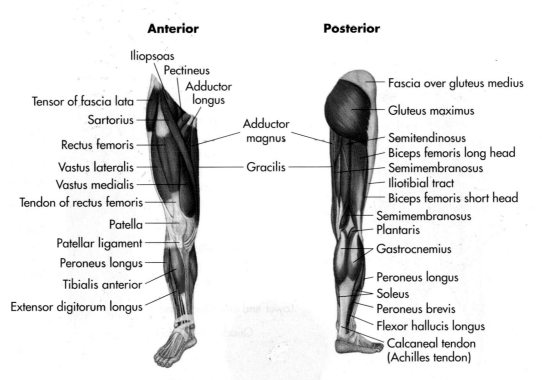

Anterior

- Iliopsoas
- Pectineus
- Adductor longus
- Tensor of fascia lata
- Sartorius
- Rectus femoris
- Vastus lateralis
- Vastus medialis
- Tendon of rectus femoris
- Patella
- Patellar ligament
- Peroneus longus
- Tibialis anterior
- Extensor digitorum longus

Posterior

- Adductor magnus
- Gracilis
- Fascia over gluteus medius
- Gluteus maximus
- Semitendinosus
- Biceps femoris long head
- Semimembranosus
- Iliotibial tract
- Biceps femoris short head
- Semimembranosus
- Plantaris
- Gastrocnemius
- Peroneus longus
- Soleus
- Peroneus brevis
- Flexor hallucis longus
- Calcaneal tendon (Achilles tendon)

PLATE 20 **Muscles of the leg.** (From Mourad LA: *Orthopedic disorders,* St Louis, 1991, Mosby.)

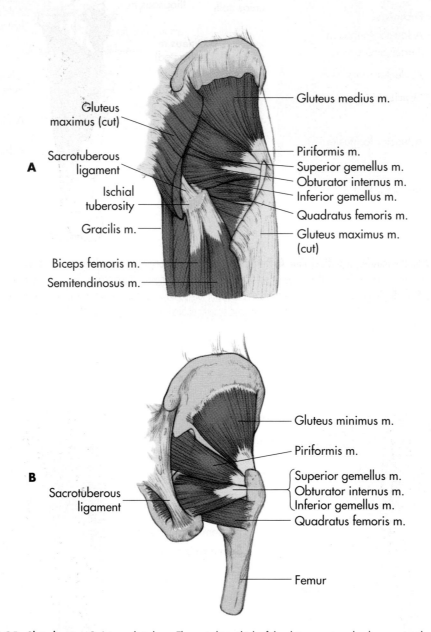

PLATE 25 Gluteal region. A, Intermediate layer. The central two thirds of the gluteus maximus has been removed, revealing some of the short rotator muscles of the gluteal region. **B,** Deep layer. The gluteus medius has been removed to reveal the more deeply placed gluteus minimus. (From Mathers LH et al: *Clinical anatomy principles,* St Louis, 1996, Mosby.)

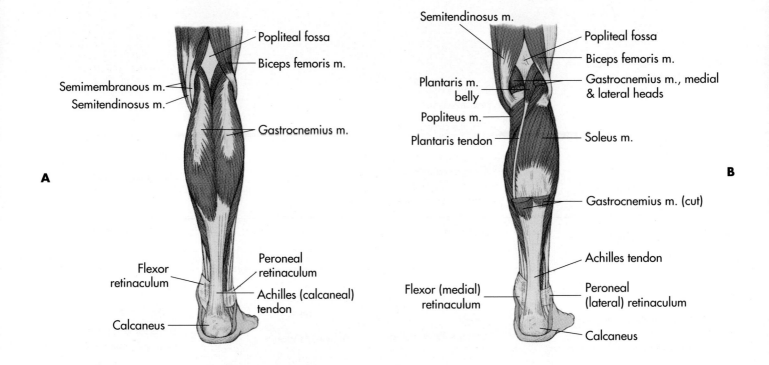

A

Popliteal fossa
Biceps femoris m.
Semimembranous m.
Semitendinosus m.
Gastrocnemius m.
Flexor retinaculum
Peroneal retinaculum
Achilles (calcaneal) tendon
Calcaneus

B

Semitendinosus m.
Popliteal fossa
Biceps femoris m.
Gastrocnemius m., medial & lateral heads
Plantaris m. belly
Popliteus m.
Plantaris tendon
Soleus m.
Gastrocnemius m. (cut)
Achilles tendon
Flexor (medial) retinaculum
Peroneal (lateral) retinaculum
Calcaneus

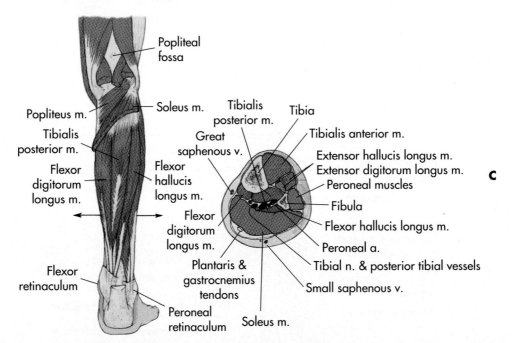

Popliteal fossa
Popliteus m.
Tibialis posterior m.
Flexor digitorum longus m.
Flexor retinaculum
Soleus m.
Flexor hallucis longus m.
Flexor digitorum longus m.
Peroneal retinaculum
Tibialis posterior m.
Great saphenous v.
Tibia
Tibialis anterior m.
Extensor hallucis longus m.
Extensor digitorum longus m.
Peroneal muscles
Fibula
Flexor hallucis longus m.
Peroneal a.
Tibial n. & posterior tibial vessels
Small saphenous v.
Plantaris & gastrocnemius tendons
Soleus m.

C

PLATE 26 Right leg muscles. A, Posterior view (superficial layer). **B,** Posterior view (middle layer). **C,** Posterior view (deep layer). With the two heads of the gastrocnemius, plantaris, and soleus all removed, we see the three deep muscles of the posterior compartment of the leg—the flexor hallucis longus, flexor digitorum longus, and tibialis posterior. On the accompanying cross-section, note the way the tibial nerve and posterior tibial vessels lie in a plane just superficial to this deepest compartment of muscles. (From Mathers LH et al: *Clinical anatomy principles,* St Louis 1996, Mosby.)

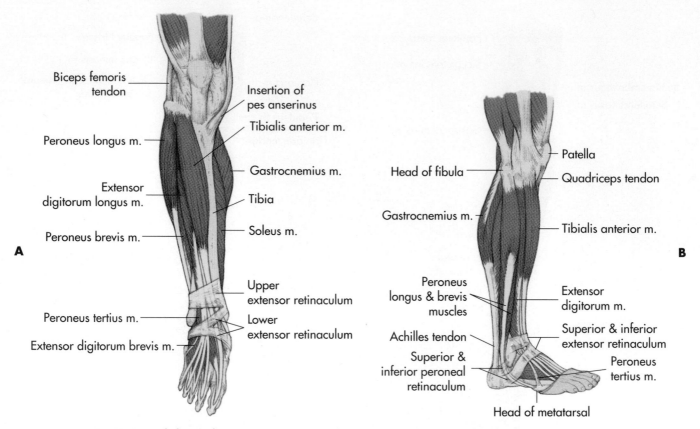

Biceps femoris tendon

Insertion of pes anserinus

Peroneus longus m.

Tibialis anterior m.

Extensor digitorum longus m.

Gastrocnemius m.

Tibia

Peroneus brevis m.

Soleus m.

A

Upper extensor retinaculum

Peroneus tertius m.

Lower extensor retinaculum

Extensor digitorum brevis m.

Head of fibula

Patella

Quadriceps tendon

Gastrocnemius m.

Tibialis anterior m.

B

Peroneus longus & brevis muscles

Extensor digitorum m.

Achilles tendon

Superior & inferior extensor retinaculum

Superior & inferior peroneal retinaculum

Peroneus tertius m.

Head of metatarsal

PLATE 27 Right leg muscles. A, Anterior view. **B,** Lateral view. (From Mathers LH et al: *Clinical anatomy principles,* St Louis, 1996, Mosby.)

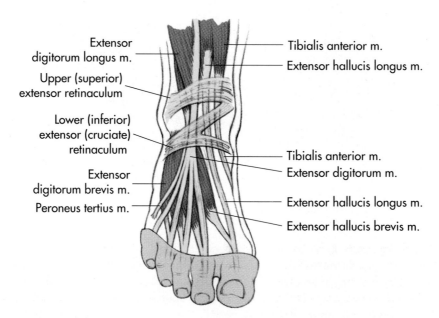

Extensor digitorum longus m.

Tibialis anterior m.

Extensor hallucis longus m.

Upper (superior) extensor retinaculum

Lower (inferior) extensor (cruciate) retinaculum

Tibialis anterior m.

Extensor digitorum m.

Extensor digitorum brevis m.

Peroneus tertius m.

Extensor hallucis longus m.

Extensor hallucis brevis m.

PLATE 28 Muscles and tendons on the dorsum of the foot, superficial view. (From Mathers LH et al: *Clinical anatomy principles,* St Louis, 1996, Mosby.)

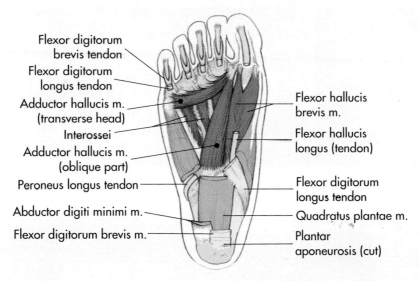

Flexor digitorum brevis tendon

Flexor digitorum longus tendon

Adductor hallucis m. (transverse head)

Interossei

Adductor hallucis m. (oblique part)

Peroneus longus tendon

Abductor digiti minimi m.

Flexor digitorum brevis m.

Flexor hallucis brevis m.

Flexor hallucis longus (tendon)

Flexor digitorum longus tendon

Quadratus plantae m.

Plantar aponeurosis (cut)

PLATE 29 **Muscles of the sole of foot, layers three and four.** (From Mathers LH et al: *Clinical anatomy principles,* St Louis, 1996, Mosby.)

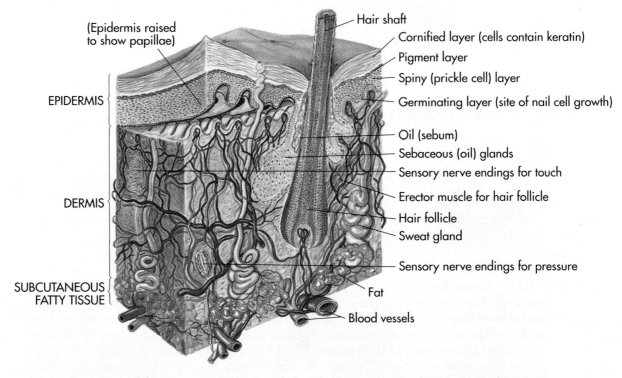

(Epidermis raised to show papillae)

Hair shaft

Cornified layer (cells contain keratin)

Pigment layer

Spiny (prickle cell) layer

Germinating layer (site of nail cell growth)

EPIDERMIS

Oil (sebum)

Sebaceous (oil) glands

Sensory nerve endings for touch

Erector muscle for hair follicle

DERMIS

Hair follicle

Sweat gland

Sensory nerve endings for pressure

SUBCUTANEOUS FATTY TISSUE

Fat

Blood vessels

PLATE 30 **Structure of skin.** (From LaFleur Brooks M: *Exploring medical language: a student-directed approach,* ed 3, St Louis, 1994, Mosby.)

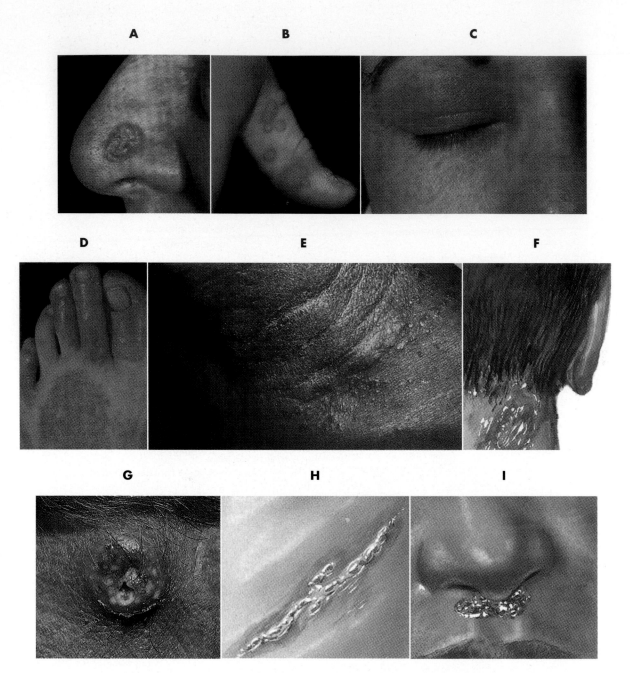

PLATE 31 Common skin disorders. NOTE: Skin problems may result from various causes such as parasitic infestations; fungal, bacterial, or viral infections; reactions to substances encountered externally or taken internally; or new growths. Many of the skin manifestations have no known cause; others are hereditary. **A,** Basal cell carcinoma. **B,** Common warts. **C,** Contact dermatitis from shampoo. **D,** Contact dermatitis from shoes. **E,** Contact dermatitis from application of Lanacane. **F,** Dermatitis. **G,** Furuncle (boil). **H,** Herpes zoster (shingles). **I,** Impetigo contagiosa. (*P* from Barkauskas VH et al: *Health and physical assessment,* ed 2, St Louis, 1998, Mosby; *B, G,* and *M* from Thibodeau GA, Patton KT: *The human body in health and disease,* ed 2, St Louis, 1997, Mosby; *F, H, I, N,* and *O* from LaFleur Brooks M: *Exploring medical language: a student-directed approach,* ed 3, St Louis, 1994, Mosby; *A* and *J* from Habif TP: *Clinical dermatology: a color guide to diagnosis and therapy,* ed 3, St Louis, 1996, Mosby; *C, D, K, L,* and *P* courtesy American Academy of Dermatology and Institute for Dermatologic Communication and Education, Schaumberg, Illinois; *E* from Zitelli BJ, Davis HW, editors: *Atlas of pediatric physical diagnosis,* ed 1, Gower Medical Publishing, 1987. By permission of Mosby International.)

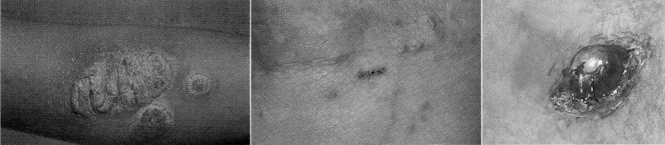

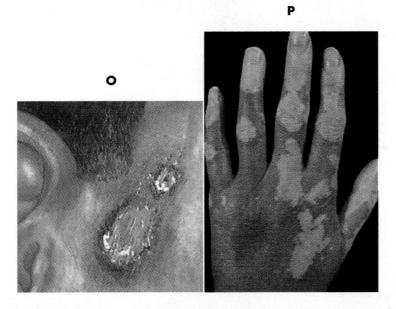

PLATE 31—cont'd   **J,** Kaposi's sarcoma. **K,** Nummular eczema. **L,** Psoriasis. **M,** Scabies. **N,** Squamous cell carcinoma. **O,** Tinea corporis (ringworm). **P,** Vitiligo.

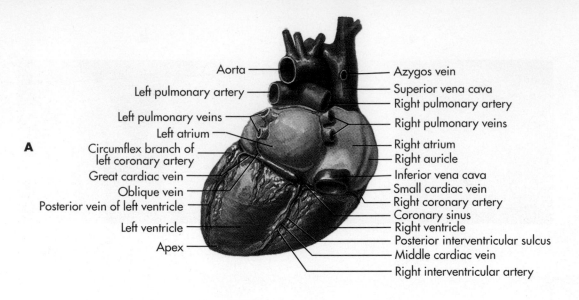

A

Aorta

Left pulmonary artery

Left pulmonary veins

Left atrium

Circumflex branch of left coronary artery

Great cardiac vein

Oblique vein

Posterior vein of left ventricle

Left ventricle

Apex

Azygos vein

Superior vena cava

Right pulmonary artery

Right pulmonary veins

Right atrium

Right auricle

Inferior vena cava

Small cardiac vein

Right coronary artery

Coronary sinus

Right ventricle

Posterior interventricular sulcus

Middle cardiac vein

Right interventricular artery

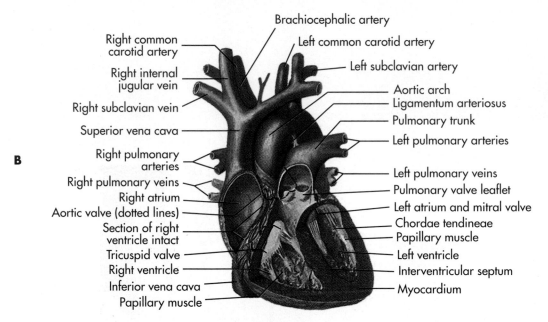

B

Brachiocephalic artery

Right common carotid artery

Right internal jugular vein

Right subclavian vein

Superior vena cava

Right pulmonary arteries

Right pulmonary veins

Right atrium

Aortic valve (dotted lines)

Section of right ventricle intact

Tricuspid valve

Right ventricle

Inferior vena cava

Papillary muscle

Left common carotid artery

Left subclavian artery

Aortic arch

Ligamentum arteriosus

Pulmonary trunk

Left pulmonary arteries

Left pulmonary veins

Pulmonary valve leaflet

Left atrium and mitral valve

Chordae tendineae

Papillary muscle

Left ventricle

Interventricular septum

Myocardium

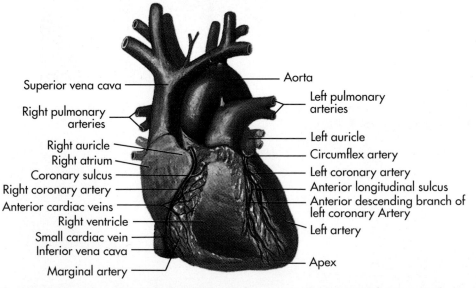

C

Superior vena cava

Right pulmonary arteries

Right auricle

Right atrium

Coronary sulcus

Right coronary artery

Anterior cardiac veins

Right ventricle

Small cardiac vein

Inferior vena cava

Marginal artery

Aorta

Left pulmonary arteries

Left auricle

Circumflex artery

Left coronary artery

Anterior longitudinal sulcus

Anterior descending branch of left coronary Artery

Left artery

Apex

PLATE 32 **A,** Posterior view of coronary vessels. **B,** Human heart in frontal section. **C,** Anterior view of coronary vessels. (From LaFleur Brooks M: *Exploring medical language: a student-directed approach,* ed 3, St Louis, 1994, Mosby.)

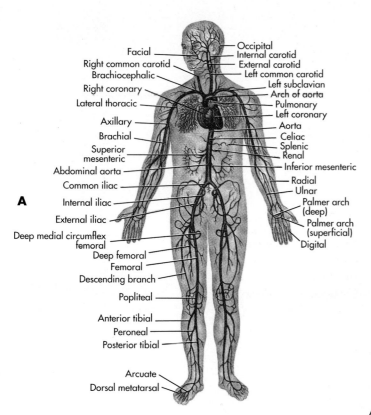

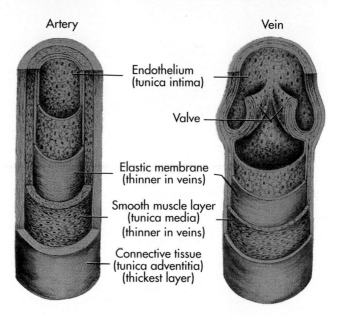

PLATE 34 Structure of arteries and veins. Note the relative thickness of the arterial walls. (From Thompson JM et al: *Mosby's clinical nursing,* ed 3, St Louis, 1993, Mosby.)

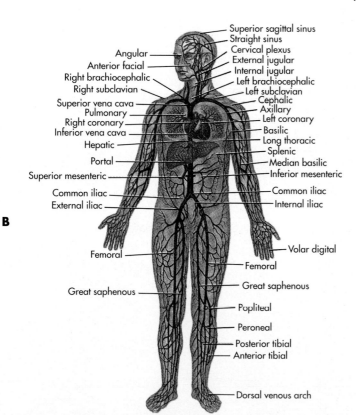

PLATE 33 Systemic circulation. **A,** Arteries. **B,** Veins. (From Seidel HM et al: *Mosby's guide to physical examination,* ed 3, St Louis, 1995, Mosby.)

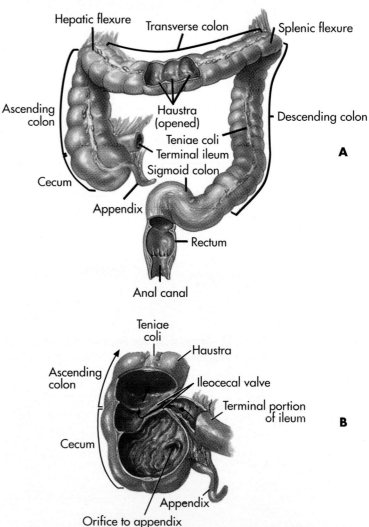

PLATE 35 A, Anatomy of large intestine showing the junction between the large and small intestines and the entry of the ileum into the cecum. **B,** Enlarged detail of cecum and terminal ileum. (From LaFleur Brooks M: Exploring medical language: a student-directed approach, ed 3, St Louis, 1994, Mosby.)

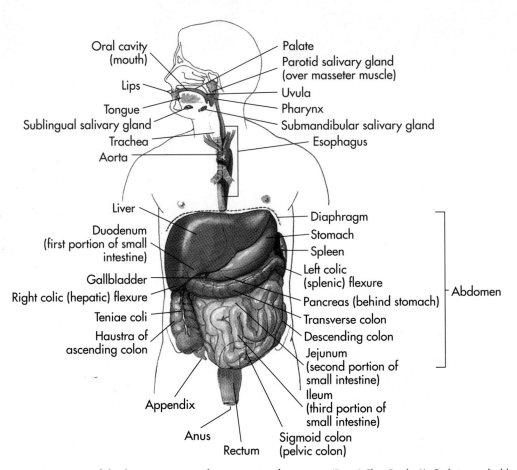

PLATE 36 Organs of the digestive system and some associated structures. (From LaFleur Brooks M: *Exploring medical language: a student-directed approach,* ed 3, St Louis, 1994, Mosby.)

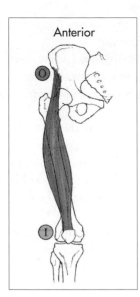

Anterior

Rectus femoris
(REK-tus FEM-or-iss)
Meaning straight or upright; related to the thigh

Function: Extends the knee joint; flexes the hip joint

Origin: Anterior inferior iliac spine; groove above the rim of the acetabulum

Insertion: Proximal border (base) of the patella and through the patellar ligament to the tuberosity of the tibia

Innervation: Femoral nerve L2 to L3 and L4

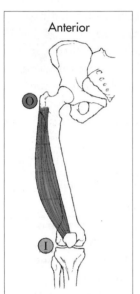

Anterior

Vastus lateralis
(VAS-tus LAT-ter-al-us)
Meaning vast or large; related to the side

Function: Extends the knee joint and exerts a lateral pull on the patella

Origin: Proximal aspect of the intertrochanteric line; greater trochanter; gluteal tuberosity; linea aspera; and lateral intermuscular septum

Insertion: Lateral border (base) of the patella and through the patellar ligament into the tuberosity of the tibia

Innervation: Femoral nerve L2 to L3 and L4

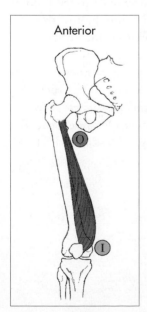

Anterior

Vastus medialis
(VAS-tus MEE-dee-al-us)
Meaning vast or large; related to the middle

Function: Extends the leg and draws the patella medially

Origin: Lower half of the intertrochanteric line; linea aspera; medial supracondylar line; medial intermuscular septum; tendon of the adductor magnus

Insertion: Medial border (base) of the patella and through the patellar ligament to the tuberosity of the tibia

Innervation: Femoral nerve L2 to L3 and L4

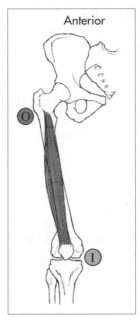

Anterior

Vastus intermedius
(VAS-tus inter-MEE-dee-us)
Meaning vast or large; among the middle

Function: Extends the knee joint

Origin: Anterior and lateral surfaces of the proximal two thirds of the body of the femur; distal one half of the linea aspera; intermuscular septum

Insertion: Deep surface of the tendon of the recti and vasti muscles; proximal border (base) of the patella and through the patellar ligament to the tuberosity of the tibia

Innervation: Femoral nerve L2 to L3 and L4

Elements common to the anterior thigh muscles

Synergists: For flexion at the hip, the synergists are the iliopsoas and pectineus; for extension of the knee, all quadriceps muscles are synergistic with one another

Antagonists:
Flexion at the hip—Extensors, primarily the gluteus maximus and hamstrings
Knee extension—Knee flexors, primarily the hamstrings, as well as the sartorius and gracilis

Trigger points:
Sartorius—Three or four areas along the belly of the muscle
Rectus femoris—Near the insertion at the pelvis
Vastus lateralis—Several locations at each attachment and in the belly of the muscle
Vastus interomedialis—Near the origin at the musculotendinous junction
Vastus medialis—In the belly of the muscle and near the attachment just above the knee

Referred pain pattern: Entire anterior thigh, with concentration at the knee

See Activity 9-61

MUSCLES OF THE ANTERIOR AND LATERAL LEG

The various muscles of the leg produce movement at the ankle joints: dorsiflexion and plantar flexion, inversion and eversion, and flexion or extension of the toes. The muscles of the anterior leg are primarily toe extensors and ankle dorsiflexors. Dorsiflexion is extremely important in preventing the toes from dragging during walking. The lateral leg muscles plantar flex and evert the foot.

The deep fascia of the leg is continuous with the fascia lata, which ensheathes the thigh and binds the leg muscles together. This construction helps prevent excessive swelling of the muscles during exercise. This same fascial sheath supports a pumping action that aids the circulation of blood and lymph; venous return flow is particularly aided. The fascia divides the leg muscles into the anterior, lateral, and posterior compartments, each with its own nerve and blood supply. The leg fascia thickens at the ankles to form the retinacula, which secure the muscle tendons in place as they cross the ankles into the feet.

Anterior Muscles

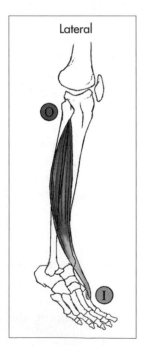

Lateral

Tibialis anterior
(TIB-ee-AL-iss)

Meaning related to the shinbone; anterior meaning before or in front

Function: Dorsiflexion of the ankle joint; assists in inversion of the foot

Origin: Lateral condyle and proximal one half of the lateral surface of the tibia; interosseous membrane; deep fascia; lateral intermuscular septum

Insertion: Medial plantar surface of the medial cuneiform bone; base of the first metatarsal bone

Innervation: Deep peroneal nerve L4 to L5 and S1

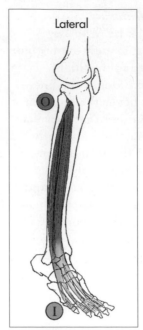

Lateral

Extensor digitorum longus
(ex-STEN-sur DIH-jih-TOR-um LONG-us)

Meaning one that stretches; of the fingers and toes; long

Function: Extends the phalanges of the second through fifth digits; assists in dorsiflexion of the ankle joint and eversion of the foot

Origin: Lateral condyle of the tibia, proximal three fourths of the anterior surface of the body of the fibula; interosseous membrane; deep fascia; intermuscular septa

Insertion: By four tendons to the second through fifth digits; each tendon divides into an intermediate slip, which is attached to the base of the middle phalanx, and two lateral slips, which are attached to the base of the distal phalanx

Innervation: Deep peroneal nerve L4 to L5 and S1

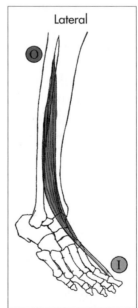

Lateral

Extensor hallucis longus
(ex-STEN-sur HAL-uh-kiss LONG-us)

Meaning one that stretches; relating to the big toe; long

Function: Extends the metatarsophalangeal joint of the great toe; also assists in inverting the foot and dorsiflexing the ankle joint

Origin: Middle half of the anterior surface of the fibula, adjacent interosseous membrane

Insertion: Base of the distal phalanx of the great toe

Innervation: Deep peroneal nerve L4 to L5 and S1

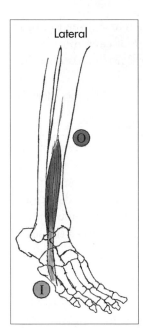

Lateral

Peroneus tertius
(per-oh-NEE-us TER-she-us)
Meaning related to the pin or
fibula; the third
Function: Dorsiflexes the
ankle joint; everts the foot
Origin: Distal one third of the
anterior surface of the fibula; interosseous membrane;
intermuscular septum
Insertion: Dorsal surface of
the base of the fifth
metatarsal bone
Innervation: Deep peroneal
nerve L4 to L5 and S1

**Elements common to the
anterior muscles**
Synergists: Tibialis anterior,
digitorum longus, peroneus tertius, and extensor
hallucis longus are synergistic for dorsiflexion
Antagonists:
Eversion and inversion—Tibialis anterior, digitorum longus
Dorsiflexion—Gastrocnemius, soleus, peroneus
longus and brevis, flexors of the toes, tibialis
posterior

Trigger points: In the belly of each muscle
Referred pain pattern: Down the leg to the ankle and
into the toes

See Activity 9-62

Lateral Muscles

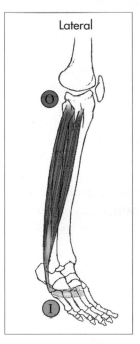

Lateral

Peroneus longus
(per-oh-NEE-us LONG-us)
Meaning related to the pin or
fibula; long
Function: Everts the foot;
assists in plantar flexion of
the ankle joint
Origin: Lateral condyle of the
tibia; head and upper two
thirds of the lateral surface of the fibula; intermuscular septa; adjacent
deep fascia
Insertion: Lateral side of the
base of the first metatarsal
bone and the medial
cuneiform bone
Innervation: Superficial peroneal nerve L4 to L5 and S1

ACTIVITY 9-62

- Draw and color the anterior leg muscles (the tibialis anterior, the extensor digitorum longus, the extensor hallucis longus, and the peroneus tertius) in the space provided.
- Label the origin and insertion points: *O,* for the origin, *I,* for the insertion.
- Place an **X** on the trigger points.
- Palpate these muscles; identify the attachment points and the belly of the muscle.
- Move these muscles on yourself.

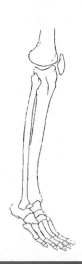
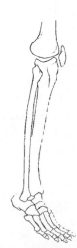
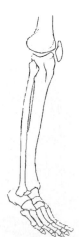
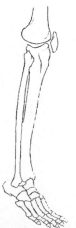

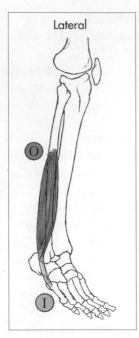

Lateral

Peroneus brevis
(per-oh-NEE-us BREV-us)
Meaning related to the pin or
   fibula; smaller
Function: Everts the foot;
   assists in plantar flexion of
   the ankle joint
Origin: Distal two thirds of
   the lateral surface of the
   fibula and adjacent intermuscular septum
Insertion: Tuberosity at the
   base of the fifth metatarsal
   bone on the lateral side
Innervation: Superficial peroneal nerve L4 to L5 and
   S1
**Elements common to the
lateral muscles**

Synergist: Eversion—extensor digitorum longus
Antagonists:
   Eversion—Tibialis anterior and posterior, exten-
      sor hallucis longus, flexor hallucis longus
   Plantar flexion—Dorsiflexors of the anterior leg

ACTIVITY 9-63

- Draw and color the lateral leg muscles (the peroneus longus and the per-
  oneus brevis) in the space provided.
- Label the origin and insertion points: *O,* for the origin, *I,* for the insertion.
- Place an **X** on the trigger points.
- Palpate these muscles; identify the attachment points and the belly of
  the muscle.
- Move these muscles on yourself.

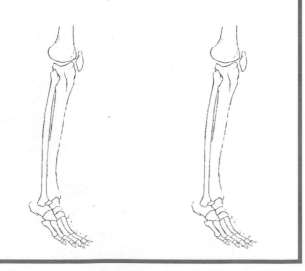

Trigger points: Located at the origin and insertion near
   the musculotendinous junction of each muscle
Referred pain pattern: To the lateral malleolus and the
   heel

See Activity 9-63

POSTERIOR LEG MUSCLES

The posterior leg muscles plantar flex the foot and
flex the toes. Plantar flexion lifts the entire weight of
the body to allow a person to stand on tiptoe and provides the necessary forward thrust for walking and
running. (Plantar flexion is a very powerful movement.) The popliteus muscle, which crosses the knee,
is important in unlocking the extended knee in
preparation for flexion.

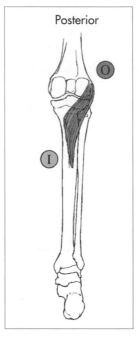

Posterior

Popliteus (pop-LIT-ee-us)
Meaning hollow of the knee
Function:
   With origin fixed—
      Medially rotates the
      tibia on the femur at the
      beginning of flexion;
      flexes the knee joint
      (non–weight bearing)
   With insertion fixed—
      Laterally rotates the
      femur on the tibia;
      flexes the knee joint
      (weight bearing) and in
      this function essentially
      unlocks the knee for
      flexion
Origin: Anterior end of the
   groove on the lateral
condyle of the femur; oblique popliteal ligament
Insertion: Triangular area above the soleal line on the
   posterior surface of the tibia, as well as the fascia
   covering its surface
Innervation: Tibial nerve L4 to L5 and S1
Synergists: Medial hamstrings, sartorius, gracilis for
   medial rotation
Antagonist: Biceps femoris
Trigger points: Belly of the muscle
Referred pain pattern: To the back of the knee

See Activity 9-64

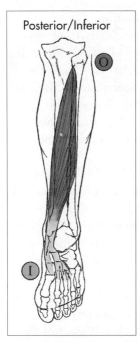

Posterior/Inferior

Tibialis posterior
(TIB-ee-AL-iss)
Meaning related to the shin-
    bone; coming after or
    behind
Function: Inversion of the
    foot; assists in plantar
    flexion of the ankle joint
Origin: Posterior surface of
    the interosseous mem-
    brane; lateral portion of
    the posterior surface of
    the tibia; proximal two
    thirds of the medial sur-
    face of the fibula; inter-
    muscular septa
Insertion: Tuberosity of the
    navicular bone; calca-
    neous; three cuneiforms
    and the cuboid; bases of the
second through fourth metatarsal bones
Innervation: Tibial nerve L5 to S1

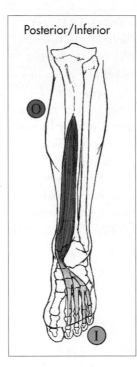

Posterior/Inferior

Flexor digitorum longus
(FLEKS-or
DIH-jih-TOR-um LONG-us)
Meaning to bend; related to
    the fingers or toes; long
Function: Flexes the joints of
    the second through fifth
    digits; assists in plantar
    flexion of the ankle joint
    and inversion of the foot
Origin: Middle two thirds of
    the posterior surface of
    the body of the tibia and
    the fascia covering the tib-
    ialis posterior
Insertion: Bases of the distal
    phalanges of the second
    through fifth digits
Innervation: Tibial nerve L5 to
    S1 and S2

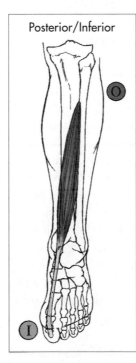

Posterior/Inferior

Flexor hallucis longus
(FLEKS-or HAL-uh-kiss
LONG-us)
Meaning to bend; related to
    the big toe; long
Function: Flexes the joints of
    the great toe; plantar
    flexes the ankle joint and
    inverts the foot
Origin: Lower two thirds of
    the posterior surface of the
    fibula; interosseous mem-
    brane; adjacent intermus-
    cular septum and fascia
Insertion: Plantar aspect of
    the base of the distal pha-
    lanx of the great toe
Innervation: Tibial nerve L5 to
    S1 and S2

ACTIVITY 9-64

- Draw and color the popliteus in the space provided.
- Label the origin and insertion points: *O*, for the origin, *I*, for the insertion.
- Place an **X** on the trigger points.
- Palpate this muscle; identify the attachment points and the belly of the muscle.
- Move this muscle on yourself.

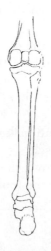

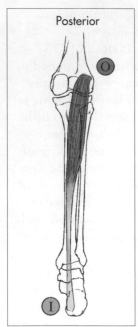

Posterior

Plantaris (plan-TAR-iss)
Meaning sole of the foot
Function: Plantar flexes the
ankle joint; assists in flexion of the knee joint
Origin: Lower part of the lateral supracondylar line of
the femur; oblique
popliteal ligament
Insertion: Posterior medial
part of the calcaneous
with the calcaneal tendon
Innervation: Tibial nerve L4 to
L5 and S1

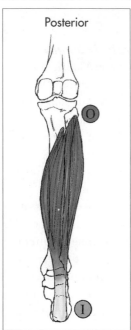

Posterior

Soleus (SOL-ee-us)
Meaning sandal or sole of
the foot
Function: Plantar flexes the
ankle joint and stabilizes
the leg over the foot
NOTE: Because of its large
venous sinuses, tough fascial
covering, and vein structure,
the soleus is an effective mus-
culovenous pump that functions as a second heart, especially during strenuous running and jumping activities
Origin: Back of the head and
upper one fourth of the
posterior surface of the
fibula; soleal line and middle one third of the medial
border of the tibia; fibrous band between the
tibia and the fibula
Insertion: With the gastrocnemius (Achilles) tendon
into the posterior surface of the calcaneous
Innervation: Two branches from the tibial nerve L5
to S1 and S2

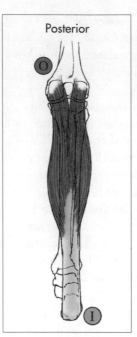

Posterior

Gastrocnemius
(GAS-troe-NEEM-ee-us)
Meaning belly and shin or leg
Function: Plantar flexes the
ankle joint; assists in flexion of the knee joint;
involved in maintaining
balance in static standing
Origin:
Medial head—Upper pos-
terior part of the medial
condyle of the femur;
capsule of the knee joint
Lateral head—Lower part
of the supracondylar
line and lateral condyle
of the femur; capsule of
the knee joint
Insertion: Middle part of the
posterior surface of the calcaneous via the calcaneal (Achilles) tendon
Innervation: Tibial nerve S1 to S2

**Elements common to the posterior leg
muscles**
Synergists:
Plantar flexion—Gastrocnemius, soleus, plantaris,
peroneus longus and brevis, flexor hallucis
longus, flexor digitorum longus, tibialis posterior
Knee flexion—Gastrocnemius, hamstrings, grac-
ilis, sartorius, popliteus
Antagonists:
Plantar flexion—Tibialis anterior, extensors of the
toes
Knee flexion—Quadriceps group
Trigger points:
Gastrocnemius—In the belly of the muscle and at
the attachment near the knee in each head of
this muscle
Soleus—Near both the origin and the insertion
Plantaris—In the belly of the muscle at the back
of the knee
Tibialis posterior—Belly of the muscle nearer the
knee
Flexor digitorum and hallucis longus—In the
belly of each muscle
Referred pain pattern: Down the posterior leg to the
heel and the sole of the foot into the plantar surface of the toes

See Activity 9-65

MUSCLES OF THE FOOT

The muscles of the sole of the foot help flex, extend, abduct, and adduct the toes; they also work with the tendons of the leg muscles to support the arches of the foot. These muscles are numerous, their arrangement is complex, and their actions are interdependent.

Dorsal Aspect

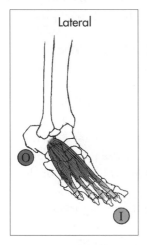

Lateral

Extensor digitorum brevis

(ex-STEN-sur DIH-jih-TOR-um BREV-us)
Meaning to stretch; related to the fingers or toes; short
NOTE: The most medial portion of the extensor digitorum brevis inserts into the dorsal surface of the base of the proximal phalanx of the great toe and is sometimes called the *extensor hallucis brevis* muscle
Function: Extends metatarsophalangeal joint of the first toe and extends the interphalangeal and metatarsophalangeal joints of the second through fourth toes

Origin: Distal and lateral surfaces of the calcaneous; lateral talocalcaneal ligament; inferior extensor retinaculum
Insertion: First tendon into the dorsal surface of the base of the proximal phalanx of the great toe; lateral sides of the tendons of the extensor digitorum longus to the second, third, and fourth toes
Innervation: Deep peroneal nerve L5 to S1 and S2

Plantar, Superficial Layer

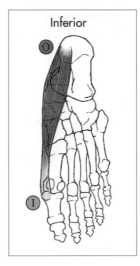

Inferior

Abductor hallucis

(ab-DUCK-tur HAL-uh-kiss)
Meaning to lead away from; big toe
Function: Abducts and assists in flexion of the metatarsophalangeal joint of the great toe
Origin: Medial process of the calcaneal tuberosity; flexor retinaculum; plantar aponeurosis; adjacent intermuscular septum

ACTIVITY 9-65

- Draw and color the tibialis posterior, the flexor digitorum longus, the flexor hallucis longus, the plantaris, the soleus, and the gastrocnemius in the space provided.
- Label the origin and insertion points: *O,* for the origin, *I,* for the insertion.

- Place an **X** on the trigger points.
- Palpate these muscles; identify the attachment points and the belly of the muscle.
- Move these muscles on yourself.

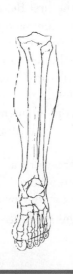
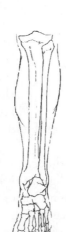
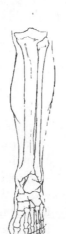
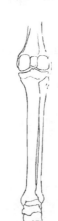
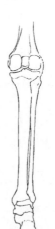
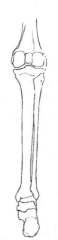

Insertion: Medial side of the base of the proximal
  phalanx of the great toe
Innervation: Medial plantar nerve L5 to S1 and S2

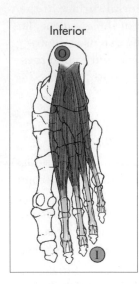

Flexor digitorum brevis
(FLEKS-or DIH-jih-TOR-um
BREV-us)
Meaning to bend; related to
  fingers or toes; short
Function: Flexes the proximal
  interphalangeal joints and
  assists in flexion of the
  metatarsophalangeal joints
  of the second through fifth
  toes
Origin: Medial process of the
  calcaneal tuberosity; plantar aponeurosis; adjacent
  intermuscular septa
Insertion: Sides of the middle
of the second through fifth toes
Innervation: Medial plantar nerve L5 to S1 and S2

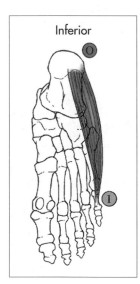

Abductor digiti minimi
(ab-DUCK-tur DIH-jih-tee
MIN-ih-mee)
Meaning to lead away from;
  related to the fingers or
  toes; smallest
Function: Abducts and assists
  in flexing the metatar-
  sophalangeal joint of the
  fifth toe
Origin: Lateral process of the
  calcaneal tuberosity; plantar aponeurosis; intermuscular septum
Insertion: Lateral side of the
  base of the proximal phalanx of the fifth toe
Innervation: Lateral plantar nerve S1 to S2

Plantar, Second Layer

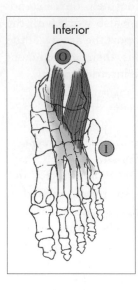

Quadratus plantae
(kwad-RATE-us PLAN-tie)
Meaning square shaped; for
  the sole of the foot
Function: Modifies the line of
  pull of the flexor digitorum longus and assists in
  flexion of the second
  through the fifth digits
Origin:
  Medial head—Medial sur-
    face of the calcaneous;
    medial border of the
    long plantar ligament
  Lateral head—Lateral
    inferior surface of the
calcaneous; lateral border of the plantar surface of the calcaneus and lateral border of the
  long plantar ligament
Insertion: Lateral margin of the flexor digitorum
  longus tendon
Innervation: Lateral plantar nerve S1 to S2

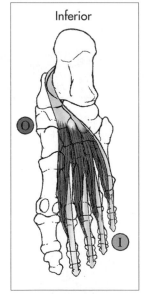

Lumbricales
(LUM-brih-kals)
Meaning earthworms
Function: Flex the metatar-
  sophalangeal joints and
  extend the interphalangeal
  joints of the second
  through the fifth digits
Origin:
  First—From the medial
    side of the first flexor
    digitorum longus tendon
  Second—From adjacent
    sides of the first and
    second flexor digitorum
    longus tendons
  Third—From adjacent
    sides of the second and third flexor digitorum
  longus tendons
  Fourth—From adjacent sides of the third and
  fourth flexor digitorum longus tendons
Insertion: With the tendons of the flexor digitorum
  longus into the base of the terminal phalanges of
  the second through fifth toes

Innervation:
First—Medial plantar nerve
Second through fourth—Deep branch of the lateral plantar nerve S1 to S2

Plantar, Third Layer

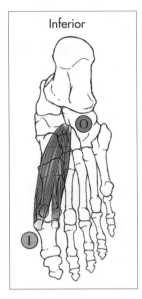

Inferior

Flexor hallucis brevis
(FLEKS-or HAL-uh-kiss BREV-us)
Meaning to bend; big toe; short

Function: Flexes metatarsophalangeal joint of the great toe

Origin: Medial aspect of the plantar surface of the cuboid bone; lateral cuneiform bone; and from the tendon of the tibialis posterior

Insertion: Medial and lateral sides of the base of the proximal phalanx of the great toe

Innervation: Medial plantar nerve L5 to S1 and S2

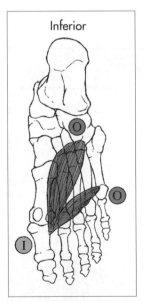

Inferior

Adductor hallucis (ad-DUCK-tur HAL-uh-kiss)
Meaning to lead toward; big toe

Function: Adducts and assists in flexion of the metatarsophalangeal joint of the great toe

Origin:
Oblique head—Bases of the second, third, and fourth metatarsal bones; sheath of the tendon of the peroneus longus
Transverse head—Plantar metatarsophalangeal ligament of the third, fourth, and fifth digits; deep transverse metatarsal ligament of the sole

Insertion: Lateral sides of the base of the proximal phalanx of the great toe

Innervation: Deep branch of the lateral plantar nerve S1 to S2

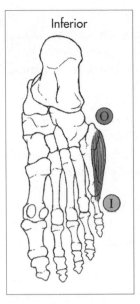

Inferior

Flexor digiti minimi brevis
(FLEKS-or DIH-jih-tee MIN-ih-mee BREV-us)
Meaning to bend; related to the fingers and toes; smallest; short

NOTE: Occasionally, some of the deeper fibers of the flexor digiti minimi brevis reach the lateral part of the distal half of the fifth metatarsal bone; this sometimes is described as a distinct muscle, the opponens digiti minimi

Function: Flexes the metatarsophalangeal joint of the fifth toe

Origin: Medial part of the plantar surface of the base of the fifth metatarsal bone; sheath of the peroneus longus

Insertion: Lateral side of the base of the proximal phalanx of the fifth toe

Innervation: Superficial branch of the lateral plantar nerve S1 to S2

Plantar, Fourth Layer

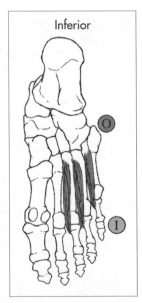

Inferior

Plantar interossei
(plan-TAR INT-er-OSS-ee-ee)
Meaning sole of the foot; between or among the bones

Function: Adduct the third, fourth, and fifth toes toward an axis through the second toe; assist in flexion of the metatarsophalangeal joints of the third through fifth toes

Origin: Three plantar interossei arise from the base and medial sides of the bodies of the third, fourth, and fifth metatarsals

Insertion: Medial sides of the bases of the proximal phalanges of the same toes; aponeuroses of the extensor digitorum longus tendons

Innervation:

First and second—Deep branch of the lateral plantar nerve

Third—Superficial branch of the lateral plantar nerve S1 to S2

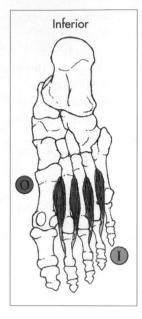

Inferior

Dorsal interossei (door-SAL INT-er-OSS-ee-ee)

Meaning on or near the back; between or among the bones

Function: Abduct the second, third, and fourth toes from a longitudinal axis through the second toes; also assist in flexion of the metatarsophalangeal joints of the second through the fourth digits

Origin: Each arises via two heads from adjacent sides of the metatarsal bones, between which they are placed

Insertion: Base of the first phalanx; aponeuroses of the extensor digitorum longus tendon; first to medial side of the second toes; remaining three to the lateral sides of the second through fourth toes

Innervation:

First, second, and third—Deep branch of the lateral plantar nerve

Fourth—Superficial branch of the lateral plantar nerve S1 to S2

Elements common to the muscles of the foot

Synergists: The long and short extensors and flexors of the toes work together with the lumbricales and the interossei

Antagonists: In this complex network, in which a muscle can be synergistic with one function and antagonistic with another, the role of antagonist depends on the function; generally, flexors oppose extensor, adductors oppose abductors, and vice versa

Trigger points: Several areas concentrated in the belly of each muscle

Referred pain pattern: The entire foot with areas concentrated at the large toe, the ball of the foot, and the heel

See Activity 9-66

ACTIVITY 9-66

- Draw and color the muscles of the foot in the space provided.
- Label the origin and insertion points: *O,* for the origin, *I,* for the insertion.
- Place an **X** on the trigger points.

- Palpate these muscles; identify the attachment points and the belly of the muscle.
- Move these muscles on yourself.

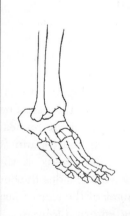
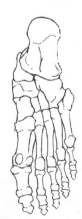
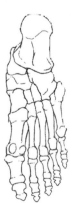
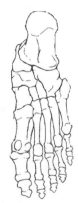
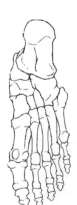

Pathologic Conditions

MECHANISMS OF DISEASE

Whenever the myofascial system (muscles and associated connective tissue) is stressed, a fairly predictable sequence of events occurs (Chaitow, 1996):

1. Causal factors (e.g., congenital factors or predisposition, overuse, misuse, abuse and disuse of the body, postural stress, chronic stressful emotional states) and reflex factors (e.g., trigger points) can lead to increased muscle tension and retention of metabolic wastes.
2. Increased tension leads to localized ischemia and edema.
3. Pain results.
4. Pain increases tension or spasm, which increases pain.
5. Inflammation or chronic irritation may result.
6. Neurologic reporting stations in tense tissue bombard the central nervous system with information, which leads to hyperactivity.
7. Macrophages and fibroblasts are activated.
8. Connective tissue production increases, with increasing shortening of fascia.
9. Because fascia is continuous throughout the body, any distortions in one area could create distortions elsewhere, affecting structures supported by or attached to the fascia, including the nerves, muscles, lymph, and blood vessels.
10. Changes occur in the muscular tissues, leading to chronic hypertension and ultimately to fibrotic changes. Increased tension in a muscle causes inhibition of the antagonist muscles and facilitation in the synergists.
11. Chain reactions in myotatic units occur. Typically, muscles used for posture shorten, and muscles used for motion weaken.
12. Sustained increases in muscle tension cause ischemia in tendinous areas, and areas of periosteal (bone) pain develop.
13. Abnormal biomechanics and body-wide compensatory patterns develop.
14. Joint restriction or imbalance, or both, develop, and fascial shortening and immobility increase.
15. Trigger points develop.
16. Generalized fatigue develops as a result both of wasted energy used to maintain unproductive patterns and of an interrupted sleep pattern.
17. Sympathetic arousal is heightened, generalizing the pattern.
18. Immune response is inhibited, and more serious systemic problems may develop.

Intervention focuses on reversing this process and supporting resourceful compensation patterns that develop in response to chronic problems.

MAJOR MUSCULAR DISORDERS

As you might expect, muscle disorders, or myopathies, generally disrupt the normal movement of the body. In mild cases these disorders vary from inconvenient to slightly troublesome. Severe muscle disorders, however, can impair the muscles used in breathing—a life-threatening situation.

Medications

Pathologic conditions of the muscles are treated pharmacologically with antibiotics. Inflammation is eased with both steroidal and nonsteroidal antiinflammatory medications. Spasm and hypertonic muscles are soothed with muscle relaxants; pain is treated with analgesics. Sleep restoration and support of other restorative processes sometimes are assisted by low-dose antidepressants.

These drugs may be either prescription or over-the-counter medications, herbal or homeopathic substances. Any form of medication or herbal remedy may have effects on the client that need to be taken into consideration when developing a treatment plan. Consideration also must be given to the interaction between soft tissue and movement therapies and the effects of medication. The intensity of pressure and the duration and amount of stretch applied to the tissues are affected by many medications used to treat muscle dysfunction.

Anytime infection is present and is being treated with antibiotics, the system already is stressed. Therapeutic methods are used to support the healing process by promoting general relaxation but are to be performed gently so as not to place additional demand on the system to respond. When antiinflammatory drugs are used, methods that produce therapeutic inflammation are to be avoided. Muscle relaxants interfere with the normal feedback systems of the stretch and tension receptors; because this protective mechanism is interrupted by these medications, care must be taken with any type of lengthening or stretching methods. Because analgesics interfere with the normal pain response, feedback from the client may be inaccurate. Intensity levels and duration need to be adjusted.

Soft tissue and movement methods can support the use of these medications, helping to make them more effective. In some instances the dosage of medication can be reduced or the medication can be replaced by soft tissue and movement therapies. Ice applications can support and sometimes reduce the use of analgesics and antiinflammatory drugs. Because all medications have side effects, the ability to take smaller doses of medication for short durations is beneficial. Any change in medication use must be set in place and carefully monitored by the prescribing health care provider.

SPECIFIC DISORDERS

Stress-Induced Muscle Tension and Headache

Stress-induced muscle tension can result in myalgia, or muscle pain; stiffness in the neck and back often accompanies stress-induced headaches. The contracted muscles exert pressure on the nerves and blood vessels in the area, causing the pain, which is a dull, persistent ache with feelings of tightness around the head, temples, forehead, and occipital areas. The headache often is less intense in the morning and worsens as the day goes on.

INDICATIONS CONTRAINDICATIONS

For Soft Tissue and Movement Therapies

Various strategies are used to treat stress-induced muscle tension headaches, including massage and other forms of soft tissue work, biofeedback, relaxation training, exercise, and stretching methods. Chronic patterns often indicate connective tissue shortening. Headaches respond best to whole-body therapy, which not only addresses the immediate areas but also relaxes the entire body.

Muscle Strain

Injury to skeletal muscles from overexertion or trauma can result in muscle strain. Muscle strains involve overstretching or tearing of muscle fibers. Although the inflammation may subside in a few hours or days, repair of damaged muscle fibers usually takes weeks, and some damaged muscle cells may be replaced by fibrous tissue, forming scars.

INDICATIONS CONTRAINDICATIONS

For Soft Tissue and Movement Therapies

Direct work over the area of injury is contraindicated regionally until all signs of inflammation have dissipated. The use of ice and gentle range of

motion can support healing. Methods to manage distortion in posture resulting from compensation in the rest of the body are helpful.

Contusion

Minor trauma to the muscles may cause a muscle bruise, or contusion, that involves local internal bleeding and inflammation. Severe trauma to a skeletal muscle may cause a crush injury that damages the affected muscle tissue and releases the muscle fiber contents into the bloodstream. This can be life-threatening, because the reddish muscle pigment myoglobin can accumulate in the blood and cause kidney failure.

INDICATIONS CONTRAINDICATIONS

For Soft Tissue and Movement Therapies

Direct work over the area of injury is regionally contraindicated until all signs of inflammation have dissipated.

Muscle Infections

Several bacteria, viruses, and parasites may infect muscle tissue, often producing local or widespread myositis (muscle inflammation). Trichinosis, which is caused by a parasite, is an example of such an infection. The muscle pain and stiffness that sometimes accompany influenza are other examples of myositis.

Poliomyelitis

Poliomyelitis is a viral infection of the nerves that control skeletal muscle movement. The disease can be asymptomatic; however, it often causes paralysis that may progress to death. Virtually eliminated in the United States through an effective vaccine, polio nonetheless still affects millions around the world who have not been vaccinated.

More common is the occurrence of postpolio syndrome in people who had polio years before. The symptoms are weakness, fatigue, intolerance to cold, and general, aching pain.

INDICATIONS CONTRAINDICATIONS

For Soft Tissue and Movement Therapies

For postpolio syndrome, general constitutional approaches seem to work best to aid in overall pain reduction and restoration of the sleep pattern. Any form of therapy that causes therapeutic inflammation, including intense exercise and stretching programs, should be avoided.

Myositis Ossificans

Myositis ossificans involves an inflammatory process that stimulates the formation of osseous tissue in the fascial components of muscles. It may occur with no apparent cause or may occur secondary to a fracture or contusion. The onset of muscle pain is gradual.

INDICATIONS **CONTRAINDICATIONS**

For Soft Tissue and Movement Therapies

Treatment is regionally contraindicated in myositis ossificans.

Tendinitis and Tenosynovitis

Tendinitis is the inflammation of a tendon; tenosynovitis is the inflammation of a tendon sheath. Causes include trauma, overuse, and systemic inflammatory disease such as rheumatoid arthritis. Tendinitis is most common in the tendons crossing the shoulder, elbow, hip, knee, and ankle. Calcific tendinitis is a degenerative process in the tendon associated with the deposit of calcium salts. Early diagnosis and treatment are important.

INDICATIONS **CONTRAINDICATIONS**

For Soft Tissue and Movement Therapies

Any methods that could increase the inflammatory response are contraindicated for areas of inflammation. In the acute phase, the use of ice and gentle movement are indicated. Chronic conditions may benefit from methods that elongate the connective tissue structures, relieving friction in the area.

Cramps/Spasms

Cramps are painful muscle spasms or involuntary twitches. Cramps involve the whole muscle; spasms involve individual motor units within a muscle. Cramps often result from mild myositis or fibromyositis, but they can be a symptom of any irritation or of an electrolyte imbalance. Clonic spasms alternate contraction and relaxation in the muscle. Tonic spasms, or tetany, are sustained muscle contractions usually caused by disorders of the central nervous system.

Cramps and spasms may seem benign, but they can be symptomatic of more severe underlying conditions. If no logical reason for the cramps or spasms can be found or if they occur frequently, the client should be referred for a diagnosis.

INDICATIONS **CONTRAINDICATIONS**

For Soft Tissue and Movement Therapies

Simple cramps or spasms can be managed either by firmly pushing the belly of the muscle together or by initiating reciprocal inhibition, which involves placing the origin and insertion of the cramping muscle close together and then contracting the antagonist. The muscle is lengthened gently after the cramp or spasm has subsided.

Flaccidity and Spasticity

A muscle with decreased tone is flaccid; a muscle with excessive tone is spastic.

INDICATIONS **CONTRAINDICATIONS**

For Soft Tissue and Movement Therapies

Flaccid or spastic muscles often are associated with motor neuron disorders. The reason for the change in tone determines the appropriateness of soft tissue or movement therapy. These conditions differ from general muscle tension or weakness in that the dysfunction has a physical cause rather than a functional one.

Contracture

Contracture is the chronic shortening of a muscle, especially the connective tissue component. Volkmann's ischemic contracture occurs in the upper or lower extremity when the blood supply is cut off. It can be caused by tight casts, tourniquets, fractures, dislocations, or vascular spasms. The ischemia can lead to fibroses and can result in the contracture of the muscles, tendons, and fascia.

INDICATIONS **CONTRAINDICATIONS**

For Soft Tissue and Movement Therapies

Gentle, slow intervention using connective tissue methods and stretching may improve contractures. Applying soft tissue and movement methods may prevent or slow the development of a contracture. The reason for the contracture must be considered in developing a treatment plan for managing this condition.

Muscular Dystrophy

The term *muscular dystrophy* encompasses a group of disorders characterized by atrophy of skeletal muscles with no malfunction of the nervous system. The muscle protein dystrophin declines or is lacking. Some forms of muscular dystrophy can be fatal.

The most common form of muscular dystrophy is Duchenne's muscular dystrophy (DMD), also called *pseudohypertrophy* (meaning false muscle growth) because the atrophy of muscle is masked by excessive replacement of muscle by fat and fibrous tissue. DMD usually begins with mild leg muscle weakness that progresses rapidly to include the shoulder muscles.

The first signs of DMD become apparent at about 3 years of age, and the child usually is severely affected within 5 to 10 years. Death from respiratory or cardiac muscle weakness often occurs by the time the individual is 21 years old.

Many pathophysiologists believe that DMD is caused by a missing fragment in the X chromosome, although other factors may be involved. DMD occurs primarily in boys. Because girls have two X chromosomes and boys only one, genetic diseases involving X chromosome abnormalities are more likely to occur in boys. This is true because girls with one damaged X chromosome may not exhibit an X-linked disease if the other X chromosome is normal.

Some less devastating forms of muscular dystrophy are fascioscapulohumeral dystrophy, which affects the fascia and shoulder girdle muscles, and limb-girdle dystrophy, which affects the pelvic and shoulder girdle muscles.

INDICATIONS CONTRAINDICATIONS

For Soft Tissue and Movement Therapies

Careful intervention may slow the atrophy process. Passive and active range of motion methods not only directly affect the muscles and joints but also aid in the circulation and elimination processes. Abdominal massage may help with constipation. Methods that cause any inflammation should be avoided.

Myasthenia Gravis

Myasthenia gravis is an autoimmune disease in which the immune system attacks muscle cells at the neuromuscular junction and interferes with the action of acetylcholine. Nerve impulses from the motor neurons are then unable to stimulate the affected muscle fully.

Myasthenia gravis is a chronic disease characterized by muscle weakness, especially in the face and throat. Most forms of this disease begin with mild weakness and chronic muscle fatigue in the face, then progress to wider muscle involvement. When severe muscle weakness causes immobility in all four limbs,

the condition is called a *myasthenic crisis*. A person in myasthenic crisis is in danger of dying of respiratory failure because of weakness of the respiratory muscles.

INDICATIONS CONTRAINDICATIONS

For Soft Tissue and Movement Therapies

General constitutional methods are indicated. As with any autoimmune disease, the practitioner should avoid stressing the system and should work toward general restorative processes that reduce pain, support sleep, and create a overall sense of well-being.

Hernia

Hernias can be subcategorized into several types. Weakness of abdominal muscles is the usual cause of a hernia, or protrusion, of an abdominal organ (commonly the small intestine) through an opening in the abdominal wall. The most common type, the inguinal hernia, occurs when the hernia extends down the inguinal canal, often into the scrotum or labia. Males experience this most often, and it can occur at any age. Women may experience a femoral hernia below the groin, often caused by changes that occur during pregnancy.

A reducible hernia is one in which the protruding organ can be manipulated back into the abdominal cavity, either naturally, by lying down, or by manual reduction through a surgical opening in the abdomen. A "strangulated" hernia is one in which the hernia is not reducible, and blood flow to the affected organ (e.g., the intestine) is blocked, which may result in obstruction and gangrene. The individual usually experiences pain and vomiting, and immediate surgical repair is required.

INDICATIONS CONTRAINDICATIONS

For Soft Tissue and Movement Therapies

Treatment with a hernia is regionally contraindicated, and referral is indicated for initial diagnosis or for any change in a hernia.

Torticollis

Torticollis, or wry neck, involves a spasm or shortening of one of the sternocleidomastoid muscles. The condition may be congenital (e.g., caused by the fetal position or by a birth injury), acute (associated with cold or flu symptoms), or chronic (resulting from emotional stress, trauma, or infection).

INDICATIONS **CONTRAINDICATIONS**

For Soft Tissue and Movement Therapies

Management of torticollis with soft tissue and movement therapies involves relaxing the neck, releasing trigger points, stretching the contracted muscles, and improving range of motion. It is important to avoid pressure on the vessels under the sternocleidomastoid muscle.

Whiplash

Whiplash is an injury to the soft tissues of the neck caused by sudden hyperextension or flexion (or both) of the neck. The most common cause is an automobile accident, resulting in pain, swelling, stiffness, and spasm in the shoulders and neck. In extension injuries, the muscles most likely to be injured are the sternocleidomastoid, scalenes, infrahyoid, suprahyoid, levator scapulae, longus colli, suboccipitals, and rhomboids. In flexion injuries, the muscles most likely to be injured are the trapezius, splenius capitis, and semispinalis capitis. A side injury affects the sternocleidomastoid, suboccipitals, and levator scapulae, and the splenius capitis and cervicis. Vestibular system damage of the inner ear may result in dizziness, nausea, vomiting, headache, and gait problems.

INDICATIONS **CONTRAINDICATIONS**

For Soft Tissue and Movement Therapies

Direct intervention during the acute phase is contraindicated unless closely supervised by a physician or other qualified health professional. Soft tissue and movement methods are valuable as part of rehabilitation in the subacute phase and can help restore function if the condition is chronic. Extension injury is the more severe and requires careful intervention.

Dupuytren's Contracture

The first sign of a Dupuytren's contracture is a thickened plaque overlying the tendon of the ring finger and occasionally the little finger at the level of the distal palmar crease. The skin in this area puckers, and a thickened, fibrotic cord develops between the palm and the finger. Flexion contracture of the fingers may increase gradually.

INDICATIONS **CONTRAINDICATIONS**

For Soft Tissue and Movement Therapies

Treatment is regionally contraindicated if methods increase symptoms.

Rotator Cuff Tear

Repeated impingement, overuse, or other conditions may weaken the rotator cuff and eventually cause partial or complete tears. The condition is more common after age 40. Prior injury may increase the likelihood of a tear. Symptoms include weakness, atrophy of the supraspinatus and infraspinatus muscles, pain, and tenderness. With a complete tear of the supraspinatus tendon, active abduction at the glenohumeral joint is severely impaired. An attempt to abduct the arm instead produces a characteristic shoulder shrug.

INDICATIONS **CONTRAINDICATIONS**

For Soft Tissue and Movement Therapies

Work on myofascial tears is contraindicated. However, soft tissue and movement therapies may be indicated in the rehabilitative process and as part of a supervised treatment protocol. Compensatory patterns can be managed or improved with these methods.

Shin Splints

Shin splints are an inflammation of the proximal portion of any of the musculotendinous structures originating from the lower part of the tibia. Pain is associated with movement, and stress fractures are a common cause.

INDICATIONS **CONTRAINDICATIONS**

For Soft Tissue and Movement Therapies

Soft tissue approaches may be beneficial as long as they do not increase inflammation and a stress fracture has been ruled out.

Anterior Compartment Syndrome

The anterior compartment of the leg is surrounded by a tough fascial sheath containing the tibialis anterior, the extensor digitorum longus, the extensor hallucis longus, and the peroneus tertius muscles, as well as nerves and blood vessels. Any condition that increases pressure in this compartment interferes with blood flow and compresses the nerves. The person usually has a tight feeling in the calf, as well as pain, numbness, and tingling. Overuse, repetitive stress, and accelerated growth of the muscles are common causal factors.

INDICATIONS **CONTRAINDICATIONS**

For Soft Tissue and Movement Therapies

Treatment is regionally contraindicated unless supervised by the diagnosing or treating health care provider. Soft tissue methods may soften the connective tissue sheath, relieving some of the pressure, but they also could aggravate the inflammatory process. Massage methods can relieve fluid congestion, but by enhancing circulation, they also could increase blood flow to the area, thus increasing the pressure. Elevation and ice may help.

Plantar Fasciitis

Plantar fasciitis is an inflammation of the plantar fascia and surrounding myofascial structures. The disorder is caused by excessive stress on the foot, especially near the attachment of the fascia to the calcaneus. The stress causes calcium to be deposited at the site, and often a spur forms. Pain in the heel is worse when the person is moving, and dorsiflexion increases the pain.

INDICATIONS CONTRAINDICATIONS

For Soft Tissue and Movement Therapies

Acute-phase plantar fasciitis responds to rest and ice. After the inflammation has diminished, soft tissue methods that address the connective tissue and judicial use of stretching are beneficial. NOTE: If the client is taking antiinflammatory or pain medication, feedback mechanisms will be inaccurate.

Fibromyalgia

Fibromyalgia is a syndrome with symptoms of widespread pain or aching, persistent fatigue, generalized morning stiffness, nonrestorative sleep, and multiple tender points. The symptoms often are found in conjunction with headaches, irritable bladder, dysmenorrhea, cold sensitivity, Raynaud's phenomenon, restless legs, atypical patterns of numbness and tingling, and complaints of weakness. The onset usually is gradual, often following prolonged exposure to damp cold, a bacterial or viral infection, or prolonged physical or emotional stress. Chronic fatigue syndrome also may be present.

A disrupted sleep pattern, coupled with the dysfunction of myofascial repair mechanisms, seems to be a factor. Treatment protocols are aimed at sleep restoration and a gradual rebuilding of the myofas-

cial system. Diet and lifestyle changes, moderate exercise, and various forms of complementary therapies and body/mind approaches are beneficial. If necessary, low-dose antidepressants often can help restore sleep patterns.

INDICATIONS CONTRAINDICATIONS

For Soft Tissue and Movement Therapies

General constitutional approaches seem to work best to aid in symptomatic pain reduction and restoration of the sleep pattern. Any form of therapy that causes therapeutic inflammation, including intense exercise and stretching programs, should be avoided until healing mechanisms in the body are functioning. When exercise programs are introduced, the process needs to be gentle and slow. If tender points have been injected with antiinflammatory medications, anesthetics, or other substances, do not massage over the area.

Acquired Metabolic and Toxic Myopathies

Acquired metabolic myopathies often occur secondary to disorders of the endocrine system. Nutritional and vitamin deficiency, especially protein deficiency and lack of vitamins C, D, and E, may lead to myopathy.

Toxic myopathies are related to certain drugs and chemicals. Corticosteroid therapy may cause steroid-induced muscle weakness. An excessive alcohol intake can result in break down of striated muscles, which can affect the skeletal and other muscles.

INDICATIONS CONTRAINDICATIONS

For Soft Tissue and Movement Therapies

Treatment for these types of myopathy usually is not contraindicated, as long as the therapeutic approaches are general and focus on supporting body restoration and the healing processes. Regional avoidance of steroid injection sites is indicated.

Soft tissue and movement approaches can support detoxification efforts, because circulation is enhanced by these methods. Care must be taken in toxic conditions not to tax an already overloaded system. The general therapeutic approach of "less is more," over a longer period, is indicated.

Summary

This chapter has taken an in-depth look at the muscular system. Individual muscles have been explored, and the interdependent nature of muscular action has been mapped in each muscle's synergist and antagonist pattern. Common trigger points and their referred pain patterns were identified. The progression of pathologic conditions in muscle dysfunction was discussed, as were the indications and contraindications for soft tissue and movement therapies for specific muscle-related dysfunctions.

The larger picture of dynamic movement is explored in the next chapter, where all the parts—bones, joints, and muscles—are seen as a functioning unit, which is more than the sum of its parts.

WORKBOOK SECTION

WORKBOOK SECTION

1. List and describe the functions of muscles.

_____

_____

_____

_____

_____

_____

_____

_____

_____

_____

_____

_____

_____

_____

_____

2. List and describe the three types of muscles.

_____

_____

_____

_____

_____

_____

_____

_____

_____

_____

_____

_____

3. List and describe the three types of skeletal muscle fibers.

_____

_____

_____

_____

_____

_____

_____

_____

_____

_____

_____

_____

_____

4. List and describe the four components of myotatic units.

_____

_____

_____

_____

_____

_____

_____

_____

_____

_____

_____

FILL IN THE BLANK

An agonist is a muscle that causes or controls joint motion through a specified plane of motion and is also known as a primary or _____ (1) mover.

The _____ (2) occurs when a muscle contraction is initiated and all of the muscle fibers contract to their full ability, or they do not contract at all.

An _____ (3) is a muscle that usually is located on the opposite side of the joint from the agonist and that has the opposite action.

Contractility is the ability of a muscle to _____ (4) forcibly with adequate stimulation.

_____ (5) forms a coarse sheet of fibrous connective tissue that binds muscles into functional groups and forms partitions, called *intermuscular septa,* between muscle groups.

Dynamic force produces _____ (6) in or of an object.

Elasticity is the ability of a muscle to recoil and resume its original resting length after being _____ (7).

_____ (8) is the ability of a muscle to receive and respond to a stimulus.

_____ (9) is the ability of a muscle to be stretched or extended.

A _____ (10) contracts to stabilize an area, enabling another limb or body segment to exert force and move.

The insertion is the most movable part of a muscle, or the part that attaches _____ (11) from the midline or center of the body.

Maximal stimulus is the point at which all the motor units of a muscle have been recruited and the muscle is unable to _____ (12) in strength.

A _____ (13) consists of the muscle fibers innervated by a single motor neuron.

The _____ (14) is the part of a muscle considered the least movable, or the part that attaches closest to the midline or center of the body.

Oxygen debt is the extra amount of oxygen that must be taken in to convert _____ (15) to glucose or glycogen.

_____ (16) force applied to an object does not produce movement.

Synergist muscles aid or assist the action of the agonists but are not primarily responsible for the action; synergists are also known as _____ (17) muscles.

The _____ _____ (18) is the stimulus at which the first observable muscle contraction occurs.

Tone is a state of slight _____ (19) in all skeletal muscle that enables the muscle to respond to stimulation.

A trigger point, as described by Dr. Janet Travell, is a _____ (20) locus within a taut band of skeletal muscle, located in the muscular tissue or its associated fascia, or both. The spot is painful on compression and can evoke characteristic _____ (21) pain and autonomic phenomena.

PROBLEM SOLVING

Read the problem presented. There is no correct answer; rather, the exercise is intended to assist the student in developing the analytic and decision-making skills necessary in a professional practice.

1. Identify the facts presented in the information.
2. Identify the possibilities ("what if" statements) or develop your own possibilities that relate to the facts.
3. Evaluate each possibility in terms of the logical cause and effect and pros and cons.
4. Consider the feelings of the people involved.
5. Write down each in the space provided.
6. Develop your solution by answering the question posed.

PROBLEM

Bodywork professionals focus on the muscular system as they work with clients. Therefore thinking in terms of individual muscles certainly seems logical when working with assessment...or is it? This chapter described the way muscles work in functional units. Muscles are controlled by the nervous system. Connective tissue is a huge component of muscles. Muscle tension increases with sympathetic arousal, as is seen in the fight-or-flight response. Is it possible that bodywork really has very little to do with muscle tissue?

Many testing processes focus extensively on the functional aspect of individual muscles and very little on the more systemic effects of bodywork. This situation may influence the curriculum at schools that teach bodywork therapies. One wonders if such an education may overemphasize the study of individual muscles and underemphasize the nervous system, endocrine system, and systemic homeostatic processes. The study of muscles is important. It is true that functional patterns of movement are really understood only when the practitioner has a solid comprehension of the components of movement—the bones, the joints, the connective tissue, and the muscles. It also is true that the major benefits of massage are based in the systems of control.

QUESTION

In this age of "too much to know," what learning is necessary to function as a health professional?

FACTS

1. Bodywork professionals focus on the muscular system.

2. _____

   _____

3. _____

   _____

POSSIBILITIES

1. Curricula at schools that teach bodywork therapies may be influenced by examination requirements.

2. _____

   _____

3. _____

   _____

LOGICAL CAUSE AND EFFECT

1. Important areas of study are not covered effectively because of lack of time.

2. _____

   _____

3. _____

   _____

IMPACT ON PEOPLE

1. Students may be frustrated with studying information that seems less important.

2. _____

   _____

3. _____

   _____

In this age of "too much to know," what learning is necessary to function as a health professional?

_____

_____

_____

PROFESSIONAL APPLICATION

What additional knowledge base would one need to work stress-induced muscle tension and headache soft tissue and movement therapies? Where might a practitioner find this information and get additional training?

_____

_____

_____

_____

_____

_____

_____

_____

_____

_____

_____

_____

_____

_____

_____

_____

_____

FURTHER STUDY

Using a comprehensive anatomy and physiology text (see Works Consulted list at the back of this book), find the chapter that pertains to the information presented in this chapter. As a study guide, locate the information presented in this text and then elaborate by writing a paragraph of additional information on each of the following topics.

1. Force

_____

_____

_____

_____

_____

_____

_____

2. Motor points

_____

_____

_____

_____

_____

_____

_____

3. Repair of muscle

_____

_____

_____

_____

_____

_____

_____

4. Cardiac muscle

_____

_____

_____

_____

_____

_____

_____

5. Smooth muscle

_____

_____

_____

_____

_____

_____

_____

Answer Key

1. Muscles produce movement, generate heat, maintain posture, and stabilize joints.

   All three types of muscle tissue provide the movement necessary for survival. Skeletal muscle moves the limbs. Skeletal, cardiac, and smooth muscle all produce movements such as those involved in breathing, heartbeat, digestion, and elimination.

   The relative constancy of the body's internal temperature could not be maintained in a cool external environment if not for the "waste" heat generated by muscle tissue during contraction.

   Maintenance of a relatively stable body posture is the primary function of the skeletal muscular system. The dynamic tension of muscle contraction opposes the forces of gravity.

   Stability of the joint structures is an often overlooked function of muscle. Especially in the more mobile joints, which by nature have a loose structural design, the dynamic contraction of muscles surrounding the joint provides external stability, supporting the structures of the joint proper.

2. Skeletal, cardiac, and smooth muscle

   Skeletal muscle fibers are long, cylindric, tapered cells that have cross-striations caused by the contractile structure inside. Skeletal muscles contain white, red, and intermediate muscle fibers. Each individual muscle fiber is wrapped by several different layers of connective tissue.

   Cardiac muscle is found in only one organ of the body, the heart. Cardiac muscle fiber does not taper, as does skeletal muscle fiber, but instead forms strong, electrically coupled junctions (intercalated disks) with other fibers. Cardiac muscles form a continuous contractile band around the heart.

   Smooth muscle comprises small, tapered cells with single nuclei. Because the myofilaments are not organized into sarcomeres, they have more freedom of movement and can contract a smooth muscle fiber to shorter lengths than can be done in skeletal and cardiac muscle.

3. White (fast twitch) fibers contract more rapidly and forcefully, are larger than red fibers, and belong to larger motor units that fire when the nervous system demands rapid, powerful motion. They do not require much oxygen to contract and are considered anaerobic. White fibers fatigue quickly.

   Red (slow twitch) fibers are smaller, contract more slowly and weakly, and belong to smaller motor units that respond during slower, delicate movements. Red fibers contain much larger quantities of myoglobin, require the presence of oxygen for contraction, and are considered aerobic. They do not fatigue quickly and can hold a contraction for a relatively long period.

   Intermediate fibers combine the qualities of both red and white fibers, allowing a rapid, moderately forceful contraction and providing moderate fatigue resistance.

4. Agonists: Muscles that cause or control joint motion through a specified plane of motion

   Synergists: Muscles that aid or assist the action of the agonists

   Antagonists: Muscles that usually are located on the opposite side of the joint from the agonist and have the opposite action

   Fixators (stabilizers): Muscles that surround the joint or body part and contract to fixate or stabilize the area to enable another limb or body segment to exert force and move

FILL IN THE BLANK

1. prime
2. all-or-none response
3. antagonist
4. shorten
5. Deep fascia
6. movement
7. stretched
8. Excitability
9. Extensibility
10. fixator
11. farthest

12. increase
13. motor unit
14. origin
15. lactic acid
16. Static
17. guiding
18. threshold stimulus
19. contraction
20. hyperirritable
21. referred

Chapter 10

Biomechanics Basics

CHAPTER OUTLINE

KEY TERMS

Center of gravity An imaginary midpoint or center of the weight of a body or object; it is where the body or object could balance on a point

Concentric contraction The action of a prime mover or agonist where a muscle develops tension as it shortens to provide enough force to overcome resistance

Eccentric contraction The action of an antagonist where a muscle lengthens while under tension and changes in tension to control the descent of the resistance; eccentric contractions may be thought of as controlling movement against gravity or resistance and are described as negative contractions

Effort The force applied to overcome resistance

Gait The rhythmic and alternating motions of the legs, trunk, and arms resulting in the propulsion of the body

Gait cycle Subdivided into the stance phase and swing phase, this cycle begins when the heel of one foot strikes the floor and continues until the same heel strikes the floor again

Isometric contraction The action of the prime mover that occurs when tension develops within the muscle but no appreciable change occurs in the joint angle or the length of the muscle; movement does not occur

Isotonic contraction The action of the prime mover that occurs when tension is developed in the muscle while it either shortens or lengthens

Lever A solid mass such as a crowbar or a person's arm that rotates around a fixed point called the *fulcrum;* the rotation is produced by a force applied to a lever at some distance from the fulcrum

Biomechanics

Biomechanics is the study of mechanical principles and actions applied to living bodies. Because the human body may be acted on by a variety of forces that can lead to movement, rest, or stress, it is important that the soft tissue and movement therapist have a basic understanding of biomechanical principles. Understanding these principles helps us in both the assessment and observation of the body and in clinical reasoning methods used to set up treatment plans.

Those who deal with the specific and rehabilitative analysis of human movement such as physical therapists, occupational therapists, and athletic trainers undertake extended studies to address problems with biomechanics or develop specific training protocols. These professionals are excellent to use for referring clients who have movement problems beyond the basics presented in this textbook.

Movement is a fundamental characteristic of human behavior. It is accomplished by contraction of skeletal muscles acting within a system of levers and pulleys formed by bones, tendons, and ligaments.

Muscles have properties permitting a large range of function to meet various demands; these demands may require the coordination of complex interactions. Sometimes muscles are required to function for long periods without fatiguing, and at other times muscles must provide maximal effort for only a few seconds. Movement is a desirable quality but so is stability in maintaining posture. Muscles must shorten to provide range of movement at joints, yet they must generate enough power to move a load at each end of the range. The fine control of muscle contraction over a wide range of lengths, tensions, speeds, and loads is accomplished by the nervous system.

As discussed in Chapter 9, muscles differ in fiber type depending on the function of the muscle. Compared with red fibers, white fast-twitch fibers contract more rapidly and forcefully, are larger, and belong to larger motor units that fire when the nervous system demands rapid, powerful motion. They do not require much oxygen to contract and are considered anaerobic. They fatigue quickly. Red twitch fibers are smaller, contract more slowly and with less strength, and belong to smaller motor units that respond during slower delicate movements. Red fibers contain much larger quantities of myoglobin, require the presence of oxygen for contraction, and are considered aerobic. They do not fatigue quickly and can hold a contraction for a relatively long period. Intermediate fibers combine the qualities of both red and white fibers to allow a rapid, moderate force contraction and moderate fatigue resistance.

TYPES OF MUSCLE CONTRACTION

Because muscles are made of a variety of fiber types, they can contract in different ways depending on the demand. Muscle contractions are classified as isometric or isotonic.

Isometric Contraction

An **isometric contraction** occurs when tension develops within a muscle but no appreciable change occurs in the joint angle or the length of the muscle. In other words, no movement occurs. Isometric contractions are static contractions because large amounts of tension develop in the muscle to maintain the joint angle in a relatively static or stable position. Fixing or stabilizing a proximal joint so that a distal joint can move is an example of the way isometric contractions are used in the body. Isometric contractions maintain upright posture.

Isotonic Contraction

An **isotonic contraction** occurs when tension develops in the muscle while it either shortens or lengthens. Isotonic contractions are dynamic contractions because the varying degrees of tension in the muscle cause the joint angles to change. Isotonic contractions produce movement. Isotonic muscle contractions can be classified as either *concentric* or *eccentric* on the basis of whether shortening or lengthening occurs.

In a **concentric contraction** the muscle develops tension as it shortens, and the contraction develops enough force to overcome any applied resistance. Concentric contractions cause movement against gravity or resistance and are described as being positive contractions. Concentric contractions occur as the angle of the joint decreases. An example is the biceps curl, in which a weight is lifted toward the shoulder by bending the elbow.

Eccentric contractions take place when the muscle lengthens while under tension and changes in tension to control the descent of the resistance. Eccentric contractions control movement with gravity or resistance and are described as negative contractions. Eccentric contractions happen as an antagonist pattern lengthens in a controlled fashion in response to a concentric contraction. The muscle

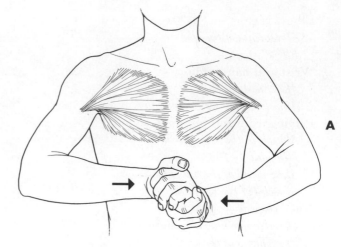

FIGURE 10-1 A, Isometric exercise. Muscle activity with no change in length. No work is performed. (From Greenstein GM: *Clinical assessment of neuromusculoskeletal disorders,* St Louis, 1997, Mosby.)

slowly yields to resistance, allowing itself to be stretched. Eccentric contractions occur as the angle of a joint increases. The amount of tension may increase or decrease, depending on the weight of the object providing the resistance to gravity. An example is the reverse of the aforementioned biceps curl such as when a weight is lowered from the shoulder by extending the elbow. The triceps, which is the prime mover, is doing some of the work while the eccentric contraction of the biceps keeps the movement under control. If the object is light, the biceps decreases in tension as it extends. If the weight is substantial, the biceps increases in tension (Figure 10-1, *A* to *C*).

CENTER OF GRAVITY

The concept of "center" has many meanings. In Eastern thought the importance of being centered is often expressed as being present in the moment and responding resourcefully to each unfolding second of life.

In biomechanical terms the concept of center refers to the center of gravity. The **center of gravity** is the midpoint, or center, of the weight of a body or object. It is where the body or object would balance on a point.

There is no anatomic center of gravity. The position of the center of gravity depends on the arrangement of the body segments and changes with every movement. The center of gravity is just as situational as being centered in terms of Eastern thought, and the principles are similar. Whether centered in biome-

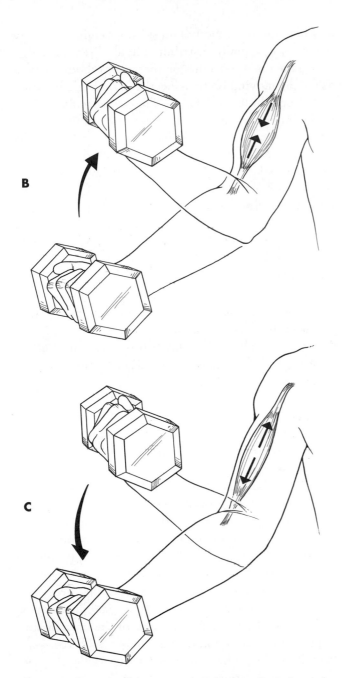

FIGURE 10-1—cont'd B, Concentric muscle activity. Muscle shortens during tension production. **C,** Eccentric muscle activity. Muscle lengthens during tension production.

chanical terms or in life, we have the ability to respond resourcefully to each event as it happens. Any loss of biomechanical stability such as occurs with a missing limb or altered posture will not only alter the total body weight distribution but also the center of gravity. Most of us can understand the way losses in life change our sense of center and reveal our human potential to alter, accommodate, and adjust to change.

Accumulated postural or movement alterations can stress the entire system, initiating a change process that can progress toward dysfunction. Although each alteration may seem to be appropriate to the moment, the accumulation of the chain reaction of change can become too much and the system breaks under the inefficient function. The sense of center is lost. Understanding biomechanics helps us to be able to reverse the degeneration process and move toward efficient functioning.

FORCE

Force causes change. Forces either push or pull on an object in an attempt to affect motion or shape. The human body moves under the influence of and is affected by both internal and external forces. Within the body, forces are mainly produced by the contraction of muscles. External forces acting on the body include gravity and forces generated by the interaction with external objects such as lifting a box or managing an umbrella in the wind. Soft tissue and movement therapies attempt to alter body function by exerting external force to generate internal forces that then effect change in the homeostatic mechanisms of the body.

Force is the product of mass times acceleration. Mass is the amount of matter or material substance that forms or composes a body. For our purposes, weight and mass can be seen as the same. The weight times the speed or acceleration determines the amount of force. A light feather floating softly down to touch our arm exerts less force than a bowling ball thrown down an alley.

The following elements influence or are related to force:

Pressure—Pressure is the amount of force on a specific area.
Inertia—Inertia is the reluctance of matter to change its state of motion. It can be understood as the lack of desire to shut off the TV and begin doing the reading in this text. Many of us waste energy going to the refrigerator, looking out the window, or listening to the conversations of others as we try to study. Because force is required to change inertia, any activity that is carried out at a steady pace, in a consistent direction, will conserve energy. Any irregularly paced or multidirectional activity will be costly to energy reserves. A movement example is handball, which is more fatiguing than dancing. There is a pearl of wisdom in the understanding of

force acting on matter to change motion. Starts and stops and juggling many different tasks at one time is fatiguing and stressful. Life lived at a steady pace with a sense of direction or purpose conserves, focuses, and supports effectiveness.

Acceleration—Acceleration is the rate of change in speed. To begin to move the body and attain speed, a strong muscular force is generally necessary. Weight (mass) coupled with the influence of gravity affects speed and acceleration during physical movements. It takes more muscle force to accelerate a 200-pound adult than a 100-pound child. Acceleration occurs in the same direction as the force that caused it. The change in acceleration is directly proportional to the force causing it and inversely proportional to the mass of the body. This means that a large force will provide a greater degree of acceleration than a small force. Given the same amount of force, more acceleration will occur on a light body than on a heavy one.

Newton's law of reaction says that for every action, there is an opposite and equal reaction. As we place force on the floor by walking over it, the floor provides an equal resistance back in the opposite direction to the soles of our feet. It is easier to walk on a wood floor than on a sandy beach because of the difference in the reaction of the two surfaces. The wood floor resists the weight and pushes back, making walking easier, whereas the sand dissipates the force and requires more effort with each step.

BALANCE, EQUILIBRIUM, AND STABILITY

Balance is the ability to control equilibrium. The two types of balance are static, or still, balance and dynamic, or moving, balance. *Equilibrium* refers to a state of zero acceleration where no change occurs in the speed or direction of the body. Equilibrium may be either static or dynamic. If the body is at rest or completely motionless, it is in static equilibrium. Dynamic equilibrium occurs when all of the applied and internal forces acting on the moving body are in balance, resulting in movement with no change in speed or direction. For us to control equilibrium to achieve balance, we need to maximize stability.

Stability is the resistance to change in the body's acceleration or the resistance to the disturbance of the body's equilibrium. Stability may be enhanced by determining the body's center of gravity and changing it appropriately. The center of gravity is the point

at which all of the body's mass and weight is equally balanced or equally distributed in all directions.

Balance is important for the resting body as well as for the moving body. Kinesthetic physiologic functions contribute to balance. The semicircular canals of the inner ear, vision, touch, pressure, and proprioceptive sense all provide balance information. The body is in a constant dynamic state of adjustment to maintain balance, reflecting dynamic homeostasis.

Balance Principles

Basic principles of balance have application in a very broad sense. The following principles speak not only of a body in balance but also of a balanced life, if applied to a social or personal realm:

A person is balanced when his center of gravity falls within the base of support.

A person is balanced in direct proportion to the size of the base of support. The larger the base of support, the more balance.

A person is balanced depending on his weight or mass. The greater the weight, the more balance.

A person's balance depends on the height of the center of gravity. The lower the center of gravity, the more balance.

A person's balance depends on where his center of gravity is in relation to the base of support. If the center of gravity is near the edge of the base, less balance is present. However, in anticipation of an oncoming force, stability may be improved by placing the center of gravity nearer the side of the base of support expected to receive the force.

In anticipation of an oncoming force, stability may be increased by enlarging the size of the base of support in the direction of the anticipated force.

Equilibrium may be enhanced by increasing the friction between the body and the surface it contacts.

Rotation around an axis is easier to balance. A bike that is moving is easier to balance than a bike that is stationary (Thompson, Floyd, 1994)(Activity 10-1).

Posture

The postural muscles help us to maintain our upright position in gravity. This is an awesome task because the center of gravity constantly changes with each movement. When we lie down, we relieve the postural muscles of this task.

Walking is an activity in which a person moves his body into and out of balance with each step. When standing and while walking, our center of gravity is

Draw a picture to illustrate each of the principles of balance.

A person is balanced when his center of gravity falls within the base of support.

A person is balanced in direct proportion to the size of the base of support. The larger the base of support, the more balance.

A person is balanced depending on his weight or mass. The greater the weight, the more balance.

A person's balance depends on the height of the center of gravity. The lower the center of gravity, the more balance.

A person's balance depends on where his center of gravity is in relation to the base of support. If the center of gravity is near the edge of the base, there is less balance. However, when anticipating an oncoming force, stability may be improved by placing the center of gravity nearer the side of the base of support expected to receive the force.

In anticipation of an oncoming force, stability may be increased by enlarging the size of the base of support in the direction of the anticipated force.

Equilibrium may be enhanced by increasing the friction between the body and the surface it contacts.

Rotation around an axis is easier to balance. A bike that is moving is easier to balance than a bike that is stationary.

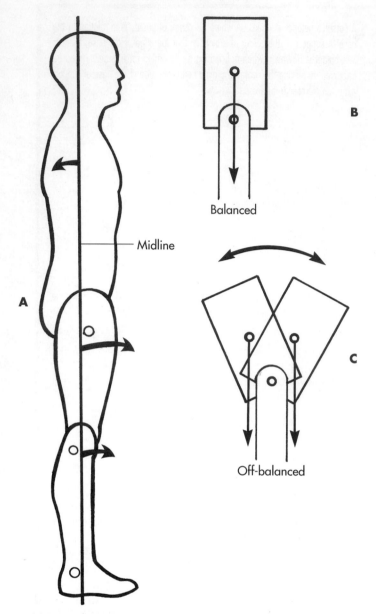

FIGURE 10-2 A, In normal relaxed standing, the leg and trunk tend to rotate slightly off the midline of the body but maintain a counterbalance force. Balance is achieved in **B** and not in **C.** Any time the trunk moves off this midline balance point, the body must compensate. (From Fritz S: *Mosby's fundamentals of therapeutic massage,* St Louis, 1995, Mosby.)

and, because of its weight, this movement takes the whole body with it. Effort is needed at the beginning of the action. Once started, movement takes on a life of its own.

The same principle can be applied to a moving car. A car needs the most power when it starts off from a stationary position and relatively little energy to keep it going at a constant speed. Our amazing bodies help us move, not by requiring increased force but by using our head to initiate the movement. "Lead all movement with your head" is more than just a biomechanically correct statement (Figure 10-2)!

LEVERS AND FULCRUMS

We need force to generate a motion in a straight line and produce rotation or angular motion. This is often achieved with the use of a lever, which helps a given effort move a heavier load or move a load farther than could otherwise be done. A **lever** is a rigid bar or mass that rotates around a fixed point called the *axis of rotation* or *fulcrum.* Rotation is then produced by a force applied to a lever at some distance from the fulcrum. The locomotion system of the human body may be considered a series of interconnected levers. In the forearm the radius and ulna can be viewed as a lever, with the elbow joint as the fulcrum (Figure 10-3).

A force applied to a lever to overcome resistance is called the **effort.**

In the forearm during elbow flexion against resistance, the effort is the force exerted by the muscles. The applied force, or effort, can be used to move a resistance or load such as when lifting a box.

In the body, joints are the fulcrums and bones are the levers. The effort is provided by muscle contraction and is applied at the muscle attachment points on a bone. The load that is moved includes the bone, the overlying tissues, and anything else you are trying to move with that particular lever, such as your bookbag.

Regardless of the type, all levers follow the same basic principles:

Effort nearer to the load than to the fulcrum produces mechanical disadvantage.

Effort farther from the load than from the fulcrum produces mechanical advantage.

In lever systems that operate at a mechanical disadvantage, force is lost but speed is gained.

In lever systems that operate at a mechanical advantage are slower, more stable, and are used where strength is a priority.

located in our pelvis at the upper sacral region anterior to the second sacral vertebra. Our head is balanced on top of the spine and the center of gravity for the head is in front of the ear by the cheek. The exact location of the center of gravity varies.

The pivot point for movement of the head is behind the center of gravity. This means that posterior occipital and cervical muscles must exert force to hold the head up. The benefit to this is that to begin forward movement, all a person has to do is relax the muscles at the back of the head. The head will move forward

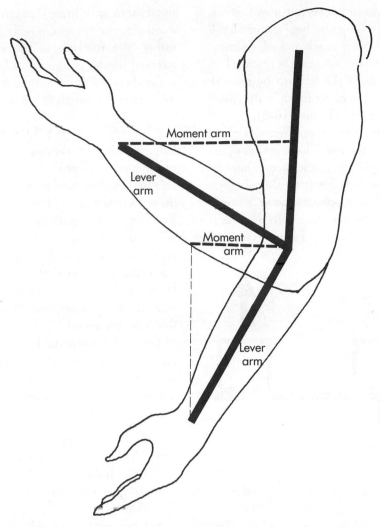

FIGURE 10-3 A lever is a rigid body that moves around a fixed axis. The lever arm will remain the same throughout the movement, but the moment arm for the lever may change as the lever moves. (From Roberts SL, Falkenburg SA: *Biomechanics: problem solving for functional activity,* St Louis, 1992, Mosby.)

Three types of levers exist: first class, second class, and third class.

In first-class levers the effort is applied at one end of the lever and the load is at the other with the fulcrum somewhere between them. Seesaws, scissors, and crowbars are familiar examples of first-class levers. Use of a first-class lever occurs when you lift your head off your chest. Some first-class levers in the body operate at a mechanical advantage when the effort is farther from the joint than the load and is less than the load to be moved. But other muscles operate at mechanical disadvantage when the effort is closer to the joint and greater than the load to be moved (Figure 10-4).

In second-class levers the effort is applied at the end of the lever and the fulcrum is located at the other end with the load at some intermediate point

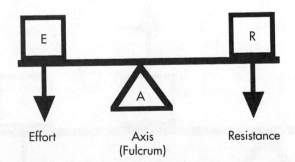

FIGURE 10-4 A first-class lever has its axis of motion between the force of effort and the force of resistance. (From Roberts SL, Falkenburg SA: *Biomechanics: problem solving for functional activity,* St Louis, 1992, Mosby.)

between them. A wheelbarrow is an example of this type of lever. Second-class levers are uncommon in the body and the best example of their use is standing on your toes. Joints forming the ball of the foot act together as the fulcrum. The load is the entire body weight. The calf muscles inserted into the calcaneus exert the effort, pulling the heel upward. All second-class levers in the body work at a mechanical advantage because the muscle insertion is always farther from the fulcrum than is the load to be moved. Second-class levers are levers of strength, with speed and range of motion sacrificed (Figure 10-5).

In third-class levers the effort is applied at a point between the load and the fulcrum. These levers operate with greater speed and always at a mechanical disadvantage. Tweezers or forceps provide this type of leverage. Most of the body operates with a third-class lever system that permits a muscle to be inserted very close to a joint, allowing rapid extensive

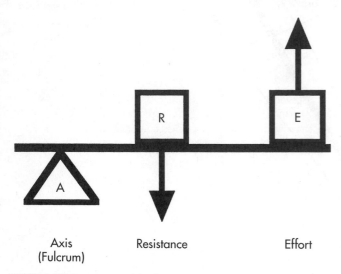

Axis
(Fulcrum)   Resistance   Effort

FIGURE 10-5 In a second-class lever the force of resistance lies between the axis of movement and the force of effort. (From Roberts SL, Falkenburg SA: *Biomechanics: problem solving for functional activity,* St Louis, 1992, Mosby.)

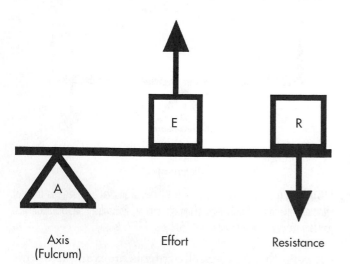

Axis
(Fulcrum)   Effort   Resistance

FIGURE 10-6 A third-class lever has its force of effort lying between the axis and the force of resistance. (From Roberts SL, Falkenburg SA: *Biomechanics: problem solving for functional activity,* St Louis, 1992, Mosby.)

movement with little shortening of the muscle. As an example, the biceps muscle of the arm provides the effort, the fulcrum is the elbow, and the force is exerted on the proximal radius. The load to be lifted is the distal forearm and anything carried in the hand or over the forearm (Figure 10-6).

WALKING/GAIT

Locomotion, or walking, is the act of moving from one place to another. Gait is the means of achieving this action. Despite years of scientific study we still do not know exactly how we stand upright and walk. The question remains as to how much of locomotion is innate and how much is learned. Humans are certainly driven to walk. Most authorities agree that both the urge and the "hard-wiring" for bipedal (two-leg) locomotion is born in us, and the coordination of all the components necessary to accomplish the task is learned.

Controlling bipedal locomotion is not an easy task. Reflexive coordination by the central nervous system is an essential part of the walking pattern. The central nervous system coordinates muscles to generate the locomotion pattern through the following actions:

- Producing appropriate propulsive forces
- Modulating changes in the center of gravity
- Coordinating multilimb trajectories
- Adapting to changing conditions and joint positions
- Coordinating visual, auditory, vestibular, peripheral afferent information, and the viscoelastic properties of muscles

Understanding these reflex patterns is an important part of understanding gait. Because most reflex actions involve a great many reflex arcs, local stimulation of a small number of receptors leads to a large number of outgoing impulses to muscles and glands. The result is a widespread and generalized reflex response. Most reflexes are polysynaptic, using many sensory neurons, interneurons, and motor neurons. Breaking down these complex patterns is often difficult but can be a clinical necessity if we are to understand the automatic and sometimes perpetuating responses of both dysfunctional and functional reflex patterns that interact in the body's ongoing attempt to maintain homeostasis. This process can be simplified with an understanding of gait and posture.

When we walk, peripheral receptors in our joints and muscles detect changes in muscle length and force, joint position, and weight-bearing status of the limbs. The relationship between the walk and the independent use of the arm/hand complex depends on the task and environment. Watching toddlers as they start to walk clearly reveals that from the very beginning, walking is counterbalanced by activity of the arms and hands. It is this counterbalancing action that becomes important in understanding the complex system of reflex control of gait patterns.

Normal Adult Walking Cycle

Simply stated, we walk around on two legs comprised of three segments each: the thigh, shank (lower leg), and the foot. On top of our legs are the trunk, head, and arms. The whole arm unit is used as a counterbalance and for momentum and moves opposite the leg movement. This pattern is linked by the contralateral reflex arc mechanism.

Flexion and extension of the hip joints cause some rotation in the lumbar spine, and to keep the head facing forward, the thorax and cervical spine rotate in the opposite direction. This action is coordinated by reflex patterns that coordinate upright posture in gravity and righting reflexes that keep the eyes on a level plane and the head oriented to the trunk. Reciprocal movements of the upper and lower limbs occur with the right upper limb flexing at the shoulder joint simultaneous with flexion at the left hip joint. Normally, the shoulder joint starts to flex or extend slightly before the same movement is seen in the elbow joint. These movements again serve to keep the head and trunk oriented and counterbalance the body weight in gravity.

🖐 PRACTICAL APPLICATION

Dysfunctional patterns can often be traced through these basic reflex principles. For example, a client complains of a stiff left shoulder. He cannot remember how he hurt the area but can remember walking around an amusement park with a blister on his right heel. This dysfunctional pattern may be the result of a change in gait, developed from an alteration in the reciprocal counterbalancing pattern, which eventually led to the shoulder pain. The shoulder difficulty may be relieved by addressing neuromuscular tension patterns in the right leg and hip. Many such patterns could develop. A bodywork practitioner, paying attention to the reflex pattern operating in the body, could more effectively manage this type of soft tissue dysfunction.

Gait Cycle

Gait is defined as the rhythmic and alternating movement of the legs along with the trunk and the arms, which results in the propulsion of the body mass. Gait is an automatic function coordinated by both innate and learned reflexes. Muscles certainly work together to produce movement, but it is interesting to note that in large portions of the gait cycle little or no muscle activity occurs in the most of the muscle groups, pointing to the energy-efficient nature of walking.

A **gait cycle** is the period during which a complete sequence of events takes place; it begins when the heel of one foot strikes the floor. The gait cycle is subdivided into the stance phase and swing phase. The stance phase occurs when the limb under consideration is in contact with the floor. In walking, there is always a period of time when both feet are in contact with the floor; this is called *double stance*. The swing phase occurs when the foot is not in contact with the floor.

In the average walking pattern the stance phase takes about 60% of the gait cycle and the swing phase about 40%. As the speed of walking, or cadence, increases, the length of time in the stance phase decreases. Double stance time increases with slow walking.

The components of the stance phase are: Heel strike, foot flat, midstance, heel-off, and toe-off (Figure 10-7, *A* to *E*).

The components of the swing phase are acceleration, midswing, deceleration, and arm swing (Figure 10-8, *A* to *D*).

Heel strike = Initial contact

Hip	25° Flexion	Hip extensors eccentrically
Knee	0°	Quadriceps concentrically
Ankle	0°	Tibials concentrically

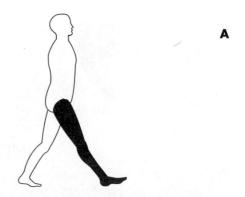

A

FIGURE 10-7 A, Components of the stance phase.

Foot Flat = Loading Response

Hip   26° Flexion   Hip extensors eccentrically and hip abductors isometrically

Knee   15° Flexion   Quadriceps eccentrically

Ankle   10° Plantar flexion   Pretibials eccentrically

B

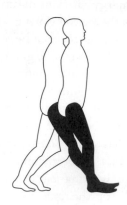

Midstance = Midstance

- The body (center of gravity) reaches its highest point in the gait cycle

Hip   0°   Hip abductors isometrically

Knee   0°   Quadriceps concentrically initially, then no muscle activity

Ankle   0°   Plantar flexors (calf) eccentrically

C

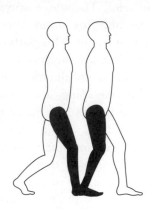

Heel-Off = Terminal Stance

Hip   20° Hip hyperextension   No muscle activity

Knee   0°   No muscle activity

Ankle   10° Dorsiflexion   Plantar flexors (calf) eccentrically

D

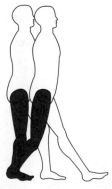

Toe-Off = Preswing

Hip   0°   Adductor longus

Knee   40° Knee flexion   No muscle activity

Ankle   20° Plantar flexion   Plantar flexors concentrically initially, then no muscle activity

E

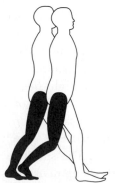

FIGURE 10-7—cont'd **B** to **E,** Components of the stance phase.

Acceleration = Initial swing

Hip	15° Hip flexion	Hip flexors concentrically
Knee	60° Knee flexion	Knee flexors concentrically
Ankle	10° Plantar flexion	Tibials concentrically

A

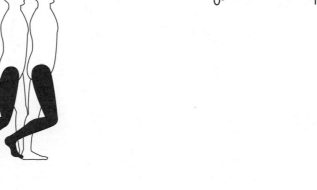

Midswing = Midswing

25° Hip flexion	Hip flexors concentrically initially, then hamstrings eccentrically
25° Knee flexion	Knee extension is created by momentum a gravity and short head of biceps femoris control rate of knee extension through e control
0°	Tibials concentrically

B

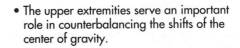

Deceleration = Terminal swing

Hip	25° Flexion	Hamstrings eccentrically
Knee	0°	Quadriceps concentrically to insure knee extension and hamstrings are active eccentrically to decelerate the leg
Ankle	0°	Tibials concentrically

C

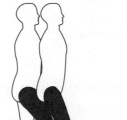

Arm swing

- The upper extremities serve an important role in counterbalancing the shifts of the center of gravity.

- A reciprocal arm swing is seen in a mature gait (e.g., the left arm swings forward as the right leg swings forward and vice versa).

- As the shoulder girdle advances, the pelvis and limb trail behind. With each step, this is reversed.

D

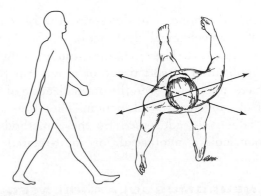

FIGURE 10-8 **A** to **D,** Components of the swing phase.

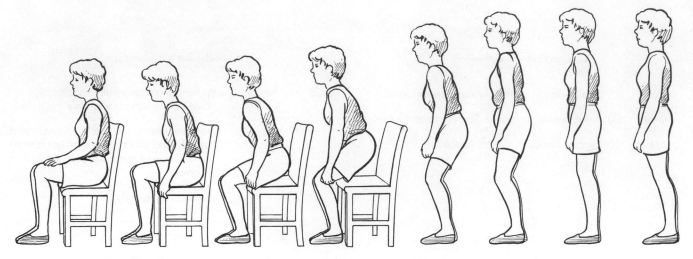

FIGURE 10-9   Sit-to-stand viewed laterally. (From Gillen G, Burkhardt A: *Stroke rehabilitation: a function-based approach*, St Louis, 1998, Mosby.)

Consideration also needs to be given to moving from a seated to standing position and bending to pick up an object on the floor. It is important to squat down to pick up an object as opposed to bending over at the hip joint and then lifting up. Bending over puts an enormous strain on the back. Half the body weight is being moved in addition to the weight of the object being lifted.

When in the seated position, moving to a standing position begins by leaning forward at the hips and leading with the head. The momentum carries the body forward into a semisquat. The leg muscles are used to lift into a standing position (Figure 10-9).

Biomechanical Dysfunction

Differential diagnosis to determine the causal factors of biomechanical dysfunction is beyond the scope of this text. The modalities studied in the specific application of soft tissue or movement therapies have much to offer in the normalization of some types of movement dysfunction. The three areas most effectively addressed by these methods are neuromuscular, myofascial, or joint-related dysfunction.

NEUROMUSCULAR-RELATED DYSFUNCTION

Neuromuscular-related dysfunction manifests as a breakdown or confusion in the nervous system inter-

action with muscle activity. Neuromuscular dysfunction can develop in many forms, including the following:

- Neurotransmitter fluctuations
- Hypermuscular or hypomuscular activity
- Increased tension in individual motor units or the entire muscle
- Hypersensitivity or hyposensitivity in the proprioceptive feedback loop and reflex arcs
- Central nervous system processing difficulties

The myotatic unit becomes disrupted with patterns of overly tense muscles and corresponding weakened or reciprocally inhibited muscles. All of these patterns can be reduced to two: regional postural muscular imbalance and nonoptimal motor function.

Regional Postural Muscular Imbalance

Muscles and muscle groups have constant muscular tone, which is neurologically defined by related segments of the spinal cord. Some muscles have higher tone, such as those that support the vertical position of the body, and others are necessary for the most important functions such as eating and breathing. This balance of tone between muscle groups is regulated by the central nervous system. As a result of a different pathologic processes, this regulation is disturbed. Most often, the tone of postural muscles, which have greater tone to begin with, is increased and so the imbalance appears.

Nonoptimal Motor Function

Every human being, as a result of his individual form, creates an optimal motor function and carriage (how the body is held and moves) unique to that person's body. *Optimal motor function* defines the degree of mobility that the body needs to operate in the most economical way. When all goes well, movement usually proceeds normally. With the appearance of pathologic changes, however, motor function changes as well. Carriage is disturbed, joint mobility becomes limited, tissues and joints are altered, and the tone-strength balance in the tissues is altered. This person spends more energy performing normal movements, which causes him to fatigue more quickly. The change of the optimal motor function influences the work of the viscera, which in turn influences the condition of the muscles and joints, and in turn alters motor function and carriage even further. Thus a vicious circle appears, in which the worsening of different processes negatively contributes to each process.

MYOFASCIAL-RELATED DYSFUNCTION

Connective tissue changes occur as function is altered or as the result of trauma, including microtrauma from accumulated overuse. Most often connective tissue loses hydration and therefore its viscous and plastic qualities result in shortening and reduced pliability. Connective tissues can also become overstretched and lax, reducing their ability to function as dynamic elements of stabilization.

JOINT-RELATED DYSFUNCTION

Joint-related dysfunction can be capsular (in the capsule itself) or noncapsular. The most common noncapsular pattern is the functional block, which is the reversible limitation of range of movement that occurs as a result of change in connective tissue after long-term muscle spasms. The muscle spasm first appears as a reflex defense mechanism against painful movement in an affected jointed area. Immobility of the joint increases stagnation of tissues, which leads to more pain, resulting in the development of the pain-spasm-pain cycle.

Contributing factors to functional block development include the following:

- Holding a weight that is too heavy for too long
- Constant loading on the spine such as occurs during work situations that demand long-term sitting
- Powerful effort such as used in lifting during sport or work

- Passive overstretching such as holding a heavy weight in the hand causing development of functional block in the shoulder joint
- Reflex influences on muscles near joints
- Long-term immobility such as when wearing a cast or when bedridden

PRACTICAL APPLICATION

Functional block may be successfully treated by massage (relaxation and pain management), mobilization (repeated passive movement and traction), muscle energy techniques (various forms of active muscle contraction followed by muscle lengthening), and stretching programs.

The powerful influences of soft tissue and movement modalities accelerate complex self-regulating processes in the direction of normalization and balance. Any soft tissue modality influences the body's systems, tissues, and viscera mechanically and reflexively. Soft tissue and movement modalities improve blood circulation, decrease chronic muscle tension, normalize range of motion of the joint, and rebuild proper proprioception.

The body perceives any technique first as a tactile perception because the skin's surface is altered by various degrees, depending on the character of the methods. Secondly, soft tissue and movement modalities alter the degree of muscle tension. Proprioceptors of the deep tissues report to the central nervous system regarding the condition of muscle tension, capillary pressure, and blood pressure of muscles and vessels.

Warmth is produced in the tissues. This heat acts as a thermal stimulant that signals the sympathetic and parasympathetic systems to cause vasodilation or vasoconstriction.

Chemical substances such as histamine and acetylcholine are formed in the tissues. Histamine stimulates the discharge of adrenaline. These substances are carried with the blood throughout the body, altering circulation, influencing the functions of inner organs (viscera), speeding up nerve impulses, mobilizing the immune system, normalizing blood pressure, and stimulating muscle activity.

All these signals create the central nervous system's reaction. The goal is to generate, through soft tissue and movement methods, the stimulation required to generate self-regulating mechanisms, allowing the body to self-correct and restore dynamic balance or homeostasis.

Biomechanical Assessment

To make decisions about the type or combination of modalities to use to restore balance in the biomechanical mechanisms, information must be gathered. This is assessment.

Assessment defines mobility through passive movements of the affected parts and observation of a distortion in these movements. In addition, muscle testing and defining the functional relationships of muscles is performed. During the client interview, any changes in body movement patterns are investigated.

In postural imbalance some postural muscles are shortened and their antagonists are weakened. Motor function is altered as a result. Postural imbalance often manifests itself as lumbar and cervical hyperlordosis. But it could also lead to other changes in the spine and joints of the limbs as well. These changes often play a pathogenic role in movement.

Three degrees of postural imbalance of muscles may occur:

First degree—Shortening or weakening of some muscles or the formation of local changes in tension or connective tissue in these muscles

Second degree—Moderately expressed shortening of postural muscles and weakening of antagonist muscles

Third degree—Clearly expressed shortening of postural muscles and weakening of antagonist muscles with the appearance of specific, nonoptimal movement

To determine appropriate therapeutic intervention it is very important to define which muscles are shortened and which are weakened. Local functional block, local hypermobility or hypomobility and postural imbalance all lead to changes in motor function, which is accompanied by joint, muscular, and nervous system disorders of temporary or chronic duration. Three degrees of distorted motor function exist:

First degree—For usual and simple movements, a person has to use additional muscles from different parts of the body. As a result, movement becomes uneconomical and labored.

Second degree—Moderately peculiar postures and movements of some parts of the body are present. Postural and movement distortion begin to occur.

Third degree—Significantly expressed peculiarity in postures and movement occurs. Increased postural and movement distortions result.

All these pathobiomechanical disturbances may occur in all age groups. On the basis of the three degrees of distorted motor function, three stages exist in the development of postural and movement pathology:

Stage 1, functional tension—At this stage, a person tires more quickly than normal. This fatigue is accompanied by some functional block in the first- or second-degree limitation of mobility, painless local myodystonia (changes in muscle tension), postural imbalance in the first or second degree, and nonoptimal motor function of the first degree.

Stage 2, functional stress—This stage is characterized by a feeling of fatigue from moderate activity, discomfort, slight pain, and the appearance of singular or multiple functional block and any degree of limited mobility. Functional block may be either painless or result in first-degree pain; it may be accompanied by local hypermobility.

Functional stress is also characterized by reflex vertebral-sensory dysfunction, local myodystony, myodystrophy (fascial/connective tissue changes), and regional postural imbalance. It is also accompanied by distortion of motor function in the first or second degree.

Stage 3, connective tissue changes in the musculoskeletal system—The reasons for connective tissue changes are overloading, disturbances of tissue nutrition, microtraumas, microhemorrhages, and other endogenous (inside the body) and exogenous (outside the body) factors. Hereditary predisposition is also a consideration. In the third stage, osteochondrosis of the spine may appear as a single or multiple functional block, local hypermobility and instability of several vertebral motion segments, hypomobility, widespread painful muscle tension and fascial and connective tissue changes in the muscles, regional postural imbalance in the second or third degree in many joints, and temporary nonoptimal motor function with second- or third-degree distortion. Visceral disturbances may be present (Gurevich, 1992).

✋ PRACTICAL APPLICATION

Stage 1 functional tension can often be managed effectively by soft tissue and movement modalities and by practitioners with training equivalent to 500 to 1000 hours that includes an understanding of the information presented in this text and technical training in their chosen modality. Working with stage 2 and 3 functional stress and connective tissue changes usually requires increased training and proper supervision within a multidisciplinary approach.

SPECIFIC BIOMECHANICAL ASSESSMENT

The clinical reasoning process is essential when assessing for biomechanical function and developing intervention (treatment) plans. For review of the clinical reasoning process, refer to Chapter 3.

Intervention plans need to work toward the client's goals. It is important to relate benefit derived from the modalities to daily function. For example, a plan based on the client goal of more effective shoulder movement would read as follows:

Improved shoulder movement would be encouraged with the use of weekly therapeutic massage and daily yoga practice. Client indicates that more effective shoulder movement could result in increased golf performance and the reduction of shoulder stiffness after the game.

A plan based on efficient biomechanical movement would be focused toward the development of reestablishing or supporting effective movement patterns.

Biomechanically efficient movement is smooth, bilaterally symmetric, and coordinated, with an easy, effortless use of the body. During assessment, noticeable variations need to be considered.

Each jointed area has a movement pattern. The movement is a product of the entire mechanism, including bones; joints; ligaments; capsular components and design; tendons; muscle shapes and fiber types; interlinked fascial networks; nerve distribution; myotatic units of prime movers, antagonists, synergists, and fixators; bodywide counterbalancing reflexes including positional and righting reflexes of vision and the inner ear; circulatory distribution; general systemic balance; and nutritional influences. If a dysfunction is identified, causal factors can be from any one or a combination of these elements. Often a multidisciplinary diagnosis is necessary to identify clearly the interconnected nature of the pathologic condition.

When a movement pattern is assessed as normal, it indicates that all parts are functioning as in a well-orchestrated song.

Assessment also identifies areas of resourceful and successful compensation. These compensation patterns occur when the body has been required to adapt to some sort of trauma or repetitive use pat-

tern. *Resourceful compensation* is not to be eliminated, but instead supported. Permanent adaptive changes, although not as efficient as optimal functioning, are the best pattern the body can develop in response to an irreversible change in the system.

The following sections of this chapter explore movement assessments by jointed areas. *For the bodywork student now, finally, all that has been studied begins to come together in a functional process.*

When assessing a movement pattern, two types of information are obtained in one assessment:

First, when a jointed area moves into flexion and the joint angle is decreased, the prime mover, synergists, and fixators concentrically contract and antagonists eccentrically contract while lengthening. Bodywide stabilization patterns also come into play to assist in allowing the motion. Resistance, applied to load the prime mover groups and synergists, is used to assess for neurologic function of strength and, to a lesser degree, endurance as the contraction is held for a period of time.

At the same time, the antagonist pattern or the tissues that are lengthened when positioning for the functional assessment can be assessed for increased tension patterns or connective tissue shortening. Dysfunction will show itself in range of motion by restricting the movement pattern. When placing a jointed area into flexion, the extensors are assessed for increased tension or shortening. When the jointed area moves into extension, the opposite becomes the case. The same holds for adduction and abduction, internal and external rotation, plantar and dorsal flexion, and so on.

Resistance (pressure against) of load applied to the muscles is focused at the end of the lever system. For example, when assessing the function of the shoulder, resistance is focused at the distal end of the humerus, not at the wrist. When assessing extension of the hip, resistance is placed at the end of the femur. When assessing flexion of the knee, resistance is placed at the distal end of the tibia.

Stabilization is essential to assess movement patterns accurately. Only the area being assessed is allowed to move. Movement in any other part of the body needs to be stabilized. A stabilizing force is usually applied by the therapist. As one hand applies resistance, the other provides the stabilization. Sometimes the client can provide the stabilization. Some modalities use straps to provide stabilization. The easiest way to identify the area to be stabilized is to move the area to be assessed through the range of motion. At the end of the range some other part of the body will begin to move: this is the area of stabilization. Return the body to a neutral position. Provide the appropriate stabilization and begin the assessment procedure.

Range of motion of a joint is measured in degrees. A full circle is 360 degrees. A flat horizontal line is 180 degrees. Two perpendicular lines (as in the shape of a capital *L*) create a 90-degree angle. Various ranges of motion are possible. For example, when the range of motion of a joint allows 0 to 90 degrees of flexion, anything less is hypomobile and anything more is hypermobile. A great degree of variability exists among individuals as to the actual normal range of motion; the degrees provided are general guidelines (Figure 10-10).

In the section *Biomechanics by Region,* specific assessment protocols are provided for the body. In actual professional practice, the practitioner picks and chooses which assessments to perform on the basis of the client's goals and intervention processes.

NOTE: During assessments, muscles should be able to hold against appropriate resistance without strain or pain from the pressure. The position should be easy to assume and comfortable to maintain for a short duration, from 10 to 30 seconds. Contraindications to this type of assessment include joint and disc dysfunction, acute pain, recent trauma, and inflammation.

General Guidelines to Assist the Clinical Reasoning Process
Guidelines include the following:

- If an area is hypomobile, consider tension or shortening in the antagonist pattern as a possible cause.
- If an area is hypermobile, consider instability of the joint structure or muscle weakness in the antagonist pattern or prime mover pattern as a possible cause.
- If an area cannot hold against resistance, consider weakness in the muscles of the prime mover and synergist pattern and tension in the antagonist pattern as possible causes.
- If pain occurs on passive movement, consider joint capsular dysfunction and nerve entrapment syndromes as possible causes.
- If pain occurs on active movement, consider muscle and fascial involvement as a possible cause.
- Always consider bodywide reflexive patterns, as discussed in the section on gait, as possible causes.

The following guidelines also are important:

- The movement patterns should be the same or very similar bilaterally.
- Opposite movement patterns should be able to be assumed easily.
- Bilateral asymmetry, pain, weakness, inability to assume the isolation position or move into the opposite position, or fatigue may indicate dysfunction.
- Intervention or referral depends on the severity of the condition and whether the dysfunction is joint related, neuromuscular related, or myofascial related.

Biomechanics by Region

TRUNK AND THORAX REGION

Biomechanics of the trunk and thorax are unique because of the complexity of the vertebral column, comprised of 24 intricate and complex articulating vertebrae and 31 pairs of spinal nerves. Vertebral motion is greatest where the articulating surfaces and discs are large.

Spinal or Vertebral Movements
Movement depends on a finely integrated system of muscles that are either deep—composed of numerous

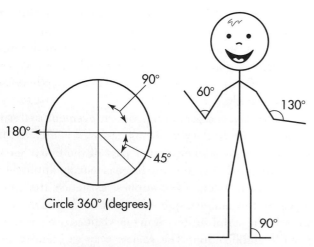

FIGURE 10-10 Degrees of range of motion.

Resources used in the development of the assessment protocols in this portion of the text include Hislop, 1995.

small bundles that attach from vertebra to vertebra—or superficial—arranged in large broad sheets.

Descriptions of spinal or vertebral movements are often preceded by the name given to the region of movement. For example, flexion of the trunk at the lumbar spine is known as lumbar flexion, and extension of the neck is often referred to as cervical extension. Movement of the head between the cranium and the first cervical vertebra is called *capital movement*. Movements occurring among the other cervical vertebrae are called *cervical movements*. These motions usually occur together.

The five spinal movements are as follows (Activity 10-2):

Spinal flexion—Spinal flexion is anterior movement of the spine. In the cervical region the head moves toward the chest. In the thoracic and lumbar regions the thorax moves toward the pelvis.

Spinal extension—Spinal extension is posterior movement of the spine to return from flexion. In the cervical spine the head moves away from the chest. The thorax moves away from the pelvis.

Lateral flexion (side bending)—Lateral flexion occurs in the cervical region when the head moves laterally toward the shoulder. In the thoracic and lumbar regions the thorax moves laterally toward the pelvis. Movement can be to the left or right.

Reduction—Reduction is the return movement from lateral flexion to neutral.

Spinal rotation (left or right)—Spinal rotation is the rotary or twisting movement of the spine in the horizontal plane. In the cervical region the chin rotates from neutral toward the shoulder. In the thoracic and lumbar regions the thorax rotates to one side.

As explained previously, each pair of vertebrae constitute a vertebral motion segment, the basic movable unit of the back. Except for the atlantoaxial joint formed by the first two cervical vertebrae, little movement is possible between any two vertebrae. The amount of movement varies depending on the shape of the vertebrae, the thickness of the intervertebral disk—with thicker discs providing greater mobility—and any rib articulations. However, the cumulative effect of the movements from several adjacent vertebrae allows for substantial movements within a given area. Most of the spinal column movement occurs in the cervical and lumbar regions. Of course, some thoracic movement occurs, but it is slight compared with that of the neck and low back.

Rotation screws the superior vertebra down into the adjacent vertebrae, compressing the disc. Prime mover muscles contract while the contralateral muscles lengthen. Ligament structures are twisted or move into torsion.

In flexion the anterior muscles contract, the posterior muscles lengthen, the superior vertebra tilts toward the front, and the discs are compressed anteriorly and expand posteriorly while the nucleus moves slightly to the back. The superior articular facets slide forward on the inferior ones. The posterior ligaments are stretched and the anterior ligaments are slack.

In extension, just the opposite occurs. The posterior muscles contract and anterior muscles lengthen. The superior vertebra tilts toward the back. The disc is compressed posteriorly and expands anteriorly, and the nucleus moves slightly to the front. The articular facets are pressed together. The anterior liga-

ACTIVITY 10-2

From a standing position, slowly move your head into flexion. Then follow with your cervical region, thoracic region, and lumbar region, each moving into flexion. Pay attention to the limitation of each region and notice the increased range of motion as each area is brought into play. Now move into extension following the same pattern. Repeat this activity for lateral flexion and rotation on both sides. In the space provided describe the experience.

Example

I noticed that it was difficult to isolate head flexion by itself.

Your Turn

ments are stretched, and the posterior ligaments slacken. Lateral flexion follows the same pattern (Figure 10-11) (Activity 10-3).

Head/Neck Region

It is hard to believe that the neck, a small portion of our body, can be so complex and have such precise performance.

The neck connects to the head in the thorax. It contains the C1 to C7 cervical vertebrae, spinal cord, 32 muscles, ligaments, pharynx, larynx, trachea, thyroid, esophagus, lymph glands, hyoid bone, blood vessels, and spinal nerves.

The cervical vertebrae allow the head and neck to be moved into flexion, extension, lateral flexion, and rotation. Combinations of these movements are also possible. The relatively small bodies and thick discs of the cervical vertebrae tend to increase mobility. Side-bending is somewhat restricted by the rectangular shape of the vertebral bodies. The atlas and axis (C1 and C2) form a pivot joint that allows the head and C1 to rotate almost 90 degrees, such as in a "no" motion. The short spinous processes of C3 to C6 allow for good extension of the head and neck.

Intervertebral discs make up approximately 25% of the height of the cervical spine. The ligaments connecting the occiput to the atlas are dense and broad. These ligaments protect the entrance of the spinal cord through the foramen magnum into the skull. The atlantoaxial (C1 and C2) joint is almost totally dependent on ligamentous structure. The cervical spine from C2 to C7 is reinforced by anterior and posterior longitudinal ligaments. These ligaments limit the amount of flexion and extension.

The body moves and is balanced at certain points throughout our form. Two of these movement segments fall within the head/neck area; one at the atlas and skull, and one at C6 to C7. (The other locations are T12/L1, L4/L5/S1, acetabulum/hips, knees, and ankles.)

All muscles that act on the head insert on the skull. Those that are anterior to the coronal midline are termed *capital flexors*. Those muscles that lie behind the coronal midline are termed *capital extensors*. Their center of motion is in the atlantooccipital or atlantoaxial joints.

Muscles that act on the cervical spine are attached to the skull and the cervical and thoracic vertebrae, sternum, clavicle, ribs, and scapula. Most movement occurs at C6 to C7.

The muscles of the erector spinae group are considered stabilizers of the spinal column. The deep muscles extend, rotate, laterally flex, and stabilize the cervical region. All the muscles serve to maintain the correct position of the head and spine while we are walking, sitting, and so on. They are physiologically adapted to work in relays so that they do not fatigue under normal conditions.

The sternocleidomastoid is primarily responsible for flexion and rotation of the head and neck. Extension, particularly extension and rotation, involves the splenius muscles together with the erector spinae and the upper trapezius muscles. The neck extensors, trapezius, scalenes, sternocleidomastoid, and levator scapulae are all considered to be major postural muscles in the body. This is a taxing responsibility for them even when the body has good posture and no pathologic condition is present. Many

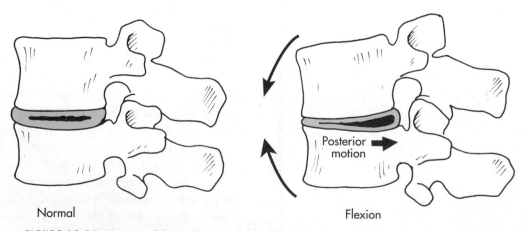

FIGURE 10-11   Movement of the spine from a position of extension into flexion causes the nucleus to move in a posterior direction. (From Shankman GA: *Fundamental orthopedic management for the physical therapist assistant,* St Louis, 1997, Mosby.)

muscles of the neck are called on to assist in breathing if incorrect breathing patterns exist.

Thoracic Vertebral Column Region

The thoracic vertebrae are structured to articulate with the ribs, with stability as the main function of this region. This area does not move extensively, but small movements at the facet joints are ongoing with the breathing process.

A few large extrinsic muscles and numerous small intrinsic muscles are found in this area. The largest muscle is the erector spinae (sacrospinalis), which extends on each side of the spinal column from the pelvic region to the cranium.

The erector spinae muscles function best when the pelvis is held up in front, thus pulling them down slightly in back. This lowers the origin of the erector spinae and makes them more effective in keeping the spine straight. As the spine is held straight, the ribs are raised, thus fixing the chest high and consequently making the abdominal muscles more effective in holding the pelvis up in front and flattening the abdominal wall.

Lumbar Vertebral Column Region

The five lumbar vertebra are the most massive of the spinal column. They carry a large share of the upper body weight, balancing the torso on the sacrum. The combined unit of the vertebrae and discs in the upright position forms the lumbar spinal curve. The lumbar vertebral discs are strong, short, and thick. The ligaments provide stability in all directions. This is the most frequently injured area of the back.

The lumbar vertebral group has less mobility than the cervical region but more than the thoracic region. Because of the absence of ribs and the shape of the spinous processes, the lumbar spine is freer in flexion and extension. Rotation, however, is limited by the amount of tension created in the surrounding ligaments and anulus fibrosis of the disks.

Motions of the lumbar spine include flexion, extension, lateral flexion, and rotation. More motion takes place at L5/S1 (the lumbosacral junction) than at L1/L2.

The angle formed between L5 and S1 is called the *lumbosacral angle.* This angle is approximately 41 degrees in the normal individual. This is typically a neutral position in that no erector spinae force needs to be exerted as a counterbalance. When special conditions exist such as obesity, pregnancy, abdominal muscle weakness, wearing high heels, foot pronation, and poor posture, this angle is undesirably increased and can lead to lumbar pain and dysfunction (Figure 10-12).

Abdominal muscles initiate flexion, while the erector spinae resist flexion. Intrinsic muscles of the back

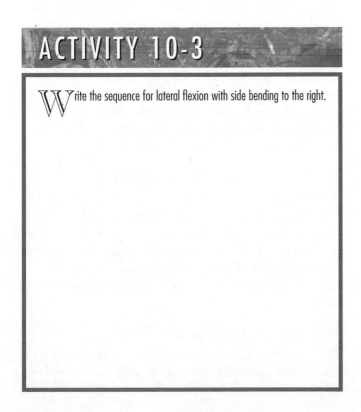

ACTIVITY 10-3

Write the sequence for lateral flexion with side bending to the right.

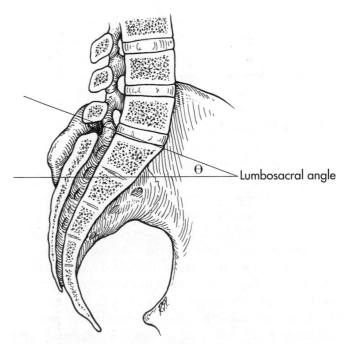

FIGURE 10-12 The lumbosacral angle. (From Malone TR, McPoil T, Nitz AJ: *Orthopedic and sports physical therapy,* ed 3, St Louis, 1997, Mosby.)

Lumbosacral angle

θ

provide extension, while the abdominal muscles (mainly rectus abdominis) resist. Lateral bending occurs in conjunction with spinal rotation. Ipsilateral structures tend to relax, while contralateral structures resist. Lumbosacral rotation takes place with a variety of complex tension and relaxation patterns. Rotation is limited by the straight, posteriorly oriented spinous processes.

Abdomen Region

Abdominal muscles do not extend from bone to bone, but attach into tendinous bands and an aponeurosis (fascia) around the rectus abdominis area. The abdominal muscles are the rectus abdominis, external oblique abdominal, internal oblique abdominal, and transversus abdominis.

The rectus abdominis muscle controls the tilt of the pelvis and the consequent curvature of the lower spine. By holding the pelvis up in front, it makes the erector spinae muscle more effective as an extensor of the spine and makes the hip flexors such as the iliopsoas more effective.

The internal oblique abdominal muscles run diagonally in the direction opposite to that of the external oblique muscles. The left internal oblique muscle causes rotation to the left, and the right internal oblique muscle causes rotation to the right. In rotary movements the internal oblique muscle and the opposite side external oblique muscle always work together.

The transversus abdominis is the chief muscle of forced expiration and, together with the rectus abdominis, external oblique abdominal, and internal oblique abdominal muscles, is effective in helping to hold the abdomen flat.

Thorax Region

As covered in Chapter 7, the skeletal foundation of the thorax is formed by 12 pairs of ribs, the manubrium, the body of the sternum, and the xiphoid process. Breathing is a major function of the thorax. Breathing involves inspiration, or inhaling, and expiration, or exhaling. The primary muscles of inspiration are the diaphragm and the external intercostal.

During quiet respiration, the diaphragm may act alone, or a slight rhythmic activity may occur in the scalenus anterior and medius and in the intercostals. In deep inspiration the action of the primary muscles is increased and the sternocleidomastoid and scalenes assist in raising the ribs. Forced inspiration involves any muscles that stabilize or elevate the

shoulder girdle to elevate the ribs directly or indirectly.

Expiration is primarily passive as relaxation of the prime movers and the weight of gravity pulls the rib cage down. The primary muscles of expiration are the internal intercostals. Forced expiration involves muscles that force the rib cage down (quadratus lumborum) or compress the abdominal cavity (oblique and transverse abdominals), forcing the diaphragm upward.

Two different types of breathing patterns exist: diaphragmatic and thoracic. Diaphragmatic, or abdominal, breathing is the natural way to breathe and can be seen in infants and sleeping adults. Air is inhaled deep into the lungs by the contraction of the diaphragm, flattening its dome shape and resulting in negative pressure in the lungs, which fill with air to equalize the pressure. The diaphragm then relaxes, and the air is expelled out of the lungs by its upward movement. Diaphragmatic breathing is even and relaxed.

Thoracic, or chest, breathing is common in people with anxiety or other emotional distress. Anxious people may experience breath holding, hyperventilation, constricted breathing, shortness of breath, or fear of passing out. Thoracic breathing is seen in people who wear restrictive clothing, hold in their abdominal muscles, or lead sedentary or stressful lives. Chest breathing is often shallow, irregular, and rapid. When air is inhaled, the chest expands and the shoulders rise to take in air. Dysfunctional patterns can develop if the accessory muscles of respiration (scalenes, sternocleidomastoid, serratus posterior superior, levator scapulae, rhomboids, abdominals, and quadratus lumborum) are constantly being used for regular breathing when forced inhalation and expiration are not required (Activity 10-4).

SHOULDER REGION

Remarkably, the complicated framework of the shoulder is not only extremely mobile but also provides a secure and stable immovable point for specific actions such as lifting, thrusting, shoving, and pushing heavy objects. This region consists of the shoulder girdle and the shoulder, or glenohumeral joint.

Shoulder Girdle Region

The shoulder girdle is made up of the scapula and clavicle (which generally move as a unit) and associated soft tissues. The clavicle has two synovial gliding joints.

In this activity, you will be working with a partner to assess individual movement patterns, normal function, and possible dysfunction in each other. One of you is to first isolate the specified movement patterns on each side of your partner, one side at a time, and assess for normal function by applying a gentle pressure opposite to the action of the isolation position. The body is to be stabilized so that only the isolated area is moving. In some instances the ability to assume the position and maintain it indicates normal function. Muscles should be able to hold against gravity or the applied pressure without strain or pain. The position itself should be easy to assume and comfortable to maintain for a short duration, from 10 to 30 seconds. The bilateral movement patterns should be the same. The opposite movement pattern should also be able to be done easily. Dysfunction may be indicated by bilateral asymmetry, pain, weakness, fatigue, and inability to assume the isolation position or move into the opposite position. Intervention or referral depends on the severity of the condition and whether the dysfunction is neuromuscular, myofascial, or joint related.

NOTE: Do not perform these assessments if contraindications exist. Contraindications to this type of assessment include joint and disc dysfunction, acute pain, recent trauma, and inflammation.

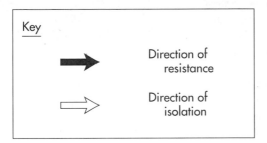

Key

→ Direction of resistance

⇨ Direction of isolation

TRUNK EXTENSION

Assesses for strength and endurance in the isolation position and tension or shortening in the flexion pattern.

Muscles involved

Erector spinae (sacrospinalis) group—Iliocostalis, longissimus spinalis
Splenius (cervicis, capitis)
Semispinalis
Multifidus

Range of motion

Thoracic spine—0 to 0 degrees
Lumbar spine—0 to 25 degrees

Position of client

Prone, with hands clasped behind head; client may hold hands behind back

Isolation and assessment

Client extends the lumbar spine until the head and chest are raised from the table
Ability to perform test indicates normal function
No resistance pressure is required

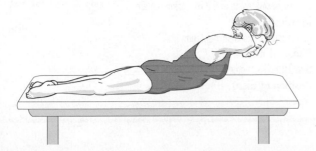

TRUNK FLEXION

Assesses for strength and endurance in the isolation position and tension or shortening in the extension pattern

Muscles involved

Rectus abdominis
Internal and external obliques
Psoas major and minor

Range of motion

0 to 50 degrees (beyond 50 degrees, any additional flexion comes from pelvic rotation)

Position of the client

Supine, with hands clasped behind head or crossed in form and placed on shoulders, knees bent, feet flat
NOTE: Client is not to lift head with hands

Isolation and assessment

Client tucks chin to chest and brings shoulders toward thighs
Ability to clear scapulae from the table indicates good function
No resistance pressure is needed

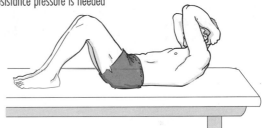

Trunk rotation

Assesses for strength and endurance in the isolation position and tension or shortening in the contralateral pattern

Muscles involved

External obliques
Internal obliques
Latissimus dorsi
Rectus abdominis
Deep back muscles (unilateral test)

Range of motion

0 to 45 degrees

Position of client

Supine, with knees bent and feet flat, with hands clasped across chest or held beside ears
NOTE: Client is not to lift head with hands

Isolation and assessment

Client slowly flexes and rotates trunk to one side. After returning to supine position, movement is repeated on opposite side. Ability to clear scapulae from the table indicates good function.
Right shoulder to left knee tests right external obliques and left internal obliques. Left shoulder to right knee tests the left external obliques and right internal obliques.

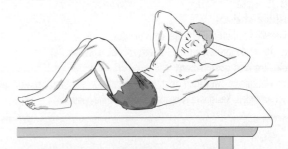

Continued

ACTIVITY 10-4—cont'd

ELEVATION OF THE PELVIS (MORE CORRECTLY KNOWN AS LATERAL TILT)

Assesses for strength and endurance in the isolation position and tension or shortening in the contralateral pattern

Muscles involved

Quadratus lumborum

Latissimus dorsi

Internal abdominal obliques

Iliocostalis lumborum

Range of motion

Not applicable

Position of client

Prone with hip and lumbar spine in extension, hip slightly abducted, feet off end of table; the client grasps the edges of the table to provide stabilization during resistance

Isolation and assessment

Client brings iliac crest toward ribs on one side

Resistance is applied to lower leg to pull hip down

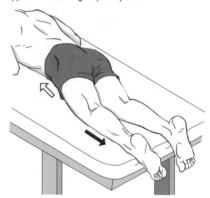

CAPITAL EXTENSION

Assesses for strength and endurance in the isolation position and tension or shortening in the flexion pattern

Muscles involved

Rectus capitis posterior major

Rectus capitis posterior minor

Longissimus capitis

Obliquus capitis superior

Obliquus capitis inferior

Splenius capitis

Semispinalis capitis

Range of motion

0 to 25 degrees

Position of client

Prone with head off end of table, arms at sides

NOTE: Do not do this test if client has cervical disk problems

Isolation and assessment

Client lifts chin up away from chest, as if beginning to nod "yes"; cervical spine is not extended. Resistance is applied to back of the head.

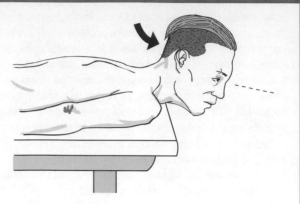

CERVICAL EXTENSION

Assesses for strength and endurance in the isolation position and tension or shortening in the flexion pattern

Muscles involved

Longissimus cervicis

Semispinalis cervicis

Iliocostalis cervicis

Splenius capitis and cervicis

Range of motion

0 to 25 degrees

Position of client

Prone, with head off end of table, arms along sides

NOTE: Do not do this test if client has cervical disk problems

Isolation and assessment

Client extends neck by lifting head toward ceiling

No resistance is needed

Ability to hold head up against gravity indicates normal function

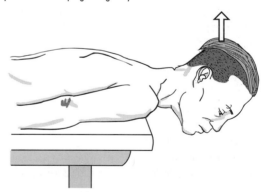

CAPITAL FLEXION

Assesses for strength and endurance in the isolation position and tension or shortening in the extension pattern

Muscles involved

Rectus longus and capitis anterior

Range of motion

0 to 10 or 15 degrees

Position of client

Supine

NOTE: Do not do this test if client has cervical disk problems

Isolation and assessment

Client tucks chin into neck as in nodding "yes"

Head remains on table

No motion should occur at the cervical spine

No resistance is needed

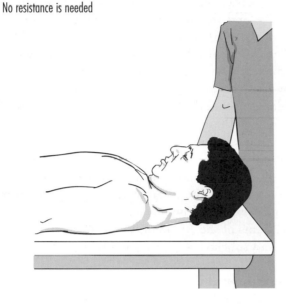

CERVICAL FLEXION

Assesses for strength and endurance in the isolation position and tension or shortening in the extension pattern

Muscles involved

Scalenus anterior, medius, posterior

Sternocleidomastoid

Longus colli

Range of motion

0 to 35 or 45 degrees

NOTE: Women usually have greater cervical lordosis than men, so it is likely that they could have a greater arc of motion

Position of client

Supine, with arms at sides

Head supported on table

NOTE: Do not do this test if client has cervical disk problems

Isolation and assessment

Client lifts head off table and tucks chin

This is a weak muscle group so no resistance is needed

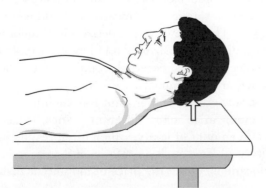

CERVICAL ROTATION

Assesses for strength and endurance in the isolation position and tension or shortening in the contralateral pattern

Muscles involved

Sternocleidomastoid

Rectus capitis posterior major

Obliquus capitis inferior

Longissimus capitis

Range of motion

0 to 45 or 55 degrees

Two separate actions will be tested

Position of client

Supine

Begin with head supported on table and turned to one side

Isolation and assessment

Client lifts head off table without any additional rotation

Returns to start position

Repeats on other side

No resistance pressure is needed

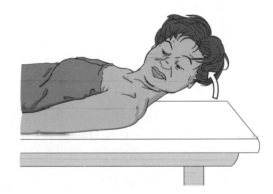

Position of client

Supine, with cervical spine in neutral flexion and extension

Begin with head supported on table and turned to one side

Isolation and assessment

Client rotates head to neutral (nose facing ceiling) against resistance

Make sure client does not lift head off table

Repeat on opposite side

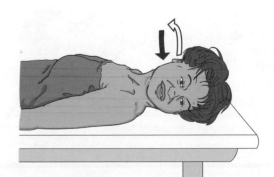

Continued

The sternoclavicular joint is medial, and the acromio-clavicular joint is lateral. When analyzing scapulothoracic movements, it is important to realize that the scapula moves on the rib cage because the joint motion actually occurs at the sternoclavicular joint and to a lesser extent at the acromioclavicular joint.

The movements of the sternoclavicular (SC) joint include elevation, depression, rotation, protraction, and retraction. For full abduction to occur, the clavicle must rotate 50 degrees posteriorly. Movement at the joint occurs indirectly as a result of scapular movement. The characteristics of the joint are indirectly influenced by the movement of the glenohumeral joint. Although no direct muscular attachments cross this joint, several muscles have indirect influence on the movement, especially the pectoralis major, subclavius, sternocleidomastoid, sternothyroid and sternohyoid, scalenus medius and posterior, and upper trapezius.

The acromioclavicular (AC) joint contributes very little to scapular movement because its joint surfaces do not allow much angular movement. A rotary and hingelike motion takes place at this joint chiefly with elevation of the arm above the horizontal plane. The S shape of the clavicle provides the extra motion during elevation of the arm.

The scapulae rotate at the AC joint at the beginning of scapular movement. Of the approximately 60 degrees that scapular movement contributes to the elevation of the arm, about 30 degrees occurs at the SC joint and the remaining 30 degrees occurs from the combined effects of clavicular rotation, which causes the clavicular joint surfaces to face upward, and the acromioclavicular movement that occurs at the AC joint.

The AC joint allows widening and narrowing of the angle between the clavicle and the scapula (from above). Narrowing occurs during protraction; widening occurs during retraction. It also allows for rotation of the scapula upward, when the inferior angle moves away from the midline, or downward, when the inferior angle moves toward the midline. The AC joint also allows rotation of the scapula in such a way that the inferior angle swings anteriorly and posteriorly. Although no muscles directly cause movements of the AC joint, the deltoid, upper trapezius, and subclavius muscles indirectly affect it.

Glenohumeral Joint

The shoulder, or glenohumeral joint, includes the scapula, humerus, and associated soft tissue. The only attachment of the shoulder joint to the axial skeleton is the clavicle at the sternoclavicular joint.

The glenohumeral joint is a ball-and-socket joint and is the articulation between the glenoid fossa of the scapula and the head of the humerus. Movements of the shoulder joint are many and varied. This extremely mobile joint allows adduction, abduction, flexion, extension, hyperextension, horizontal adduction and abduction, and lateral and medial rotation of the humerus.

It is unusual to have movement of the humerus without scapula movement. Much of the movement of the scapula is related to movement at the glenohumeral joint. When the humerus is flexed and abducted, the scapula is elevated, rotated upward, and abducted. Adduction and extension of the humerus results in depression, rotation downward, and adduction of the scapula. The scapula is abducted with humeral internal rotation and horizontal adduction. Scapula adduction accompanies external rotation and horizontal abduction of the humerus.

Because the shoulder joint has such a wide range of motion in so many different planes, it also has a certain amount of laxity, which often results in instability problems such as rotator cuff impingement or dislocations. Often the price of mobility is instability.

ACTIVITY 10-4—cont'd

MUSCLES OF QUIET INSPIRATION

Muscles involved
Diaphragm
Intercostals

Position of client
Supine

Isolation and assessment
Client inhales with maximal effort and holds maximal inspiration
Then pressure is applied to abdomen just below the rib cage (avoid pressure on xiphoid process)

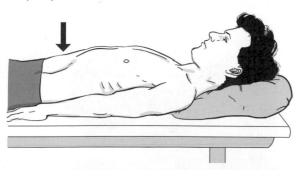

The concept that the more mobile a joint is, the less stable it is and that the more stable it is, the less mobile it is applies generally throughout the body but especially in the shoulder joint.

An important, protective fibroosseous arch over the glenohumeral arch is formed by the coracoacromial ligament, together with the acromion (or the lateral end of the clavicle articulating directly with the acromion and indirectly with the coracoid process through the coracoclavicular ligaments) and coracoid process. This arch forms a secondary restraining socket for the humeral head, preventing superior dislocation or displacement of the humeral head.

At the brim of the glenoid fossa is a fibrocartilaginous ring called the *glenoid labrum* that adds stability and substance to this relatively shallow and mobile articulation.

The glenoid labrum merges with several ligaments and tendons to form the joint capsule of the glenohumeral joint. Tendons that connect at this joint are from the muscles of the *s*ubscapularis, *i*nfraspinatus, *t*eres minor, and the *s*upraspinatus, also known as *SITS*, or rotator cuff muscles, because they contribute to the rotation of the humerus. In reality, numerous muscles and tendons intersect the glenohumeral joint, and because of their attachment points, they contribute to the stability of the joint through their tension and lines of pull. The deltoid forms a hood over the small muscles that closely surround the joint and acts as a shock absorber to protect the joint from impact.

The deep fascia covering the deltoid, known as the *deltoid aponeurosis*, is a fibrous layer that covers the outer surface of the muscle. It is thick and strong behind, where it is continuous with the infraspinatus fascia, and thinner over the rest of the muscle. In front, the deltoid aponeurosis is continuous with the fascia covering the pectoralis major; behind, with the fascia covering the infraspinatus; above, it is attached to the clavicle, the acromion, and spine of the scapula; below, it is continuous with the deep fascia of the arm. This extensive fascial network provides dynamic stability.

Scapulothoracic Junction

The scapulothoracic junction meets the criteria of a joint in that it allows the scapula to glide over the ribs and is separated by muscle, fascia, and bursae. It is not a true synovial joint because it does not have regular synovial features and its movement is totally dependent on the sternoclavicular and acromioclavicular joints. Even though scapular movement occurs as a result of motion at the SC and AC joints, the scapula can be described as having a total range of 25 degrees of abduction-adduction, 60 degrees of upward-downward rotation, and 55 degrees of elevation-depression. A very large subscapular bursal sheet and fat pad enhance the gliding of this junction.

In analyzing shoulder girdle movements, it is often helpful to focus on a specific bony landmark such as the inferior angle (posteriorly), glenoid fossa (laterally), and acromion process (anteriorly). All of the following movements have their pivotal point where the clavicle joins the sternum at the sternoclavicular joint. Movements of the shoulder girdle can be described as movements of the scapula.

Movements of the Scapula

Abduction (protraction) — Movement of the scapula laterally away from the spinal column

Adduction (retraction) — Movement of the scapula medially toward the spinal column

Upward rotation — Turning the glenoid fossa upward and moving the inferior angle superiorly and laterally away from the spinal column

Downward rotation — Returning the inferior angle medially and inferiorly toward the spinal column and the glenoid fossa to its normal position

Elevation — Upward or superior movement, as in shrugging the shoulders

Depression — Downward or inferior movement, as in returning to normal position

Movements of the Glenohumeral Joint

Abduction — Lateral movement of the humerus out to the side and away from the body

Adduction — Movement of the humerus medially toward the body from abduction

Flexion — Movement of the humerus anteriorly

Extension — Movement of the humerus posteriorly

Horizontal adduction (flexion) — Movement of the humerus in a horizontal or transverse plane toward and across the chest

Horizontal abduction (extension) — Movement of the humerus in a horizontal or transverse plane away from the chest

External rotation — Movement of the humerus laterally around its long axis away from the midline

Internal rotation — Movement of the humerus medially around its long axis toward the midline

The shoulder joint and shoulder girdle work together in carrying out upper extremity activities.

Table 10-1 shows a pairing of shoulder girdle and shoulder joint movements (Activity 10-5).

Shoulder Girdle Muscles

Five muscles are primarily involved in shoulder girdle movements. To avoid confusion, it is helpful to group the muscles of the shoulder girdle separately from the shoulder joint. All five shoulder girdle muscles have their origin on the axial skeleton, with their insertion located on the scapula or clavicle. Shoulder girdle muscles do not attach to the humerus nor do they cause actions of the shoulder joint. The shoulder girdle muscles are essential in providing dynamic stability of the scapula so that it can serve as a base of support for shoulder joint activities.

The trapezius muscle fixates the scapula for deltoid action by preventing the glenoid fossa from being pulled down when the arms lift objects. The muscle is used strenuously when lifting with the hands, as in picking up a heavy wheelbarrow. The trapezius must prevent the scapula from being pulled downward such as when an object is held overhead or a person is carrying an object that is resting on the tip of his shoulder.

Shrugging the shoulder calls the levator scapulae muscle into play, along with the upper trapezius muscle.

The rhomboid muscle fixes the scapula in adduction/retraction when the muscles of the shoulder joint adduct or extend the arm. The trapezius and rhomboid muscles work together to produce adduction, with slight elevation of the scapula. To prevent this elevation, the latissimus dorsi muscle is called into play. The serratus anterior muscle is used in movements drawing the scapula forward with slight upward rotation. It works along with the pectoralis

major muscle in actions such as throwing a baseball. A winged scapula condition indicates a definite weakness of the serratus anterior.

The pectoralis minor muscle is used, along with the serratus anterior muscle, in true abduction (protraction) without rotation. When true abduction of the scapula is necessary, the serratus anterior draws the scapula forward with a slight upward rotation and the pectoralis minor pulls forward with slight downward rotation. The two pulling together give true abduction. These muscles will be seen working together in most movements of pushing with the hands.

Glenohumeral Joint Muscles

Muscles of the glenohumeral joint contribute to more than one action when the humerus is in a sequence of movement. The muscles involved in flexion of the shoulder and glenohumeral joint cross the joint anteriorly. The primary flexors are the pectoralis major, anterior deltoid, and coracobrachialis. Synergists to flexion are the biceps brachii and the subscapularis.

In extension of the glenohumeral joint, when movement is not resisted in any way, gravity is the

TABLE 10-1 SHOULDER JOINT

SHOULDER JOINT	SHOULDER GIRDLE
Abduction	Upward rotation
Adduction	Downward rotation
Flexion	Elevation/upward rotation/protraction
Extension	Depression/downward rotation/retraction
Internal rotation	Abduction (protraction)
External rotation	Adduction (retraction)
Horizontal abduction	Adduction (retraction)
Horizontal adduction	Abduction (protraction)

ACTIVITY 10-5

Slowly and deliberately move your scapula and glenohumeral joint through each of the movement patterns just described. Identify the interplay between the shoulder girdle movements and the shoulder joint movements. Pay attention to the limitation of each region and notice the increase in range of motion as each area is brought into play. In the space provided describe the experience.

Example

I noticed that it was confusing to attempt to isolate scapular movements by themselves.

Your Turn

prime mover, with the flexor muscles eccentrically contracting to control the action of extension. When resistance occurs, the posterior muscles of the glenohumeral joint go to work, specifically the teres major, latissimus dorsi, and sternocostal pectoralis. Synergists for extension are the posterior deltoid, particularly when the humerus is externally rotated, and the triceps brachii (long head) when the elbow is flexed.

Two primary movers are involved in abduction of the glenohumeral joint: the middle deltoid and supraspinatus. Both muscles intersect the shoulder superior to the glenohumeral joint. The supraspinatus begins the movement of abduction for approximately the first 110 degrees. The middle deltoid is active from approximately 90 degrees to 180 degrees. To counteract superior dislocation, the infraspinatus, subscapularis, and teres major contract to control the action of the middle deltoid.

Adduction of the glenohumeral joint is another movement in which, if no resistance occurs, gravity is the prime mover, with the abductors as the antagonist controlling the speed of the motion. With resistance, the principal adductors are the latissimus dorsi, teres major, and pectoralis major sternal, all positioned inferior to the glenohumeral joint. The synergists are the biceps (short head) and triceps (long head).

Medial rotation of the humerus is a result of the subscapularis and teres major as the prime movers. Both insert to the anterior aspect of the humerus. Synergists to medial rotation are the pectoralis major, anterior deltoid, latissimus dorsi, and biceps brachii (short head).

Muscles inserting into the posterior aspect of the humerus generate the lateral rotation, specifically the infraspinatus and teres minor.

Horizontal adduction is the result of the actions of anterior muscles, which include the anterior deltoid, pectoralis major, and coracobrachialis. The synergist to horizontal adduction is the biceps brachii (short head).

Horizontal abduction is affected by the middle and posterior deltoid, infraspinatus, and teres minor, muscles located on the posterior aspect of the joint. The synergists to horizontal abduction are the teres major and latissimus dorsi (Activity 10-6).

ACTIVITY 10-6

In this activity, you will be working with a partner to assess individual movement patterns, normal function, and possible dysfunction in each other. One of you is to first isolate the specified movement patterns on each side of your partner, one side at a time, and assess for normal function by applying a gentle pressure opposite the action of the isolation position. The body is to be stabilized so that only the isolated area is moving. In some instances the ability to assume the position and maintain it indicates normal function. Muscles should be able to hold against gravity or the applied pressure without strain or pain. The position itself should be easy to assume and comfortable to maintain for a short duration, from 10 to 30 seconds. The bilateral movement patterns should be the same. The opposite movement pattern should also be able to be done easily. Dysfunction may be indicated by bilateral asymmetry, pain, weakness, fatigue, and inability to assume the isolation position or move into the opposite position. Intervention or referral depends on the severity of the condition and whether the dysfunction is neuromuscular, myofascial, or joint related.

NOTE: Do not perform these assessments if contraindications exist. Contraindications to this type of assessment include joint and disk dysfunction, acute pain, recent trauma, and inflammation.

Before starting scapular motion assessments, do a visual assessment of your partner to check for variations in position and symmetry. Asymmetry often shows with one shoulder or scapula higher, especially in those who carry briefcases, purses, or babies on one side.

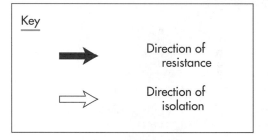

Key

→ Direction of resistance

⇨ Direction of isolation

Working with your partner, determine the position of the scapulae at rest and whether the two sides are symmetric. The normal scapula lies close to the rib cage with the vertebral border nearly parallel and from 1 to 3 inches lateral to the spinous processes. The inferior angle is tucked in. If the inferior angle of the scapula is tilted away from the rib cage, check for tightness of the pectoralis minor and weakness of the trapezius.

The most prominent abnormal posture of the scapula is "winging," in which the vertebral border tilts away from the rib cage, a sign of serratus weakness.

Within the total arc of 180 degrees of shoulder forward flexion, 120 degrees is glenohumeral motion and 60 degrees is scapular motion. Because these movements are not isolated, it is more correct to say that the glenohumeral and scapular motions coexist after 60 degrees and up to 150 degrees.

Continued

ACTIVITY 10-6—cont'd

Passively raise your partner's test arm in forward flexion completely above his head to determine scapular mobility. The scapula should start to rotate at about 60 degrees, although considerable individual variation exists.

Check that the scapula basically remains in its rest position at ranges of shoulder flexion less than 60 degrees with some variation among individuals. If the scapula moves as the glenohumeral joint moves below 60 degrees, that is, within this range they move as a unit, limited glenohumeral motion is evident, but the scapula may move through a complete or even excessive range.

From greater than 60 degrees and to about 150 or 160 degrees in both active and passive motion, the scapula moves in concert with the humerus.

SCAPULAR ABDUCTION (PROTRACTION)

Assesses for strength and endurance in the isolation position and tension or shortening in the scapular adduction pattern

Muscles involved

Serratus anterior

Pectoralis minor

Range of motion

Reliable values are not available

Position of client

Seated, with legs over end or side of table

Hands at sides on top of table

Isolation and assessment

Client flexes straight arm to approximately 130 degrees as resistance is applied to arm just above the elbow to push arm down

Scapula should not wing out

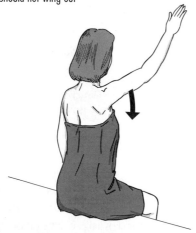

SCAPULAR ADDUCTION (RETRACTION)

Assesses for strength and endurance in the isolation position and tension or shortening in the scapular abduction pattern

Muscles involved

Trapezius (middle fibers)

Rhomboid major and minor

Latissimus dorsi

Range of motion

Reliable values are not available

Position of client

Seated with legs over edge of table

Shoulder is abducted to 90 degrees and externally rotated

Elbow is flexed to a right angle and held at shoulder level

Isolation and assessment

Client horizontally abducts arm to adduct the scapula, while resistance is applied to the posterior arm above the elbow to push the arm into horizontal adduction

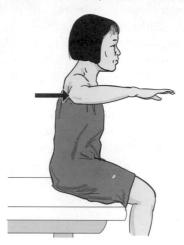

SCAPULAR ELEVATION

Assesses for strength and endurance in the isolation position and tension or shortening in the scapular depression pattern

Muscles involved

Trapezius (upper fibers)

Levator scapulae

Rhomboid major and minor

Range of motion

Reliable values are not available

Position of client

Seated, with legs over side of table and arms relaxed

Isolation and assessment

Client lifts shoulders toward ears, as in shrugging, while resistance is given to push the shoulders down

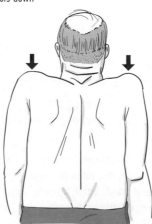

ACTIVITY 10-6—cont'd

SCAPULAR UPWARD ROTATION WITH ABDUCTION

Assesses for strength and endurance in the isolation position and tension or shortening in the scapular downward rotation pattern

Muscles involved

Upper and lower trapezius

Anterior serratus

Pectoralis minor

Range of motion

Reliable values are not available

Position of client

Seated, with legs over table, arms resting at sides

Isolation and assessment

Client flexes shoulder forward to 90 degrees with no rotation or horizontal movement while resistance is applied to arm just above elbow to push it down

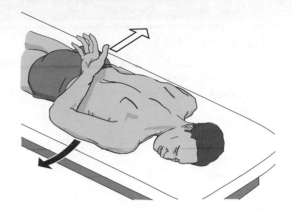

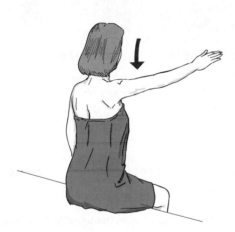

SCAPULAR DEPRESSION WITH ADDUCTION AND DOWNWARD ROTATION

Assesses for strength and endurance in the isolation position and tension or shortening in the scapular elevation and upward rotation pattern

Muscles involved

Lower trapezius

Lower anterior serratus

Levator scapula

Rhomboid major and minor

Latissimus dorsi

Range of motion

Reliable values are not available

Position of client

Prone

Head may be turned to either side for comfort

Internally rotate shoulder, flex elbow, and adduct arm across back

Hand rests on low back near waist

Isolation and assessment

Client further adducts arm by attempting to touch the opposite side

Resistance is applied to the medial side of upper arm to pull it away from the body

SHOULDER FLEXION

Assesses for strength and endurance in the isolation position and tension or shortening in the shoulder extension and adduction pattern

Muscles involved

Deltoid (anterior and middle)

Supraspinatus

Pectoralis major (upper)

Coracobrachialis

Biceps brachii

Subscapularis

Range of motion

0 to 180 degrees

Position of client

Seated with knees bent off table, arms at sides, elbows slightly flexed, forearm pronated

Isolation and assessment

Client flexes shoulder to 90 degrees without rotation or horizontal movement, as resistance is applied to upper arm above elbow to push arm down

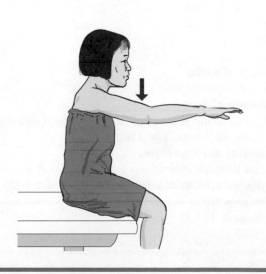

Continued

ACTIVITY 10-6—cont'd

SHOULDER EXTENSION

Assesses for strength and endurance in the isolation position and tension or shortening in the shoulder flexion pattern

Muscles involved

Latissimus dorsi

Deltoid (posterior)

Teres major

Triceps brachii (long head)

Range of motion

0 to 45 degrees

Position of client

Prone, with arms at sides and shoulder internally rotated (palm up)

Elbow remains extended throughout isolation

Isolation and assessment

Client lifts arm off table and holds

Resistance is applied to posterior arm above elbow to push it down

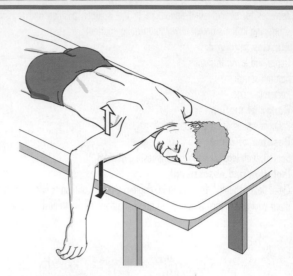

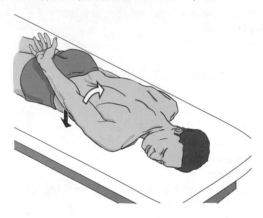

SHOULDER HORIZONTAL ABDUCTION

Assesses for strength and endurance in the isolation position and tension or shortening in the shoulder horizontal adduction pattern

Muscles involved

Deltoid (posterior fibers)

Infraspinatus

Teres minor

Range of motion

0 to 90 degrees (beginning at 90 degrees flexion)

Position of client

Prone with shoulder abducted to 90 degrees, elbow flexed, upper arm supported on table, and forearm off edge of table

Isolation and assessment

Client horizontally (posteriorly) abducts shoulder (lifts elbow toward ceiling) while resistance is applied to the posterior arm above elbow to push arm down

SHOULDER HORIZONTAL ADDUCTION

Assesses for strength and endurance in the isolation position and tension or shortening in the shoulder horizontal abduction pattern

Muscles involved

Pectoralis major

Deltoid (anterior fibers)

Range of motion

0 to 40 degrees when starting from a position of 90 degrees of forward flexion

Position of client

Supine

Shoulder abducted to 90 degrees, upper arm supported on table and elbow flexed to 90 degrees

Isolation and assessment

Client horizontally abducts arm to move it across the chest while resistance is applied to medial side of upper arm above elbow to push it down

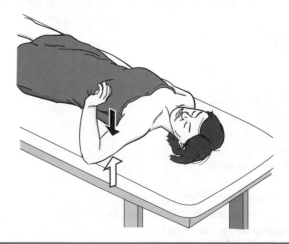

ELBOW REGION

The elbow is considered a relatively stable joint with firm osseous support and is comprised of three articulations: the humeroulnar joint, humeroradial joint, and radioulnar joint. It is a uniaxial hinge joint that moves only in one plane along a single axis. Its action is flexion/extension. The elbow is capable of moving from 0 degrees of extension to approximately 145 to 150 degrees of flexion.

After the elbow flexes beyond 20 degrees, its bony stability is somewhat unlocked, allowing for more side-to-side laxity. In flexion, the stability of the elbow depends on the lateral or radial collateral ligament with most of the work by the medial or ulnar collateral ligament.

The radioulnar joint is classified as a trochoid or pivot-type joint. The radial head rotates around its location at the proximal ulna. This rotary movement is accompanied by the distal radius rotating around the distal ulna. The radial head is maintained in its joint by the annular ligament. The radioulnar joint can supinate approximately 80 to 90 degrees from the neutral position. Pronation varies from 70 to 90 degrees.

Practically any movement of the upper extremity will involve the elbow and radioulnar joints. Quite often, these joints are grouped together because of their close anatomic relationship. Radioulnar joint motion may be incorrectly attributed to the wrist joint because it appears to occur there. However, with close inspection, the elbow joint and its movements may be clearly distinguished from those of the radioulnar joints, just as the radioulnar movements may be distinguished from those of the wrist.

When the arm is in an anatomic extended position, the upper arm and forearm's longitudinal axes form a valgus angle at the elbow joint known as the *carrying*

ACTIVITY 10-6—cont'd

SHOULDER EXTERNAL OR LATERAL ROTATION

Assesses for strength and endurance in the isolation position and tension or shortening in the shoulder internal or medial rotation pattern

Muscles involved

Infraspinatus

Teres minor

Deltoid (posterior)

Range of motion

0 to 90 degrees

Position of client

Prone, with head turned toward test side

Shoulder is abducted to 90 degrees with upper arm fully supported on table, elbow flexed, and forearm hanging over edge of table

Isolation and assessment

Client moves forearm upward toward the level of the table keeping upper arm on table while resistance is applied to distal forearm above wrist to push it down

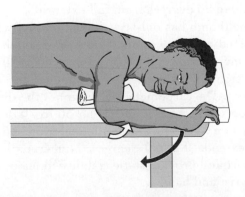

SHOULDER INTERNAL ROTATION

Assesses for strength and endurance in the isolation position and tension or shortening in the shoulder external or lateral rotation pattern

Muscles involved

Subscapularis

Pectoralis major

Latissimus dorsi

Teres major

Deltoid (anterior)

Range of motion

0 to 80 degrees

Position of client

Prone with shoulder abducted to 90 degrees, upper arm supported on table, elbow flexed, and forearm hanging over edge of table

Examiner stabilizes upper arm

Isolation and assessment

Client moves forearm through internal rotation (backward and upward) as resistance is applied to forearm above wrist to push down

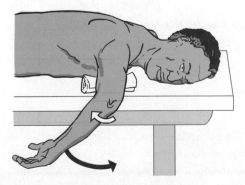

angle; this angle approximates 5 degrees in men and between 10 and 15 degrees in women. Anatomically, the carrying angle is designed to fit closely into the waist depressions immediately superior to the iliac crest. The carrying angles should be bilaterally symmetric.

The olecranon fossa of the humerus, which receives the olecranon of the ulna during extension, is filled with fat and covered by a portion of the triceps muscle and aponeurosis.

The cubital fossa is defined by the brachioradialis laterally and the pronator teres medially with the biceps tendon, brachial artery, median and musculocutaneous nerves passing through this area. The biceps tendon is a taut, long structure that is medial to the brachioradialis muscle, and the pulse of the brachial artery can be palpated medial to the biceps tendon.

Movements of the Elbow (Activity 10-7)

Flexion — Movement of the forearm to the shoulder by bending the elbow to decrease its angle

Extension — Movement of the forearm away from the shoulder by straightening the elbow to increase its angle

Pronation — Internal rotary movement of the radius on the ulna that results in the hand moving from the palm-up to the palm-down position

Supination — External rotary movement of the radius on the ulna that results in the hand moving from the palm-down to the palm-up position

ACTIVITY 10-7

Slowly and deliberately move your humeroulnar joint, humeroradial joint, and radioulnar joint through each of the movement patterns described. In the space provided describe the experience.

Example

I noticed that it took less effort to pronate than to supinate.

Your Turn

Elbow Muscles

The elbow flexors are the biceps brachii, brachialis, and brachioradialis. The triceps brachii is the primary elbow extensor, assisted by the anconeus. The pronator group consists of the pronator teres, pronator quadratus, and brachioradialis. The brachioradialis also assists with supination, which is mainly controlled by the supinator muscle and the biceps brachii (Activity 10-8).

WRIST AND HAND REGION

The joints of the wrist, hand, and fingers are often taken for granted, even though the fine motor characteristics of this area are essential in skilled activities requiring precise functioning of the wrist and hand. Anatomically and structurally, the human wrist and hand have highly developed, complex mechanisms capable of a variety of movements. The amazing diversity of motion is a result of the arrangement of the 29 bones, more than 25 joints, and more than 30 muscles (of which 15 are intrinsic muscles with both origin and insertion found inside the hand). This complexity may be simplified by relating the functional anatomy to the major actions of the joints: flexion, extension, abduction, and adduction of the wrist and hand.

The wrist joint allows flexion, extension, abduction, and adduction. Wrist motion occurs primarily between the distal radius and the proximal carpal row, consisting of the scaphoid, lunate, and triquetrum. The joint allows 70 to 90 degrees of flexion and 65 to 85 degrees of extension. The wrist can abduct 15 to 25 degrees and adduct 25 to 40 degrees.

Each finger has three joints. In these joints, 0 to 40 degrees of extension and 85 to 100 degrees of flexion are possible. The proximal interphalangeal joint, classified as a hinge joint, can move from full extension to 90 to 120 degrees of flexion. The distal interphalangeal joints, also classified as hinge joints, can flex 80 to 90 degrees from full extension.

The thumb has only two joints, both of which are classified as hinge joints. The metacarpophalangeal joint moves from full extension into 40 to 90 degrees of flexion. The interphalangeal joint can flex 80 to 90 degrees. The carpometacarpal joint of the thumb is a unique saddle-type joint having 50 to 70 degrees of abduction. It can flex approximately 15 to 45 degrees and extends 0 to 20 degrees. Numerous ligaments support and provide static stability to many joints of the wrist and hand.

ACTIVITY 10-8

In this activity you will be working with a partner to assess individual movement patterns, normal function, and possible dysfunction in each other. One of you is to first isolate the specified movement patterns on each side of your partner, one side at a time, and assess for normal function by applying gentle pressure opposite to the action of the isolation position. The body is to be stabilized so that only the isolated area is moving. In some instances the ability to assume the position and maintain it indicates normal function. Muscles should be able to hold against gravity or the applied pressure without strain or pain. The position itself should be easy to assume and comfortable to maintain for a short duration, from 10 to 30 seconds. The bilateral movement patterns should be the same. The opposite movement pattern should also be able to be done easily. Dysfunction may be indicated by bilateral asymmetry, pain, weakness, fatigue, and inability to assume the isolation position or move into the opposite position. Intervention or referral depends on the severity of the condition and whether the dysfunction is neuromuscular, myofascial, or joint related.

NOTE: Do not perform these assessments if contraindications exist. Contraindications to this type of assessment include joint and disk dysfunction, acute pain, recent trauma, and inflammation.

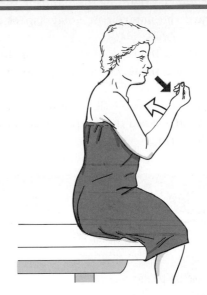

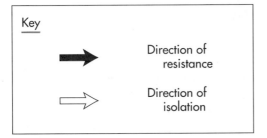

Key

→ Direction of resistance

⇨ Direction of isolation

ELBOW FLEXION

Assesses for strength and endurance in the isolation position and tension or shortening in the elbow extension pattern

Muscles involved

Biceps brachii—short head

Brachialis

Brachioradialis

Pronator teres

Range of motion

0 to 150 degrees

Position of client

Seated, with arms at sides

Three separate muscles can be isolated depending on position of forearm:

Biceps brachii—forearm in supination

Brachialis—forearm in pronation

Brachioradialis—forearm in midposition between pronation and supination

Client's forearm is flexed to 90 degrees and examiner stabilizes at elbow

Isolation and assessment (all three forearm positions)

Client flexes elbow through range of motion while resistance is applied to distal forearm

ELBOW EXTENSION

Assesses for strength and endurance in the isolation position and tension or shortening in the elbow flexion pattern

Muscles involved

Triceps brachii

Anconeus

Range of motion

0 to 180 degrees

Position of client

Standing or seated with arm to be tested able to extend without touching table

Forearm is flexed and examiner stabilizes at elbow

Isolation and assessment

Client extends elbow to end of available range without extending shoulder

Resistance is applied at wrist to prevent the action

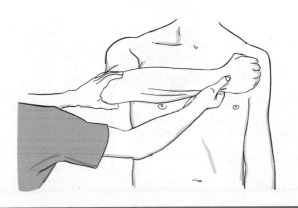

Continued

Movements of the Wrist and Hand (Activity 10-9)

Flexion—Moving the palm of the hand or the phalanges toward the anterior or volar aspect of the forearm

Extension—Moving the back of the hand or the phalanges toward the posterior or dorsal aspect of the forearm

Abduction (radial flexion)—Movement of the thumb side of the hand toward the lateral aspect or radial side of the forearm

Adduction (ulnar flexion)—Movement of the little finger side of the hand toward the medial aspect or ulnar side of the forearm

Opposition—Movement of the thumb across the palmar aspect to oppose any or all of the phalanges

Muscles of the Wrist and Hand

The extrinsic muscles of the wrist and hand may be grouped according to function and location. The wrist flexor-pronator muscle group includes the pronator teres, flexor carpi radialis, flexor carpi

---

ACTIVITY 10-8—cont'd

FOREARM SUPINATION

Assesses for strength and endurance in the isolation position and tension or shortening in the pronation pattern

Muscles involved

Supinator

Biceps brachii

Range of motion

0 to 90 degrees

Position of client

Seated, arm at side and elbow flexed to 90 degrees; forearm in neutral or mid-position

Examiner stabilizes at elbow with one hand and grasps forearm above wrist with other hand

Isolation and assessment

Client supinates the forearm until the palm faces the ceiling while examiner resists motion

FOREARM PRONATION

Assesses for strength and endurance in the isolation position and tension or shortening in the supination pattern

Muscles involved

Pronator teres

Pronator quadratus

Flexor carpi radialis

Range of motion

0 to 80 degrees

Position of client

Seated with arm at side and elbow flexed to 90 degrees; forearm in neutral position

Examiner stabilizes at elbow with one hand and grasps forearm at wrist with other hand

Isolation and assessment

Client pronates the forearm until the palm faces downward while examiner resists motion of supination

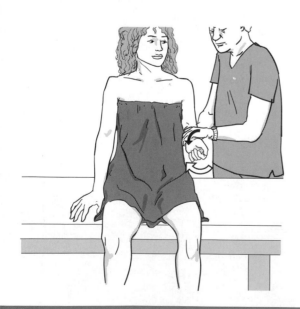
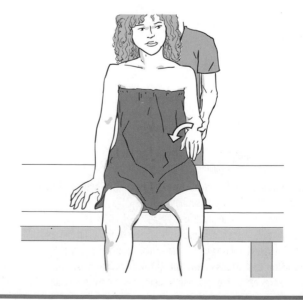

ulnaris, and palmaris longus. All the wrist flexors generally have their origins on the anteromedial aspect of the proximal forearm and medial epicondyle of the humerus, whereas their insertions are on the anterior aspect of the wrist and hand.

The wrist extensors include the extensor carpi radialis longus, extensor carpi radialis brevis, and extensor carpi ulnaris muscles. The wrist extensors generally have their origins on the posterolateral aspect of the proximal forearm and lateral humeral epicondyle, and their insertions are located on the posterior aspect of the hand and wrist.

The wrist abductors include the flexor carpi radialis, extensor carpi radialis longus, extensor carpi radialis brevis, abductor pollicis longus, extensor pollicis longus, and extensor pollicis brevis. These muscles generally cross the wrist joint anterolaterally and posterolaterally to insert on the radial side of the hand. The flexor carpi ulnaris and extensor carpi ulnaris adduct the wrist and cross the wrist joint anteromedially and posteromedially to insert on the ulnar side of the hand.

Another nine muscles function primarily to move the phalanges but are also involved in wrist joint actions because they originate on the forearm and cross the wrist. These muscles are generally weaker in their actions on the wrist. The flexor digitorum superficialis and flexor digitorum profundus are finger flexors, and they also assist in wrist flexion along with the flexor pollicis longus, which is a thumb flexor. The extensor digitorum, extensor indicis, and extensor digiti minimi are finger extensors and also assist in wrist extension, along with the extensor pollicis longus and extensor pollicis brevis, which extend the thumb. The abductor pollicis longus abducts the thumb and assists in wrist abduction.

Intrinsic hand muscles have their origin and insertion within the hand. They are primarily responsible for fine and precise movements of the fingers and thumb. Those acting on the thumb, located in the thenar eminence, include the opponens pollicis, abductor pollicis brevis, and flexor pollicis brevis. Those acting on the little finger are the opponens digiti minimi, abductor digiti minimi, and flexor digiti minimi brevis. These muscles are located in the hypothenar eminence. Acting with the thenar muscles, they function in opposition, allowing effective grasping movements.

The lumbricales flex the metacarpophalangeal joint and extend the interphalangeal joints. The dorsal and palmar interossei muscles are involved with adduction and abduction of the fingers. The adductor and abductor pollicis muscles adduct and abduct the thumb. With these actions the hand is able to hold and manipulate small objects such as a pencil (Activity 10-10).

ACTIVITY 10-9

Slowly move your wrist and fingers through the movement patterns described. Isolate wrist action from finger action. Combine as many different wrist, finger, and thumb actions as possible and notice the endless combinations. In the space provided describe the experience.

Example

I can make my hand dance.

Your Turn

PELVIC GIRDLE AND HIP JOINT REGION

The pelvis consists of two bones and three joints. The bones are the coxal bones, made up of the ilium, ischium, pubis, and sacrum. The three joints are the two sacroiliac articulations and the symphysis pubis.

Motion in the Pelvic Girdle

The pelvic girdle functions as one unit with all three bones moving at all three joints. It is influenced by the lower extremities, the vertebral column, and the trunk. The unit moves around a vertical axis. In a movement to the left, the symphysis turns left of the midline, the right coxal is turning forward, the left coxal turns backwards, and the sacrum turns a little to the left. The reverse happens when rotating to the right.

ACTIVITY 10-10

In this activity, you will be working with a partner to assess individual movement patterns, normal function, and possible dysfunction in each other. One of you is to first isolate the specified movement patterns on each side of your partner, one side at a time, and assess for normal function by applying a gentle pressure opposite to the action of the isolation position. The body is to be stabilized so that only the isolated area is moving. In some instances the ability to assume the position and maintain it indicates normal function. Muscles should be able to hold against gravity or the applied pressure without strain or pain. The position itself should be easy to assume and comfortable to maintain for a short duration, from 10 to 30 seconds. The bilateral movement patterns should be the same. The opposite movement pattern should also be able to be done easily. Dysfunction may be indicated by bilateral asymmetry, pain, weakness, fatigue, and inability to assume the isolation position or move into the opposite position. Intervention or referral depends on the severity of the condition and whether the dysfunction is neuromuscular, myofascial, or joint related.

NOTE: Do not perform these assessments if contraindications exist. Contraindications to this type of assessment include joint and disk dysfunction, acute pain, recent trauma, and inflammation.

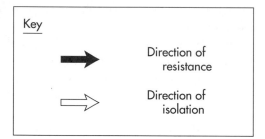

Key

→ Direction of resistance

⇨ Direction of isolation

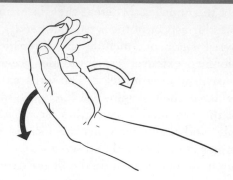

WRIST EXTENSION
Assesses for strength and endurance in the isolation position and tension or shortening in the flexion pattern
Muscles involved
Extensor carpi radialis longus
Extensor carpi radialis brevis
Extensor carpi ulnaris
Extensor digitorum
Extensor digiti minimi
Extensor indicis
Extensor pollicis longus
Range of motion
0 to 85 degrees
Position of client
Seated, with elbow flexed as needed; forearm pronated while arm is supported on table
Isolation and assessment
Client hyperextends wrist while examiner resists action
Client's thumb and fingers stay relaxed

WRIST FLEXION
Assesses for strength and endurance in the isolation position and tension or shortening in the extension pattern
Muscles involved
Flexor carpi radialis
Flexor carpi ulnaris
Palmaris longus
Abductor pollicis longus
Flexor digitorum superficialis
Flexor pollicis longus
Flexor digitorum profundus
Range of motion
0 to 80 degrees
Position of client
Seated with elbow flexed if needed and the forearm supinated while supported on its dorsal surface on a table
Wrist position is neutral
Isolation and assessment
Client flexes the wrist while examiner resists action
Make sure client's thumbs and fingers are relaxed

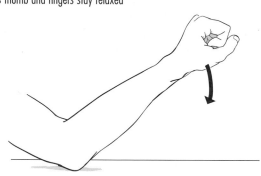

FLEXION OF FINGERS
Assesses for strength and endurance in the isolation position and tension or shortening in the finger extension pattern
Muscles involved
Lumbricales
Dorsal interossei
Palmar interossei
Flexor digitorum superficialis
Flexor digitorum profundus

ACTIVITY 10-10—cont'd

Range of motion

0 to 100 degrees

Position of client

Seated, elbow flexed, forearm supinated and supported on a table, wrist in neutral

Wrist is maintained in neutral

Begin with metacarpophalangeal (MP) joints fully extended and interphalangeal (IP) joints flexed

Each finger is to be isolated separately

Isolation and assessment

Client flexes the MP joint (bends knuckles) and extends the IP (finger) joints while examiner resists MP flexion

Make sure client does not flex IP joint

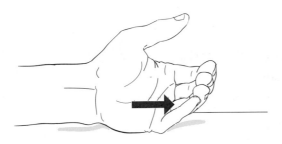

FINGER EXTENSION

Assesses for strength and endurance in the isolation position and tension or shortening in the finger flexion pattern.

Muscles involved

Extensor digitorum

Extensor indicis

Extensor digiti minimi

Range of motion

0 to 15 degrees

Position of client

Seated, with forearm in pronation and supported on a table; wrist in neutral

Isolation and assessment

No resistance needed

Ability to perform isolation indicates normal function

Extensor digitorum—Client extends MP joints (all fingers simultaneously), allowing the IP joints to be in slight flexion

Extensor indicis—Client extends the MP joint of the index finger

Extensor digiti minimi—Client extends the joint of the fifth digit

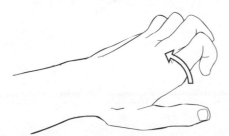

FINGER ABDUCTION

Assesses for strength and endurance in the isolation position and tension or shortening in the finger adduction pattern

Muscles involved

Dorsal interossei

Abductor digiti minimi

Range of motion

0 to 20 degrees

Position of client

Seated, with forearm pronated and supported, wrist in neutral

Fingers are abducted (separated) and MP joints remain neutral

Isolation and assessment

Each finger is isolated separately while resistance is given near distal end of finger to push it together with other fingers

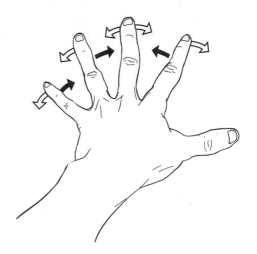

Dorsal interossei:

Abduction of ring finger toward little finger (includes abductor digiti minimi)

Abduction of middle finger toward ring finger

Abduction of middle finger toward index finger

Abduction of index finger toward thumb

FINGER ADDUCTION

Assesses for strength and endurance in the isolation position and tension or shortening in the finger abduction pattern

Muscles involved

Palmar interossei

Range of motion

0 to 20 degrees

Position of client

Seated, with elbow flexed, forearm pronated and supported, wrist in neutral, and fingers extended and adducted (together)

MP joints are neutral

Isolation and assessment

Fingers are tested separately, middle finger is not tested because it has no palmar interossei muscle

Continued

ACTIVITY 10-10—cont'd

Resistance is given near distal end of finger to pull it away from other fingers
Adduction of little finger is toward ring finger
Adduction of ring finger is toward middle finger
Adduction of index finger is toward middle finger
Adduction of thumb is toward index finger

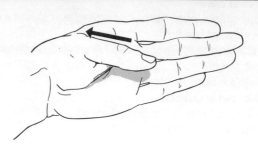

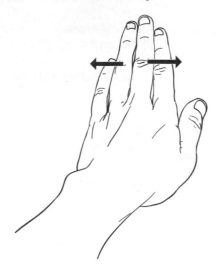

THUMB ADDUCTION, FLEXION, AND MEDIAL ROTATION

Assesses for strength and endurance in the isolation position and tension or shortening in the thumb extension pattern
Thumb extensors are extrinsic muscles
The thumb has 0 to 20 degrees of extension

Muscles involved

Flexor pollicis brevis
Flexor pollicis longus
Adductor pollicis

Range of motion

MP flexion—0 to 50 degrees
IP flexion—0 to 80 degrees
Adduction—0 to 70 degrees

Position of client

Seated, with forearm supinated and supported; wrist in neutral
Carpometacarpal (CMC) joint and IP joints neutral
Thumb in adduction

Isolation and assessment

Client flexes the MP joint of the thumb to slide thumb across palm while resistance to pull thumb back is given between CMC and IP joints
IP joint does not flex

THUMB OPPOSITION

Muscles involved

Opponens pollicis
Opponens digiti minimi

Range of motion

0 to 70 degrees

Position of client

Seated, with forearm supinated and supported, wrist in neutral, and thumb in palmar abduction
Opponens pollicis—Apply resistance for the opponens pollicis at the head of the first metacarpal in the direction of lateral rotation, extension, and adduction

Isolation and assessment

Client medially rotates and flexes thumb toward little finger while little finger flexes and rotates toward thumb so pads of digits touch (not tips of digits)
The examiner applies resistance on palmar surface of thumb and fifth metacarpal to bring them apart

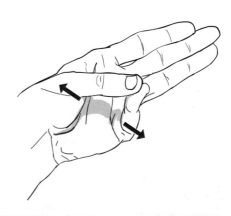

The pelvic girdle moves back and forth within three planes for a total of six different movements. To avoid confusion, it is important to analyze the pelvic girdle activity to determine the exact location of the movement.

All pelvic girdle rotation results from motion at the right hip, left hip, or lumbar spine. Although it is not essential for movement to occur in all three of these areas, it must occur in at least one for the pelvis to rotate in any direction. Even though the sacroiliac (SI) joints are synovial joints, they permit very little movement and even fuse in many people later in life. This general reduction of motion is related to degenerative changes such as osteoarthritis.

Four groups of ligaments form the main bond that keeps the ilium and sacrum in close approximation. Stability of the SI joints is crucial because they maintain support for a large portion of the body's weight. More movement (therefore less stability) is present in the sacroiliac joints of women, who have smaller and flatter surfaces involving only the first two sacral vertebra, than in men, who have longer, more concave surfaces involving the first three sacral vertebra.

When weight is shifted from one leg to the other while standing, the symphysis may show an upward/downward motion of 2 mm. During pregnancy the symphysis may separate from 5 to 9 mm.

During normal walking, motions involve the entire pelvic girdle and both hip joints. When the pelvic girdle rotates forward, hip flexion occurs; when it rotates backward, hip extension occurs. The symphysis pubis serves as the axis for the rotation. Jogging and running result in faster and greater range of these movements.

Muscular attachments to the pelvic girdle are extensive, but no muscles directly influence the sacroiliac joint. Indirect actions come from the abdominal muscles, which insert on the superior aspect of the pelvic girdle and are joined by the quadratus lumborum.

Six groups of hip and thigh muscles are attached to the pelvic girdle and lower extremities. These hip muscles highly influence the movement of the two coxal bones within the pelvic girdle. Anterior to the SI joint are two very important muscles, the psoas and piriformis.

The psoas crosses over the anterior aspect of the SI joint and goes from the lumbar region to insert into the lesser trochanter of the femur. The right and left piriformis originate from the anterior surface of the sacrum, pass through the sciatic notch, and insert into the greater trochanter of the femur. Muscle imbalance of any of these groups can adversely affect pelvic function.

The pelvic girdle is thought to be of importance within the craniosacral system. Theory indicates that the sacrum has a mobility between the two coxals as part of the craniosacral rhythm. Any changes or alteration in biomechanical function of the pelvic girdle can negatively influence the craniosacral mechanism; the reverse is also true.

Because the pelvis is the supporting base of the spine, dysfunctions in its joints have a great effect on the lumbar spine. Sacroiliac pain is felt as a dull ache, usually in the bones above the buttock on one side. Because the nerves in that region are not very specific, pain caused by the SI joint can also be felt in the groin, back of the thigh, and lower abdomen.

One of the most common dysfunctions occurs when leaning forward to lift some heavy object, instead of going into the bent-knee position. If the abdominals are strong and support the anterior pelvis, stabilizing the trunk to maintain a more or less constant balance between the trunk and the pelvis, no dysfunction happens. But if the abdominal muscles and the sacrotuberous ligaments are weak, dysfunction and pain could occur.

Hip Joint

Except for the glenohumeral joint, the hip joint is one of the most mobile joints of the body, largely because of its multiaxial arrangement. Unlike the glenohumeral, the hip joint's bony architecture provides a great deal of stability, resulting in relatively few hip joint dislocations. An extremely strong and dense ligamentous capsule reinforces the joint, especially the anterior portion.

Because of individual differences, some disagreement exists about the exact range of each movement in the hip joint, but the ranges are generally 0 to 130 degrees of flexion, 0 to 30 degrees of extension, 0 to 35 degrees of abduction, 0 to 30 degrees of adduction, 0 to 45 degrees of internal rotation, and 0 to 50 degrees of external rotation.

Movements of the Hip Joint

Anterior and posterior pelvic rotations occur in the sagittal or anteroposterior plane, whereas right and left lateral rotation occur in the lateral or frontal plane. Right transverse (clockwise) rotation and left transverse (counterclockwise) rotation occur in the horizontal or transverse plane of motion.

Anterior pelvic rotation—Anterior movement of the upper pelvis; the iliac crest tilts forward in a sagittal plane

Posterior pelvic rotation—Posterior movement of the upper pelvis; the iliac crest tilts backward in a sagittal plane

Left lateral pelvic rotation—In the frontal plane the left pelvis moves superiorly in relation to the right pelvis, either the left pelvis rotates upward or the right pelvis rotates downward

Right lateral pelvic rotation—In the frontal plane the right pelvis moves superiorly in relation to the left pelvis; either the right pelvis rotates upward or the left pelvis rotates downward

Left transverse pelvic rotation—In a horizontal plane of motion the pelvis rotates to the body's left; the right iliac crest moves anteriorly in relation to left iliac crest, which moves posteriorly

Right transverse pelvic rotation—In a horizontal plane of motion the pelvis rotates to the body's right; the left iliac crest moves anteriorly in relation to right iliac crest, which moves posteriorly

Hip flexion—Movement of the femur straight anteriorly toward the pelvis

Hip extension—Movement of the femur straight posteriorly away from the pelvis

Hip abduction—Movement of the femur laterally to the side away from midline

Hip adduction—Movement of the femur medially toward the midline

Hip external rotation—Rotary movement of the femur laterally around its longitudinal axis away from the midline

Hip internal rotation—Rotary movement of the femur medially around its longitudinal axis toward the midline

The lumbar spine, hip joint, and pelvic girdle work together in carrying out lower extremity activities. Table 10-2 shows a comparison of pelvic girdle, lumbar spine, and hip joint movements (Activity 10-11).

Muscles of the Hip Joint

At the hip joint are six two-joint muscles that have one action at the hip and another at the knee. The muscles usually involved in hip and pelvic girdle motions depend largely on the direction of the movement and the position of the body in relation to the earth and its gravitational forces. In addition, it should be noted that the body part that moves the most will be the part least stabilized. For example, when standing on both feet and contracting the hip flexors, the trunk and pelvis will flex anteriorly; but when lying supine and contracting the hip flexors, the thighs will move forward into flexion on the stable pelvis. In another example, the hip flexor muscles are used in moving the legs toward the trunk, but the extensor muscles are used eccentrically when the pelvis and trunk move downward slowly on the femur and concentrically when the trunk is raised on the femur such as rising to the standing position.

In the downward phase of the knee-bend exercise, the movement at the hips and knees is flexion. The muscles involved primarily are the hip and knee extensors in eccentric contraction.

The iliopsoas muscle provides powerful actions such as raising the legs from a supine position on the floor. Its origin in the lower back tends to move the lower back anteriorly, or, in the supine position, pulls the lower back up as it raises the legs. For this reason, lower back problems are often felt with this activity because leg raising is primarily hip flexion, not abdominal action. Strong abdominals prevent

TABLE 10-2 PELVIC GIRDLE, LUMBAR SPINE, AND HIP JOINT MOVEMENTS

PELVIC ROTATIONS	LUMBAR SPINE MOTION	RIGHT HIP MOTION	LEFT HIP MOTION
Anterior rotation	Extension	Flexion	Flexion
Posterior rotation	Flexion	Extension	Extension
Right lateral rotation	Right lateral flexion	Adduction	Abduction
Left lateral rotation	Left lateral flexion	Abduction	Adduction
Right transverse rotation	Left lateral rotation	Internal rotation	External rotation
Left transverse rotation	Right lateral rotation	External rotation	Internal rotation

lower back strain by pulling up on the front of the pelvis and thus flattening the back.

The sartorius, a two-joint muscle, is effective as both a hip and knee flexor. It is weak when both actions occur at the same time. When the knees are extended, the sartorius becomes a more effective hip flexor.

The rectus femoris muscle pulls from the anterior inferior iliac spine of the ilium to rotate the pelvis anteriorly. Only the abdominal muscles can prevent this from occurring. In older adults the pelvis may be permanently tilted forward. The relaxed abdominal wall does not hold the pelvis up, and therefore an increased lumbar curve results. The rectus femoris muscle is a powerful extensor of the knee when the hip is extended but is weak when the hip is flexed.

The pectineus tends to rotate the pelvis anteriorly. The abdominal muscles pulling up on the pelvis in front counteract this tilting.

The tensor fasciae latae muscle is used when flexion and internal rotation take place. This muscle also aids in preventing external rotation of the femur as it is flexed by other flexor muscles.

Typical action of the gluteus medius and gluteus minimus muscles is seen in walking. As the weight of the body is shifted to one leg, these muscles prevent the opposite hip from sagging. Weakness in the gluteus medius and gluteus minimus can result in what is known as the *Trendelenburg gait.*

With this weakness, the individual's opposite hip will sag on weight bearing because the hip abductors cannot maintain proper alignment. As the body ages, the gluteus medius and gluteus minimus muscles tend to lose their effectiveness. Walking loses its easy spring and becomes more labored.

The gluteus maximus muscle comes into action when movement between the pelvis and the femur approaches and goes beyond 15 degrees of extension. As a result, it is not used extensively in ordinary walking. It is important in extension of the thigh with external rotation.

The six deep lateral rotator muscles—piriformis, gemellus superior, gemellus inferior, obturator externus, obturator internus, quadratus femoris—provide powerful movements of external rotation of the femur. Standing on one leg and forcefully turning the body away from that leg is accomplished by contraction of these muscles.

The hamstrings (semitendinosus, semimembranosus, and biceps femoris), together with the gluteus maximus muscle, are used in the extension of the thigh when the knees are straight. These muscles are used in ordinary walking as extensors of the hip and allow the gluteus maximus to relax in the movement. When the trunk is bent forward with the knees straight, the hamstring muscles have a powerful pull on the rear pelvis and tilt it down in back. If the knees are flexed when this movement takes place, the work is done chiefly by the gluteus maximus muscle.

The adductor brevis, adductor longus, adductor magnus, and gracilis all provide powerful movement of the thighs toward each other (Activity 10-12).

ACTIVITY 10-11

Slowly and deliberately move your joints through each of the movement patterns described. Identify the interplay between the hip movements and the pelvic girdle movements, paying close attention to the secondary movement of the pelvic girdle during hip movement. In the space provided, describe the experience.

Example

I could feel the rotation at the symphysis pubis when I walked if I placed my fingers on the joint.

Your Turn

KNEE REGION

The knee joint is the largest and most complex joint in the body. It is primarily a hinge joint. The combined functions of weight bearing and locomotion place considerable stress and strain on the knee joint. The ligaments provide static stability to the knee joint, and contractions of the quadriceps and hamstrings produce dynamic stability.

The knee includes the articulation of the femur and tibia and the patella, which covers it anteriorly. The knee acts as part of a chain with the lumbar spine, hip, and ankle. Weight-bearing forces normally bisect the

ACTIVITY 10-12

In this activity, you will be working with a partner to assess individual movement patterns, normal function, and possible dysfunction in each other. One of you is to first isolate the specified movement patterns on each side of your partner, one side at a time, and assess for normal function by applying gentle pressure opposite to the action of the isolation position. The body is to be stabilized so that only the isolated area is moving. In some instances the ability to assume the position and maintain it indicates normal function. Muscles should be able to hold against gravity or the applied pressure without strain or pain. The position itself should be easy to assume and comfortable to maintain for a short duration, from 10 to 30 seconds. The bilateral movement patterns should be the same. The opposite movement pattern should also be able to be done easily. Dysfunction may be indicated by bilateral asymmetry, pain, weakness, fatigue, and inability to assume the isolation position or move into the opposite position.

Intervention or referral depends on the severity of the condition and whether the dysfunction is neuromuscular, myofascial, or joint related.

NOTE: Do not perform these assessments if contraindications exist. Contraindications to this type of assessment include joint and disk dysfunction, acute pain, recent trauma, and inflammation.

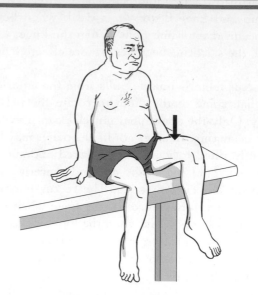

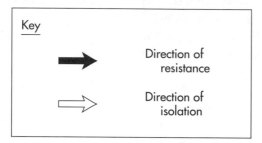

Key

➡ Direction of resistance

⇨ Direction of isolation

HIP FLEXION

Assesses for strength and endurance in the isolation position and tension or shortening in the hip extension pattern

Muscles involved

Psoas major
Iliacus
Rectus femoris
Sartorius
Tensor fasciae latae
Lectineus
Adductor brevis
Adductor longus
Adductor magnus

Range of motion

0 to 130 degrees

Position of client

Seated, with knees bent with thighs fully supported on table and feet hanging over the edge
Client may use arms for stability

Isolation and assessment

Client flexes hip through full range while examiner applies resistance on anterior thigh above knee to push leg down

HIP EXTENSION

Assesses for strength and endurance in the isolation position and tension or shortening in the hip flexion pattern

Muscles involved

Gluteus maximus
Semitendinosus
Semimembranosus
Biceps femoris (long head)

Range of motion

0 to 30 degrees

Position of client

Prone, with arms overhead or abducted to hold sides of table
Place pillows under hips to help flex hips for start position

Isolation and assessment

Client extends hip through entire available range of motion while knee is extended
Entire leg should clear table
Resistance is applied to posterior thigh above knee to push leg down

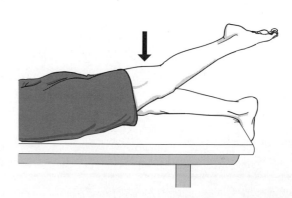

ACTIVITY 10-12—cont'd

HIP ABDUCTION

Assesses for strength and endurance in the isolation position and tension or shortening in the hip adduction pattern

Muscles involved

Gluteus medius

Gluteus minimus

Tensor fasciae latae

Gluteus maximus (upper fibers)

Range of motion

0 to 35 degrees

Position of client

Side-lying on nontest side, hip and knee flexed for stability

Hip is slightly extended on leg to be tested

Isolation and assessment

Client abducts hip through range of motion leading with heel to prevent flexing or rotating the hip

Resistance is applied to lateral aspect of thigh above knee to push leg down

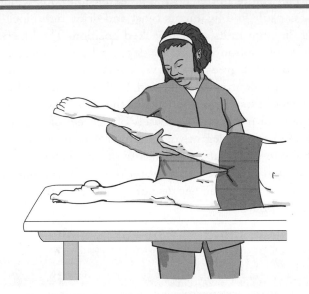

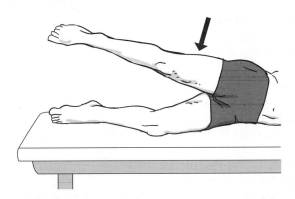

HIP ADDUCTION

Assesses for strength and endurance in the isolation position and tension or shortening in the hip abduction pattern

Muscles involved

Adductor magnus

Adductor brevis

Adductor longus

Pectineus

Gracilis

Range of motion

0 to 15 to 30 degrees

Position of client

Side-lying on test side with uppermost limb in 25 degrees of abduction, supported by the examiner

The therapist cradles the leg with the forearm, the hand supporting the limb on the medial surface of the table

Isolation and Assessment

Client adducts hip until the lower limb contacts the upper one

No resistance is needed

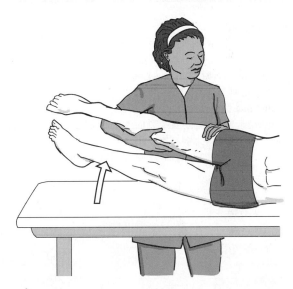

HIP EXTERNAL OR LATERAL ROTATION

Assesses for strength and endurance in the isolation position and tension or shortening in the hip internal or medial rotation pattern.

Muscles involved

Obturator externus

Obturator internus

Quadratus femoris

Piriformis

Gemellus superior

Gemellus inferior

Gluteus maximus

Sartorius

Range of motion

0 to 45 degrees

Continued

knee even though it has a slight valgus angulation. A slight hyperextension of both knees when standing is normal (more in females). The extension ends when the capsule and ligaments twist and draw tight, locking the joint in its closed-packed position. The knee's range of motion is 5 to 10 degrees hyperextension, 135 to 150 degrees flexion with soft tissue of the calf and thigh limiting flexion, and 10 degrees internal or external tibial rotation. With the knee flexed 30 degrees or more, approximately 30 degrees of internal rotation and 45 degrees of external rotation can occur. The external rotation of the tibia toward the end of extension and internal rotation during beginning of flexion is automatic because of the shape of the articulating bones.

The quadriceps pull the patella in line with the femur. The patellar tendon pulls it in line with the tibia. The Q angle is the angle formed by these two pulls. The tension from the quadriceps and patellar tendon plus the anterior projection of the lateral femoral condyle and the deep patellar groove in the femur hold the patella in place during flexion. As the muscle contracts, the patella moves out of the groove and lateral, and the Q angle decreases. The lateral femoral condyle and the contraction of the vastus medialis muscle help prevent lateral dislocation of the patella. This is particularly important for a female because the broader pelvis causes a greater Q angle and a stronger lateral pull (Figure 10-13).

ACTIVITY 10-12—cont'd

Position of client
Seated, with hips flexed but not rotated
Patella in line with anterior superior interior spine (ASIS)
Examiner stabilizes outer thigh above knee
Trunk is supported by placing hands at sides

Isolation and assessment
Client externally rotates hip by bringing the sole of the foot toward the opposite calf while resistance is applied to inner ankle
Caution must be taken to avoid knee stress with resistance

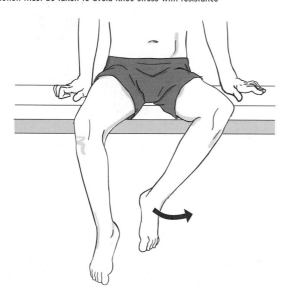

HIP INTERNAL OR MEDIAL ROTATION
Assesses for strength and endurance in the isolation position and tension or shortening in the lateral or external hip rotation pattern

Muscles involved
Gluteus minimus
Gluteus medius
Tensor fasciae latae

Range of motion
0 to 50 degrees

Position of client
Seated, with hips flexed, patella in line with ASIS
Arms at sides to support the trunk
Examiner stabilizes medial thigh just above knee

Isolation and assessment
Client internally rotates hip turning sole of foot to the side and bringing the knee toward the opposite leg while examiner applies resistance to outer ankle, avoiding knee strain

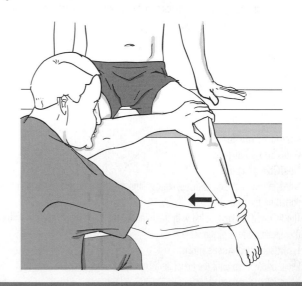

The superior tibiofemoral joint aids the knee in supporting one sixth of the body weight. It glides anteriorly during knee flexion and rotates with ankle dorsiflexion. Joint dysfunctions such as hypomobility can lead to lateral knee, leg, or ankle pain.

Other Major Knee Components

Two cartilaginous menisci partially fill the space between the tibia and femur's articulating surfaces. Both menisci are thicker on the periphery than in the center margin. They move with the tibia during flexion or extension and with the femur in rotation. Menisci improve weight distribution by increasing the contact area between the two long bones. They act as shock absorbers by spreading the stress over the articulating surfaces, decreasing friction and cartilage wear. They are part of the knee's "locking" mechanism, which prevents hyperextension by directing the movement of the articulating condyles.

The medial (tibial) collateral ligament (MCL) is a strong, broad triangular strap that attaches to the femur's medial epicondyle. It helps prevent anterior tibial displacement on the femur. The lateral collateral ligament (LCL) is shorter and more rounded than the MCL. It is located between the biceps femoris tendon externally and the popliteus tendon internally. It does not attach to the lateral meniscus. Its fibers are tight, especially during knee extension, tibial adduction, and lateral rotation. It helps to protect the lateral aspect of the knee from varus stress.

The MCL and LCL twist in relationship with each other to protect the knee externally from excessive tibial rotation and extension. The cruciate ligaments are the main rotary stabilizers and cross each other within the capsule. These ligaments are vital in maintaining the anterior, posterior, and rotary stability of the knee joint. They aid the rolling and gliding movements of the tibia on the femur and are rotary guides for the "screw-home" locking mechanism of the knee.

The screw-home mechanism occurs with rotary movement of the knee. This rotary motion occurs, not as a result of muscle action, but from joint and menisci structure. The articular surface of the medial femoral condyle is longer than that of the lateral condyle. In addition the **C** shape of the medial meniscus allows the medial tibial condyle to rotate around the femoral condyle. The lateral meniscus is shaped like an **O** and holds the lateral tibial condyle more securely against the femoral condyle and does not allow motion. As a result of these structural features, the medial condyle of the tibia rotates on the femur during the last 15 degrees of knee extension in an external direction in the non–weight-bearing position. In the weight-bearing position, the femur medially rotates on the tibia when the knee is fully extended. This action locks the knee into extension, which allows us to stand without using muscle action but instead supported on the ligaments at the hip. This saves energy and allows individuals to stand for extended periods without fatigue. The popliteus muscle unlocks the knee to begin flexion.

The knee joint is well supplied with synovial fluid from a synovial cavity, which lies under the patella and between the surfaces of the tibia and the femur. Commonly, this synovial cavity is called the "capsule of the knee." More than 10 bursae are located in the knee, some of which are connected to the synovial cavity. Bursae are located where they can absorb shock or prevent friction.

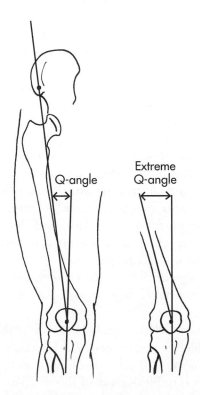

FIGURE 10-13 The quadriceps angle (Q-angle) is measured from the ASIS through the axis of the patella and distally to the insertion of the patellar tendon on the tibial tubercle. (From Shankman GA: *Fundamental orthopedic management for the physical therapist assistant,* St Louis, 1997, Mosby.)

Movements of the Knee

Flexion and extension of the knee occur in the sagittal plane, whereas internal and external rotation occur in the horizontal plane (Activity 10-13).

Flexion—Bending or decreasing the angle of the knee; characterized by the heel moving toward the buttocks

Extension—Straightening or increasing the angle of the knee

External rotation—Rotary motion of the lower leg laterally away from the midline

Internal rotation—Rotary motion of the lower leg medially toward the midline

Muscles of the Knee

The muscles that flex and medially rotate the knee are the hamstrings, sartorius, gracilis, and popliteus. The popliteus muscle is the only flexor of the leg found only at the knee. All other flexors are two-joint muscles. Two-joint muscles are most effective when either origin or insertion is fixed by the contraction of the muscles that prevent movement in the direction of the pull. All the hamstring muscles, as well as the rectus femoris, are biarticular (two-joint) muscles.

The popliteus provides posterolateral stability to the knee and assists the medial hamstrings in internal rotation of the lower leg at the knee. The plantaris and gastrocnemius assist flexion.

The quadriceps extend the knee. All quadriceps muscles attach to the patella and by the patellar tendon to the tibial tuberosity. All these muscles are superficial and palpable except the vastus intermedius, which is under the rectus femoris. It is generally desired for this muscle group to be 25% to 33% stronger than the hamstring muscle group (knee flexors).

The tensor fascia latae helps flexion and extension. The semimembranosus and semitendinosus (medial hamstrings) muscles are assisted by the popliteus in internally rotating the knee, whereas the biceps femoris (lateral hamstrings) is responsible for knee external rotation (Activity 10-14).

ANKLE AND FOOT REGION

The ankle joint is made up of the talus, distal tibia, and distal fibula. The ankle joint allows approximately 50 degrees of plantar flexion and 15 to 20 degrees of dorsiflexion. Greater range of dorsiflexion is possible when the knee is flexed, which reduces the tension of the biarticular gastrocnemius muscle.

Inversion and eversion, although commonly thought to be ankle joint movements, technically occur in the subtalar and transverse tarsal joint. These joints combine to allow approximately 20 to 30 degrees of inversion and 5 to 25 degrees of eversion. Minimal movement occurs within the remainder of the intertarsal and tarsometatarsal arthrodial joints.

The complexity of the foot is evidenced by the 26 bones, 19 large muscles, many small (intrinsic) muscles, and more than 100 ligaments that make up the structure of the foot. The bones of the foot connect with the upper body's bony structure through the fibula and tibia. Body weight is transferred from the tibia to the talus and calcaneous.

Support and propulsion are the two functions of the foot. Proper functioning and adequate development of the muscles of the foot, and the practice of proper foot mechanics are essential for everyone. In our modern society, foot trouble is one of our most common ailments. Poor foot mechanics begun in early life invariably lead to foot discomfort in later years.

The metatarsophalangeal (MP) joint of the great toe flexes 45 degrees and extends 70 degrees, whereas the interphalangeal (IP) joint can flex from 0 degrees of full extension to 90 degrees of flexion. The MP joints of the four lesser toes allow approximately 40 degrees of flexion and 40 degrees of extension. The MP joints also adduct minimally. The proximal interphalangeal (PIP) joints in the lesser toes flex from 0 degrees of extension to 35 degrees of flexion. The distal interpha-

ACTIVITY 10-13

Slowly and deliberately move your joints through each of the movement patterns described. In the space provided, describe the experience.

Example

I could feel the rotation of my knee during the last phase of extension and noticed how solid it felt when the screw-home mechanism kicked in.

Your Turn

ACTIVITY 10-14

I n this activity, you will be working with a partner to assess individual movement patterns, normal function, and possible dysfunction in each other. One of you is to first isolate the specified movement patterns on each side of your partner, one side at a time, and assess for normal function by applying gentle pressure opposite to the action of the isolation position. The body is to be stabilized so that only the isolated area is moving. In some instances the ability to assume the position and maintain it indicates normal function. Muscles should be able to hold against gravity or the applied pressure without strain or pain. The position itself should be easy to assume and comfortable to maintain for a short duration, from 10 to 30 seconds. The bilateral movement patterns should be the same. The opposite movement pattern should also be able to be done easily.

Dysfunction may be indicated by bilateral asymmetry, pain, weakness, fatigue, and inability to assume the isolation position or move into the opposite position. Intervention or referral depends on the severity of the condition and whether the dysfunction is neuromuscular, myofascial, or joint related.

NOTE: Do not perform these assessments if contraindications exist. Contraindication to this type of assessment include joint and disk dysfunction, acute pain, recent trauma, and inflammation.

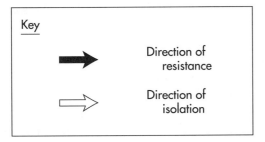

Key

→ Direction of resistance

⇨ Direction of isolation

KNEE FLEXION

Assesses for strength and endurance in the isolation position and tension or shortening in the extension pattern

Muscles involved

Biceps femoris

Semitendinosus

Semimembranosus

Popliteus

Gastrocnemius

Range of motion

0-150 degrees

Position of client

Prone, with limbs straight and toes hanging over the edge of the table

Examiner applies light to moderate counterpressure to hamstrings

Isolation and assessment

Client flexes knee through full range, keeping thigh in contact with table

Resistance is gradually applied to posterior leg proximal to ankle joint after knee reaches 45 degrees to straighten leg

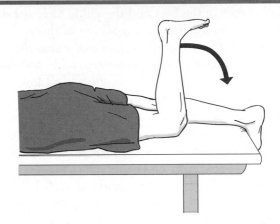

KNEE EXTENSION

Assesses for strength and endurance in the isolation position and tension or shortening in the flexion pattern

Muscles involved

Rectus femoris

Vastus intermedius

Vastus lateralis

Vastus medialis

Range of motion

0-135 degrees

May extend 10 degrees beyond 0 in those with hypertension

Position of client

Seated, with hips flexed and small pillow under thigh to maintain 90 degrees of hip flexion

Client grasps table edge for stabilization while examiner places one hand on distal anterior thigh

Isolation and assessment

Client extends knee through available range of motion as examiner applies resistance to distal end of anterior leg to bend it at the knee

Do not allow the client to hyperextend the knee or lift thigh off table

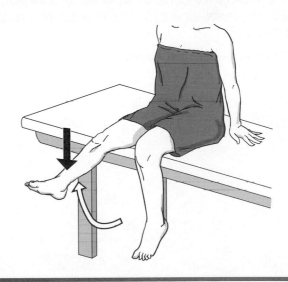

langeal (DIP) joint flexes 60 degrees and extends 30 degrees. Much variation exists from joint to joint and person to person in all of these joints.

Ligaments in the foot and the ankle have the difficult task of maintaining the position of the arches in the foot. The foot has three longitudinal arches: the medial and lateral and the transverse arch. Individual long arches vary from high, medium, and low, but a low arch is not necessarily a weak arch.

The medial longitudinal arch is located on the medial side of the foot and extends from the calcaneus to the talus, the navicular, the three cuneiforms, and the proximal ends of the three medial metatarsals. The lateral longitudinal arch is located on the lateral side of the foot and extends from the calcaneus to the cuboid and proximal ends of the fourth and fifth metatarsals. The transverse arch extends across the foot from one metatarsal bone to the other. A vast network of fascia in the sole of the foot supports the arches. Plantar fascia with the muscles provides the spring to the arch structure.

Movements of the Ankle and Foot (Activity 10-15)

Dorsiflexion—Movement of the top of the ankle and foot toward the anterior tibial bone; accomplished by the extensor muscles of the ankle

ACTIVITY 10-15

Slowly and deliberately move your ankle and then your toes through the movement patterns. Then move the ankle and toes together and differentiate between extrinsic (muscles with attachment outside the foot proper) and intrinsic (muscles with all attachments within the foot proper) muscle activity.

In the space provided describe the experience.

Example

It was hard to isolate the intrinsic muscle.

Your Turn

Plantar flexion—Movement of the ankle and foot away from the tibia; accomplished by the flexor muscles of the ankle

Eversion—Turning the ankle and foot outward, away from the midline; weight on the medial edge of the foot

Inversion—Turning the ankle and foot inward, toward the midline; weight on the lateral edge of the foot

Toe flexion—Movement of the toes toward the plantar surface of the foot

Toe extension—Movement of the toes away from the plantar surface of the foot

Muscles of the Ankle and Foot

The large number of muscles in the ankle and foot may be grouped according to location and function. In general, the muscles located on the anterior of the ankle and foot are the dorsal flexors. Those to the posterior are plantar flexors. Muscles that are everters are located more to the lateral side, and the invertors are located medially. The muscular strength patterns are not balanced. Plantar flexion is dominant over dorsiflexion, and inversion dominates eversion.

The gastrocnemius muscle is more effective as a knee flexor if the foot is elevated and more effective as a plantar flexor of the foot if the knee is held in extension. You can observe this when someone sits too close to the wheel when driving a car. When the knees are bent, the muscle becomes an ineffective plantar flexor, and the person finds it difficult to depress the brakes.

The soleus muscle is one of the most important plantar flexors of the ankle. This is especially true when the knee is flexed. When the knee is slightly flexed, the effect of the gastrocnemius is reduced, thereby placing more work on the soleus.

The tibialis posterior muscle pulls down from the underside and contracts to invert and plantar flex the foot. Use of the tibialis posterior in plantar flexion and inversion gives support to the longitudinal arch of the foot.

Passing down the back of the lower leg under the medial malleolus and then forward, the flexor digitorum longus muscle draws the four lesser toes down into flexion toward the heel as it plantar flexes the ankle. It is very important in helping other foot muscles maintain the longitudinal arch.

Pulling from the underside of the great toe, the flexor hallucis muscle may work independently of the flexor digitorum longus muscle or with it.

The peroneus longus muscle passes behind and beneath the lateral malleolus and under the foot from the outside to under the inner surface. Because of its line of pull, it is a strong everter and assists in plantar flexion. When the peroneus longus muscle is used effectively with the other ankle flexors, it helps support the transverse arch as it flexes.

The peroneus brevis muscle passes down behind and under the lateral malleolus to pull on the base of the fifth metatarsal. It is a primary everter of the foot and assists in plantar flexion. In addition, it aids in maintaining the longitudinal arch as it depresses the foot.

The tibialis anterior muscle holds up the inner margin of the foot. However, as it contracts, it dorsiflexes the ankle and is used as an antagonist to the plantar flexors of the ankle. The tibialis anterior is forced to contract strongly when a person ice skates or walks on the outside of the foot. It strongly supports the long arch in inversion.

Strength is necessary in the extensor digitorum longus muscle to maintain balance between the plantar and the dorsal flexors. The strength of the ankle is evident when the gastrocnemius, soleus, tibialis posterior, peroneus longus, peroneus brevis, digitorum longus, flexor digitorum brevis, and flexor hallucis longus muscles are all used effectively in walking.

Intrinsic Muscles of the Foot

The intrinsic muscles of the foot have their origin and insertion on the bones within the foot. Four layers of these muscles are found on the plantar surface of the foot. These muscles are involved with dorsiflexion and plantar flexion of the toes (Activity 10-16).

ACTIVITY 10-16

In this activity, you will be working with a partner to assess individual movement patterns, normal function, and possible dysfunction in each other. One of you is to first isolate the specified movement patterns on each side of your partner, one side at a time, and assess for normal function by applying gentle pressure opposite to the action of the isolation position. The body is to be stabilized so that only the isolated area is moving. In some instances the ability to assume the position and maintain it indicates normal function. Muscles should be able to hold against gravity or the applied pressure without strain or pain. The position itself should be easy to assume and comfortable to maintain for a short duration, from 10 to 30 seconds. The bilateral movement patterns should be the same. The opposite movement pattern should also be able to be done easily.

Dysfunction may be indicated by bilateral asymmetry, pain, weakness, fatigue, and inability to assume the isolation position or move into the opposite position. Intervention or referral depends on the severity of the condition and whether the dysfunction is neuromuscular, myofascial, or joint related.

NOTE: Do not perform these assessments if contraindications exist. Contraindications to this type of assessment include joint and disk dysfunction, acute pain, recent trauma, and inflammation.

PLANTAR FLEXION

Assesses for strength and endurance in the isolation position and tension or shortening in the dorsiflexion pattern.

Muscles involved
Gastrocnemius
Soleus
Flexor digitorum longus
Flexor hallucis longus
Plantaris
Tibialis posterior

Range of motion
0 to 50 degrees

Position of client
Gastrocnemius—Prone, with ankle dorsiflexed off end of table and knees extended
Soleus—Prone, with knee flexed and ankle dorsiflexed

Isolation and assessment (both positions)
Client plantar flexes ankle through the available range of motion while examiner applies resistance to posterior calcaneus or sole of foot to push foot into dorsiflexion

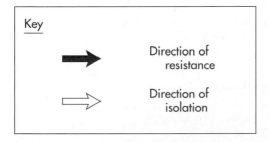

Key

➡ Direction of resistance

⇨ Direction of isolation

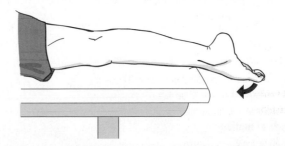

Continued

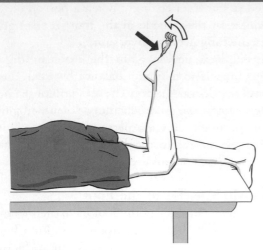

FOOT DORSIFLEXION

Assesses for strength and endurance in the isolation position and tension or shortening in the plantar flexion pattern

Muscles involved

Tibialis anterior

Peroneus tertius

Extensor digitorum longus (extensor of lesser toes)

Extensor hallucis longus (greater toe extensor)

Range of motion

0 to 20 degrees

Position of client

Supine with leg straight

Isolation and assessment

Client dorsiflexes ankle, keeping toes relaxed and resistance is applied to pull foot into plantar flexion

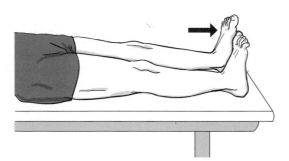

FOOT INVERSION

Assesses for strength and endurance in the isolation position and tension or shortening in the eversion pattern

Muscles involved

Tibialis anterior

Tibialis posterior

Flexor digitorum longus (flexor of lesser toes)

Flexor hallucis longus (great toe flexor)

Gastrocnemius (medial head)

Range of motion

0 to 30 degrees

Position of client

Supine or side-lying on test side with ankle in neutral position

Isolation and assessment

Client inverts foot through available range of motion as resistance is applied to medial edge of forefoot to pull into eversion

Client keeps toes relaxed

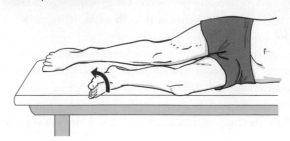

FOOT EVERSION

Assesses for strength and endurance in the isolation position and tension or shortening in the inversion pattern

Muscles involved

Peroneus longus

Peroneus brevis

Peroneus tertius

Extensor digitorum longus

Range of motion

0 to 25 degrees

Position of client

Supine or side-lying on nontest side with ankle in neutral position

Isolation and assessment

Client everts foot through full range while resistance is applied to lateral edge of foot to pull into inversion

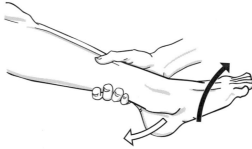

TOE FLEXION

Assesses for strength and endurance in the isolation position and tension or shortening in the extension pattern

Muscles involved

Flexor digitorum longus

Flexor digitorum brevis

Flexor hallucis longus

Flexor hallucis brevis

Flexor digiti minimi brevis

Lumbricales

Interossei (dorsal and plantar)

Range of motion

Great toe—0 to 45 degrees

Lateral four toes—0 to 40 degrees

Position of client

Supine with foot and ankle in neutral position

Examiner stabilizes metatarsals

First layer (most superficial)—Adductor hallucis, flexor digitorum brevis, abductor digit quinti

Second layer—Quadratus plantae, lumbricales (four)

Third layer—Flexor hallucis brevis, flexor digiti quinti brevis, adductor hallucis

Fourth layer (deepest)—Interossei (seven)

Summary

This chapter has presented the basic principles of biomechanics.

Three main biomechanical dysfunctional patterns were discussed with intervention suggestions and referral recommendations. An assessment protocol for biomechanical function was practiced.

The concepts in this chapter may seem complex and at times difficult to understand. Comprehending how all the aspects of movement work together requires knowledge and the development of an understanding of the relationship of the pieces to function. Sometimes it is just too much to know, and being able to use reference texts effectively is helpful.

Many students find themselves lost in the terminology of all the pieces: the bones, ligaments, names of the joints, action of movement, names of the muscles, and directions for isolation. When this happens, slow down and move with the words. The entire unit has been about movement. Movement is best understood by moving. Continue to look up the definitions of the words that are confusing. Persist in understanding biomechanical concepts.

Balance and center may be the most important concepts of all. Remember, the importance of being centered is often expressed as being present in the moment and responding resourcefully to each unfolding second of life.

ACTIVITY 10-16—cont'd

Isolation and assessment
Great toe is tested separately from lateral four toes
Client flexes great toe while examiner applies light resistance to plantar surface of proximal phalange to push into extension
Client flexes four toes while examiner applies light resistance to plantar surface of proximal phalanges to push into extension

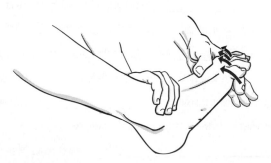

TOE EXTENSION
Assesses for strength and endurance in the isolation position and tension or shortening in the flexion pattern
Muscles involved
Extensor digitorum longus
Extensor digitorum brevis
Extensor hallucis longus

Range of motion
Great toe—0 to 70 degrees
Lateral four toes—0 to 40 degrees
Position of client
Supine with foot and ankle in neutral position
Examiner stabilizes metatarsals
Isolation and assessment
Great toe is tested separately from lateral four toes
Client extends great toe while examiner applies light resistance to dorsal surface of proximal phalange to pull into flexion
Client extends four toes while examiner applies light resistance to dorsal surface of proximal phalanges to pull into flexion

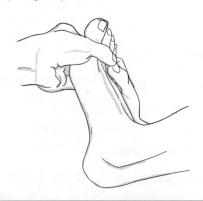

WORKBOOK SECTION

1. Explain the basic principles of balance.

_____

_____

_____

_____

_____

_____

_____

_____

_____

2. Describe the steps in the normal adult walking cycle.

_____

_____

_____

_____

_____

_____

_____

_____

_____

_____

3. Identify the three main biomechanical dysfunctional patterns.

_____

_____

_____

FILL IN THE BLANK

_____ (1) is the study of mechanical actions as applied to living bodies. _____ (2) is a fundamental characteristic of human behavior accomplished by the contraction of skeletal muscles acting within a system of levers and pulleys.

An_____ (3) contraction occurs when tension is developed within the muscle but no appreciable change occurs in the joint angle or length of the muscle. Movement does not occur.

_____ (4) contractions occur when tension is developed in the muscle while it either shortens or lengthens.

In a_____ (5) contraction, the muscle develops tension as it shortens, and the contraction occurs when the muscle has enough force to overcome the applied resistance._____ (6) contractions take place when the muscle lengthens while under tension and continue as the muscle gradually changes in tension to control the descent of the resistance.

In biomechanical terms, the concept of center refers to the _____ (7), the midpoint or center of weight of a body or object. Any loss of biomechanical _____ (8) such as what occurs with a missing limb or altered posture, will not only alter the total body weight distribution but the center of gravity as well.

External forces acting on the body include_____ (9) and those forces generated by the interaction with _____ (10) such as lifting a box or managing an umbrella in the wind. Soft tissue and movement therapies attempt to alter body function by exerting _____ (11) force to generate _____ (12) forces, which then affect change in the homeostatic mechanisms of the body.

_____ (13) is the reluctance of matter to change its state of motion. Any irregularly paced or multidirectional activity will be very costly to energy reserves.

_____ (14) may be defined as the rate of change in velocity. It occurs in the same direction as the force that caused it.

_____ (15) is the ability to control equilibrium. Equilibrium refers to a state of zero acceleration in which no change occurs in the speed or direction of the body. _____ (16) equilibrium occurs when the body is at rest or completely motionless.

_____ (17) equilibrium occurs when all of the applied on internal forces acting on the moving body are in balance, resulting in movement with unchanging speed or direction.

_____ (18) is the resistance to change in the body's acceleration or the resistance to the disturbance of the body's equilibrium.

PROBLEM SOLVING AND PROFESSIONAL APPLICATION EXERCISE

Design an assessment form. On this form, list each of the activity assessments in this chapter and provide room for your responses. As you develop this form, consider how you would use it to organize the information in this chapter as you take a physical assessment. Possibilities for design of the form include a checklist or a silhouette drawing providing areas that can be marked to indicate function and dysfunction during the assessment process. You may come up with a different idea. Be creative. However, be sure to develop a comprehensive form to use as a tool that will remind you of the information in this chapter as you work professionally with a client. (The activity assessments begin with the section on Biomechanics by Region, starting with the Trunk and Thorax.)

FURTHER STUDY

Using a comprehensive anatomy and physiology text (see Works Cited list at the back of this text), identify chapters pertaining to the information presented in this chapter. As a study guide, locate the information presented in this text and then elaborate by writing a paragraph of additional information on each of the following:

Center of gravity

_____

_____

_____

_____

_____

_____

_____

_____

_____

Levers

_____

_____

_____

_____

_____

_____

_____

_____

_____

Gait

_____

_____

_____

_____

_____

_____

_____

_____

Answer Key

1. A person has balance when the center of gravity falls within the base of support. A person has balance in direct proportion to the size of the base of support. The larger the base of support, the more balance. A person has balance depending on the weight or mass. The greater the weight, the more balance.
   A person has balance depending on the height of the center of gravity. The lower the center of gravity, the more balance. A person has balance depending on where the center of gravity is in relation to the base of support. The balance is less if the center of gravity is near the edge of the base. However, when anticipating an oncoming force, stability may be improved by placing the center of gravity nearer the side of the base of support expected to receive the force. In anticipation of an oncoming force, stability also may be increased by enlarging the size of the base of support in the direction of the anticipated force. Equilibrium may be enhanced by increasing the friction between the body and the surface it contacts. Rotation about an axis is easier to balance. A bike that is moving is easier to balance than a bike that is stationary.

2. Human beings move about on two legs comprised of three segments each: the thigh, shank, and foot. Atop the two legs is the trunk, head, and arm unit. The arm unit is used as a counterbalance and for momentum and moves opposite the leg movement. This pattern is linked in the contralateral reflex arc mechanism. Flexion and extension of the hip joints cause some rotation in the lumbar spine; to keep the head facing forward, the thorax and cervical spine rotate in the opposite direction. This action is coordinated by reflex patterns that coordinate upright posture in gravity and righting reflexes that keep the eyes on a level plane and the head oriented to the trunk. Reciprocal movements of the upper and lower limbs occur with the right upper limb flexing at the shoulder joint simultaneous with flexion at the left hip joint. Normally the shoulder joint starts to flex or extend slightly before the same movement is seen in the elbow joint. These movements again serve to keep the head and trunk oriented and counterbalance the body weight in gravity.

3. Neuromuscular, myofascial, or joint related.

FILL IN THE BLANK

1. Biomechanics
2. Movement
3. isometric
4. Isotonic
5. concentric
6. Eccentric
7. center of gravity
8. stability
9. gravity
10. external forces
11. external
12. internal
13. Inertia
14. Acceleration
15. Balance
16. Static
17. Dynamic
18. Stability

Section Four

The Rest of the Body

CHAPTER 11 THE INTEGUMENTARY, CARDIOVASCULAR, LYMPHATIC, AND IMMUNE SYSTEMS
CHAPTER 12 THE RESPIRATORY, DIGESTIVE, URINARY, AND REPRODUCTIVE SYSTEMS

Any health care professional must have a comprehensive knowledge of the body to understand the ways in which the mechanisms of health and disease function and support or disrupt the homeostatic balance of a well-tuned organism. However, just as with any discipline, such study involves both specialized knowledge and general knowledge.

Although all parts of the body are equally important, to the soft tissue and movement therapist, the areas of principal concern are the systems of control and movement. This specialized knowledge has been covered in the first three sections. This section, in Chapter 11, presents an overview of the integumentary system, the cardiovascular and lymphatic systems, and the functions of immunity. In Chapter 12, the respiratory, digestive, and urinary and reproductive systems are presented. The areas of most concern to the soft tissue and movement process are dealt with in more detail. Because learning does not end, but evolves, one layer on another, further study of these areas, using a comprehensive anatomy and physiology textbook, is recommended once the more basic information has been absorbed.

The text *Basic Health Care Terminology*, by R. W. Williams (see Works Consulted), was used as a pattern for this section. It contains clear, concise descriptions of the body's systems. Although the information has been adapted, paraphrased, and focused to serve the particular audience of soft tissue and movement therapy students, the text is recommended as a useful adjunct to this study.

This section is divided into two chapters, each with four main topic areas. Each topic area contains a Clinical Reasoning Activity, described on p. 448.

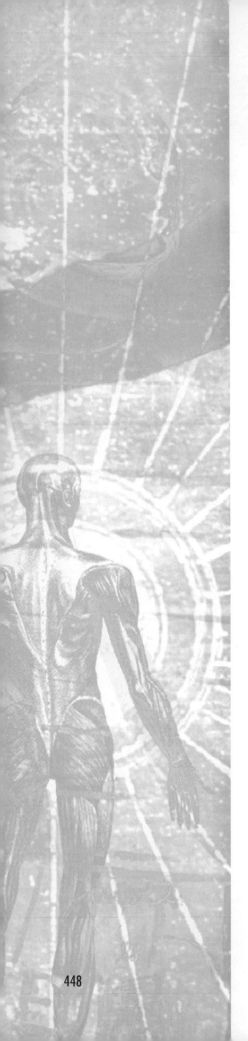

Clinical Reasoning Activities

At the end of each topic area, the student is asked to decide on one or more primary methods of therapeutic intervention and to use the clinical reasoning model to justify the effectiveness of the soft tissue or movement method (or methods) she chose in supporting balanced functioning of each system involved.

This same approach can be used to justify the use of a particular modality when dealing with disease or dysfunction. Students must be able to explain and justify the ways in which soft tissue and movement therapies are beneficial in supporting optimum function and how these same modalities can support a return to health if pathology exists.

In completing the Clinical Reasoning Activities, the student will need to refer to other sections of this text. Section Two, Systems of Control, will be particularly useful. The student also will need knowlege of the soft tissue or movement approach being justified. Reference texts dealing with those areas will be helpful.

These exercises, when well thought out, should help the student understand the connection between what is done (the modality) and what is effected (the change in physiology). Since what is done (the modality) depends on where it is done (the anatomy), putting all the pieces together in an explanation of the benefits of soft tissue or movement modalities will help the student not only to understand the process but also to educate others.

The following list of treatment modalities provides only examples for each category; it is not an exhaustive compilation. It is presented to help the student recognize the different types of soft tissue and movement approaches.

- Soft tissue approaches: Therapeutic (Swedish) massage, reflexology, muscle energy technique, shiatsu, acupressure, trigger point therapy, myofascial release, and rolfing
- Subtle energy approaches: Polarity, therapeutic touch, applied kinesiology, Touch for Health, Reiki, and Zero Balancing
- Movement approaches: Yoga, tai chi, dance, and all forms of therapeutic exercise and movement therapy
- Body/mind methods: Progressive relaxation, self hypnosis, autogenic training, biofeedback, and meditation

The Clinical Reasoning Activities are presented in the following format.

Modality: _____

1. **What are the facts?**
    a. Which system is involved, and which structures of that system can be reached directly and indirectly?

b. Which of these structures are most affected by this modality?

c. Which physiologic functions are affected by this approach?

d. When the treatment is applied, what changes in function will result in

(1) this system

(2) the whole body

e. What is considered normal or balanced function?

f. How are the functions of this system related to the body's homeostasis?

g. What has worked and has not worked?

h. Where could you find information that would support the use of this modality as a therapeutic intervention?

i. What research is available to support the use of the therapeutic intervention?

j. How does the intervention support a healthy state?

k. Under which pathologic or dysfunctional conditions is the intervention most likely to be beneficial?

2. **What are the possibilities?**

a. What do the data suggest?

b. What are the reasons for using the proposed methods?

c. What are the possible interventions?

d. List at least three applications of this modality that would affect both the structure and function of the system involved.

e. What are other ways to look at the situation?

f. What other methods could provide similar benefits?

3. **What is the logical outcome of the therapeutic intervention?**

a. What would be the logical progression of the symtom pattern, contributing factors, and current behavior?

b. What are the benefits and drawbacks of each intervention suggested?

c. What are the costs in terms of time, resources, and finances?

d. What is likely to happen if this modality is not used?

e. What is likely to happen if this modality is used?

4. **For the intervention proposed, what would be the impact on the people involved, specifically the client, the practitioner, and other professionals working with the client?**

a. How does each of the people involved (including, besides those named above, the client's family and support system) feel about the possible interventions?

b. Does the practitioner feel qualified to work with the situation and apply the identified modality to the particular situation?

c. Does a feeling of cooperation and agreement exist among all those involved, and how would the practitioner recognize this feeling?

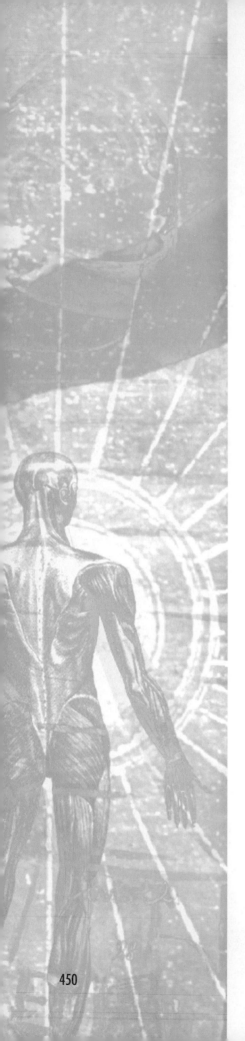

Justification

Using the information developed in the clinical reasoning model, present a clear, concise statement of the ways in which the particular soft tissue or movement modality would be beneficial, either in supporting the particular body system in a healthy condition or as part of a treatment plan for a pathologic or dysfunctional condition. Use the information gathered by answering the above questions to develop a brief summary of the effective use of the modality for this system.

Example of the Clinical Reasoning Process Used to Create a Justification Statement: In the following example, this process is applied to the muscular system.

Modality: _Therapeutic massage_

1. **What are the facts?**
   a. Which system is involved, and which structures of that system can be reached directly or indirectly

   The muscles and associated connective tissue are involved, along with various nerves and sensory receptors. The circulation to the muscles is affected as well.

   b. Which of these structures are most affected by this modality?

   Proprioceptors, connective tissue

   c. Which physiologic functions are affected by this approach?

   Muscle tension patterns, connective tissue viscosity

   d. When the treatment is applied, what changes in function will result in
   (1) this system

   Muscle tension patterns and reflexes may be restored to balanced function if imbalances exist. Connective tissue may normalize, usually by softening, although specific methods can be used to firm lax connective tissue.

   (2) the whole body

   The whole body usually relaxes, and restorative processes are supported.

   e. What is considered normal or balanced function?

   The muscles maintain posture, produce movement, stabilize joints, and generate heat efficiently without wasting energy. The muscles should be able to respond to activation of the sympathetic portion of the autonomic nervous system and then return to a relaxed state.

   f. How are the functions of this system related to the body's homeostasis?

   The pumping action of muscle contraction supports blood and lymph circulation. Maintenance of a constant internal heat is an important part of muscle action. Support of posture and joint stability provides internal space for internal organs and efficient operation without restriction. Movement is used to obtain air and food and to ensure survival.

g. What has worked or has not worked?

Many different forms of massage produce beneficial results for the muscles. The basic approaches include compression, lifting, kneading, tapping, and horizontal gliding, along with various forms of active and passive movement and muscle contraction methods. The intensity and duration of massage applications depend on the desired results. However, the benefits of extremely painful methods may be diminished by activation of the body's defensive mechanisms.

h. Where could you find information that would support the use of this modality as a therapeutic intervention?

Textbooks, research institutes, and various medical, nursing, physical therapy, chiropractic, and bodywork journals; professional organizations; clinical application by other professionals; the Internet

i. What research is available to support the use of the therapeutic intervention?

Greenman P: Principles of manual medicine, ed 2, Baltimore, 1996, Williams & Wilkins.

Yates J: Physiological effects of therapeutic massage and their application to treatment, Vancouver, 1990, British Columbia Massage Therapist Association.

Leon Chaitow: Although not a researcher, this author effectively translates research into useful application.

j. How does the intervention support a healthy state?

The various types of sensory stimulation provided by massage result in alteration of the nervous system control mechanisms toward more balanced function. The more mechanical normalization of associated connective tissue supports pliability and stability of the muscles.

k. Under which pathologic or dysfunctional conditions is the intervention most likely to be beneficial?

Increased or decreased muscle tension from daily mechanical and emotional stress. Management of pain resulting from such alterations. Compression on nerves or vessels from increased muscle tension and the resulting pain and dysfunction.

2. **What are the possibilities?**

a. What do the data suggest?

The data suggest (1) normal muscle function that needs support to maintain health, (2) the development of muscle problems that could readily be reversed, restoring the system to health, or (3) a serious pathologic condition that requires several interventions.

b. What are the reasons for using the proposed method?

Therapeutic massage could relax the muscles, reduce pain, increase both blood and lymph circulation, increase nutrition to the muscles, and encourage repair of muscles.

c. What are the possible interventions?

Bodywork, exercise, medications, meditation, yoga, therapeutic massage, physical therapy, acupuncture, and biofeedback

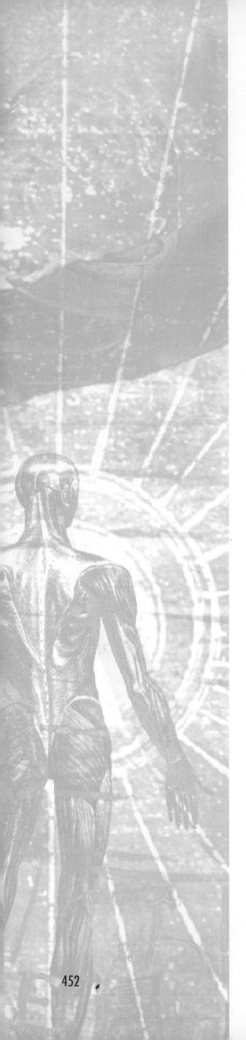

d. List at least three possible applications of this modality that would affect both the structure and function of this system.

Compression spreads muscle fibers, affects proprioception, and increases circulation. The "tense, relax, and lengthen" technique affects reflex mechanisms. Tapping at the muscle tendon strengthens muscles through its effect on the tendon organ.

e. What are other ways to look at the situation?

The muscle symptoms could be a reflection of a neurologic pathologic condition; medications may be influencing the muscle; or emotional armoring in the muscles may provide effective coping patterns.

f. What other methods could provide similar benefits?

Various form of aerobic exercise; stretching programs (e.g., yoga); physical therapy; and medications

3. **What is the logical outcome of the therapeutic intervention?**

a. What is the logical progression of the symptom pattern, contributing factors, and current behaviors?

Increased muscle tension is a waste of energy and a common source of pain, and it often interferes with sleep. Any long-term sleep interference affects the body's restorative processes. More serious pathologic conditions could result from the increased levels of stress.

b. What are the benefits and drawbacks of the intervention suggested?
Benefits:

Massage is pleasurable, often easily accepted by the client, and effective in short-term symptom control of muscle dysfunction.

Massage can replace or reduce the use of palliative types of medication such as muscle relaxants and analgesics.

Drawback:

Massage is not curative and requires continual maintenance intervention to support benefits.

c. What are the costs in terms of time, resources, and finances?

Compared with other interventions, massage is cost effective even for long-term intervention. Weekly or biweekly 1-hour sessions can produce results. A maintenance schedule, once goals have been achieved, can be less intensive and therefore less costly. Massage professionals are easily found in most areas. Home and office care often are available.

d. What is likely to happen if this modality is not used?

Muscle tension probably would increase and the symptoms worsen. More serious pathologic conditions could develop.

e. What is likely to happen if this modality is used?

Daily stress management and support for healthy function of the muscle system would be achieved, and use of over-the-counter or prescription medications would be reduced.

4. **For the intervention proposed, what would be the impact on the people involved, specifically the client, the practitioner, and other professionals working with the client?**

   a. How does each of the people involved (including, besides those named above, the client's family and support system) feel about the possible intervention?

   Touch intervention can be very nurturing to many clients; however, those with various forms of touch trauma may not have predictable responses to the intense duration of touch in the form of massage. Health care professionals are still confused about the benefits and applications of massage. The practitioner may have issues of countertransference with the client that would need to be addressed.

   b. Does the practitioner feel qualified to work with the situation and apply the identified modality to the particular situation?

   Depending on the practitioner's training and the client's therapeutic goals, as well as the support of other health care or training professionals, most situations can be addressed effectively with some sort of massage intervention. The more complex the situation, the more support and training are required.

   c. Does a feeling of cooperation and agreement exist among all those involved, and how would the practitioner recognize this feeling?

   Support and cooperation depend on shared knowledge and the ability to educate in the benefits of massage. Free exchange of information, with the client's permission, and the client's willingness to participate would indicate cooperation.

NOTE: The previous questions stimulate thought processes and support more effective information gathering. The information is then evaluated, organized, and condensed to form a short, concise, and valid justification statement.

Justification

Therapeutic massage provides a pleasurable, easily accessible, cost-effective approach to support function of the muscular system by increasing circulation and waste removal from the muscles, by maintaining normal connective tissue structures, by encouraging appropriate neuromuscular interaction, and by enhancing general restorative functions.

Muscle tension and pain syndromes can be managed more effectively using massage as a treatment method because the general benefits listed above are important in the treatment of these conditions. Massage can provide some of the same short-term benefits as medication without the side effects.

Chapter 11

The Integumentary, Cardiovascular, Lymphatic, and Immune Systems

CHAPTER OUTLINE

CHAPTER OBJECTIVES

After completing this chapter, the student should be able to perform the following:

- List and describe the components of the integumentary system.
- Describe the function of the integumentary system.
- Describe two main concerns with integumentary pathologic conditions.
- List and describe the components of the cardiovascular system.
- List and describe the components of blood.
- Describe the function of the cardiovascular system.
- List and describe the components of the lymphatic system.
- List and describe the components of lymph.
- Describe the function of the lymphatic system.
- Define immunity.
- Explain the difference between nonspecific and specific immunity.
- Describe and explain the implementation of Universal Precautions.
- Justify the effectiveness of soft tissue and movement modalities in supporting health maintenance for the integumentary, cardiovascular, lymphatic, and immune systems.

KEY TERMS

Arterioles (Ar-TEER-ee-oles) The smallest arteries.

Arteriosclerosis (ar-tee-ree-o-skle-RO-sis) A term meaning *hardening of the arteries;* it refers to arteries that have become brittle and have lost their elasticity.

Artery (AR-ter-ee) A blood vessel that transports either oxygenated blood from the heart to the body or deoxygenated blood from the heart to the lungs.

Atherosclerosis (ath-er-o-skle-RO-sis) A condition in which fatty plaque is deposited in medium and large arteries.

Atrium (AY-tree-um) One of the two small, thin-walled, upper chambers of the heart; the right and left atria are separated by a thin interatrial septum.

Blood A thick, red fluid that provides oxygen, nourishment, and protection to the cells and carries away waste products. Whole blood consists of two components: the formed cellular elements and the liquid plasma. Blood is a form of connective tissue.

Blood pressure The measurement of pressure exerted by the heart on the walls of the blood vessels. The highest pressure exerted is called systolic pressure, which results when the ventricles are contracted. Diastolic pressure, the lowest pressure, results when the ventricles are at rest. Blood forced into the aorta during systole sets up a pressure wave that travels down the arteries. The wave expands the arterial wall, and the expansion can be palpated by pressing the artery against tissue; the waves constitute the pulse rate.

Capillary (KAP-I-lair-ee) One of the small blood vessels found between arteries and veins that allow the exchange of gases, nutrients, and waste products. The walls of capillaries are very thin, allowing molecules to diffuse easily.

Coronary (KOR-o-nair-ee) ***arteries*** The arteries that supply oxygenated blood to the heart muscle itself; they are located in grooves between the atria and ventricles and between the two ventricles.

Dermatitis (der-mah-TIE-tis) A general term for acute or chronic skin inflammation characterized by redness, eruptions, edema, scaling, and itching. The three main types are atopic dermatitis, seborrheic dermatitis, and contact dermatitis. Eczema is a form of dermatitis.

Dermis (DER-mis) The inner layer of skin; it contains collagen and elastin fibers, which provide much of the structure and strength of the skin and is much thicker than the epidermis.

Epidermis (ep-i-DER-mis) The outer, or top, layer of skin, which is made up of sublayers called *strata*. The epidermis contains no nerves or blood vessels.

Heart The pump of the cardiovascular system; it is hollow, cone-shaped, and about the size of a fist; it is located in the mediastinum of the thoracic cavity. The myocardium is the heart muscle itself, the endocardium is the thin inner lining, and the epicardium is the outer membrane.

Heart valves Four sets of valves that keep the blood flowing in the correct direction through the heart.

Immunity Resistance to disease, which is provided by the body through specific or nonspecific immunity. The immune system is a functional system rather than an organ system in the anatomic sense. The most important immune cells are lymphocytes and macrophages. The key to immunity is the body's ability to distinguish self from nonself.

Integument (in-TEG-yoo-ment) The skin and its appendages: hair, sebaceous and sweat glands, nails, and breasts.

Lymph (limf) A clear, interstitial tissue fluid that bathes the cells. Lymph contains lymphocytes, which provide immune response; it also returns plasma proteins that have leaked out through capillary walls, and it transports fats from the gastrointestinal system to the bloodstream.

Lymph nodes Small, round structures distributed along the network of lymph vessels that provide a filtering system for removing waste products and transferring them to the bloodstream for removal to the spleen, intestines, and kidneys for detoxification. Lymph nodes are centers for lymphocyte production. Their main function is to prevent bacteria and viruses from gaining access to the bloodstream. Generally clustered at the joints for assistance in pumping when the joint moves, they are especially numerous in the axillae, groin, and neck and along certain blood vessels of the pelvic, abdominal, and thoracic cavities.

Pericardium (Pair-i-KAR-dee-um) A double membranous, serous sac surrounding the heart. The pericardium secretes a lubricating fluid to prevent friction from the movement of the heart.

Plasma (PLAZ-mah) A thick, straw-colored fluid that makes up about 55% of the blood.

Superficial fascia The subcutaneous tissue that composes the third layer of skin; it consists of loose connective tissue and contains fat or adipose tissue.

Tumor Also referred to as a *neoplasm*, a tumor is a growth of new tissues that may be benign (nonthreatening or noncancerous) or malignant (cancerous).

Universal Precautions Safety measures established in 1987 by the Centers for Disease Control and Prevention (CDC); they were instituted to prevent the spread of bacterial and viral infections by setting up specific methods of dealing with human fluids and waste products. Universal Precautions protect both client and practitioner from pathogens.

Veins Blood vessels that collect blood from the capillaries and transport it back to the heart; 75% of the blood of the body is in the venous system. Larger veins often contain a set of valves, which ensure that blood flows in the correct direction to the heart and also prevent backflow.

Ventricles (VEN-tri-kul) The two large, lower chambers of the heart; they are thick walled and separated by a thick interventricular septum.

Venules (VEN-yools) The smallest veins.

The Integumentary System

PHYSIOLOGY OF TOUCH

The skin is the most sensitive of our organs and is the home for touch receptors of the nervous system. Touch is the fifth sense, and along with taste, vision, smell, and hearing, it expands on the ways we experience our world. It is the first sense to develop in the embryo, and the need for touch remains throughout our lives. Soft tissue and movement therapists touch, and the skin is our contact point (Figure 11-1); therefore we must understand the effects of skin stimulation.

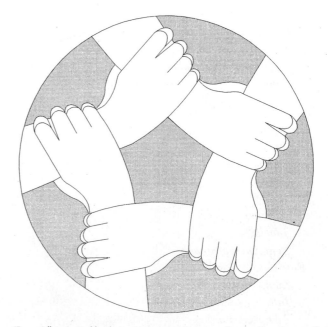

(From Gillen G, Burkhardt A: *Stroke rehabilitation: a function-based approach*, St Louis, 1998, Mosby.)

Touch is the most important and yet the most neglected of our senses. We can survive without sight, hearing, taste, and smell, but without the ability to feel, we are in constant danger (Figure 11-2). A complete loss of the sense of touch can cause psychotic breakdown. A lack of touch in infants can cause death from marasmus (wasting away). Sensory stimulation is essential to well-being at all stages of life, and touch is a necessary component. Touch deprivation leads to a diminishment of the neuroendocrine chemicals necessary for well-being because touch stimulates the production of chemicals in the body. Touch-deprived individuals frequently develop inappropriate forms of sensory stimulation or abusive or addictive behavior (often food or drugs) in an attempt to stimulate the production of chemicals the body needs.

The ability to feel is a survival mechanism. Millions of sensory receptors in the skin alert us to danger through variations in temperature, vibration, and pressure. Touch informs us of differences in texture, shape, resistance, and tension. About one third of the 5 million or so sensory receptors are in the skin of our hands. The fingertips have more than 1000 nerve endings per square inch, and the lips and tongue have even more.

Different types of touch are identified by different receptors in the skin. The degree of pressure in light touch as opposed to deep touch is sensed by different receptor mechanisms and can evoke entirely different responses. A slow, light touch can relay compassion or intimacy. A deeper slow touch can evoke relaxation or security, whereas an abrupt touch startles and alerts. Touch can evoke pleasure, which we seek, and pain or discomfort, which we avoid. Each of these sensations triggers the manufacture and release of neurochemicals. (See Chapters 4 through 6).

What more intimate form of communication is there than touch? It is even reflected in our language: "That was a touching experience," "What you said touched me," "You hurt my feelings," "Let's keep in

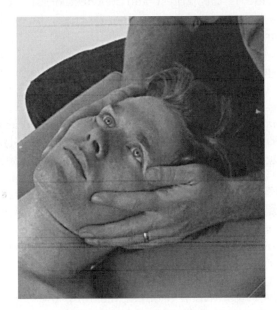

FIGURE 11-1 (Modified from D'Ambrogio KJ, Roth GB: *Positional release therapy: assessment and treatment of musculoskeletal dysfunction,* St Louis, 1997, Mosby.)

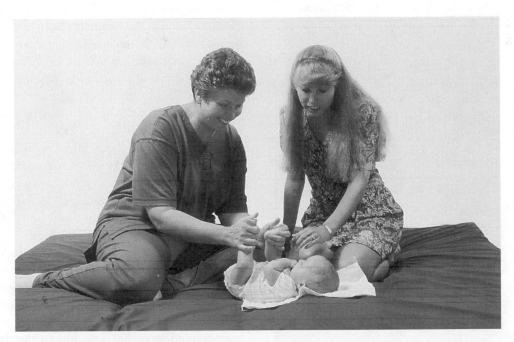

FIGURE 11-2 (From Fritz S: *Mosby's fundamentals of therapeutic massage,* St Louis, 1995, Mosby.)

touch." The qualities of touch—nurturing, angry, parental, fearful, sexual, happy, comforting, playful—are somehow understood by the neuropathways of the skin. How amazing (Activity 11-1)!

STRUCTURE OF THE INTEGUMENT

The word **integument** means covering. The integumentary system, which covers our bodies, is made up of the skin and its appendages: hair, sebaceous glands, sweat glands, nails, and breasts (Activity 11-2). Some of the major functions of the integumentary system are as follows:

- Protecting the internal organs and structures from trauma, sun exposure, chemicals, and water loss

ACTIVITY 11-1

This exercise is done with a partner. Your partner sits quietly with her eyes closed through the entire exercise while you think of a time when you were nurturing, angry, parental, fearful, happy, comforting, playful, and so on. Hold the thought in your mind while you touch your partner on the forearm with your hand. See if your partner can guess what emotion is being expressed.

Repeat the exercise, only this time deliberately attempt to communicate each of the emotions listed (nurturing, angry, parental, fearful, happy, comforting, playful, and so forth), using the touch of your hand on your partner's forearm. See if your partner can identify the emotion being expressed. Then change roles. Finally, describe the experience in the space provided.

NOTE: Remember that the touch is limited to using your hand on your partner's forearm.

Example It was difficult to distinguish between a nurturing touch and a comforting touch. When touching my partner, I found it easy to communicate playfulness but difficult to communicate parental feelings. I did not like keeping my eyes closed while I was touched but found it easier to touch someone else if she could not see me.

Your Turn

- Assisting in immunity by preventing the entry of bacteria and viruses
- Synthesizing vitamin D when exposed to ultraviolet rays of the sun
- Detecting the stimuli sensed as touch, temperature, pain, and pressure
- Regulating body temperature
- Excreting sweat and salts and secreting sebum

Skin

The skin is the largest and heaviest organ of the body. It is composed of two major layers: the epidermis and the dermis.

The **epidermis,** the outer layer of the skin, contains no nerves or blood vessels. It consists of sublayers called *strata*. Most areas have four layers; areas subject to pressure or friction such as the palms and the soles, have five layers. In all areas the outermost layer is the stratum corneum. This layer is made up of 20 to 30 layers of flat, keratin-filled, dead cells that continuously shed and are replaced from the layer below. The innermost layer is the stratum basale, which produces a continuous supply of new cells. As the new cells develop and mature, they move up through the other layers until they reach the top and are shed, a process that takes about 2 to 3 weeks. This lowest layer also contains melanocytes, which produce melanin, the pigment that colors our skin. Keratin is produced in the epidermis by keratinocytes. Keratin is the fibrous protein that protects our skin and makes it waterproof.

The **dermis,** the inner layer of our skin, is much thicker than the epidermis. The dermis is composed of dense connective tissue that contains collagen and elastin fibers, which provide much of the structure and strength of our skin. The fibers are arranged in such a manner that the skin can be moved in many directions. Stretch marks are caused when these fibers are overstretched. The top layer of the dermis forms into ridges and presses up into the epidermis to create our fingerprints. Hair, sebaceous and sweat glands, and nails originate in the dermis and also push upward through the epidermis. Blood vessels and nerves are found in the dermis.

Subcutaneous tissue, consisting of loose connective tissue and fat (adipose) tissue, is found below the dermis. This layer, known as the **superficial fascia,** sits above the muscle and bone. It is not actually a part of the integument, but because it contains loose connective tissue that attaches to the dermis, it usually is described with the integumentary system. The adipose tissue insulates and provides padding; its distribution varies in men and women and is affected by hereditary factors.

The appendages of the skin are special structures that perform a variety of functions.

Hair

Hair protects the skin and orifices of the body, keeps us warm, and assists in our sense of touch. It is found all over the body except on the palms of the hands, the soles of the feet, the palmar and plantar surfaces of the digits, the lips, the nipples, and portions of the external genitalia. Some parts of the body appear hairless but actually have very fine hair. Hair is composed of dead cells that have become keratinized, or hardened. Hair follicles, which include the hair root and connective tissue, hold the hair in place. A root hair plexus is a nerve that is stimulated each time the hair is moved. Tiny muscles, called *erector pili,* are attached to hair follicles and cause the hair to stand on end at times. When this happens, the body is more sensitive to changes in air pressure and more alert to movement as a possible sign of danger. It is thought that one reason energy forms of bodywork are effec-

tive is that the near touch and gentle movements stimulate the root hair plexus to provide sensory stimulation.

Nails

Toenails and fingernails are hard, keratinized cells that protect the ends of the digits and assist us in grasping. The *lunula* is the crescent-shaped white area at the base of the nail. The nail actually grows from the lunula; it is white because the blood vessels are covered with connective tissue and do not show. The clear, visible portion of the nail is the *nail body.*

Sebaceous (Oil) Glands

Most oil glands are connected to hair follicles by small ducts. They can be found over most of the body except on the palms and soles. By secreting an oily substance known as *sebum,* the oil glands prevent dehydration, soften the skin and hair, and slow the growth of bacteria. The secretion of sebum is stimulated by the release of hormones, primarily androgens. If the sebum builds up and blocks the oil gland, a whitehead can form. If the sebum dries and makes

ACTIVITY 11-2

In Figure 11-3, write the names of the integumentary structures listed below next to the matching number in the illustration. Color each part after you have labeled it.

1. Pore
2. Hair
3. Sebaceous gland
4. Fibrous tissue
5. Sweat gland
6. Nerves
7. Fat cells
8. Hair follicle
9. Blood vessels
10. Erector muscle
11. Subcutaneous layer
12. Dermis
13. Epidermis
14. Nail
15. Lunula

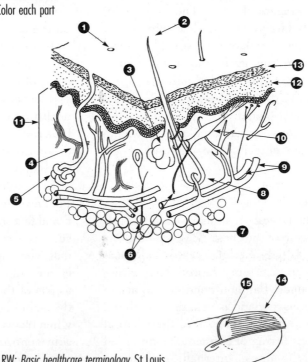

FIGURE 11-3 (From Williams RW: *Basic healthcare terminology,* St Louis, 1995, Mosby.)

contact with oxygen, it forms a blackhead. Acne is a bacterial inflammation of the sebaceous glands.

Sweat Glands

Known also as *sudoriferous glands*, sweat glands are found in most areas of the body. Most are located on the forehead, palms, and soles. The sweat glands are classified into types according to their structure and location; the two main types are the eccrine glands and the apocrine glands.

The eccrine glands, which are the most common, are responsible for the moisture that appears on the body's surface when body temperature rises, particularly during physical activity. The functions of the eccrine glands are to cool the body and provide minor elimination of metabolic waste. Sweat is 99% water. Sweating is regulated by the sympathetic division of the autonomic nervous system. Heat-induced sweating tends to begin on the forehead and then spread to the rest of the body. Emotionally induced sweating, stimulated by fright, embarrassment, or anxiety, begins on the palms and in the axillae and then spreads to the rest of the body.

The apocrine glands, which are located in areas of body hair, discharge their secretions when a person is under stress. They begin to work during puberty. The apocrine glands differ from the eccrine glands in that the apocrine secretion is thicker and has a stronger odor. Apocrine glands are located primarily in the axillary and anogenital areas. The exact function of these glands has yet to be determined, but because they are stimulated during sexual arousal and phases of the menstrual cycle, they may be similar to the sexual scent glands in other animals.

Ceruminous glands are modified apocrine glands found in the external ear canal. They secrete a sticky substance called *cerumen*, or earwax, that prevents foreign material from entering the ear and repels insects.

Mammary Glands

More commonly called *breasts*, mammary glands develop in the pectoral region of the chest. Developmentally, the mammary glands are modified apocrine sweat glands. The breasts are accessory reproductive structures in the female but are flat, nonfunctional organs in the male. Each mammary gland is contained within a rounded, skin-covered breast anterior to the pectoral muscles of the thorax. A ring of pigmented skin called the *areola* surrounds the nipple. Internally, each mammary gland consists of 15 to 25 lobes located around the nipple. The lobes are padded and separated from each other by fibrous connective tissue and fat. Ligaments attach the breast to the underlying muscle fascia and to the overlying skin, providing support. During lactation, glandular alveoli produce milk, which collects in lobules within the lobes and passes through lactiferous ducts to the nipple.

Skin Color

Skin color is created by combinations of pigments in the skin and in the blood flowing through the skin. These pigments are melanin, carotene, and hemoglobin.

Melanin, which is found in the epidermis, ranges in color from yellow to black. Melanin makes up most of our skin color. All of us have the same number of melanocytes, or melanin-producing cells, but the amount of melanin produced depends on genetic factors and exposure to ultraviolet light. Melanin is a natural sunscreen that protects us from ultraviolet (UV) rays by darkening our skin; this is a form of homeostasis. Freckles, moles, age spots, and actinic keratoses result from increases in the melanin concentration or from changes in melanocytes.

Carotene is a yellow pigment found in the dermis that naturally gives the skin of some individuals a yellow tint. If plant foods containing carotene make up a large part of a person's diet, carotene can accumulate in the skin and adipose tissue and give the skin a temporary yellow or orange color, especially on the face and the palms.

Hemoglobin is the oxygen-carrying red pigment molecule in the blood. In people with fair skin, the color of the hemoglobin shows through as pink.

The color of the skin can be an indicator either of health or of a pathologic condition. For example, a blue tint to the skin can be caused by cyanosis, a condition caused by defective or deficient oxygenation of the blood.

Skin color is also influenced by emotional stimuli. Pallor, or whiteness of the skin, may be due to emotional factors. A decrease in the amount of hemoglobin such as is seen in anemia may be suspected in individuals who appear pale. Sometimes the lack of rosy color is due only to opaqueness of the epidermis. As much as 5% of the blood in our bodies can be contained in the skin. During sympathetic autonomic activation, when blood is needed by the muscles, the vessels of the skin contract to move the blood out. Sudden pallor may be caused by stressful situations such as those provoking anger or fear. Excessive redness may be caused by embarrassment (blushing), an increase in body temperature or fever, hypertension, inflammation, allergy, rosacea, or hormonal fluctuations.

A yellow-gold color to the skin may result from jaundice or liver disorders. A bronze or metallic hue often is a sign of Addison's disease, a hypofunction of the adrenal cortex. Black and blue marks on the skin, or bruises, are the result of blood leaving the blood vessels and clotting in the surrounding tissues. Most commonly caused by trauma or injury, constant bruising may indicate a vitamin C deficiency or hemophilia.

PRACTICAL APPLICATION

Observation of a person's skin color and changes in the appearance, texture, and suppleness of the skin and the appendages can provide information about changes in a person's health status. Because soft tissue practitioners touch the skin more than any other professional, they should be especially observant of the skin and its appendages, which can be indicators either of dysfunction or of improved health.

PATHOLOGIC CONDITIONS

Pathologic conditions of the integument give rise to two main concerns related to impairment of the skin's structural integrity. The first concern is loss of the skin's protection of internal structures. The second concern is loss of the skin's ability to prevent the pathogens of contagious disease from entering the body. Observing the Universal Precautions, guidelines established by the Centers for Disease Control and Prevention (CDC), and proper sanitation methods maintains the security of the skin and its protective barriers. Pathologic conditions of the skin, especially sores, rashes, and changes in color and texture (see Color Plate 31), can be indicators of more serious systemic disease, and the client should be referred to a physician for diagnosis.

INDICATIONS/CONTRAINDICATIONS

For Soft Tissue and Movement Therapies

Soft tissue and movement therapies usually are not contraindicated, but local avoidance of the affected area is necessary. Most skin disorders can be irritated by localized touch. Therapy is contraindicated if the skin is inflamed or if the condition is contagious or transmissible through touch. Malignancy is a contraindication unless the therapy is supervised by the appropriate medical personnel.

Corn

A corn is a painful, conical thickening of skin over bony prominences of the feet caused by continual pressure and friction on normally thin skin. When corns are located in moist areas, such as between the toes, they are called *soft corns*.

Callus

A callus is an area of thickened, hardened skin, like a corn, that develops in an area of friction or a region of recurrent pressure. A callus involves skin that normally is thick such as the sole of the foot or the palm of the hand and usually is painless. If a callus is painful, an underlying plantar wart may be present.

Ulcer

An ulcer is a round, open sore of the skin or mucous membrane. It results from tissue damage that accompanies inflammation, infection, or malignancy.

Neurotrophic ulcer

Neurotrophic ulcers develop at pressure point areas on the feet when pain sensation is diminished or absent, as in diabetic neuropathy. Although often deep and infected, these ulcers are painless. Callus formation around the ulcer, like the ulcer itself, results from chronic pressure.

Decubitus ulcer

A decubitus ulcer is an open sore that develops primarily over the bony areas of the heels and hips of those who are immobile, bedridden, or in a wheelchair. Continuous pressure on the skin diminishes or stops circulation, and the tissue dies.

Bacterial Infections

Impetigo

Impetigo is an acute, highly contagious, bacterial skin infection usually found on the face. It is characterized by small, red spots that develop into vesicles, which become filled with pus, burst, and develop a thick, yellow crust.

Cellulitis

Cellulitis is a rapidly spreading, acute bacterial infection of the skin usually found in the lower extremities. Bacteria enter through damaged skin or as a result of complications of diabetes or poor circulation. Symptoms include redness, heat, swelling, and pain.

Acne

Acne vulgaris is the common form of acne. It is a chronic inflammation of the sebaceous glands and hair follicles caused by the interaction of bacteria, sebum, and sex hormones. It is most common at puberty and may recur in women during menopause. It can produce blackheads, whiteheads, cysts, pustules, and inflamed nodules.

Fungal Skin Infections

Dermatophytosis: tinea (ringworm)

More commonly known as *ringworm,* tinea is a group of common fungal infections contracted by touching contaminated items or an infected person's skin. The types of tinea are named by their location on the body. *Tinea corporis* appears on the nonhairy portions of the skin as fast-growing, reddish, elevated lesions surrounded by a dry and scaly or moist and crusty raised, ringlike border, which gives it the "ringworm" appearance. *Tinea pedis,* or athlete's foot, is marked by blisters and cracking of the skin between the toes and on the ball of the foot. *Tinea cruris,* or jock itch, is ringworm of the pubic area.

Candidiasis

Candidiasis is an infection of the skin or mucous membranes, most often caused by the organism *Candida albicans.* Red, scaly patches may appear in the creases of the axillae and groin and under the breasts, as well as between the fingers and toes. Associated candidal infections can occur in the ear, the vagina, and the mouth (thrush). *C. albicans* is a common cause of diaper rash in infants.

Viral Skin Infections

Warts

A wart is a benign growth of the keratin-producing cells of the epidermis and mucous membranes caused by the human papilloma virus (HPV). Warts are transmitted through direct contact. The *common wart* (verruca vulgaris) has a rough, elevated surface and is found mainly on the hands and fingers of children and young adults. *Filiform warts* are longer, slender growths on the face, neck, and axillae. *Periungual warts* are found around the nails of the fingers and toes. *Flat warts* are flesh colored and form when several warts spread, through scratching or shaving. *Plantar warts* have rough surfaces and are located in the thickened skin of the sole of the foot. They may be mistaken for a callus but often have small, dark spots, which calluses do not. Normal skin lines stop at the wart's edge.

Cold sores

Cold sores are infections caused by the herpes simplex virus (HSV). Outbreaks of herpes simplex virus type I consist of painful, fluid-filled blisters found on or near the mouth or nose. As with all herpes viruses, the virus remains dormant in the nerves of the body until resistance is low, at which time it travels down the nerve to cause the eruption. All of the herpes viruses are very contagious.

Parasitic Skin Infections

Scabies

Scabies is a contagious skin disease characterized by intense itching that is caused by a microscopic, parasitic mite that burrows under the epidermis. It can attack any area of the body, but the parts most susceptible are the finger webs, anterior wrist, elbows, axillary region, areolae of the breasts, genitals, and lower buttocks. The parasite is transmitted by skin-to-skin contact with human beings or pets or by direct contact with contaminated items.

Lice

Lice are parasites, and three types affect human beings. Head lice (pediculosis capitis) are the most common type. They are found mainly on the scalp and sometimes in the eyebrows and eyelashes and cause intense itching. Outbreaks generally occur among schoolchildren. The bite of the body louse (pediculosis corporis) leaves visible, itchy, red spots primarily on the shoulders, buttocks, and abdomen. Genital lice (pediculosis pubis; crab lice) usually are found in the pubic area and are transmitted during sexual activity or contact with contaminated bedding.

Miscellaneous Skin Disorders

Alopecia

Alopecia is hair loss or baldness on parts or all of the body. Alopecia can be caused by aging, genetic predisposition, local diseases, chemotherapy, stress, or nutritional imbalances. Androgens seem to play a part in hair loss. Male-pattern baldness features hair loss on the forehead and top of the head, whereas female-pattern baldness involves thinning of the hair in the frontal and parietal regions.

Burns

The term *burn* refers to cells that are destroyed or inflamed as a result of heat, chemicals, radiation, or electricity. Fluid loss or secondary bacterial infection can occur as a consequence of the tissue damage.

Burns are classified by the depth of damage and are identified by degree.

In a *first-degree burn*, only the epidermis sustains injury. Signs and symptoms can include redness, mild stinging or pain, and mild swelling. These burns usually heal within a matter of days or weeks. A mild sunburn is a first-degree burn.

In a *second-degree burn*, both the epidermis and dermis are damaged. Besides redness and moderate to intense pain and swelling, blisters usually develop. In deeper burns the tissues may be white because of damage to the vascular supply. Second-degree burns can take 6 weeks to a few months to heal and often leave scars.

In a *third-degree burn*, the epidermis and entire dermis are severely damaged or destroyed. Damage to nerves can interrupt pain signals in the actual area of the burn. The skin may appear white, black, or charred, and no blisters form. Dehydration and infection may occur as a result of the loss of the protective barrier. A third-degree burn develops scars and may require a skin graft and a long healing period.

Dermatitis and eczema

Dermatitis is a general term for an acute or chronic skin inflammation characterized by redness, eruptions, edema, scaling, and itching. The term *eczema* often is used interchangeably with dermatitis, but many medical references limit the designation dermatitis to conditions caused by internal factors. Three major types of dermatitis have been recognized.

Atopic dermatitis. Atopic dermatitis is caused by an allergy or hypersensitivity, most commonly caused by pollens, cosmetics, or foods. It often is associated with other hypersensitivity disorders. Symptoms include inflammation, oozing and crusting, and intense itching.

Seborrheic dermatitis. Seborrheic dermatitis is a chronic condition that manifests with inflammation, scales, and crusting. The skin may be dry or greasy. The adult form of seborrheic dermatitis is a mild form of dandruff, most commonly seen at the eyebrows and on the scalp as a dry or greasy scaling. Cradle cap is the associated childhood form. Genetic predisposition, weather, stress, and some neurologic diseases may be risk factors.

Contact dermatitis. Contact dermatitis is caused by sensitivity to a substance that damages or irritates the skin such as poison ivy, a medication, cosmetics, or rubber. It may be marked by blisters or itchy, flaky skin.

Psoriasis

Psoriasis is a common, chronic skin disease characterized by reddened skin covered by dry, silvery scales. It most often is found on the scalp, elbows, knees, back, or buttocks.

Rosacea

Rosacea is a chronic skin problem in which the small blood vessels of the forehead, cheeks, and nose become dilated. It may affect a small area or the entire face. Eye inflammation (conjunctivitis) may develop. Rosacea may lie dormant for a time and then be activated by stress, infection, hot or spicy food, sunlight, or physical activity.

Scleroderma

Scleroderma (systemic sclerosis) is an autoimmune disorder of the connective tissue characterized by inflammation and overproduction of collagen. This results in scarring, which causes the tissues to stiffen and compress the capillaries, thus diminishing or halting blood flow. The disease usually appears in people between 30 and 50 years of age and affects women more often than men. It is found primarily in the skin and tissues surrounding the esophagus. Characteristics include increased joint stiffness, muscle weakness, swelling of the fingers, and skin-thickening collagen deposits. Besides the integument, collagen deposits can invade many of the body's systems such as the gastrointestinal tract, reducing the absorption of nutrients, and the lungs, diminishing respiratory effectiveness. Hypersensitivity to cold in the fingers, toes, ears, and nose (Raynaud's syndrome) may be present. In the most serious cases, heart and lung failure may occur.

Urticaria

Urticaria, or hives, is a condition of localized skin eruptions (wheals) in the dermis caused by allergy, exposure to heat or cold, or an emotional reaction. Urticaria may be accompanied by local pruritus (itching).

Vitiligo

Vitiligo is a disease marked by loss of skin pigmentation in irregular patches. It usually affects exposed areas of the skin in people under 30 years of age who have a family history of the disease.

Benign Tumors and Growths

A **tumor,** which also is referred to as a *neoplasm,* is a growth of new tissue. Tumors may be benign (i.e., nonthreatening or noncancerous) or malignant (cancerous).

Mole

A mole, or nevus, is a benign, pigmented skin growth formed of melanocytes.

Skin tag

A skin tag is a small, soft, flesh-colored or pigmented benign growth found on the neck or in the axillary or groin region.

Lipoma

A lipoma is a benign tumor formed from mature fat cells. It appears as a soft, movable, subcutaneous nodule typically found on the trunk, forearms, or neck.

Seborrheic keratosis

A seborrheic keratosis is a slightly raised skin lesion most commonly seen on the chest, back, neck, and face. These benign growths usually appear in middle-aged and elderly individuals as light brown or black flat areas. They may grow quickly and can be mistaken for moles or warts.

Angioma

An angioma is a benign tumor composed of blood or lymph vessels. Angiomas are common in newborns and usually disappear during childhood.

Sebaceous cyst

A sebaceous cyst is a slow-growing, benign tumor caused by the blockage of a sebaceous gland. It contains keratin, sebum, and hair follicle cells.

Malignant Skin Tumors

Skin cancer is the most common of all malignancies. Most skin cancers appear on the head, neck, and other areas frequently exposed to the sun. Too much sun exposure damages the skin by causing the elastin fibers to clump, leading to leathery skin and wrinkling. Immune function may be temporarily depressed, and deoxyribonucleic acid (DNA) is altered, leading to skin cancer. Three types of malignancy can occur.

Basal cell carcinoma

Basal cell carcinoma, the most common form of skin cancer, is associated with ultraviolet (UV) exposure. Basal cell carcinoma grows slowly and is the easiest type to treat successfully when recognized early.

Squamous cell carcinoma

Squamous cell carcinoma, also related to UV exposure, makes up one third of all skin cancers. Like basal cell carcinoma, it is best treated in the earlier stages, before it metastasizes. People with fair skin, blond or red hair, and chronic skin inflammation who are exposed to the sun or who suffered sun damage when young are more at risk for basal and squamous cell carcinoma.

Malignant melanoma

Malignant melanoma is the least common and the most dangerous of the skin cancers. It is not directly connected to sun exposure. Because it spreads rapidly, it must be identified and treated quickly. The memory device for identifying a melanoma is *ABC: a*symmetry, *b*order irregularity, and *c*olor change. Most melanomas are not evenly round; rather, they have an irregular border with a white, blue, or red edge and turn color to brown or black. Moles are especially susceptible to transformation into melanomas.

Breast Disorders

Fibrocystic disease

Fibrocystic disease is the most common disorder of the breast. It involves the growth of small, lumpy cysts, which develop as a result of changes in the milk-producing glands. It affects about 50% of women. No treatment is necessary, but because the incidence of breast cancer is higher in these women, recommendations on breast self-examination and the frequency of mammograms must be addressed individually by health care providers.

Breast cancer

Breast cancer is the leading cause of cancer deaths in women, with the peak incidence occurring in the early menopausal age group. Most women develop a painless, firm lump, often in the upper outer quadrant. In one form of breast cancer, no lump develops. The diagnosis is made using low-voltage soft tissue radiographs, called *mammograms*, and by fine needle biopsy. The standard medical treatment is based on many factors, including the size of the lump, the patient's age and physical condition, and the involvement of lymph nodes and other tissues. Muscle tissue and lymph nodes are removed when metastasis has occurred.

Surgical intervention consists of one of the following procedures: a lumpectomy (removal of the tumor), a simple mastectomy (removal of the breast only), a radical mastectomy (removal of the breast, pectoralis major and minor muscles, and the axillary lymph nodes), an extended radical mastectomy (in addition to the above, removal of the internal mammary lymph nodes near the sternum), or a modified radical mastectomy (removal of the breast and axillary lymph nodes, preserving the pectoralis major muscle). Radiation therapy, chemical therapy (chemotherapy), and hormone therapy are other methods of intervention, which may be used alone or in conjunction with surgery.

Although the number of men who develop breast cancer is extremely small, lumps and changes in the tissues of a man's breast cannot be ignored, and such a client should be referred to a physician for examination.

Anatomic and physiologic problems after a mastectomy. When the pectoralis major muscle is removed, some flexion and adduction of the arm is lost. The anterior part of the deltoid, as well as the coracobrachialis and the long head of the biceps, may be developed to help with flexion.

Loss of lymphatic channels in the axillae causes obstruction of lymph flow from the arm, and localized edema develops. Elevation of the arm and use of a special sleeve to provide compression are helpful. Mild cases may be helped by massage (Activity 11-3).

ACTIVITY 11-3

As soft tissue and movement therapists, we must be able to explain and justify the therapeutic value of the work we do. The following activity will help you develop the skills needed to explain the effectiveness of various modalities to clients and other health care professionals. Use the clinical reasoning model that follows to accomplish this task; an example of that model is provided in the Section Four opener, p. 450. Your focus should be the primary modality or modalities you would apply to the integumentary system.

Modality/modalities

1. **What are the facts?**
   a. Which system is involved, and which structures of that system can be reached directly or indirectly?

   b. Which of these structures are most affected by this modality?

   c. Which physiologic functions are affected by this approach?

   d. When the treatment is applied, what changes in function will result in
      (1) This system

      (2) The whole body

   e. What is considered normal or balanced function?

   f. How are the functions of this system related to the body's homeostasis?

Continued

g. What has worked or has not worked?

2. **What are the possibilities?**

h. Where could you find information that would support the use of this modality as a therapeutic intervention?

a. What do the data suggest?

b. What are the reasons for using the proposed methods?

i. What research is available to support the use of the therapeutic intervention?

c. What are the possible interventions?

j. How does the intervention support a healthy state?

d. List at least three applications of this modality that would affect both the structure and function of this system.

k. Under which pathologic or dysfunctional conditions is the intervention most likely to be beneficial?

e. What are other ways to look at the situation?

f. What other methods could provide similar benefits?

d. What is likely to happen if the modality is not used?

3. What is the logical outcome of therapeutic intervention?

a. What would be the logical progression of the symptom pattern, contributing factors, and current behaviors?

e. What is likely to happen if the modality is used?

b. What are the benefits and drawbacks of each intervention suggested?
Benefits:

4. For the Intervention proposed, what would be the impact on the people involved, specifically the client, practitioner, and other professionals working with the client?

a. How does each of the people involved (including, besides those named above, the client's family and support system) feel about the possible interventions?

Drawbacks:

c. What are the costs in terms of time, resources, and finances?

b. Does the practitioner feel qualified to work with the situation and apply the identified modality to the particular situation?

Continued

ACTIVITY 11-3—cont'd

c. Does a feeling of cooperation and agreement exist among all those involved, and how would the practitioner recognize this feeling?

Justification

Using the information developed in the clinical reasoning model, present a clear, concise statement of the ways in which the particular soft tissue or movement modality would be beneficial, either in supporting the particular body system in a healthy condition or as part of a treatment plan for a pathologic or dysfunctional condition. Based on the above information, give a brief summary of the effectiveness of the modality for this system.

The Cardiovascular System

The cardiovascular system is a transport system composed of the heart, blood vessels, and blood. The heart is the pump that sends the oxygen and nutrient-rich blood out to the body via the strong arteries and arterioles. The blood leaves the capillaries and enters the tissues. Deoxygenated blood and metabolic wastes leave the tissues, reenter the capillaries, and pass through the venules and veins on their way to the lungs, liver, and kidneys. Carbon dioxide is eliminated by the lungs, and other waste products are altered or eliminated by the liver and kidneys.

HEART

The **heart** is the major organ of the cardiovascular system (Figure 11-4). It is a hollow, muscular pump about the size of a clenched fist that is located in the mediastinum, the space between the lungs. The narrow, rounded point of the cone-shaped heart lies just behind the sternum, and the broader, flat base extends slightly to the left of center, near the fifth rib. The **pericardium** is a sac that surrounds the heart. It secretes a lubricating fluid that prevents friction from the movement of the heart. It also maintains the heart's location within the thoracic cavity.

The myocardium is the actual heart muscle that makes up the thickest part of the heart and generates the contractions. The outer membrane of the heart is called the *epicardium.* The endocardium is the smooth, thin, inner lining of the heart. The blood actually slides along the endocardium as it flows through the heart.

The heart is divided into four chambers. The two small, thin-walled upper chambers are the atria, known separately as the left **atrium** and the right atrium. They are separated by the interatrial septum. The two larger, lower chambers are the left and right **ventricles**. Their thick walls are separated by the interventricular septum. The atria and ventricles are separated by a fibrous structure, the skeleton of the heart.

Heart Valves

Created from the folds of the endocardium and maintained within the skeleton of the heart are the **heart valves,** four sets of valves that regulate the flow of blood through the heart. Atrioventricular (AV) valves allow blood to flow into the ventricles but keep it from returning to the atria. Strings of connective tissue known as *chordae tendineae* actually connect between the ventricle wall and the valves to help close the valve without letting it collapse into the atria. The bicuspid, or mitral, valve is located between the left atrium and the left ventricle; the tricuspid valve is found between the right atrium and the right ventricle.

Semilunar valves control the blood flow out of the ventricles into the aorta and pulmonary arteries and prevent any backflow of blood into the ventricles. The aortic valve is found between the left ventricle and the aorta, and the pulmonary valve is between the pulmonary artery and the right ventricle. These valves open in response to pressure generated when the blood leaves the ventricle. They close when blood pools in small pockets of the cusps of the valves and pushes the valves closed.

Blood Vessels

The term *great vessels* refers to the large blood vessels entering or leaving the heart that transport blood to the lungs and the rest of the body. There are three great vessels:

Aorta—The artery that carries oxygen and nutrients to the body and the heart

Pulmonary trunk—The artery that carries blood to the lungs to release carbon dioxide and take in oxygen

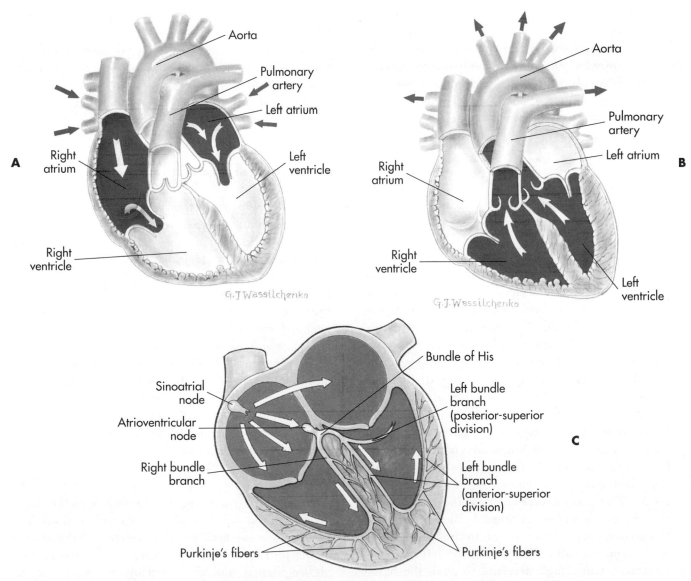

FIGURE 11-4 **A,** Blood flow during diastole. **B,** Blood flow during systole. **C,** Cardiac conduction. (From Canobbio MM: *Cardiovascular disorders,* St Louis, 1990, Mosby.)

Superior vena cava—The vein that returns poorly oxygenated blood to the right atrium from the upper venous circulation

Other major blood vessels include the following:

Inferior vena cava—The vein that returns oxygen-poor blood from the lower venous circulation to the right atrium

Pulmonary veins—The four veins, two from each lung, that bring oxygen-rich blood to the left atrium

Blood Supply to the Heart

The two **coronary arteries,** which originate from the base of the aorta, supply oxygenated blood to the heart muscle. Coronary veins follow parallel to the arteries and return the blood to the right atrium via the coronary sinus. Both types of coronary vessels run in grooves between the atria and ventricles and between the two ventricles. If either of the coronary arteries is unable to supply sufficient blood to the heart muscle, a heart attack occurs. The most common site of a heart attack is the anterior or inferior part of the left ventricle.

Blood Flow Through the Heart

Blood moves into and out of the heart in a well-coordinated and precisely timed rhythm. For examination purposes, it can be divided into the following stages.

Stage 1—Oxygen-poor blood from the body enters the superior and inferior vena cavae and flows into the right atrium. When the right atrium is full, it empties through the tricuspid valve into the right ventricle.

Stage 2—The right ventricle, when full, contracts and pushes blood through the pulmonary valve into the pulmonary artery. This artery divides into the left and right pulmonary arteries and takes the blood to both lungs (these are the only arteries in the body that carry oxygen-poor blood). Four pulmonary veins leave the lungs carrying oxygen-rich blood back to the left atrium (these are the only veins in the body that carry oxygen-rich blood).

Stage 3—This process takes place at the same time as the process described in Stage 1. Blood leaves the left atrium and passes through to the left ventricle via the mitral valve. When full, the left ventricle contracts, using high pressure to push the blood through the aortic valve into the aorta and descending aorta and to all parts of the body except the lungs. The walls of the left ventricle are thicker to provide the extra strength needed to pump blood out to the entire body.

Heart Pump

The heart has its own built-in rhythm. Not only can each cardiac cell contract without nerve stimulus, the heart can contract even if removed from the body. The autonomic nervous system can affect the rate of the rhythm and the force of contraction through sympathetic and parasympathetic activation.

Both atria contract while both ventricles are relaxed. When the atria relax, the ventricles contract. This synchronization leads to the sequence of events known as the *cardiac cycle.* It consists of one heartbeat, or diastole, which is the relaxation of the ventricles during filling, and systole, the contraction of the ventricles as they empty.

Although the heart has an atrial diastole and systole, the stronger ventricular actions are used for identification.

Our heart rate is identified by the number of cardiac cycles that occur in 1 minute. In the average healthy person, that works out to be 60 to 70 cycles, or beats, per minute.

The coordinated rhythm of the heart is initiated by the built-in electrical system in the sinoatrial (SA) node, which sets the pace of the heart rate. The signal originates in the right atrium and travels to the left atrium, causing the atria to contract. At the precise moment the atria have completed their contraction, the signal travels through the AV bundle to the right ventricle and into the left ventricle, causing the ventricles to contract. The rhythm can be checked through an electrocardiogram (ECG or EKG), which monitors the electrical changes in the heart. A portable ECG machine, known as a Holter monitor, can measure the heart signals over a 24-hour period. If difficulty with the electrical system in the SA node develops, a device known as a pacemaker can be implanted to assist or take over initiation of the signal.

Heart Sounds

Heart sounds can be heard through a stethoscope. Closure of the valves produces two main sounds. The first is a low-pitched "lubb" generated by the closing of the mitral and tricuspid valves. The second is a higher-pitched "dubb" caused by the closing of the aortic and pulmonary valves. Extra sounds such as those resulting from faulty valves are referred to as murmurs. Valves usually are quiet as they open.

Blood Volume and Flow

Cardiac output is the amount of blood pumped by the left ventricle in 1 minute. The average output under normal conditions is 5 to 6 liters of blood. In order to pump more oxygen and nutrients to the cells during exercise and in times of stress, output may rise to 20 liters or more. The speed of the blood flow is fastest in arteries, moderate in veins, and slowest in capillaries. This allows for exchange of nutrients and waste products between tissues and blood.

Entrainment

Entrainment is the coordination or synchronization to a rhythm. It was first presented in Chapter 2. Research at the Institute of HeartMath and other facilities indicates that the heart rhythm tends to be the guide that the other body rhythms follow. The heart rate, respiratory rate, and thalamus synchronization combine to support the entrainment process, and the other, more subtle, body rhythms follow. Most meditation processes or relaxation methods create an environment for this entrainment to occur.

The heart is seen as the seat of love and the home of emotions relating to relationships. The heart is the symbol of love on valentine cards. We speak of how a person's heart can be broken with loss and grief. We have lost heart when we give up hope. We have a big heart when we are compassionate and nurturing. Is it possible that the strong rhythm of the heart, of which we easily can become conscious, also brings us awareness of how experience affects us? The heart rate and strength of contraction can change in a moment in response to the demands of life. Living aware of our hearts is a way to live aware of our response to experience.

VASCULAR SYSTEM

The vascular system is the other part of the cardiovascular system. It consists of blood vessels that carry blood from the heart to the lungs and body tissues and back to the heart in a continuous cycle. A blood vessel that transports blood from the heart is called an **artery.** Arteries eventually branch off into smaller and smaller arteries, the smallest of which are called **arterioles.** A **capillary** is one of the

ACTIVITY 11-4

Label Figure 11-5 by writing the names of the arteries listed below next to the matching number in the illustration.

1. Right common carotid
2. Brachiocephalic
3. Aorta
4. Celiac
5. Renal
6. Radial
7. Deep femoral
8. Peroneal
9. Left external carotid
10. Left subclavian
11. Brachial
12. Mesenteric
13. Abdominal aorta
14. External iliac
15. Femoral
16. Popliteal
17. Anterior tibial

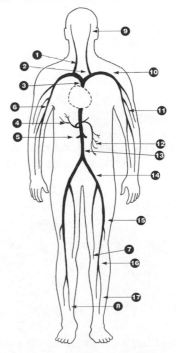

FIGURE 11-5 (From Williams RW: *Basic healthcare terminology,* St Louis, 1995, Mosby.)

tiny blood vessels located between the arterioles and the **venules,** the smallest of the veins. The veins get larger and larger as they get closer to the heart. The largest veins return blood to the right atrium of the heart.

Arteries

The body has three types of arteries (Activity 11-4):

1. Elastic arteries are the large arteries capable of undergoing passive stretching. They have thick walls and recoil when the ventricles relax, which maintains pressure to move the blood. The aorta and pulmonary artery are elastic arteries.
2. Muscular arteries constitute most of the arteries in the body. These are small to medium arteries that distribute blood to all tissues by contracting or dilating to control blood flow.
3. Arterioles are the smallest arteries, with a diameter of less than 0.5 mm. They also constrict or dilate to control the amount of blood entering capillaries.

🖐 PRACTICAL APPLICATION

Soft tissue and movement therapists can increase arterial blood flow in two ways. By stimulating sympathetic autonomic functions, the heart rate is increased, providing more push to the blood in the arteries. This is a reflexive, indirect method that involves the use of homeostatic mechanisms to maintain balance. Modalities of touch and movement can be structured to be stimulating to the sympathetic autonomic nervous system. In general, the methods used are brisk and involve active contraction of the muscles coupled with an increased respiratory rate.

Arterial blood flow also can be increased mechanically through the pump and tube mechanism of the cardiovascular system. Arteries are pliable muscular tubes that carry blood (a fluid) under pressure from the heart pump. If the tube is crimped or closed, pressure builds between the pump (the heart) and the barrier, like water behind a dam. When the barrier is removed, the buildup of pressure provides an

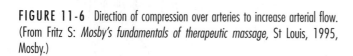

FIGURE 11-6 Direction of compression over arteries to increase arterial flow. (From Fritz S: *Mosby's fundamentals of therapeutic massage,* St Louis, 1995, Mosby.)

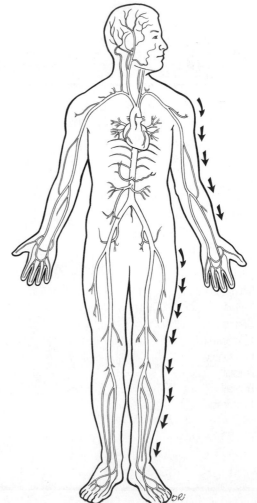

initial extra push to the fluid. Compression over more superficial arteries to close off the flow of blood temporarily results in the same phenomenon. Back pressure builds, and when the compression is released, the blood pushes forward with more force than would have been available from the heart action alone. The compression against the arteries is applied to the legs and arms to assist peripheral circulation. The rhythm of compression and release is a rate of about 60 beats per minute, to coincide with the heart rhythm. The increase in blood flow is temporary, and in healthy individuals with adequate blood flow, the effect may be negligible (Figure 11-6).

Veins

Veins collect blood from the capillaries and transport it back to the heart. At any given time, the venous system contains 75% of the blood of the body. Veins are under less pressure than arteries. Their walls contain fewer muscle cells and are not as elastic as the walls of arteries. The walls of the smaller veins actually collapse when blood leaves and inflate when blood flows through. The larger veins contain valves that keep the blood flowing in one direction. The

veins of the legs contain more valves than the veins of the arms to help fight the effects of gravity and prevent blood from pooling in the feet. Some of the more superficial veins in our hands and arms are visible. All superficial veins empty into the deeper veins. The deeper veins usually are found near arteries.

Proper venous return of blood is necessary for the heart to have sufficient blood for normal cardiac output. Factors that affect venous return include the following (Activity 11-5):

Valves—Valves close in the veins to prevent backflow and pooling of blood. Improperly working valves can cause blood to back up and remain in the venous system.

Muscular pump—Muscle contractions help push venous blood toward the heart.

Gravity—Standing in one position for a long time is detrimental to venous return because blood in the veins below the heart must constantly overcome gravity to return to the heart.

Respiratory pump—During inhalation and exhalation, movement of the diaphragm and intercostal muscles helps move blood through the venous system.

ACTIVITY 11-5

Label Figure 11-7 by writing the names of the veins listed below next to the matching number in the illustration.

1. Right internal jugular
2. Right external jugular
3. Right subclavian
4. Brachial
5. Hepatic
6. Basilic
7. Renal
8. Radial
9. Ulnar
10. Femoral
11. Anterior tibial
12. Inferior vena cava
13. Mesenteric
14. Common iliac
15. Great saphenous
16. Small saphenous

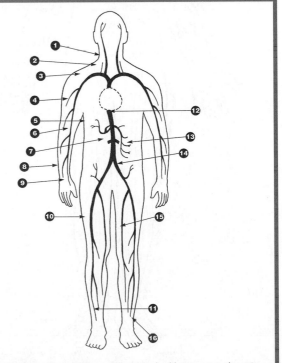

FIGURE 11-7 (From Williams RW: *Basic healthcare terminology*, St Louis, 1995, Mosby.)

PRACTICAL APPLICATION

The principles affecting venous return can be incorporated into soft tissue and movement approaches to encourage venous return flow:

- Muscular pump—Rhythmic contraction and relaxation of the muscles during movement encourages venous return flow.
- Massage—Stroking over the veins toward the heart passively moves blood in the veins. This method is particularly effective in the limbs.
- Gravity—Positioning the limbs higher than the heart passively assists venous return flow.
- Respiratory pump—Slow, deep diaphragmatic breathing in conjunction with the modality used enhances venous return flow.

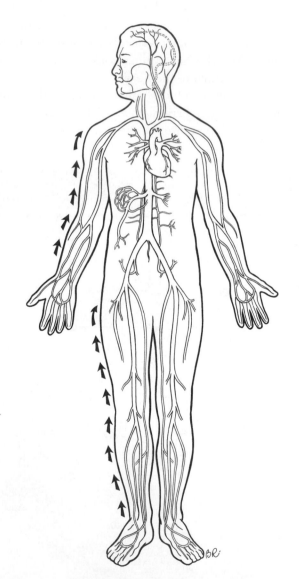

FIGURE 11-8 Direction of effleurage strokes to facilitate venous flow. (From Fritz S: *Mosby's fundamentals of therapeutic massage*, St Louis, 1995, Mosby.)

Rhythmic contraction of the muscles can be provided by having the person move her limbs through a complete range of motion against movement resistance in a contract-and-relax rhythm of about 60 cycles per minute. Next, short strokes (1 or 2 inches long) are applied over the veins toward the heart at sufficient pressure to push the blood in the superficial veins. The limbs are then placed in a supported position above the heart for gravity to assist the return flow while the client is encouraged to relax and breathe deeply (Figure 11-8).

Capillaries

The exchange of gases, nutrients, and waste products occurs in the capillaries, which branch out into all of the body's tissues. Their walls are very thin and are made of loose connective tissue, which allows easy diffusion of molecules.

Blood Pressure and Pulse

The amount of pressure exerted by the blood on the walls of the blood vessels is called **blood pressure.** The maximal pressure, called *systolic pressure,* occurs when the ventricles contract. Diastolic pressure occurs when the ventricles relax. Blood forced into the aorta during systole sets up a pressure wave that travels along the arteries. The wave expands the arterial wall, and the expansion can be palpated by pressing the artery against tissue. The number of waves is known as the pulse, which is a direct reflection of the heart rate.

The pulse rate is measured when a person is at rest; it may be regular or irregular, strong or weak. An irregular pulse commonly is found with atrial fibrillation and premature contractions. A strong pulse is seen with hyperthyroidism, a weak one with shock and myocardial infarction. A resting heart rate over 100 beats per minute is known as tachycardia; a heart rate below 50 or 60 beats per minute is known as bradycardia (Figure 11-9).

PRACTICAL APPLICATION

The pulses can be monitored during assessment. In general, the pulses should feel bilaterally equal. Should differences be noted, the client should be referred for diagnosis. The pulse rate ranges from 50 to 70 beats per minute while resting. A rate much slower or faster indicates a need for referral. If the general intent of the therapy session is stress management focused toward relaxation with parasympathetic predomination, the pulse rate would slow somewhat over the duration of the session. The opposite would be true if the goal was increased arousal of the sympathetic system to energize the client.

Blood pressure is regulated by sympathetic nerves to the arterioles. Normally, arterioles are in a state of partial constriction, called *arteriole tone.* Stimulation of the sympathetic system causes further arteriolar constriction and an increase in blood pressure. Nonstimulation results in a decrease in blood pressure. With hypertension, the sympathetic system is in a state of continuous stimulation, resulting in constant high blood pressure.

Blood pressure is measured with a sphygmomanometer, a cloth-covered rubber bag that is wrapped around the arm over the brachial artery. Blood pressure is highest during contraction of the heart (systole), the systolic blood pressure. It is lowest when the heart is relaxing (diastole), the diastolic pressure. As the vessels become more and more remote from the heart, the systolic and diastolic pressures merge into one pressure. When the vessels change from arteries to arterioles to capillaries to venules to veins, the pressure gets lower and lower,

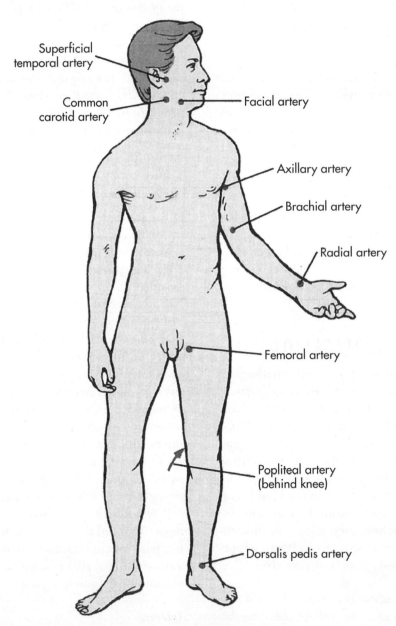

FIGURE 11-9 Pulse points. Each pulse point is named after the artery with which it is associated. (From Thibodeau GA, Patton KT: *The human body in health and disease,* St Louis, 1992, Mosby.)

until in the large veins there may be no pressure at all or a negative pressure. This is why, when drawing venous blood, one has to pull back on the syringe.

Blood pressure is recorded as millimeters of mercury (mm Hg), which refers to how many millimeters of mercury are displaced by the changes in pressure. The first number is the systolic pressure, and the second number is the diastolic pressure. When the pressure is recorded, only the numbers are written; the unit of measure mm Hg usually is dropped.

Normal blood pressure range

Blood pressure depends on the person's size. The average newborn has a blood pressure of 90/60; at 15 years of age, the average blood pressure is about 120/60. An average, healthy young adult has a blood pressure of 120/80. Generally, a blood pressure under 100/60 is considered hypotension; a pressure over 140/90 is considered hypertension. The blood pressure changes under various conditions, and a single reading should never be used as a final determinant.

Consider these facts:

- A systolic increase is seen in temporary conditions such as anxiety and exercise.
- Hypertension involves an increase in both the systolic and diastolic pressures.
- Hypotension is a decrease in the systolic and diastolic pressures. It is an important manifestation of shock, which is the result of an inadequate blood supply to vital organs.

✋ PRACTICAL APPLICATION

Stress management programs include methods of movement and moderate aerobic exercise, stretching programs, massage, and other forms of soft tissue methods. Although they initially elevate blood pressure, when continued, they activate parasympathetic quieting responses such as slow, deep breathing and progressive relaxation and therefore tend to have a normalizing effect on the blood pressure. These methods are classified as nonspecific constitutional approaches; they allow the homeostatic mechanisms to reset to a more effective functional pattern when disruption has occurred.

Medulla and Baroreceptors

In the medulla of the brain, the cells of the reticular formation regulate three vital signs: heart rate, blood pressure, and respiration. They work in conjunction with signals from the various nerve centers in the

body. One type of nerve center in the cardiovascular system is the baroreceptor.

Baroreceptors are stretch receptors in the carotid arteries, the aorta, and nearly every large artery of the neck and thorax. When blood pressure increases, arteries stretch. The baroreceptors transmit signals about sudden, brief changes in blood pressure such as when we change position. When blood pressure is elevated for a long period, the baroreceptor reflex resets to the new blood pressure level.

When blood pressure suddenly drops, the frequency of signals from the baroreceptors declines. This sets off a response in the cardioregulatory center of the medulla that increases sympathetic stimulation and decreases parasympathetic stimulation, resulting in an increase in the heart rate. This raises the blood pressure. Conversely, when blood pressure increases, the signal increases and the medulla changes its output to slow the heart rate and blood pressure by increasing parasympathetic signals. This is another example of how a negative feedback system works in the body.

✋ PRACTICAL APPLICATION

Stimulation of baroreceptors during soft tissue work could affect blood pressure. The blood pressure could drop, and the client may be lightheaded and show other signs of low blood pressure.

Names of Specific Arteries and Veins

The names of most arteries and veins are derived from the anatomic structure they serve. The femoral artery and the femoral vein, for example, are found close to the femur, where these blood vessels serve the tissue of the upper and lower leg. The renal artery is so named because it exits the abdominal aorta and enters the kidney. The renal vein exits the kidney and enters the inferior vena cava. Arteries and veins are found on both sides of the body and are identified as either right or left (e.g., the right common carotid artery and the left common carotid artery).

The following is a list of the main arteries and veins. Many of them change names as they enter into and pass through certain areas of the body. You may want to follow along in the Color Plates or another anatomy text to help locate each vessel.

Arteries

Main arteries of the head and neck. The arch of the aorta gives rise to three arteries; from right to left they are the brachiocephalic (or innominate) artery, the left common carotid artery, and the left subclavian artery. The subclavian veins supply the upper extremities.

The brachiocephalic artery, a short artery, becomes the right common carotid artery and the right subclavian artery.

The common carotid arteries branch at the level of the upper part of the thyroid cartilage to become the external and internal carotid arteries. The common carotid artery is an important pulse-taking artery; damage to this artery may result in a transient ischemic attack. The internal carotid artery supplies the brain; the external carotid artery supplies the face, head, and neck.

The superficial temporal artery is the cranial termination of the external carotid artery. The superficial temporal artery is a pulse-taking artery located superior and anterior to the ear.

The two vertebral arteries become the basilar artery, which helps supply the brain.

Main arteries of the upper extremity. The subclavian artery becomes the axillary artery at the clavicle.

Near the head of the humerus, the axillary artery becomes the brachial artery. The brachial artery is the main artery for measuring blood pressure. It is also a pulse-taking artery.

The brachial artery divides at the elbow region into the radial and ulnar arteries.

The ulnar artery lies deep and medial. The radial artery lies more superficial and lateral. Both arteries communicate in the hand via two deep anastomoses and a superficial and deep palmar arch.

Main arteries of the trunk. After supplying the head, neck, and upper extremity, the aorta descends posteriorly as the thoracic aorta, sending branches to the intercostal muscles as the right and left intercostal arteries.

The intercostal arteries anastomose anteriorly with the left and right internal thoracic arteries. If the aorta is damaged, the intercostal muscles, which are important in breathing, may still receive a blood supply by way of the internal thoracic arteries.

Main arteries of the abdomen. When the thoracic aorta penetrates the diaphragm, it is known as the *abdominal aorta,* which supplies the abdominal organs. The following structures, listed in a cranial to caudal direction, are the main branches of the abdominal aorta:

Celiac trunk—Supplies the stomach, spleen, and liver via the gastric, splenic, and hepatic arteries

Superior mesenteric artery—Supplies the small intestine, part of the pancreas, and half of the colon

Renal arteries—Supply the kidneys

Testicular or ovarian arteries—Supply the gonads

Inferior mesenteric artery—Supplies the remaining half of the colon to the rectum

The abdominal aorta then divides into the left and right common iliac arteries. The common iliac divides into the internal iliac artery, which supplies the pelvic organs, and the external iliac artery.

Main arteries of the lower extremity. After passing under the inguinal ligament, the external iliac artery becomes the femoral artery. The femoral artery lies superficially at the femoral triangle and then descends posteriorly through the adductor muscles. The femoral artery is an important pulse-taking artery. When the femoral artery emerges behind the knee in the popliteal region, it becomes the popliteal artery. The popliteal artery then divides to become the anterior and posterior tibial arteries.

The anterior tibial artery becomes the dorsalis pedis artery on the dorsal aspect of the foot. The dorsalis pedis is an important pulse-taking artery.

The posterior tibial artery descends behind the medial malleolus. This artery is also a pulse-taking artery, but it usually is more difficult to find than the dorsalis pedis.

Veins

Main veins of the head and neck:

Superficial—The right and left external jugular veins drain blood from the face, head, and neck. Each external jugular vein empties into a subclavian vein.

Deep—Venous drainage from the brain is accomplished by the internal jugular veins. Each internal jugular vein joins a subclavian vein to form a brachiocephalic vein.

Main veins of the upper extremity:

Superficial—Superficial veins originate on the dorsum of the hand as the dorsal venous plexus. They curve around the wrist to the ventral side as the cephalic vein, which runs along the lateral aspect of forearm and arm, going deep at the deltoid muscle, and the basilic vein, which runs along the medial aspect of forearm and arm and goes deep at the biceps muscle. The medial cubital vein is an anastomosis between the basilic and cephalic veins.

Deep—The deep veins are formed from branches in the hand and forearm. Although some individuals have a short brachial vein, most often the first main deep vein is the axillary vein. The axillary vein becomes the subclavian vein when it passes under the clavicle.

Main veins of the trunk

The subclavian vein joins the internal jugular vein to become the brachiocephalic vein. The subclavian vein is an important central vein for intravenous (IV) infusion.

Two brachiocephalic veins join to become the superior vena cava, which empties into the right atrium.

The azygous system, which lies on the posterior body wall, drains the intercostal veins. The azygous vein empties into the superior vena cava.

The inferior vena cava drains blood from the abdominal viscera into the right atrium. The digestive organs and spleen first drain into the portal vein, which empties into the liver. The following veins, listed from cranial to caudal, are branches of the inferior vena cava:

Hepatic veins from the liver
Right and left renal veins from the kidneys
Right and left testicular or ovarian veins from the gonads
Two common iliac veins (the continuation of the femoral veins)

Main veins of the lower extremity

Superficial veins of the leg begin as a dorsal venous arch on top of the foot.

The great saphenous vein ascends medially from the foot up the leg to the thigh and drains into the femoral vein. The great saphenous veins may become chronically dilated in some people and develop into varicose veins. They may then become inflamed and form blood clots, a condition known as *thrombophlebitis.*

The small saphenous vein runs laterally from the foot along the gastrocnemius muscle and drains into the popliteal vein.

The anterior tibial vein and posterior tibial vein drain into the popliteal vein.

The popliteal vein becomes the femoral vein after it passes the knee. The deep veins of the leg may become inflamed, a condition referred to as *deep vein thrombosis.* This is a more serious condition than superficial thrombophlebitis. The clot may break off and travel to the heart, then lodge in the lung as a pulmonary embolism.

BLOOD

Blood, the thick, red fluid in our bodies, is a form of connective tissue. It transports nutrients to the individual cells and removes waste products. Whole blood consists of solid formed elements and the liquid matrix, or plasma.

Red blood cells, white blood cells, and platelets are the formed elements of blood that float in the **plasma,** a thick, straw-colored fluid (Activity 11-6). Amino acids, carbohydrates, electrolytes, hormones, lipids,

ACTIVITY 11-6

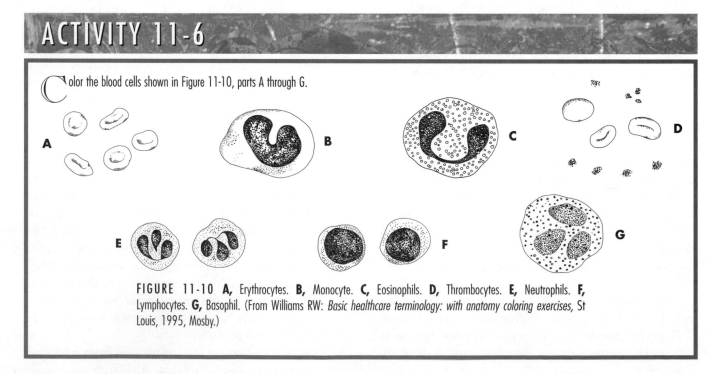

Color the blood cells shown in Figure 11-10, parts A through G.

FIGURE 11-10 **A,** Erythrocytes. **B,** Monocyte. **C,** Eosinophils. **D,** Thrombocytes. **E,** Neutrophils. **F,** Lymphocytes. **G,** Basophil. (From Williams RW: *Basic healthcare terminology: with anatomy coloring exercises,* St Louis, 1995, Mosby.)

proteins, vitamins, and waste materials are the other constituents of blood. A person who weighs 140 to 150 pounds has about 5 quarts of blood.

In an adult, blood cells are formed mainly in the marrow of the bones of the chest, vertebrae, and pelvis. Yellow marrow can convert to red marrow if the body requires increased production of blood cells. The stages of blood cell development in red marrow constitute a process called *hematopoiesis*. Blood cells originate from a common precursor cell, called the *stem cell*. Immature blood cells are blast cells. When the cells are mature, they move into the bloodstream. Blast cells may be seen in peripheral blood in leukemia because the body is sending them out even before they are mature.

Red Blood Cells

Red blood cells, also known as *erythrocytes* or *red blood corpuscles*, make up more than 90% of the formed elements in blood. They are round and have raised edges and a flattened middle. Their function is to transport oxygen to the cells and carbon dioxide away from the cells. Men have slightly more red blood cells than women, and the cells live slightly longer in men (about 120 days) than in women (110 days). The body recycles dead red blood cells; hemoglobin is used in new cells, and proteins from the dead cells are broken down into amino acids to create new blood proteins.

Because red blood cells cannot divide, they must be produced frequently to replace dead cells. A red blood cell loses its nucleus and most of its organelles during development. Red bone marrow produces enough red blood cells daily to replace dead blood cells. The body needs a proper intake and assimilation of iron, vitamin B_{12}, and folic acid to produce new red blood cells.

Erythrocytes contain an iron-protein compound known as *hemoglobin*. Oxygen binds to hemoglobin in the capillaries of the lungs and is transported to all parts of the body. A lack of oxygen or anemia can stimulate erythropoiesis, the production of red blood cells. Red blood cells also transport carbon dioxide from the tissues of the body to the lungs. An abnormal increase in red blood cells is known as *polycythemia;* an abnormal decrease is called *anemia*.

A variety of chemicals are present in red blood cells. Some of these chemicals are commonly called *factors*, which are used to identify the type of blood. The best-known grouping method is the ABO system. This system has four blood groups, A, B, AB, and O, commonly called the *blood types*. The Rh system, the most complex of all the blood grouping methods, has 42 different groups.

White Blood Cells

White blood cells are also called *leukocytes* or white blood corpuscles. Their white color is due to a lack of hemoglobin. The usual ratio of white to red blood cells is 1 to 500. The main function of the white blood cells is to protect the body from pathogens and remove dead cells and substances. White blood cells are divided into the following five groups:

Neutrophils—Neutrophils are granular leukocytes; more than half of all white blood cells are neutrophils. These cells fight disease by engulfing bacteria in a cell-eating process called *phagocytosis*. Neutrophils are very important in the body's defense against bacterial infection. A buildup of neutrophils and the debris they collect is called *pus*.

Monocytes—Monocytes are the largest of the white blood cells, yet they account for only about 6% of the total number. They also protect the body through phagocytosis. Monocytes are unique because when they leave the blood and enter the tissues, they can develop into very large phagocytic cells called *macrophages*.

Lymphocytes—Lymphocytes account for about 30% of the total number of white blood cells in the body. They produce antibodies and chemicals that are active in regulating disease, allergic reactions, and controlling tumors.

Eosinophils—About 3% of the total white blood cell count is made up of eosinophils. However, the number increases greatly with either parasitic infections or allergic reactions (e.g., hay fever). Eosinophils are capable of phagocytic activity, and they release chemicals during the inflammatory process.

Basophils—Basophils are also granular white blood cells, and they make up about 1% of the total white blood cell count. Their exact function is not yet clearly understood.

Platelets

Thrombocytes, also called *platelets*, are the smallest cellular elements of the blood. They are very important in the blood clotting process and are manufactured in the bone marrow. The normal number of platelets in human blood ranges from 240,000 to 400,000 mm^3.

Plasma

Plasma is the straw-colored liquid found in blood and lymph. It is about 90% water; the rest is nutrients, gases, and waste products. Plasma constitutes about 55% of blood. It plays a major role in the movement of water between the tissues and the blood.

Clotting

When a blood vessel is damaged, chemicals are released. Special proteins, called *clotting factors*, are activated, and they in turn form additional clotting factors. When a special protein called *fibrin* is formed, it seals the damaged blood vessels by trapping red blood cells, platelets, and fluid, to form a clot. Fibrin then anchors the clot in place. The clotting process starts the instant the blood vessel is damaged and takes only a few minutes to complete. Calcium and vitamin K are important to the success and speed of the clotting process (Activity 11-6).

PATHOLOGIC CONDITIONS

INDICATIONS CONTRAINDICATIONS

For Soft Tissue and Movement Therapies

In general, cardiovascular disease presents contraindications for soft tissue and movement therapies. If the contraindication does not arise from the disease itself, the medication taken to control the disease may pose problems. Blood thinners, for example, increase the possibility of bruising and hemorrhage. Nonetheless, soft tissue and movement modalities often are indicated as part of a supervised treatment program. The key is supervision by a qualified health care provider, because cardiovascular diseases can be complex, both in the presenting pathologic condition and the treatment protocols. The general stress management and homeostatic normalization effects of soft tissue and movement treatments are desirable for most cardiovascular difficulties as long as the treatments are supervised as part of a total therapeutic program.

Cardiovascular disease is the leading cause of death in Western societies. Cardiac arrest may occur as a result of a number of conditions, the most common being a heart attack (myocardial infarction).

Myocardial Infarction (Heart Attack)

An infarct is an area of dead tissue that results when the blood supply to that area is blocked. Most heart attacks are caused by blockage of a coronary artery by a blood clot, especially in arteries narrowed by coronary artery disease. The blocking of blood flow damages or destroys the heart muscle. The first symptom usually is a crushing pain in the center of the chest over the sternum. Pain may also occur in the arms, neck, jaw, and upper abdomen and occasionally in the back. The person also may perspire heavily and complain of dizziness, chills, or nausea. Immediate treatment is essential.

Aneurysm

An aneurysm is a permanent dilation of part of a vessel as a result of weakness or damage to its structure. Although usually the result of arteriosclerosis, an aneurysm also may be congenital or the result of inflammation. The most common sites are the aorta and the arteries of the brain.

Embolus

An embolus is a plug in the bloodstream that may consist of a blood clot (a thrombus), plaque, air or gas, fat, tumor cells, tissue, or clumps of bacteria.

Ischemia

Ischemia is a temporary deficiency or diminished supply of blood to a tissue.

Occlusion

An occlusion is a blockage of a vessel.

Thrombus

A thrombus is an intravascular clot.

Arteriosclerosis and Atherosclerosis

Arteriosclerosis, which means *hardening of the arteries,* refers to arteries that have become brittle and lost their elasticity. Arteries gradually lose elasticity as we age. If they cannot enlarge, blockage becomes more serious. Although arteriosclerosis has several causes, the most common and important is **atherosclerosis,** the deposit of fatty plaques in medium and large arteries. Often the two terms are used interchangeably, which is incorrect. In atherosclerosis, small fat deposits from cholesterol in the blood build up at stress points in the arteries. These stress points occur where the arteries branch out or incur damage. The fat combines with connective tissue sent to repair the damage and forms plaque. As this process continues, blood flow diminishes. Symptoms do not usually appear until a major blockage occurs. The body compensates by enlarging the artery, if possible. Sometimes the artery enlarges, forms an aneurysm, and ruptures. Problems also occur when the plaque breaks off and completely blocks the vessels. In the brain, this is called a *stroke.*

Countries with high-fat diets, particularly diets high in saturated fatty acids and cholesterol, have a higher incidence of atherosclerosis. Nonsurgical interventions such as modifying the diet and taking part in aerobic exercise may be able to enlarge an artery, increasing the blood flow. Also, collateral circulation may develop around the blockage as new vessels are created. Surgical interventions may include creating a bypass from blood vessels transferred from other parts of the body, excising the blockage, or enlarging the vessel.

Coronary Artery Disease

Coronary artery disease (CAD) most often is caused by arteriosclerosis, atherosclerosis, and thrombus formation in one or more of the coronary arteries. Partial occlusion causes the transient chest and arm pain of angina. Total occlusion causes the crushing or squeezing pain of infarction. Blockage of the artery diminishes the amount of oxygen and nutrients reaching the heart tissues. Among the many risk factors that contribute to CAD, some can be controlled such as diet, weight, and avoiding smoking. Treatment frequently includes the use of β-blockers and calcium channel blockers to slow the heart rate and reduce the strength of the contraction. In addition to lowering the blood pressure, calcium channel blockers dilate the coronary arteries.

Angina Pectoris

Angina pectoris is chest pain or discomfort that results when the amount of oxygen supplied to the heart declines. It is caused mainly by CAD but can also be a sign of heart disease, anemia, or hyperthyroidism. Symptoms most often occur during exertion, emotional upset, or cold weather. The pain begins in the center of the chest and often spreads to the arms, neck, or jaw. In severe cases, pain may occur when the person is at rest. The symptoms usually are relieved by rest or the use of nitroglycerin

Congestive Heart Failure

Heart failure occurs when the heart muscle weakens and cannot pump sufficient blood, when the heart valves are damaged, or as a result of hypertension or excessive demands on the heart. Blood pools in the veins and not enough reaches the heart. The heart compensates by pumping out more blood, causing even more pooling in the veins and organs. This buildup of fluid is called *congestion;* thus the condition is called *congestive heart failure* (CHF). Treatment usually includes use of a diuretic such as furosemide (Lasix) to eliminate excess fluid and reduce blood pressure.

Hypertension

Most authorities consider hypertension to be a blood pressure sustained over 140/90 mm Hg. Hypertension can be graded as mild, moderate, borderline high, or severe, depending on the diastolic reading. In most cases the cause is unknown (essential hypertension), although kidney disease and arteriosclerosis may play a role. With hypertension, continuous sympathetic stimulation constricts arterioles. Chronic untreated hypertension leads to hypertensive heart disease. The heart becomes enlarged because of the increased work of the left ventricle against arteriolar resistance, and heart failure or infarct may result. Other important complications of untreated hypertension are stroke and kidney disease.

Nondrug therapy consists of restricting salt (which reduces fluid retention), losing weight (which reduces the resistance against which the heart must pump), reducing the consumption of alcohol, avoiding smoking, and participating in stress management and aerobic exercise programs.

Medical treatment may include a diuretic, a β-blocker, a calcium channel blocker, an angiotensin-converting enzyme (ACE), or a combination of these medications as needed.

Rheumatic Heart Disease

Rheumatic fever may occur in young children after an untreated streptococcal throat infection as an immunologic response to bacterial substances remaining in the body. Besides its signature rash, other signs and symptoms include joint pain, swelling, fever, and endocarditis. If left untreated, the endocarditis may result in rheumatic heart disease, in which the inflamed heart valves, particularly the mitral valve, become deformed.

Inflammation of the Heart and Pericardium

Inflammations that affect the heart and pericardial sac are not very common. They usually follow acute or chronic viral or bacterial infections or accompany alcohol abuse or radiation therapy. The symptoms usually are mild but can lead to heart failure or arterial blockage if the condition is not treated early.

Pericarditis is an inflammation of the pericardium; myocarditis is an inflammation of the heart muscle. With endocarditis, the endocardium, heart valves, or both may be affected.

Mitral Valve Dysfunction

Although all valves may undergo some change in structure or function, the mitral valve is the one most commonly affected.

Mitral valve prolapse is a deformity in the mitral valves that may be congenital or may be the result of rheumatic fever or some other heart disease. The valve does not close completely, and blood leaks back into the left atrium. Although many people do not notice any symptoms, others may experience chest pain, palpitation, fatigue, or shortness of breath. This condition may be a factor in anxiety-related disorders.

Mitral valve stenosis is scarring that causes the parts of the valve to stick together and gradually narrow. Blood backs up in the left atrium and pressure increases, which causes blood to back up into the pulmonary veins.

Shock

Shock is a condition that results when the blood supply to vital organs becomes inadequate, causing diminished function of these organs. The blood vessels dilate rapidly, and blood pressure drops. The brain receives insufficient oxygen and can be damaged. Treatment usually consists of administration of intravenous (IV) fluids until the person's condition stabilizes and the cause can be determined.

The four main types of shock are hypovolemic shock, which is caused by loss of blood or other bodily fluids; cardiogenic shock, which results from defective heart function, meaning the heart does not pump sufficient blood; septic shock, which is caused by a bacterial infection (e.g., toxic shock syndrome), and anaphylactic shock, which results from an allergy or overreaction of the immune system.

Arrythmia

Arrythmias are conditions that affect the heart rate. The heart's rhythm may be partly or completely irregular, or it may be regular but the frequency may be too slow or too fast. Treatment may include medication, installation of a pacemaker to start the heartbeat, or use of a defibrillator to restore normal heart rhythm.

Bradycardia

In bradycardia the resting heart rate is less than 60 beats per minute. However, healthy athletes often have a heart rate between 50 and 60 beats per minute, which is not necessarily a pathologic condition in these individuals. Primary treatment, when necessary, involves administration of atropine, a parasympathetic blocking agent.

Tachycardia

In most healthy people the heart rate increases in response to extra demands on the heart such as those imposed by exercise. In tachycardia the heartbeat increases suddenly without any increase in physical or emotional stress. Treatment ranges from no intervention to administration of sympathetic blocking agents. Interventions for people with paroxysmal supraventricular tachycardia (PSVT) include interrupting the sympathetic signals by such methods as holding the breath or rinsing the face with cool water. Because stimulation of the vagus nerve slows the heart rate, the Valsalva maneuver (forced expiration against a closed airway) may help. A physician may massage the carotid baroreceptor or inject medication to reduce the heart rate.

Varicose Veins

Varicose veins result when veins stretch so much that the valves cannot close sufficiently. More women than men are affected. The condition may be congenital, it may be the result of remaining in one position (especially standing) too long, or it may be caused by obesity, pregnancy, or menopause. The great and small saphenous veins are affected most often.

Treatment includes rest, elevating the legs, wearing compression stockings, surgical removal of the vein, or sclerotherapy (injection of a saline solution into the vein).

Inflammation of Veins

The term *phlebitis* refers to inflammation of a vein caused by injury, infection, or swelling. These insults diminish blood flow, which may cause thrombic clots to develop, a condition known as *thrombophlebitis*. The superficial leg veins are the most common sites, primarily the saphenous veins. Clots also may form in the deep veins, especially in the legs and abdomen, a condition known as *deep vein thrombosis*. These clots can break off and travel to the lung, resulting in a pulmonary embolism.

NOTE: Care must be taken to avoid any form of soft tissue work over sites of thrombophlebitis or deep vein thrombosis. Systemic contraindications also may be present. Any client with unexplained leg pain must be referred for diagnosis.

Temporal Arteritis

Temporal arteritis is an inflammation of the temporal arteries, which causes pain, swelling, and tenderness.

It can also cause a decrease or loss of vision and, in severe cases, stroke.

Raynaud's Disease/Phenomenon

Both Raynaud's disease, a primary condition, and Raynaud's phenomenon, a secondary condition, are primarily circulatory disorders that affect the blood supply to the fingers and toes, and occasionally to the nose. Temporary spasms in the small arteries reduce or stop blood flow to the area, and the skin turns pale, then blue. Tissue damage or ulceration, or both, may follow. The Raynaud's disorders are aggravated by cold and emotional disturbances and often are seen in individuals with connective tissue disorders or other systemic or emotional disturbances.

Common Disorders of Blood and Body Fluids

Anemia

Anemia is a decrease in the normal number of red blood cells or in the amount of hemoglobin or iron in the blood. The various anemias are classified according to whether the cause is a loss in the number or the usability of red cells, or a decline in the production of red cells.

Sickle cell anemia. Sickle cell anemia is an inherited disease that affects mainly those who live in the Mediterranean region or in Africa or the descendants of these population groups. It is the most prevalent of the hemolytic anemias, disorders that cause premature destruction of red blood cells. In sickle cell anemia, blood cells contain hemoglobin S because of an amino acid substitution on the hemoglobin molecules. These cells collapse and, because of their abnormal shape, do not flow smoothly through the vessels and can block them. When the sickle cells block small blood vessels, multiple infarctions can result throughout the body. Common signs and symptoms are jaundice, diminished growth and development, and pain in the arms, legs and abdomen because of lack of oxygen. Death usually is caused by infection or a cerebrovascular accident. The primary treatment is symptomatic and includes administration of oxygen, blood transfusions, and use of analgesics.

Nutritional anemias. Iron deficiency anemia may result from an inability either to absorb sufficient iron in the small intestine or maintain iron levels in the blood. Pernicious anemia usually is the result of an inability to absorb vitamin B_{12}. Other nutritional anemias may be the result of folic acid deficiency or of lack of intrinsic factor in the stomach.

Bone marrow suppression. Various types of anemia result from bone marrow suppression. Marrow suppression may be seen in individuals undergoing chemotherapy or taking certain antibiotics, as a complication of radiation therapy, or in people with chronic diseases. The red blood cells may be damaged or destroyed, and the body often tries to compensate by producing new ones and sending them out before they mature. In severe cases, transfusions must be given, along with bone marrow transplantation.

Edema

Edema is the accumulation of abnormal amounts of fluid in tissue spaces. It often accompanies congestion, which is an increase in the volume of blood in dilated vessels. Common causes of edema are heart failure, kidney disease, and liver disease. Localized edema is seen with inflammation and lymphatic obstruction.

Polycythemia

Polycythemia is an increase in red cells. This condition may be normal for people living at high altitudes, where oxygen is low, because more red cells are needed to carry what little oxygen is available. The condition also may be directly related to smoking or to taking diuretics. In rare cases actual overproduction is the problem, and it must be slowed to prevent serious complications.

Thrombocytopenia

Thrombocytopenia is a decrease in platelets, which diminishes the blood's ability to clot. Common causes include blood loss, infection, cancer (especially Hodgkin's disease and leukemia), and lupus. The condition may also be a result of radiation therapy or chemotherapy. Idiopathic thrombocytopenic purpura (ITP) is an autoimmune disease in which antiplatelet antibodies are present. Common signs include easy bruising, nosebleeds, bleeding gums, and blood in the urine. Complications include cerebral hemorrhage and bleeding into nerve tissue, causing paralysis.

Hemophilia

Hemophilia is a bleeding disorder in which factor VIII, a vital clotting factor in the blood, is greatly diminished or lacking. In more than 75% of cases the disease is inherited. Although hemophilia is passed on by women, they usually have only minor bleeding problems or no symptoms. Men with hemophilia may have extended episodes of bleeding and may be susceptible to internal bleeding from minor trauma (Activity 11-7).

ACTIVITY 11-7

As soft tissue and movement therapists, we must be able to explain and justify the therapeutic value of the work we do. The following activity will help you develop the skills needed to explain the effectiveness of various modalities to clients and other health care professionals. Use the clinical reasoning model that follows to accomplish this task; an example of that model is provided in the Section Four opener, p. 450. Your focus should be the primary modality or modalities you would apply to the cardiovascular system.

Modality/modalities

1. **What are the facts?**
   a. Which system is involved, and which structures of that system can be reached directly or indirectly?

   b. Which of these structures are most affected by this modality?

   c. Which physiologic functions are affected by this approach?

   d. When the treatment is applied, what changes in function will result in

(1) This system

(2) The whole body

   e. What is considered normal or balanced function?

   f. How are the functions of this system related to the body's homeostasis?

   g. What has worked or has not worked?

   h. Where could you find information that would support the use of this modality as a therapeutic intervention?

ACTIVITY 11-7—cont'd

i. What research is available to support the use of the therapeutic intervention?

a. What do the data suggest?

b. What are the reasons for using the proposed methods?

c. What are the possible interventions?

j. How does the intervention support a healthy state?

d. List at least three applications of this modality that would affect both the structure and function of this system.

k. Under which pathologic or dysfunctional conditions is the intervention most likely to be beneficial?

e. What are other ways to look at the situation?

2. What are the possibilities?

Continued

ACTIVITY 11-7—cont'd

f. What other methods could provide similar benefits?

d. What is likely to happen if the modality is not used?

3. **What is the logical outcome of therapeutic intervention?**
   a. What would be the logical progression of the symptom pattern, contributing factors, and current behaviors?

e. What is likely to happen if the modality is used?

b. What are the benefits and drawbacks of each intervention suggested?
   Benefits:

4. **For the intervention proposed, what would be the impact on the people involved, specifically the client, practitioner, and other professionals working with the client?**
   a. How does each of the people involved (including, besides those named above, the client's family and support system) feel about the possible interventions?

   Drawbacks:

c. What are the costs in terms of time, resources, and finances?

b. Does the practitioner feel qualified to work with the situation and apply the identified modality to the particular situation?

The Lymphatic System

The lymphatic system comprises the spleen, thymus, and tonsils; the lymph channels, ducts, and nodes; and lymph and lymphocytes. It is a one-way system that begins in the tissues and ends when it reaches the blood vessels. It helps the body maintain homeostasis by collecting accumulated tissue fluid and returning it to the blood circulation. The lymphatics play an active part in the body's immune defenses by filtering out and destroying foreign substances and microorganisms. It also plays an active role in digestion by absorbing fats from the small intestine (Figure 11-11).

LYMPH

Lymph is a clear interstitial tissue fluid that bathes the cells. This fluid is released by the cells during normal metabolic processes. Lymph contains less protein and far fewer red and white blood cells than does blood plasma. It restores plasma proteins to the bloodstream and transports absorbed fats from the gastrointestinal system to the bloodstream.

LYMPH VESSELS, NODES, AND ORGANS

Lymph Vessels

The tiny lymph capillaries are open-ended channels located in tissue spaces of the entire body except for the brain, spinal cord, and cornea. They join to form larger lymph vessels that look like veins, but have thinner, more transparent walls. Like veins, they have valves to prevent back flow. The large vessels continue to merge and eventually become two main ducts called the *right lymphatic duct* and the *thoracic duct (left lymphatic duct)*. The right lymphatic duct drains the upper right half of the body and empties into the right subclavian vein. The thoracic duct drains the rest of the body and empties into the left subclavian vein.

Lymph Nodes

Lymph nodes are small, round structures located along the lymph vessels. They are generally clustered at the joints, which assists in pumping lymph through the nodes when the joint moves. The superficial lymph nodes are most numerous in the groin, axillae,

ACTIVITY 11-7—cont'd

c. Does a feeling of cooperation and agreement exist among all those involved, and how would the practitioner recognize this feeling?

Justification

Using the information developed in the clinical reasoning model, present a clear, concise statement of the ways in which the particular soft tissue or movement modality would be beneficial, either in supporting the particular body system in a healthy condition or as part of a treatment plan for a pathologic or dysfunctional condition. Based on the above information, give a brief summary of the effectiveness of the modality for this system.

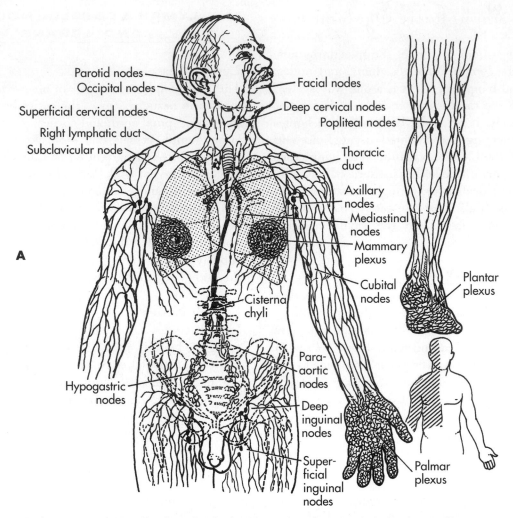

A

Parotid nodes
Occipital nodes
Superficial cervical nodes
Right lymphatic duct
Subclavicular node
Facial nodes
Deep cervical nodes
Popliteal nodes
Thoracic duct
Axillary nodes
Mediastinal nodes
Mammary plexus
Cubital nodes
Plantar plexus
Cisterna chyli
Hypogastric nodes
Para-aortic nodes
Deep inguinal nodes
Superficial inguinal nodes
Palmar plexus

FIGURE 11-11 **A,** Principal lymph vessels and nodes. (**A,** From Birmingham JJ: *Medical terminology: a self-learning text,* ed 2, St Louis, 1990, Mosby; **B,** From Seeley RR, Stephens TD, Tate P: *Anatomy and physiology,* St Louis, 1995, Mosby.)

and neck; most of the deep lymph nodes are found alongside blood vessels of the pelvic, abdominal, and thoracic cavities. All lymph passes through one or more nodes before it enters the bloodstream. As it passes, it can activate immune function. Identification of bacteria or viruses in the lymph stimulates production of lymphocytes in the nodes. The nodes also provide a filtering system that removes waste products and transfers them for detoxification in the other systems of the body. During times of infection, the additional activity in the nodes and the buildup of the microorganisms can make the nodes swollen and painful.

Spleen

The spleen, the largest of the lymphoid organs, is located near the stomach, under the diaphragm. Macrophages in the spleen filter out worn out red blood cells and destroy microorganisms in the blood. The spleen serves as a blood reservoir and can release small amounts of blood into the circulation during times of emergency or blood loss. It functions with the lymphatic system by storing lymphocytes and releasing them as part of the immune response.

Thymus

The thymus gland is a triangular-shaped gland composed of lymphoid tissue. It is located in the upper chest, above the superior vena cava and below the thyroid gland, where it lies against the trachea. This organ is most prominent in the newborn; it begins to atrophy after puberty, becoming only a small lymphoid remnant in the adult. The thymus is important in the development and maturation of certain lymphocytes and in programming them to become T-cells of the immune system.

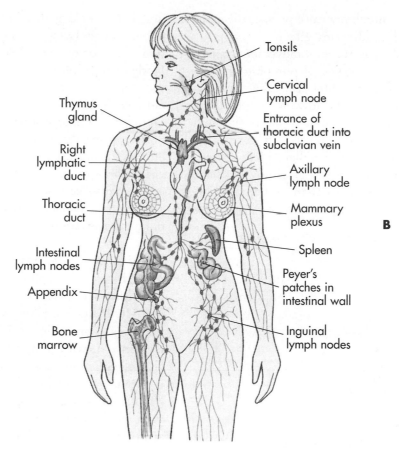

FIGURE 11-11—cont'd **B**, Major organs and vessels of the lymphatic system.

Tonsils

Lymphoid tissues located in the oral cavity and pharynx are known as *tonsils*. There are three different sets, all of which provide defense against microorganisms that enter the mouth and nose. The palatine tonsils on the sides of the throat are the set that we identify as the tonsils, whereas the pharyngeal tonsils are known as the adenoids. The third set, the lingual tonsils, are found at the side of the tongue.

Lymphatic Drainage

Movement of lymph throughout the lymphatic system is known as *lymphatic drainage,* and it begins in the lymph capillaries. Lymph movement out of the interstitial spaces and into the lymph capillaries is assisted by the pressure exerted by compression of skeletal muscles against the vessels during movement, changes in internal pressure during respiration, and the compression of lymph vessels from the pull of the skin and fascia during movement. Major lymph plexuses are found on the soles and the palms, possibly because the rhythmic pumping of walking and grasping facilitate lymphatic flow.

Current research suggests that the lymph vessels themselves may have an intrinsic pumping action. Little pressure is needed to move the fluid. The pressure provided by specially focused soft tissue methods mimics the compressive forces of movement and respiration.

PRACTICAL APPLICATION

One of the extensively documented benefits of massage is stimulation of the lymphatic system. Simple muscle tension puts pressure on the lymph vessels and may block them, interfering with efficient drainage. Soft tissue and movement modalities can normalize muscle tension. As the muscles relax, the lymph vessels open.

Lymphatic massage mechanically stimulates the flow of lymph by tracing the lymphatic routes with very light pressure on the surface of the skin. The focus of the pressure is on the dermis just below the surface layer of skin and the layer of tissue just beneath the skin and above the muscles (the superficial fascia). Little pressure is required to reach the area; too much pressure presses the capillaries closed and nullifies any effect.

Rhythmic, gentle, passive joint movement reproduces the body's normal way of pumping lymph. The client helps the process by deep, slow breathing, which stimulates lymph flow. When possible, the area being massaged should be positioned above the heart so that gravity can assist the lymph flow. Because lymph capillary plexuses are present on the bottoms of the feet, rhythmic compression on the soles also enhances lymph flow (Figure 11-12).

PATHOLOGIC CONDITIONS

Lymphomas

A lymphoma is a tumor of the lymphatic system that is almost always malignant. Most lymphomas are

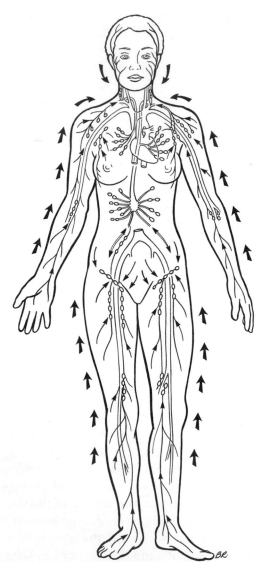

FIGURE 11-12 Direction of strokes for facilitating lymphatic flow. (From Fritz S: *Mosby's fundamentals of therapeutic massage,* St Louis, 1995, Mosby.)

first felt as enlarged, painless lymph nodes or lymphoid tissues. Lymphomas are generally divided into two categories: Hodgkin's disease and non-Hodgkin's lymphoma.

Hodgkin's disease

Hodgkin's disease is a painless swelling of the lymph nodes, primarily in the neck and groin, caused by enlarged, mutated macrophages. Radiation and chemotherapy are the primary treatment methods, and this disease has one of the highest cure rates for any form of cancer. Some individuals may require bone marrow transplantation.

Non-Hodgkin's lymphoma

Non-Hodgkin's lymphoma is any cancer of lymphoid tissue that is not classified as Hodgkin's disease. Most non-Hodgkin's lymphomas involve mutation of lymphocytes, correlation with retroviruses, or T-cell leukemia. As with Hodgkin's disease, the first symptom is swollen lymph nodes, most often in the neck, axilla, or groin. But unlike Hodgkin's disease, non-Hodgkin's lymphoma is a grouping of diverse lymphomas that may manifest very different primary and secondary symptoms. Non-Hodgkin's lymphoma often is subcategorized by grade and area of tumor involvement.

NOTE: Some forms of leukemia may be classified as lymphomas, because they involve lymphocytes. However, not all types of leukemia are disorders of the lymphoid tissues; instead, some could be classified as blood disorders.

Leukemia

Leukemia is cancer of the white blood cells. Not only does the body produce abnormal cells at a faster rate, these cells live longer. Because the cancerous cells do not have the exact same structure as a healthy white blood cell, they function differently. Leukemic cells do not perform the functions of phagocytosis. They build up and invade the body's organs, interfering with organ function. Red cell and platelet production, which takes place in the marrow, may be affected, resulting in anemia or diminished clotting ability. Brain hemorrhage and infection may follow.

Leukemia may progress rapidly (acute leukemia) or slowly (chronic leukemia). In most cases the acute forms show mostly immature blast cells, and the chronic forms show mostly mature types. Two categories of leukemia are described by the white blood cell they affect. Lymphocytic leukemia affects the cells that form into lymphocytes; myelocytic leukemia is a cancer of the cells that develop into granulocytes or monocytes. The myelocytic leukemias may also be identified by the terms *granulocytic* or *monocytic leukemia*.

The common leukemias are as follows:

Acute myelogenous leukemia—Develops rapidly and demonstrates such symptoms as an increase in infections, sores in the mouth, and an increased tendency to bruise or bleed

Chronic myelogenous leukemia—Found in young adults and most often associated with a chromosome abnormality

Acute lymphoblastic (acute lymphocytic) leukemia—Affects children, with a peak incidence at 5 years of age; frequently can be cured with chemotherapy, and complete remissions occur often

Chronic lymphocytic leukemia—Affects older people; the increase in abnormal white cells reduces the number and effectiveness of the normal white blood cells, sometimes resulting in anemia and an increase in infections; often no therapy is required unless symptoms are evident

Infectious Mononucleosis

Infectious mononucleosis is a contagious viral infection more common in teenagers and young adults. It affects the lymphocytes, causing an increase in the number and a change in the structure of some of these cells. The infection is transmitted primarily by kissing, hence its nickname, the "kissing disease." Common signs and symptoms are fever, sore throat, enlarged cervical lymph nodes, a rash, and in some, anemia. Complications include a ruptured spleen, hepatitis, encephalitis, meningitis, and depression. The primary treatment is bed rest for several weeks or months.

Lymphedema

Lymphedema is an increase of tissue fluid caused by inflammation or obstruction caused by scar tissue, parasites, or trauma. For example, after a radical mastectomy, in which axillary lymph channels are removed, arm drainage often is partly blocked and the arm swells. The primary treatment for generalized edema is cautious use of diuretics to remove the fluid. Some forms of massage are effective in the management of moderate lymphedema. External pumping sleeves that rhythmically compress the area are beneficial in chronic cases. A client with any form of edema needs to be referred for diagnosis because edema is symptomatic of many disease processes, particularly cardiovascular disease (Activity 11-8).

ACTIVITY 11-8

As soft tissue and movement therapists, we must be able to explain and justify the therapeutic value of the work we do. The following activity will help you develop the skills needed to explain the effectiveness of various modalities to clients and other health care professionals. Use the clinical reasoning model that follows to accomplish this task; an example of that model is provided in the Section Four opener, p. 450. Your focus should be the primary modality or modalities you would apply to the lymphatic system.

Modality/modalities

1. What are the facts?
   a. Which system is involved, and which structures of that system can be reached directly or indirectly?

b. Which of these structures are most affected by this modality?

c. Which physiologic functions are affected by this approach?

Continued

ACTIVITY 11-8—cont'd

d. When the treatment is applied, what changes in function will result in
   (1) This system

   (2) The whole body

e. What is considered normal or balanced function?

f. How are the functions of this system related to the body's homeostasis?

g. What has worked or has not worked?

h. Where could you find information that would support the use of this modality as a therapeutic intervention?

i. What research is available to support the use of the therapeutic intervention?

j. How does the intervention support a healthy state?

k. Under which pathologic or dysfunctional conditions is the intervention most likely to be beneficial?

ACTIVITY 11-8—cont'd

2. What are the possibilities?

a. What do the data suggest?

b. What are the reasons for using the proposed methods?

c. What are the possible interventions?

d. List at least three applications of this modality that would affect both the structure and function of this system.

e. What are other ways to look at the situation?

f. What other methods could provide similar benefits?

3. What is the logical outcome of therapeutic intervention?
   a. What would be the logical progression of the symptom pattern, contributing factors, and current behaviors?

   b. What are the benefits and drawbacks of each intervention suggested?
   Benefits:

   Drawbacks:

Continued

ACTIVITY 11-8—cont'd

c. What are the costs in terms of time, resources, and finances?

d. What is likely to happen if the modality is not used?

e. What is likely to happen if the modality is used?

4. **For the intervention proposed, what would be the impact on the people involved, specifically the client, practitioner, and other professionals working with the client?**
   a. How does each of the people involved (including, besides those named above, the client's family and support system) feel about the possible interventions?

b. Does the practitioner feel qualified to work with the situation and apply the identified modality to the particular situation?

c. Does a feeling of cooperation and agreement exist among all those involved, and how would the practitioner recognize this feeling?

Justification

Using the information developed in the clinical reasoning model, present a clear, concise statement of the ways in which the particular soft tissue or movement modality would be beneficial, either in supporting the particular body system in a healthy condition or as part of a treatment plan for a pathologic or dysfunctional condition. Based on the above information, give a brief summary of the effectiveness of the modality for this system.

The Immune System

Immunity is a complex response that networks all of the systems in our bodies to eliminate any pathogen, foreign substance, or toxic material that can be damaging to the body. The immune system is not a specific structural organ system; rather, it is a functional system (Figure 11-13). It responds in one of two ways by drawing on the structures and processes of each of the organs, tissues, and cells and the chemicals produced in them. In a nonspecific immune response, the body responds exactly the same way to all substances that are not identified as part of the body. Nonspecific response is programmed genetically in the human body. Specific immunity involves very specific responses to each identified foreign substance and calls on special memory cells to help if that invader reappears. Specific immunity can be acquired in one of two ways: through natural immunity, which is the result of natural exposure, or through artificial immunity, in which a substance is introduced into the body to stimulate the immune response.

The key to immunity is the body's ability to recognize self and nonself. The recognition of self begins during fetal development and continues throughout life. In many psychologic approaches and spiritual practices, this is also a core issue—*who am I?* When this recognition of self breaks down, the body attacks itself or fails to defend against antigens. Life tends to do the same thing when our sense of mental or spiritual self breaks down. Psychologic approaches provide structure, methodology, and professional support for the rediscovery of the self. Spiritual healing practices often provide community, ritual, and disciplines for self-understanding and self-awareness. It makes sense that knowing the self supports health.

The body must be able to identify which substances are capable of causing a threat before any type of response can be initiated. An antigen is any substance that causes the body to produce antibodies. Antigens usually are proteins identified as harmful or potentially dangerous to the body. Foreign antigens are those that come from outside the body, and self-antigens are those that come from within. An antibody is a specific protein produced to destroy or suppress antigens. Microorganisms are minute life forms that may be damaging to the body or may interfere with its function. Pathogens are microorganisms capable of producing disease.

When the immune system is operating effectively, it intelligently protects the body from most infectious microorganisms and any of the body's own cells that have turned against it, that is, cells that have overreacted in their response or that develop and grow at an unhealthy rate or by mutating (cancer). The immune system does this both directly, by cell attack, and indirectly, by releasing mobilizing chemicals and protective antibody molecules. The resulting resistance to disease is called *immunity.*

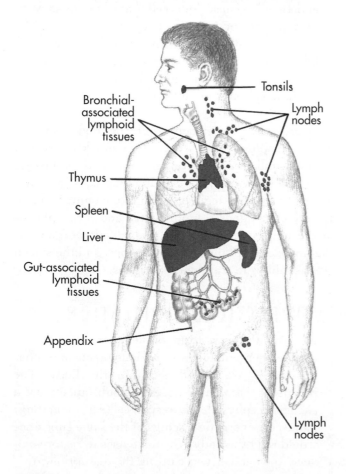

FIGURE 11-13 Organization of the immune system. Cellular constituents of the immune system are derived from bone marrow stem cells. When they maturate, these cells are released into the peripheral blood flow and subsequently populate organized tissues of the lymphoreticular system. (From Thompson JM et al: *Mosby's clinical nursing,* ed 4, St Louis, 1997, Mosby.)

NONSPECIFIC DEFENSES

Nonspecific immunity can involve actions such as sneezing or coughing to remove microorganisms from the respiratory tract. Keeping the structure of the skin intact prevents potentially damaging substances from entering the body. No matter what the substance is, the body responds in the same manner, with the same chemicals and cells mediating the actions. This general response is both a preventive measure and a first response in immune function.

Cellular response is the action of the blood cells, primarily white blood cells, that deals with pathogens. Cells such as macrophages and neutrophils begin to phagocytize, or surround and destroy, pathogens. Basophils and mast cells (from connective tissue) release chemicals that initiate inflammation. Eosinophils release chemicals that slow or stop the inflammatory response—the body's way of maintaining homeostasis.

Chemical response includes not only the chemicals released by the above-mentioned cells, but also substances found throughout the body. Our skin and mucous membranes maintain a certain degree of acidity that prevents entry of foreign pathogens. Mucus is sticky and secretes enzymes that destroy these microorganisms, and saliva, tears, and urine actually wash them out of the body. *Complements* are proteins found in blood that combine to create substances that phagocytize bacteria. *Interferon* is a protein produced by cells infected by viruses. Interferon forms antiviral proteins to help protect uninfected cells.

Inflammatory response is a sequence of events involving chemical and cellular activation that destroys pathogens and aids in the repair of tissues. For example, when a tissue is damaged, chemicals are released by basophils and mast cells. These chemicals increase the blood flow, which brings neutrophils and macrophages to the area. The phagocytic white cells, mainly macrophages, enter the tissues to destroy any bacteria. At the same time, the chemical response changes the blood vessel walls' permeability, and fibrin also can enter the tissues to repair the damage. This process continues until the damage has been repaired and all bacteria have been removed.

Sanitary practices such as hand washing support immunity by preventing exposure to pathogens.

SPECIFIC IMMUNITY

Specific immunity is the ability to recognize certain antigens and destroy them.

Lymphocytes are the cells of specific immunity, because they can recognize and destroy specific molecules and put them in memory. Memory cells are the reason that, after we have had a disease such as measles, the lymphocyte pattern set up with the first infection can respond to a second exposure and prevent reinfection. Lymphocytes develop in the following three ways:

- T-cells begin in the bone marrow and grow in the thymus. They are able to recognize antigens and respond by releasing inflammatory and toxic materials. Specialized T-cells also regulate immune responses. T4 cells release molecules that amplify the response, and T8 cells suppress the body's response. Some T-cells develop into memory cells and handle secondary response on reexposure to antigens that already have produced a primary response.
- B-cells grow and develop in the bone marrow. B-cells contain immunoglobulin, an antibody that responds to specific antigens. Some B-cells modify and become antigen nonspecific, which provides them with a greater ability to respond to bacterial and viral pathogens. Some B-cells, like T-cells, become memory cells and handle reexposure to antigens.
- A few lymphocytes do not develop the same structural or functional characteristics as the T-cells and B-cells. These "null cells" are known as *natural killer cells*, or *NK cells*. They also develop in the bone marrow and, when mature, can attack and kill tumor cells and virus-infected cells during their initial developmental stage before the immune system is activated.

Because of the structure of the body, specific defense responses can develop very quickly. Because lymph capillaries pick up proteins and pathogens from nearly all body tissues, immune cells in lymph nodes are in a strategic position to encounter a large variety of antigens. Lymphocytes and macrophages in the tonsils act primarily against microorganisms that invade the oral and nasal cavities, and the spleen acts as a filter to trap blood antigens.

PRACTICAL APPLICATION

Homeopathy is a form of health care in which minute energetic forms of various plants and other substances are introduced into the body. The premise is that if large doses of a substance cause a particular physiologic response (e.g., vomiting) minuscule energetic tracings of the same substance would rally the body's own defenses to restore balance to whatever was causing the disruption.

The concept of vaccination is similar to and may have been based on the concept of homeopathy. The difference is the strength of the product. Vaccines are weakened or killed forms of the actual pathogen, whereas homeopathic substances are "energetic forms" of the actual substance. Live vaccines can cause disease, as is seen by the symptoms babies sometimes develop when they receive their immunizations. However, both systems seek to activate and teach the body to protect and heal itself.

IMMUNE SYSTEM DYSFUNCTION

The organizational structure and responses of the immune system can break down. The imbalances that occur are immune deficiencies, hypersensitivity, and autoimmune diseases.

Immune deficiency is a condition in which the body is unable to mount the proper immune response to a pathogen. An analogy would be an office that has too much work and not enough workers to get the job done. The work piles up, the workers get farther and farther behind, and eventually the office system breaks down. Some immune deficiencies are present at birth. These congenital problems affect the development of lymphocytes and result in severe inability to respond to disease. Other immune deficiencies arise later in life such as acquired immunodeficiency syndrome (AIDS). Chronic stress also suppresses the immune system. Stress can be caused by physical mechanisms (e.g., chronic pain), other forms of chronic disease, or unresolved emotional or spiritual disturbances. When immunosuppressed, the body is more likely to be susceptible to a variety of bacterial, viral, and toxic pathogenic activity.

The immune system also can become overactive, a condition called hypersensitivity or allergy. Few people die from an allergy, but life can be made miserable. Allergy can be understood by equating the immune system's response to creating mountains out of molehills. Anaphylactic shock is the exception, and although rare, it is life-threatening. Anaphylactic shock is a severe, usually immediate reaction to a substance that causes respiratory distress, anxiety, and weakness. In extreme cases, it also can involve arrhythmia and can result in death if not treated immediately.

Autoimmune diseases occur when the body cannot distinguish self from nonself; self-antigens are treated as foreign antigens. When the recognition of self breaks down, the immune cells begin to attack the self. Some of the autoimmune diseases are multiple sclerosis, Graves' disease, rheumatoid arthritis, and juvenile diabetes.

BODY/MIND CONNECTION

The sheer power of the mind to affect the body as a whole and the general state of health is amazing. Scientists have confirmed that a witch doctor can cause death simply by telling those who believe in his powers that they are going to die. On the other hand, it has been confirmed that we can think ourselves well.

Studies of neuroimmunomodulation have discovered that left-handed people are more likely to suffer immune system disorders than are right-handed people. These studies indicate that the left hemisphere most directly controls the immune cells through the T-cell response, but that the right hemisphere enhances and modulates the response. Other investigations have shown that although the nervous and immune systems have different chemical languages, they seem to share a few of the more important chemical signals such as the opiate neuropeptides. Like neurons, many cells involved with the immune response have receptors for the opiate neuropeptides, which have long been known to influence mood and behavior. Many scientists are convinced that macrophages have receptors for these neuropeptides, which are released by pain-sensing neurons and lymphocytes. Why these cells, which are active in immunity, should respond or react to chemicals used by the nervous system to deal with pain is not fully understood. It is thought that this process may be an important link in the communication between the brain and body.

High levels of natural opiates or heroin suppress NK cell activity. During times of stress and severe depression, T-cells are depressed, which weakens the immune system and increases our susceptibly to physical illness. Hormones such as corticosteroids and epinephrine also provide chemical links between the two systems.

Immune function gradually declines as we age. Scientists do not understand this process, but studies in longevity have found a link between living vitally in the advanced years and a balanced life that includes physical activity, a simple diet, a moderate lifestyle, regular sleep and wake cycles, loving relationships, a sense of purpose or reason for being, and spiritual strength. These same factors have been shown to support the immune response and the regeneration and healing capacities of the body.

Immunity is a body-wide process. The integumentary system, especially the keratinized epithelial cells, provide a mechanical barrier, and these same cells act as an alarm system, triggering responses when the integument is breached. The skeletal system provides the bone marrow as the developmental home for the lymphocytes and macrophages. Heat from the muscle system actively initiates feverlike effects. The nervous and endocrine systems directly interact, linking the mind/body effects of the immune response through a shared chemical language. The cardiovascular system provides the travel network, lymphatic system, and filtering system. The respiratory system provides oxygen needed by immune cells, and the digestive system nourishes the immune cells and secretes acids hostile to pathogens. The urinary system eliminates waste and maintains the protective acid balance. The reproductive system works with the endocrine system to influence the process through hormone function.

The immune system is truly the body's best example of teamwork or a multidisciplinary approach, and there is a lesson to be learned here. When any one of us does not do our job, others are overtasked; in the body, this is immune deficiency. When we overreact, our hypersensitivities are unproductive and we feel miserable, wasting energy that could be better used in other ways. When we are unaware of our self (autoimmunity), not only do we attack ourselves, we also cannot combine efforts to support others. Again, energy for the common good is wasted, and a lack of self-recognition destroys us, little by little. The amazing multidimensional links of the immune system support the idea that we truly are what we think, eat, do, hate, love, breathe, support, and become. Living well in our own bodies and sharing space with all forms of life on this planet reflects the ancient spiritual wisdom of living in a balanced way with cooperation and respect.

DISEASE PREVENTION AND CONTROL

The key to preventing many diseases caused by pathogenic organisms is to prevent them from entering the body. This sounds simple enough but often is very difficult to accomplish. Following is a partial list of the ways in which pathogens can spread:

1. Environmental contact—Many pathogens are found in the environment in food, water, and soil and on various surfaces. Disease caused by environmental pathogens often can be prevented by avoiding contact with certain materials and by observing safe sanitation practices.
2. Opportunistic invasion—Nearly everyone has some potentially pathogenic organisms on their skin and mucous membranes. However, these organisms do not cause disease until they have the opportunity. Preventing opportunistic infection involves avoiding conditions that could promote infections. Changes in the pH (acidity), moisture, temperature, or other characteristics of the skin and mucous membranes often promote opportunistic infections. Cleaning and aseptic treatment of wounds helps prevent these infections.
3. Person-to-person contact—Small pathogens often can be carried in the air from one person to another. Direct contact with an infected person or with contaminated materials handled by the infected person is a common mode of transmission. The rhinovirus that causes the common cold is often transmitted in these ways. Some viruses such as those that cause hepatitis B are transmitted when infected blood, semen, or other bodily fluids enter a person's bloodstream.

Aseptic technique is the killing or disabling of pathogens on surfaces before they can spread to other people. Some common aseptic techniques are listed in Table 11-1.

Hand Washing

Proper hand washing is the single biggest deterrent to the spread of disease. Hands must be washed before and after each client contact, after blowing the nose or coughing into the hands, and after using the toilet. Hands and forearms need to be washed in hot,

TABLE 11-1 COMMON ASEPTIC TECHNIQUES

METHOD	ACTION	EXAMPLE
Sterilization	Destroys all living organisms	Pressurized steam bath, extreme temperature, radiation
Disinfection	Destroys most or all pathogens on inanimate objects but not necessarily all harmless microbes	Chemicals such as iodine, chlorine, alcohol, and soap
Isolation	Separates possibly infectious individuals or materials from uninfected people	Quarantine of affected patients; use of protective apparel while giving treatments; sanitary transport, storage, and disposal of bodily fluids and body tissues, as well as other potentially infectious materials

running water to wash away the infectious organisms. Soap or another hand washing product must be used. A clean towel must be used to dry the hands and forearms. Faucets and door handles are contaminated and should not be touched after washing the hands. The towel should be used to turn off the water and open the door.

Universal Precautions

Universal Precautions are guidelines for preventing the spread of bacterial and viral infections. They were first issued in 1987 by the Centers for Disease Control and Prevention (CDC). Health care professionals must update their information on the Universal Precautions at least yearly (updated specifications are available from the CDC).

Normal germs can be very dangerous to any immune-suppressed (i.e., sick) individual. Universal Precautions are intended to protect both the client and the practitioner from pathogens. The following is a short version of the Universal Precautions:

- Latex gloves should be worn for all cleanup procedures.
- Bleach is the cleaning agent research laboratories prefer. A mixture of 1 part bleach to 9 parts water is made, a 10% bleach solution. If blood or bodily secretions are plentiful, a stronger mixture should be used. The mixture should be made fresh each day, and any leftover solution should be disposed of at the end of the day.

Cleanup procedures for spills

Any person touching a spill of blood or other bodily substances (e.g., vomit, urine, feces) should wear latex gloves. To clean up such spills, use a 10% bleach solution (described above). Surround the spill with bleach solution and work inward with the mop or cloth, working slowly and carefully to avoid splashes or aerosols (airborne particles). A stronger bleach solution should be used if excessive amounts of blood or bodily substances are present. When the cleanup is finished, the mop head or cloth should be soaked in 10% bleach solution. Agitate (stir up) the mop head carefully to ensure that all mop surfaces are exposed to the cleaning fluid. Roll all linens away from you and bag separately from all other soiled linens. Use a double plastic bag and mark the bag *Contaminated with Body Fluids*. Wash the treatment table with a strong disinfectant solution and let it air dry.

Cleanup procedures for skin contamination

If your skin comes in contact with a contaminated substance, immediately wash the area of skin with soap and water and an antiviral agent (e.g., 10% bleach solution).

If an open wound is exposed to a contaminated substance, the wound should be flushed immediately with large amounts of hydrogen peroxide or a 10% bleach solution. *Do not use hydrogen peroxide on mucous membrane surfaces.* Also, do not use hydrogen peroxide in the mouth, eyes, vagina, anus, or urethra.

PATHOLOGIC CONDITIONS

INDICATIONS CONTRAINDICATIONS

For Soft Tissue and Movement Therapies

Soft tissue and movement approaches support immune function by supporting balanced homeostatic functions. No specific methods are used for the immune system, yet any behavior that supports wellness, including regular bodywork, supports immunity. Any modality that normalizes autonomic nervous system functions supports immunity. Certain herbs, known as adaptogens, are noted for their support of the immune system. The most common are ginseng, enchinacea, garlic, and licorice.

Any activity, including soft tissue or movement modalities, that causes the body to adapt puts stress on the system. If the client is basically healthy, she will be able to adapt without overstressing the body. However, if a client is immune suppressed, the reserves to adapt are already at the breakdown point. The intensity and duration of bodywork methods must be gauged against the body's ability to adapt, so that the stress introduced supports a return to balance and is not "the straw that breaks the camel's back." The premise of "less is more" is a wise approach for individuals with immune dysfunction.

HIV Infection and AIDS

Acquired immunodeficiency syndrome (AIDS) is caused by a dysfunction in the body's immune system. The diseases of the AIDS syndrome are caused by germs encountered in everyday life. In fact, some of these germs live permanently in small numbers inside the human body. When the immune system weakens, these germs have the opportunity to multiply freely; thus the diseases these germs cause are called *opportunistic diseases*.

The human immunodeficiency virus (HIV), which may be responsible for AIDS, is a ribonucleic acid (RNA) virus. In most RNA viruses the viral RNA directly hijacks the host cell. However, HIV is different. After it is injected into the host cell, HIV's RNA strand "writes" dual strands of viral DNA (the opposite of human cells). This backward writing is called *reverse transcription*. The newly written DNA strands then go on to hijack the cell and oversee the production of new RNA replicas. Reverse-writing viruses such as HIV are called *retroviruses*.

As a group, retroviruses can live in their hosts for a long time without causing any sign of illness. In most animals, retrovirus infections last for life. Retroviruses are not very tough; they die when exposed to heat, are killed by many common disinfectants, and usually do not survive if the tissue or blood they are in dries up. However, retroviruses have a high rate of mutation and as a result tend to evolve very quickly into new strains or varieties. HIV seems to share this and other traits with other known retroviruses.

HIV likes to replicate (live) in the lymphocytes, or T-cells. The virus's favorite target is the T4 cell. The T4 cell, also called the helper/inducer T-cell, performs a vital job in the immune system. It finds germ invaders by circulating through the bloodstream and bumping into them. On recognizing the invading germ, the T4 cell releases a chemical alarm that triggers other parts of the immune system into action.

HIV infection of the T4 cells creates a defect in the body's immune system, which may eventually cause AIDS. After HIV hijacks a T-cell, the lymphocyte stops functioning normally, although this change is not immediately apparent. Then . . . nothing happens. Evidently, very little or no viral replication takes place for an indefinite period. The HIV takeover is a quiet event.

When the T4 cell does become active, rather than functioning normally, it manufactures viral RNA strands. An infected T4 cell no longer detects invaders and triggers alarms. Eventually, the infected T4 cells begin to die, gradually reducing the T4 cell alarm network and allowing opportunistic diseases to enter and grow within the body.

Mechanics of transmission

HIV must travel from the inside of one person to the inside of another person, arriving with its RNA strands intact. Then the virus, or its intact RNA strands, must get into the new host's bloodstream and find and enter a T-cell. Once inside a host cell, HIV can prepare for replication. After replication, replica viruses infect other host cells, probably attaching to new host cells when the infected host cell collides with other cells in the bloodstream.

Viruses generally are not able to enter the body through intact skin. Therefore, viruses must enter the body through an open wound or one of a number of possible body openings. Most of these body openings contain mucous membranes, which protect most openings and passages in the human body. These membranes secrete mucus, which contains germicidal chemicals and keeps the surrounding tissues moist. Mucous membranes are found in the mouth, inside the eyelids, in the nose and air passages leading to the lungs, in the stomach, along the digestive tract, in the vagina, in the anus, and inside the "eye" of the penis. Many viruses, if placed on the surface of a mucous membrane, can travel through the membrane and enter the tiny blood vessels inside.

The mucous membranes of the eyes and mouth are often doorways into our bodies for highly infectious viruses such as the influenza virus. You can catch the influenza virus from another person in the following manner: The person coughs into his hand, you shake hands soon afterward, and then your virus-carrying hand touches your eye or mouth.

"The flu" is highly infectious because the influenza virus lives in the lungs, throat, and sinuses. For this reason the sputum of an infected person has a high concentration of viral organisms. (Sputum is the substance expelled by coughing or by clearing the throat. Concentration is the number of viral organisms per unit of volume). Coughing forces many viruses out of the lungs and into the air or onto the sick person's hand or handkerchief. The influenza virus easily crosses the mucous membrane.

The danger with HIV is very different. With HIV, the major infection sites are the bloodstream and central nervous system. Although HIV-carrying macrophages (roving white blood cells that engulf invaders but are susceptible to HIV infection) are found in the connective tissues of the lungs and in oral and mucous membranes, the number of viral organisms present does not seem great. Thus HIV is present in low concentrations, if at all, in saliva and sputum. Therefore coughing should not expel a large quantity of HIV, if any. Apparently, HIV cannot cross the mucous membrane very easily, and large concentrations of HIV probably are necessary.

HIV can be found in any bodily fluid or substance that contains lymphocytes. Substances that contain lymphocytes include blood, semen, vaginal and cervical secretions, mother's milk, saliva, tears, urine, and feces.

The presence of HIV in a substance does not necessarily mean that the substance is capable of transmitting HIV infection. All of these substances are capable, in theory, of transmitting disease, but in reality the most dangerous substances seem to be blood, semen, cervical and vaginal secretions, and perhaps feces. Despite much looking, no one has been able to find a clear-cut case of saliva causing transmission, although kissing theoretically could.

The concentration of HIV in these substances is very important when it comes to infection. The higher the concentration of viral organisms in a substance, the more likely it is that HIV can be transmitted by that substance. Below a certain concentration of organisms, the substance cannot effectively transmit HIV infection.

Hepatitis

Hepatitis is an inflammatory process and an infection of the liver caused by a virus. Hepatitis A, the less serious form, usually is transmitted by fecal contamination of food and water. It does not become chronic, and once infected, a person becomes immune to future hepatitis A infections.

Hepatitis B (HBV) is transmitted through routes similar to those for HIV. HBV may be acute or chronic. The acute symptoms are similar to those of hepatitis A, but hepatitis B is much more severe in both the chronic and acute stages. As liver cells die, liver function is impaired, and death can result.

Two types of vaccines are available for preventing hepatitis B. It is estimated that more than 1 million people in the United States are carriers of the hepatitis B virus. Hepatitis B is 100 times more contagious than HIV.

Hepatitis C accounts for 85% of the new cases of hepatitis each year. It is transmitted mostly by blood transfusions or when IV drug users share needles. This disease usually becomes chronic.

Hepatitis D infects only those who have hepatitis B, and the symptoms are more severe than other forms of hepatitis. Vaccines do not appear to be effective for hepatitis D.

Hepatitis E is transmitted through food and water contaminated with feces. It usually is a self-limited type of hepatitis that may occur after natural disasters.

The treatment for all forms of hepatitis is rest and a high-protein diet. Observance of Universal Precautions can prevent the spread of hepatitis. Obviously, all behaviors that are means of transmission for HIV and HBV must be avoided (Activity 11-9).

ACTIVITY 11-9

As soft tissue and movement therapists, we must be able to explain and justify the therapeutic value of the work we do. The following activity will help you develop the skills needed to explain the effectiveness of various modalities to clients and other health care professionals. Use the clinical reasoning model that follows to accomplish this task; an example of that model is provided in the Section Four opener, p. 450. Your focus should be the primary modality or modalities you would apply to the immune system.

Modality/modalities

1. **What are the facts?**
   a. Which system is involved, and which structures of that system can be reached directly or indirectly?

b. Which of these structures are most affected by this modality?

c. Which physiologic functions are affected by this approach?

Continued

ACTIVITY 11-9—cont'd

d. When the treatment is applied, what changes in function will result in
   (1) This system

   (2) The whole body

e. What is considered normal or balanced function?

f. How are the functions of this system related to the body's homeostasis?

g. What has worked or has not worked?

h. Where could you find information that would support the use of this modality as a therapeutic intervention?

i. What research is available to support the use of the therapeutic intervention?

j. How does the intervention support a healthy state?

k. Under which pathologic or dysfunctional conditions is the intervention most likely to be beneficial?

ACTIVITY 11-9—cont'd

2. What are the possibilities?

a. What do the data suggest?

b. What are the reasons for using the proposed methods?

c. What are the possible interventions?

d. List at least three applications of this modality that would affect both the structure and function of this system.

e. What are other ways to look at the situation?

f. What other methods could provide similar benefits?

3. What is the logical outcome of therapeutic intervention?
   a. What would be the logical progression of the symptom pattern, contributing factors, and current behaviors?

   b. What are the benefits and drawbacks of each intervention suggested?
   Benefits:

   Drawbacks:

Continued

c. What are the costs in terms of time, resources, and finances?

b. Does the practitioner feel qualified to work with the situation and apply the identified modality to the particular situation?

d. What is likely to happen if the modality is not used?

c. Does a feeling of cooperation and agreement exist among all those involved, and how would the practitioner recognize this feeling?

e. What is likely to happen if the modality is used?

Justification

Using the information developed in the clinical reasoning model, present a clear, concise statement of the ways in which the particular soft tissue or movement modality would be beneficial, either in supporting the particular body system in a healthy condition or as part of a treatment plan for a pathologic or dysfunctional condition. Based on the above information, give a brief summary of the effectiveness of the modality for this system.

4. **For the intervention proposed, what would be the impact on the people involved, specifically the client, practitioner, and other professionals working with the client?**
   a. How does each of the people involved (including, besides those named above, the client's family and support system) feel about the possible interventions?

Summary

This chapter began with a discussion of touch. This important topic certainly could be explored in more depth, because soft tissue and movement therapies depend on touch, not only for therapeutic benefit but also for the compassionate, nurturing connection between practitioner and client.

Basic anatomy, physiology, and pathologic conditions of the integumentary, cardiovascular, lymphatic, and immune systems were presented.

The justification exercises began the process of explaining and validating bodywork. Being able to justify the effectiveness of soft tissue and movement modalities in supporting health maintenance or as part of a multidisciplinary approach for pathologic conditions will become increasingly important as these methods are used by more people. Being able to explain the benefits of the modalities and the skills each professional has to offer, based on a solid foundation of anatomy and physiology, adds to professional development and supports the use of these important treatments.

WORKBOOK SECTION

1. What are some of the major functions of the integumentary system?

_____

_____

_____

_____

2. List the appendages of the skin.

_____

_____

3. What are the two main concerns with integumentary pathologic conditions?

_____

_____

4. List and describe the three types of arteries and give an example of each type.

_____

_____

_____

_____

_____

_____

_____

_____

5. List the four sets of heart valves and explain what each set does.

_____

_____

_____

_____

_____

_____

_____

_____

6. Why is venous blood return important? List factors that can affect it.

_____

_____

_____

_____

_____

_____

_____

_____

_____

7. What are the five groups of white blood cells?

_____

_____

_____

8. How is blood supplied to the heart? What happens if this supply is interrupted?

_____

_____

_____

_____

_____

_____

9. What are the normal and abnormal heart sounds, and how are they produced?

_____

_____

_____

_____

_____

_____

_____

_____

10. What are the normal ranges for blood pressure based on size and what are the terms used for high blood pressure and low blood pressure?

_____

_____

_____

_____

_____

11. What are the two main lymphatic ducts? How are they formed and into what do they empty?

_____

_____

_____

_____

_____

_____

12. What are lymph nodes and where are they found?

_____

_____

_____

_____

_____

13. What is the name of the body's defense system and in what way does it respond to threats?

_____

_____

_____

_____

_____

_____

_____

14. How is nonspecific immunity provided?

_____

_____

_____

_____

_____

FILL IN THE BLANK

The _____ (1) is made up of the skin and its appendages: hair, sebaceous glands, sweat glands, nails, and breasts.

The _____ (2) is the outer layer of skin; it consists of sublayers called *strata*. There are four or five layers of strata, depending on the location on the body.

The _____ (3), the inner layer of skin, is much thicker than the epidermis. It is composed of dense connective tissue that contains collagen and elastin fibers. The various appendages of the skin originate in the dermis and push upward through the epidermis. Blood vessels and nerves are present in the dermis but not in the epidermis. Subcutaneous tissue, which is located below the epidermis, is also called _____ _____ (4). It consists of loose connective tissue and contains fat (adipose) tissue.

The _____ _____ (5) is a transport system composed of the heart, blood vessels, and blood. It functions to bring nutrients to the tissues and remove waste products from them.

One part of the cardiovascular system, the _____ (6), is a hollow, muscular pump about the size of a closed fist. It is located in the _____ (7), the space between the lungs. The _____ (8) is a sac that surrounds the heart. It secretes a lubricating fluid that prevents friction caused by the movement of the heart.

The two small, thin-walled upper chambers of the heart are the _____ _____ (9), known separately as the right atrium and left atrium. They are separated by the thin interatrial septum. The two large lower chambers are the left and right _____ (10). Their thick walls are separated by the interventricular septum.

_____ _____ (11) is the amount of blood pumped by the left ventricle in 1 minute. The average output is 5 to 6 L of blood under normal conditions.

The _____ _____ (12) is the sequence of events in one heartbeat. It consists of diastole and systole. The average person has 60 to 70 cardiac cycles per minute. The number of cardiac cycles in 1 minute is known as the _____ _____ (13).

The vascular system is the other part of the cardiovascular system. It consists of blood vessels that carry blood from the heart to the lungs and body tissues and back to the heart in a continuous cycle. Blood vessels that transport blood from the heart are called _____(14); these branch off into smaller and smaller arteries. The smallest of the arteries are called the _____(15).

_____ (16) are the tiny blood vessels located between the arterioles and the veins. The function of the _____ (17) is to collect blood from the capillaries and transport the blood back to the heart. The smallest of the veins are the _____ (18). The veins get larger as they get closer to the heart. The largest veins return blood to the right atrium of the heart.

The amount of pressure exerted by the blood on the walls of the blood vessels is called _____ _____ (19). The maximal pressure is called _____ _____(20); this occurs when the ventricles are contracted. _____ _____ (21) occurs when the ventricles relax. Blood pressure is measured with a _____ (22), a cloth-covered rubber bag that is wrapped around the arm over the brachial artery. Blood pressure is highest during contraction of the heart (systole), which produces the systolic blood pressure. It is lowest when the heart is relaxing (diastole), which gives the diastolic pressure.

_____ (23), the thick, red fluid in our bodies, is a form of connective tissue. It transports nutrients to the individual cells and removes waste products.

The cellular substances in blood are red blood cells, white blood cells, and platelets. Blood cells float in a thick, straw-colored fluid called _____ (24). Red blood cells, also called _____(25), or red blood corpuscles, constitute more than 90% of the formed elements in blood. Their function is to transport oxygen to the cells and carbon dioxide away from the cells. White blood cells are also called _____ (26), or white blood corpuscles. Their white color is due to a lack of hemoglobin.

Thrombocytes, also called _____ (27), are the smallest cellular elements of the blood. They are very important in the blood-clotting process and are manufactured in the bone marrow. A special protein, called _____ (28), is formed to seal damaged blood vessels by trapping red blood cells, platelets, and fluid to form a clot. This protein also anchors the clot in place.

The term _____ (29) means *hardening of the arteries* and refers to arteries that have become brittle and have lost their elasticity. Although the condition has several causes, the most common and important is _____(30), the deposit of fatty plaques in medium and large arteries.

The _____ _____ (31) collects accumulated tissue fluids from the entire body and returns them to the blood circulation. This is a one-way system that begins in the tissues and ends in the blood vessels. The lymphatics work as an active part of our immunity by filtering and destroying foreign substances and microorganisms. They also play an active role in digestion by absorbing fats from the small intestine.

_____ (32) is a clear interstitial tissue fluid that bathes the cells. The tiny _____ (33) are open-ended channels found in the tissue spaces of the entire body except for the brain, spinal cord, and cornea. They join to form larger lymph vessels that look like veins, but have thinner, more transparent walls. Like veins, they have valves to prevent backflow.

_____ (34) is a complex response that networks all of the systems in the body to eliminate any pathogen, foreign substance, or toxic material that can be damaging to the body. The immune system is not a specific structural organ system, but rather a functional system.

_____ (35) are the cells of specific immunity because they recognize and destroy specific molecules and have the ability to "remember" that particular pathogen.

EXERCISE: SKIN STRUCTURE

In the cross section of the skin's structure pictured below, write the name of each component next to the corresponding letter. Color each part after you label it.

Answer Key

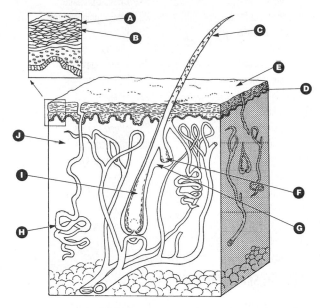

(From Williams RW: *Basic healthcare terminology,* St Louis, 1995, Mosby.)

EXERCISE: STRUCTURES OF THE HEART

In the illustration of the structures of the heart pictured below, write the name of each structure next to the corresponding letter. Color each part after you label it.

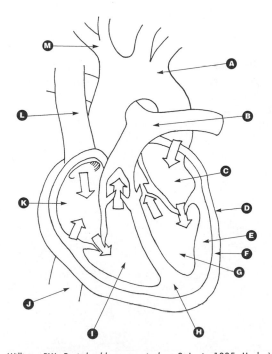

(From Williams RW: *Basic healthcare terminology,* St Louis, 1995, Mosby.)

1. The integumentary system protects the internal organs and structures from trauma, sun exposure, chemicals, and water loss; assists the immune function by preventing the entry of bacteria and viruses; synthesizes vitamin D when exposed to the ultraviolet rays of the sun; detects the stimuli sensed as touch, temperature, pain, and pressure; regulates body temperature; excretes sweat and salts; and secretes sebum.

2. Hair, sebaceous glands, sweat glands (apocrine and eccrine), nails, and breasts (mammary glands)

3. The first concern is loss of the skin's protection of internal structures. The second concern is loss of the skin's ability to prevent the pathogens of contagious disease from entering the body.

4. Elastic arteries—The large arteries capable of undergoing passive stretching. They have thick walls and recoil when the ventricles relax; this maintains pressure to move the blood. Examples include the aorta and pulmonary artery.
   Muscular arteries—The small and medium arteries that distribute blood to all tissues by contracting or dilating to control blood flow. Most of the arteries in the body are of this type.
   Arterioles—The smallest arteries; they have a diameter of less than 0.5 mm. They constrict or dilate to control the amount of blood entering capillaries.

5. Atrioventricular valves allow blood to flow into the ventricles but prevent it from returning to the atria. Semilunar valves control the blood flow out of the ventricles into the aorta and pulmonary arteries and prevent any backflow of blood into the ventricles. The aortic valve is found between the left ventricle and aorta, and the pulmonary valve is between the pulmonary artery and right ventricle. These two valves open in response to pressure generated by the blood leaving the ventricle and close when blood pools in small pockets of the cusps of the valves, pushing the valves closed.

6. If the heart is to have sufficient blood for normal cardiac output, proper venous return of blood must exist. Some factors that affect venous return include the following:
   Valves—Valves close in the veins to prevent backflow and pooling of blood. Improperly working valves can cause blood to back up and remain in the venous system.
   Muscular pump—Muscle contractions help push venous blood toward the heart.
   Gravity—Standing in one position for a long time is detrimental to venous return because blood in the veins below the heart must constantly overcome gravity to return to the heart.
   Respiratory pump—During inhalation and exhalation, movement of the diaphragm and intercostal muscles helps move blood through the venous system.

7. Neutrophils, monocytes, lymphocytes, eosinophils, and basophils

8. The two coronary arteries, which originate from the base of the aorta, supply oxygenated blood to the heart muscle. Coronary veins follow parallel to the arteries and return the blood to the right atrium via the coronary sinus. Both types of coronary vessels run in grooves between the atria and ventricles and between the two ventricles. If either of the coronary arteries is unable to supply sufficient blood to the heart muscle, a heart attack occurs. The most common site of a heart attack is the anterior or inferior part of the left ventricle.

9. Two main sounds result from the closure of the valves. The first is a low-pitched "lubb" produced by closure of the mitral and tricuspid valves. The second is a higher-pitched "dubb" caused by the closure of the aortic and pulmonary valves. Extra sounds such as those resulting from faulty valves are referred to as *murmurs.* Valves usually are quiet as they open.

10. Blood pressure depends on a person's size. The average newborn has a blood pressure of 90/60; at age 15, the average blood pressure is about 120/60. An average, healthy young adult has a blood pressure of 120/80. On average, a blood pressure over 140/90 is considered hypertension; a blood pressure under 100/60 is considered hypotension. Blood pressure changes under various conditions, and a single reading should never be used as a final determinant.

11. The large lymph vessels gradually merge and eventually become two main ducts, called the *right lymphatic duct* and the *thoracic duct* (or *left lymphatic duct*). The right lymphatic duct drains the upper right half of the body and empties into the right subclavian vein. The thoracic duct drains the rest of the body and empties into the left subclavian vein.

12. Lymph nodes are small, round structures located along the lymph vessels. They are composed of lymphatic tissue and generally are clustered at the joints, which assists in pumping when the joint moves. The superficial lymph nodes are most numerous in the groin, axillae, and neck, whereas most of the deep lymph nodes are found beside blood vessels of the pelvic, abdominal, and thoracic cavities.

13. The body's defense system is known as the *immune system;* it is not a specific structural organ system, but rather a functional system. It responds in one of two ways by drawing on the structures and processes of each of the organs, tissues, cells, and chemicals produced within. In a nonspecific immune response, the body responds exactly the same way to all substances that are not identified as part of the body. Nonspecific response is genetically programmed into the human body. Specific immunity produces very specific responses to each identified substance and calls on special memory cells to help if that substance reappears. Specific immunity can be acquired in one of two ways: through natural immunity, which is the result of natural exposure, and through artificial immunity, which involves introducing a substance into the body to stimulate the immune response.

14. Nonspecific immunity can involve actions such as sneezing or coughing to remove microorganisms from our respiratory tract. Keeping the structure of the skin intact prevents entry of potentially damaging substances into the body. No matter the substance, the body responds in the same manner, with the same chemicals and cells mediating the actions. This general response is both a prevention and a first response in immune function.

FILL IN THE BLANK

1. integument
2. epidermis
3. dermis
4. superficial fascia
5. cardiovascular system
6. heart
7. mediastinum
8. pericardium
9. atria
10. ventricles
11. Cardiac output
12. cardiac cycle
13. heart rate
14. arteries
15. arterioles
16. Capillaries
17. veins
18. venules
19. blood pressure
20. systolic pressure
21. Diastolic pressure
22. sphygmomanometer
23. Blood
24. plasma
25. erythrocytes
26. leukocytes
27. platelets
28. fibrin
29. arteriosclerosis
30. atherosclerosis
31. lymphatic system
32. Lymph
33. lymph capillaries
34. Immunity
35. Lymphocytes

EXERCISE: SKIN STRUCTURE

A. Horny tissue
B. Melanin
C. Hair
D. Epidermis
E. Skin
F. Sebaceous gland
G. Sebum
H. Sweat gland
I. Hair follicle
J. Dermis

EXERCISE: STRUCTURES OF THE HEART

A. Aorta
B. Pulmonary artery
C. Left atrium
D. Endocardium
E. Myocardium
F. Pericardium
G. Left ventricle
H. Septum
I. Right ventricle
J. Inferior vena cava
K. Right atrium
L. Superior vena cava
M. Blood vessel

Chapter 12

The Respiratory, Digestive, Urinary, and Reproductive Systems

CHAPTER OUTLINE

CHAPTER OBJECTIVES

After completing this chapter, the student should be able to perform the following:

- List and describe the components of the respiratory system.
- Describe the function of the respiratory system.
- Explain hyperventilation syndrome.
- List and describe the components of the digestive system.
- Describe the process of digestion.
- List and describe the main food groups.
- List and describe the components of the urinary system.
- Describe the function of the urinary system.
- List and describe the components of the male and female reproductive system.
- Explain the three stages of pregnancy.
- Justify the effectiveness of soft tissue and movement modalities for support of health maintenance for the respiratory, digestive, urinary, and reproductive systems.

KEY TERMS

Absorption The movement of food molecules from the digestive tract to the circulatory or lymphatic systems.

Diaphragm A dome-shaped sheet of muscle attached to the thoracic wall that separates the lungs and thoracic cavity from the abdominal cavity. As the chest cavity enlarges, the diaphragm moves downward and creates a vacuum that allows air to flow into the lungs. As the chest contracts and the diaphragm relaxes, it arches upward, helping air to flow out of the lungs.

Digestion The mechanical and chemical breakdown of food from its complex form into simple molecules.

Elimination (egestion) Removal and release of solid waste products from food that cannot be digested or absorbed.

External respiration The exchange of oxygen and carbon dioxide between the lungs and the bloodstream.

Gestation (jes-TAY-shun) The period of fetal growth from conception until birth.

Hyperventilation (hye-per-ven-ti-LAY-shun) Abnormally deep or rapid breathing in excess of physical demands.

Hyperventilation syndrome A complex set of behaviors that leads to overbreathing without a pathologic condition present. It is a functional syndrome in which all the parts are working effectively; therefore a pathologic condition does not exist. Instead, the breathing pattern is inappropriate for the situation, resulting in confused signals to the central nervous system, which sets up a whole chain of events.

Ingestion (in-JEST-chun) Taking food into the mouth.

Internal respiration The exchange of gases between the tissues and blood.

Lower respiratory tract The larynx, trachea, bronchi, and alveoli.

Lungs The primary organs of respiration, they are soft, spongy, highly vascular structures separated into the left and right lungs by the mediastinum. Each lung is separated into lobes. The right lung has three lobes: an upper, middle, and lower; the left two lobes: an upper and lower.

Peristalsis (pair-I-STAL-sis) Rhythmic contraction of smooth muscles that propel products of digestion along the tract from the esophagus to the anus.

Respiration The movement of air in and out of the lungs, the exchange of oxygen and carbon dioxide between the lungs and blood, and the exchange between blood and body tissues.

Sinus (SYE-nus) Four groups of air-filled spaces that open into the internal nose. They are located in the frontal, ethmoid, sphenoid, and maxillary bones of the skull. Sinuses are lined with mucosa and function to lighten the weight of the skull, making it easier to hold the head up, and help in the production of sound.

Thorax (THOR-aks) Also known as the *chest cavity*, it is the upper region of the torso enclosed by the sternum, ribs, and thoracic vertebrae. It contains the lungs, heart, and great vessels.

Upper respiratory tract The nasal cavity and all its structures and the pharynx.

The Respiratory System

Breathing is a sacred act. According to Biblical scripture, "God breathed into man the breath of life and man became a living soul."

Of all the basic life support systems in the body, the respiratory system is the only one under volun-

tary, as well as automatic, control. It functions to obtain the oxygen (O_2) necessary to create energy for body functions and eliminate carbon dioxide (CO_2) produced during cellular metabolism. There is considerable voluntary control over respiratory movements used most often in connection with speech. Respiration and breath are intimately connected to the expression of emotion—as in laughing or crying, the explosive burst in anger, breath holding in fear, and the sigh of relief.

In terms of vital functions the respiratory system may be considered the most important because the heart and brain require a continuous supply of oxygen to function. Apnea, the lack of spontaneous breathing, can cause irreversible brain damage if it continues for more than 3 or 4 minutes.

Respiration is the movement of air in and out of the lungs, the exchange of oxygen and carbon dioxide between the lungs and blood, and the exchange between blood and body tissues. Breathing is a mechanical action of inhalation and exhalation that draws oxygen into the lungs and releases carbon dioxide into the atmosphere.

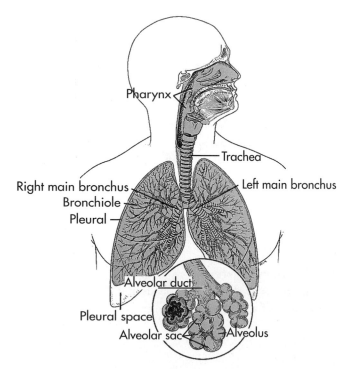

FIGURE 12-1 Pharynx, trachea, and lungs. Alveolar sacs in *inset*. (From Thibodeau GA: *Anthony's textbook of anatomy and physiology*, ed 13, St Louis, 1990, Mosby.)

External respiration is the exchange of oxygen and carbon dioxide between the lungs and the bloodstream. The exchange of gases between the tissues and blood is called **internal respiration.**

On the average, we breathe 12 times per minute. Each breath contains approximately 500 milliliters of air (about 2 cups), so in 1 hour we breathe about 360 liters, or 82 gallons, of air.

The organs of the respiratory system are divided into upper and lower regions. The **upper respiratory tract** consists of the nasal cavity, all its structures, and the pharynx; the **lower respiratory tract** is made up of the larynx, trachea, and bronchi and alveoli in the lungs (Figure 12-1).

ORGANS OF THE RESPIRATORY SYSTEM

The Nose and Nasal Cavity

The structure of the nose is divided into two parts: the external and internal portions. The lower two thirds of the external nose is composed mostly of cartilage. The upper third, or bridge of the nose, is formed from two small hard nasal bones. The tip of the nose is the apex, and the nostrils are the nares. Air enters the external nares and passes across internal nasal hairs that trap particles of dirt and other foreign material; the air then flows into the nasal cavity.

The internal nose is the continuation of the nose inside the skull and above the mouth and includes the sinuses. The roof is formed by a small portion of the frontal bone and the ethmoid and sphenoid bones, and the floor is formed by the hard palate, consisting of the maxillae and palatine bones. The internal nares are the portion of the internal nose that communicates with the throat. The nasal cavity is the actual space inside both the external and internal nose structures. It is separated into left and right sides by the septum, a partition composed of cartilage and bone. At the upper portion of the nasal cavity, three thin, curled bones, the turbinates or conchae, project inward from the two outer walls. These turbinates separate into small grooved passageways called *meatuses,* which continue to move the air. As air passes through the nasal cavity, it is warmed by small blood vessels close to the surface of the lining and moistened by the mucous membranes and secretions from the sinuses. The mucous membranes line the entire respiratory tract, and the sticky mucus traps smaller inhaled particles, helping to prevent infection. The small hairs, or cilia, that line the nasal cavity, larynx, and trachea transport these foreign particles to the throat where they are swallowed and destroyed in the stomach.

Nerve endings for the olfactory nerve lie on the upper third of both sides of the nasal septum, the olfactory region. They are stimulated by changes in gas consistency. Olfactory nerve fibers pass through small holes in the ethmoid bone to the olfactory bulb, and then to the cortex, where the impulses are interpreted as smell.

Venous areas called *swell bodies* are located on the turbinates. About every half hour, the swell bodies on one side of the nasal cavity engorge with blood, resulting in decreased air flow on that side, with good flow on the other side. Then it reverses. These periodic changes permit the inside of the nose to recover from drying. This same mechanism becomes important during sleep. When a person lies with his head to one side, the swell bodies of the lower nostril become congested. The chamber narrows and the lumen is closed. When sleeping, we only breath though one nostril at a time. The closure of the nostril then initiates movement of the head from one side to the other, which in turn causes a major movement and turning of the body. This head-body moving cycle, initiated by the nose, ensures maximal rest during sleep. A poorly functioning nose may allow the body and head to remain in one position and can cause symptoms such as backaches, numbness, cramps, and circulatory dysfunction.

The nasal septum is supplied with sensory nerves and blood vessels. Nasal reflex responses and referred phenomena are well established between the nose, ears, throat, larynx, heart, lungs, diaphragm, nervous system, and body temperature. Contained in the coordination of these various reflex patterns is the mechanism of entrainment between heart rate, breathing rate, and synchronization of other body rhythms. Most relaxation methods and methods of ritual, meditation, and many healing practices incorporate a form of structured breathing. This practical application of ordering and coordinating body rhythms seems to be able to be accomplished through the coordination of air flow through the nose.

A deviated septum is a condition in which the cartilage is bent, usually as the result of a blow to the nose, resulting in difficulty in breathing from one side of the nose. As simple as it seems, because of reflex patterns, any disruption of air flow through the nose can have body-wide effects such as disturbing sleep patterns.

Sinuses

The **sinuses** are four groups of air-filled spaces that open into the internal nose. They are located in the frontal, ethmoid, sphenoid, and maxillary bones of the skull. Sinuses are lined with mucosa and function to lighten the weight of the skull, making it easier to hold the head up, and help in the production of sound. Because the sinus mucosa communicates with the nasal cavity, sinuses are prone to the same infections as the nasal cavity.

Pharynx

The pharynx, or throat, is divided into three areas. The nasopharynx is the continuation of the nasal cavity into the throat; it transports air. The Eustachian tubes open into the nasopharynx and help equalize pressure in the head, nose, and pharynx. The oropharynx is the portion of the throat that you can see; it contains the tonsils and functions both as a passageway for food between the mouth and the esophagus and as a passageway for air between the nose, mouth, and trachea. The laryngopharynx begins at the hyoid bone and separates into the esophagus and larynx, so it functions as both a pathway for respiration and digestion. At the entrance to the larynx is a small cartilaginous flap, the epiglottis. As we swallow food, the epiglottis closes over the glottis, preventing food or fluids from entering the lungs.

Larynx

The larynx, or voice box, connects the pharynx to the trachea. Its structure consists of cartilage, ligaments, connective tissue, muscles, and the vocal cords. The cartilage provides a rigid structural framework for the larynx and trachea below, making sure that there is an open airway at all times. The thyroid cartilage, known as the Adam's apple, is located on the anterior portion of the larynx; it is larger in men. The vocal cords and the spaces between the cords are located inside the glottis.

The function of the larynx, in addition to permitting air passage to and from the lungs, is to produce sound, or phonation. The lips and the tongue create speech. As we exhale, the vocal cords vibrate to produce high or low sounds, or pitch. In high-pitch sounds the glottis is narrower and there is more tension in the vocal cords, whereas in low-pitch sounds, the glottis is more open and the vocal cords are more relaxed. Laryngitis is an inflammation of the vocal cords caused by overuse, infection, or irritation from substances such as cigarette smoke or tumors. If it affects the vocal cords, hoarseness or loss of the voice can result. If the glottis is obstructed such as with food it can be fatal. Bacterial infection of the epiglottis (epiglottitis) in children is a life-threatening but rarer cause of obstruction.

Trachea

The trachea, or windpipe, is the main airway to the lungs. It is a 4- to 5-inch long tube that begins at the glottis and ends at the junction of the two main bronchi near the level of the sternal angle. The trachea consists of 16 to 20 horseshoe-shaped rings of cartilage that have connective tissue between them. When a foreign particle enters the trachea, it is trapped by mucus and cilia, initiating the cough reflex.

The trachea branches off into two bronchi, which have the same structural framework, except that there is more smooth muscle than in the trachea. The first branches of the bronchial tubes are the right and left primary bronchi. Each main bronchus divides into two (left lung) or three (right lung) lobar bronchi.

Lungs

The two **lungs** are the primary organs of respiration. These soft, spongy, highly vascular structures are separated into the left and right lungs by the mediastinum. Each lung is separated into lobes. The right lung has three lobes: an upper, middle, and lower; the left has two lobes: an upper and lower.

The lobar bronchi, which extend from the trachea, each divide into 10 segmental bronchi, which again further divide. The amount of cartilage in each tube gradually decreases until there is none. At this point the tubes are about 1 millimeter in diameter and are known as the *bronchioles*, which terminate in the air sacs, or alveoli. The alveoli are surrounded by capillaries. This is where the internal respiratory action takes place.

The lungs are enclosed in a pleural cavity lined with two pleural membranes. One connects directly to the lung, and the other attaches to the mediastinum and inside chest wall. This cavity created by the membranes contains approximately one-half teaspoon of lubricating fluid that reduces friction between the two layers as we breathe. Increases in the amount of fluid are often seen with diseases such as lung cancer and pulmonary edema and can make breathing difficult. Pneumothorax is a condition in which air enters the pleural cavity as a result of trauma or rupture of part of the lung as a result of a penetrating injury such as from a bullet or knife, or in disease processes such as emphysema. A chest tube called a *thoracostomy tube* is inserted between the ribs and connected to a pump to remove the air. In hemothorax, blood in the pleural space is drained in a similar manner.

Diaphragm

The **diaphragm** is a dome-shaped sheet of muscle attached to the thoracic wall that separates the lungs and thoracic cavity from the abdominal cavity. As the chest cavity enlarges, the diaphragm moves downward and creates a vacuum that allows air to flow into the lungs. As the chest contracts and the diaphragm relaxes, it arches upward, helping air to flow out of the lungs.

At the entrance to the larynx is a small cartilaginous flap, the epiglottis. As we swallow food, the epiglottis closes over the glottis, preventing food or fluids from entering the lungs.

Thorax

The **thorax,** or chest cavity, is the upper region of the torso enclosed by the sternum, ribs, and thoracic vertebrae. It contains the lungs, heart, and great vessels.

NERVES AND VESSELS OF THE LUNGS AND RESPIRATORY MUSCLES

The autonomic nervous system supplies the bronchi and bronchioles. Stimulation of the vagus nerve (parasympathetic) causes contraction of the smooth muscles and narrows the diameter of the tubes (bronchoconstriction). Stimulation of sympathetic nerves initiates smooth muscle relaxation, resulting in widening of the tubes (bronchodilation).

The nerve supply to the intercostal muscles is from spinal nerves T1 to T11. The phrenic nerve originates at C3 to C5 and innervates the diaphragm. The reason that the nerve supply originates so distant is that during fetal development the diaphragm actually begins its growth in the neck and then descends from the neck to the abdomen. A broken neck that injures the spinal cord below C5 still allows the person to breathe because the diaphragm does most of the breathing. Injury to both phrenic nerves, or a spinal cord injury above C3 to C5, severely compromises breathing.

The pulmonary arteries and veins participate in the exchange of oxygen and carbon dioxide between the capillaries and alveoli. Branches of the aorta and upper intercostal arteries supply blood to most of the lung tissue. Venous drainage is from the azygous vein on the right side of the thorax, and the first intercostal vein on the left.

THE MECHANICS OF BREATHING

During the moments before we take a breath, the pressure both inside the lungs and outside the body are equal, whereas the pressure inside the pleural space is slightly lower. When we begin to inhale, the external intercostal muscles between the ribs contract, lifting the lower ribs up and out. This creates a vacuum that expands the lungs, causing the pressure inside the lungs to decrease. The diaphragm moves down, increasing the volume of the pleural cavities and decreasing their pressure even more. Elastic fibers in the alveolar walls stretch, permitting expansion of the air sacs. Air is drawn into the lungs until the pressure is equal again.

As we exhale, the pressure inside the pleural cavity increases; the external intercostals, diaphragm, and alveolar walls relax; the volume inside the lungs decreases; and the pressure in the lungs raises until it again equalizes the atmospheric pressure.

In diseases such as asthma, bronchitis, and emphysema, accessory muscles of respiration are often used. Inspiration is aided by contraction of the sternocleidomastoid and other muscles of the neck, whereas expiration is aided by the use of the internal intercostals and abdominal muscles (Figure 12-2).

Lung Volumes

Breathing in and out changes the volume of air. Four different pulmonary volumes can be measured to use as guidelines in health assessments. The tidal volume is the amount of air taken in or exhaled in a single breath during normal breathing, usually while the person is resting. The inspiratory reserve volume (IRV) is the amount of air that can be forcefully inhaled after normal tidal volume inspiration, whereas the expiratory reserve volume (ERV) is the amount of air that can be forcefully exhaled after a normal exhalation. The reserve volume is the amount of air that remains in the lungs and passageways after a maximal expiration. The vital capacity (VC) is the total of the tidal volume, IRV, and ERV. In the normal healthy adult lung, that usually varies from 3.5 to 5.5 liters.

In lung diseases such as asthma and emphysema the VC and forced expiratory reserve (FEV) amounts are

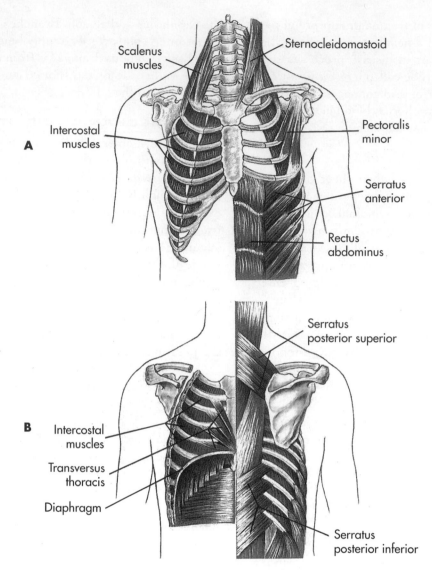

FIGURE 12-2 Muscles of respiration. **A,** Anterior view. **B,** Posterior view. (From Seidel HM et al: *Mosby's guide to physical examination,* ed 3, St Louis, 1995, Mosby.)

abnormal. A person with asthma, for example, may have a normal tidal volume and VC but decreased FEV, whereas a person with emphysema may have a normal (but often decreased) tidal volume and decreased VC and EEV. The end result is that the person cannot effectively exhale.

Transport of Oxygen and Carbon Dioxide

The exchange of oxygen and carbon dioxide takes place by diffusion. The pulmonary arteries bring oxygen-deficient blood from the right ventricle to the lungs. Carbon dioxide diffuses from the bloodstream through the capillary and alveolar membranes and is exhaled by the lungs. Oxygen diffuses in the opposite direction, from the alveoli through both membranes and into the bloodstream. The pulmonary veins return oxygen-rich blood to the left atrium.

The amount of oxygen in the blood depends on the amount of oxygen available in the atmosphere. The air in the average room is composed of the following:

Nitrogen (N_2) — 79%
Oxygen (O_2) — 20.96%
Carbon dioxide (CO_2) — 0.04%

Oxygen is transported by red blood cells in the blood as oxyhemoglobin. Red cells move into the capillaries. At the arteriole end of the capillary, O_2 leaves the red cell, then passes through the capillary membrane into the tissue fluid. It then diffuses through the tissue cell membrane to be used as fuel for cellular metabolism.

Carbon dioxide moves out of the tissue cell in the reverse direction through the same membranes into the red blood cell, where most of it is converted to bicarbonate ion (HCO_3). Bicarbonate is transported by way of the plasma to the lungs, where the process is reversed in the alveolus, and carbon dioxide is exhaled.

Control of Breathing

The respiratory center is a group of nerve cells in the medulla and pons. The center is affected by a variety of stimuli. Impulses from the cerebral cortex under voluntary control modify respiration, as do changes in the carbon dioxide content and acidity of blood and cerebrospinal fluid. Chemoreceptors, nerve cells found near the baroreceptors, are sensitive to the oxygen level and to a lesser extent to CO_2 and pH (acid/base balance) levels in the bloodstream. Two are located near the arch of the aorta (aortic bodies), and one is in each carotid artery (carotid bodies). The aortic bodies transmit impulses to the respiratory center in the medulla through the vagus nerve; the carotid bodies transmit by way of the glossopharyngeal nerve. When the concentration of oxygen in the body is low, chemoreceptors are stimulated and the respiratory rate increases.

The Respiratory Rate

The respiratory rate in adults is about 12 to 16 breaths per minute. In the newborn it is about 35, and gradually decreases to adult values at about age 20. Emotions are a powerful stimulus for respiratory changes. Fear, grief, and shock slow the rate, whereas anger and sexual arousal increase respiratory rate.

Besides being affected by emotions, changes in breathing rates can occur as a result of increased oxygen requirement from exercise, in obesity as a result of increased vessel resistance, during infections and fever because of increased energy requirements, in heart failure from decreased oxygen flow, during pain because of increased nervous stimulation, with anemia because of decreased oxygen transport, in hyperthyroidism from an increase in metabolic rate, and during emphysema and pneumothorax as a result of blockage of oxygen. Hyperpnea is fast breathing and tachypnea is rapid shallow breathing. This type of breathing can lead to acute hyperventilation or chronic overbreathing called *hyperventilation syndrome*, which causes a variety

of signs and symptoms and is discussed later in this section. Bradypnea, or slow breathing, is seen in alcohol and other depressant-drug intoxication because of the depressant action on the brain. It is also seen in increased intracranial pressure from pressure on the respiratory center and in diabetic coma.

Periods of hyperpnea alternating with periods of apnea (no breathing) are sometimes seen in the sleep of infants, particularly premature ones. These patterns also appear in brain injury and in the terminally ill.

PATHOLOGY

Asthma

Asthma is the narrowing of the small airways not related to cardiovascular disease. It presents itself as acute attacks that constrict and obstruct these airways. Asthma attacks may be triggered by allergic reactions, air pollutants, exercise, hypersensitivity to substances from work or recreation such as wood or flour, chemicals, viral infections, or an emotional upset. During an episode, the smooth muscle layer of the bronchi and bronchioles goes into spasm (constriction) and the glands of the bronchi hypersecrete mucus. The airways fill with thick mucus, and air cannot leave the lungs. Breathlessness, coughing, chest tightness, and wheezing occur as the person tries to force air out of the lungs. Arterial blood gases initially show a low amount of CO_2, a condition known as *respiratory alkalosis*. Long-term therapy may include the use of a bronchodilator, mast cell stabilizer, or corticosteroids. Antibiotics may benefit the person if the trigger is a respiratory infection.

Carbon Monoxide Poisoning

Carbon monoxide poisoning is the leading cause of gas deaths in this country. Carbon monoxide is odorless and binds to hemoglobin 210 times more readily than oxygen. Most deaths occur from smoke inhalation during fires. Some occur from automobile exhaust fumes, poorly ventilated or defective gasoline heaters, and charcoal stoves. Poisonings also occur in machine shops where ventilation is poor. Symptoms are headache, dizziness, weakness, and nausea, which occurs when the blood has about 6% to 7% carboxyhemoglobin.

Choking

Choking often happens when a person is talking while eating and inhales at the same time as swallowing. The piece of food, usually meat, obstructs the larynx. Frequently, the person is also drinking alcohol. The person starts to cough, which often dislodges the object. If not, the airway can become totally blocked. The person usually appears distressed, grasps his neck, and cannot inhale or exhale. The term *café coronary* has been applied because it often occurs in a restaurant and superficially resembles a heart attack.

Before beginning assistance, ask the person if he can speak. If he can, he is not choking.

Chronic Obstructive Pulmonary Disease

Although the processes involved in the evolution of emphysema and bronchitis are different, the end result is irreversible respiratory insufficiency, sometimes called *chronic obstructive pulmonary disease (COPD)*. In emphysema the obstruction is in the alveoli; in bronchitis it is in the bronchi. A component of each is seen in heavy smokers.

Acute bronchitis often occurs along with an upper respiratory infection, measles, or the flu. Although it is usually caused by a virus, it may also involve a bacterial infection. Symptoms include a mild fever, an increase in mucus secreted, and coughing in an attempt to loosen and remove the phlegm, which is often yellow and green. Chronic bronchitis is usually caused by prolonged irritation by cigarette smoke. The person usually has a chronic cough. As in the acute stage, sputum production increases in response to the constant irritation of the tissues. The lung tissues changes, and the person becomes less able to tolerate exercise and any activity. The cilia are damaged from the smoke, so excess mucus cannot be moved out of the airway. Wheezing noises may be heard. Treatment involves the use of bronchodilators and oxygen therapy. The condition often reverses when cigarette smoking is stopped.

In emphysema resulting from long-term irritation of the bronchi and bronchioles, mucus and pus accumulate, and the air in the alveoli becomes trapped. When the pressure exceeds the elastic limit, the alveoli become permanently ballooned out, producing the typically barrel-chested person who uses the internal intercostals as well as the abdominal and neck muscles to breathe. As it progresses, the person becomes breathless with minor exertion. Inflammation brings in more white blood cells, which break down the walls of the alveoli, which merge to form larger sacs. This results in less surface area for the internal exchanges of gases, so oxygen in the blood decreases. Emphysema is the most common cause of respiratory failure. Bronchodilators and oxygen therapy may help.

Common Cold

The common cold can be caused by one of more than 200 viruses and is easily transmitted. Usually affecting the nasal mucosa, the viruses may spread to the sinuses, pharynx, and down the respiratory tract. The person's temperature rises to eliminate the virus. Irritation in the nose and pharynx causes coughing and sneezing. Fluids and bed rest are recommended.

Croup

Croup is a viral infection in children that most often affects boys ages 3 months to 5 years. The larynx, trachea, and bronchi are red and swollen and may block the glottis. A "seal bark" cough is usually present. Sometimes a high-pitched whistling inhalation is present and the child must use his neck and abdominal muscles to breathe. Humidified air often eases the symptoms; if not, oxygen therapy may be used.

Cystic Fibrosis

Cystic fibrosis is a genetic disorder that causes abnormally thick and sticky mucus to be produced throughout the body. This mucus cannot be moved out by the cilia, so bacteria and viruses are held in instead of moving through the body. Infections develop and the smaller airways are obstructed. (See the section on the digestive system for more information.)

Drowning

In drowning, the victim both inhales and swallows water. In 10% of cases the larynx goes into spasm when the first small amount of fluid is inhaled, and asphyxia or suffocation (from lack of oxygen and an increase in carbon dioxide) takes place even with no fluid in the lungs. Survival depends mostly on the continued presence of a pulse and not necessarily on the time of immersion. Treatment in near-drowning consists of cardiopulmonary resuscitation, with oxygen given at the hospital and bicarbonate for the acidosis caused by the carbon dioxide levels.

Hayfever

Hayfever is an allergic reaction seen in people who have a sensitivity to pollen, house dust, and feathers, among other things. Nasal vessels engorge with blood and become congested. Fluid leaks from the capillaries into the tissue spaces and drains into the nasal cavity, causing a runny nose. The congestion and edema cause the irritation, sneezing, redness, and swelling seen in the weary sufferers in the spring and summer months. Treatment is with an antihistamine and decongestant.

Hiccups

Hiccups (singultus) is a sudden involuntary contraction of the inspiratory muscles, producing the sound of inspiration with the glottis closed. Most cases involve food or alcohol, are short-lived, and resolve without therapy. This is a primitive reflex, similar to yawning, coughing, sneezing, and vomiting. The reflex is designed to dislodge a foreign object. Often, sedatives and home remedies work. In prolonged cases the use of a tranquilizer may be necessary.

Hyperventilation Syndrome

Physiologists define **hyperventilation** as abnormally deep or rapid breathing in excess of physical demands. Dyspneic (no air) fear is a core factor in the cause of panic attacks.

Hyperventilation syndrome is a complex set of behaviors that leads to overbreathing in the absence of a pathologic condition. It is a functional syndrome in which all the parts are working effectively, therefore a pathologic condition does not exist. Instead, the breathing pattern is inappropriate for the situation, resulting in confused signals to the central nervous system, which sets up a whole chain of events. People experiencing this difficulty are often told that nothing is wrong, which induces further puzzlement and adds to their anxiety, or they are told to take a few deep breaths, which increases their symptoms. One review indicates that as many as 28% of patients within various medical populations may be functional hyperventilators.

Increased ventilation is a common component of fight-or-flight responses, but when our breathing increases and our actions and movements are restricted, we are breathing in excess of metabolic need. Blood levels of CO_2 fall, and symptoms may occur. As we exhale too much CO_2 too quickly, our blood becomes more acidic. These biochemical changes can cause many of the following signs and symptoms:

Cardiovascular—Palpitations, missed beats, tachycardia, sharp or dull atypical chest pain, "angina," vasomotor instability, cold extremities, Raynaud's phenomenon, blotchy flushing of blush area, capillary vasoconstriction (face, arms, hands)

Neurologic—Dizziness, unsteadiness, or instability; faint feelings (rarely actual fainting); visual disturbance (blurred or tunnel vision); headache (often migraine); paraesthesia (i.e., numbness, uselessness, heaviness, "pins and needles," burning, limbs feeling out of proportion or "not belonging"), commonly of hands, feet, or face, sometimes scalp or whole body; intolerance of light or noise; large pupils (wearing dark glasses on a dull day); sensation of faintness or giddiness

Respiratory—Shortness of breath typically after exertion, irritable cough, tightness or oppression of chest, difficulty breathing, "asthma," air hunger, inability to take a satisfying breath, excessive sighing, yawning, sniffing

Gastrointestinal—Difficulty in swallowing, dry mouth and throat, acid regurgitation, heartburn, hiatal hernia, nausea, flatulence, belching, air swallowing, abdominal discomfort, bloating

Muscular—Cramps, muscle pains (particularly occipital, neck, shoulders, between scapulae; less commonly, the lower back and limbs), tremors, twitching, weakness, stiffness, or tetany (seizing up)

Psychic—Tension, anxiety, "unreal feelings," depersonalization, feeling "out of body," hallucinations, fear of insanity, panic, phobias, agoraphobia

General—Weakness; exhaustion; impaired concentration, memory, and performance; disturbed sleep, including nightmares; emotional sweating (axillae, palms, sometimes whole body); woolly head

Cerebrovascular constriction, a primary response to hyperventilation syndrome, can reduce the oxygen available to the brain by about one half. Among the resulting symptoms are dizziness, blurring of consciousness, and possibly because of a decrease in cortical inhibition, tearfulness and emotional instability. Other effects of hyperventilation syndrome that therapists should watch for are generalized body tension and chronic inability to relax. In addition, those who hyperventilate are particularly prone to spasm (tetany) in muscles involved in the "attack posture"—they hunch their shoulders, thrust head and neck forward, scowl, and clench their teeth.

Influenza

Influenza (flu) is a common viral infection of the entire body, resulting in fever, muscle aches and weakness, backache, and cough. Primary treatment, as with most viral infections, is bed rest and fluids.

Lung Cancer

About 90% of all cases of lung cancer are caused by tobacco. Primary tumors usually develop in the bronchus and block air passage. Cancer in the lung can spread to other parts of the body. Symptoms frequently begin with cough, blood in the phlegm, wheezing, chest pain, and fever. If the tumor is large enough, there may be problems swallowing.

Diagnosis is made with a physical examination, x-ray films, and computed tomography (CT) scans.

Sleep Apnea

In the disorder known as *sleep apnea*, the person stops breathing for period of 10 seconds or more while sleeping, at least a few times per hour. Each time breathing stops, oxygen levels fall and cause the person to wake, which results in resumption of breathing. It most often occurs because of obstructed breathing, which is identified as obstructive sleep apnea (OSA). OSA results in drowsy episodes accompanied by snoring and apneic spells. OSA is more common in men, especially those who are overweight and are heavy drinkers. It is also seen in persons with enlarged tonsils, small jaws, large tongues and soft palates, and other subtle anatomic abnormalities. People taking medications such as sleeping pills can suffer from OSA because the upper airways muscles can relax too much. It appears that the tongue falls back during the non–rapid eye movement (REM) sleep and blocks the airway. Infant apnea is associated with infections that obstruct the airway; sometimes there is no identifiable cause. Sudden infant death syndrome (SIDS) may be a variation. Both central nervous system and obstructive problems may cause SIDS, but OSA seems to be an important component. Additional risk factors for SIDS include being male, low birth weight, decreased carotid body substance, and an upper respiratory infection.

Pleurisy

Pleurisy (pleuritis) is an inflammation of the pleural membrane, usually from a lung infection such as pneumonia. The inflamed membranes rub against each other, causing stabbing pain that is worse during inhalation.

Pneumonia

Pneumonia is an acute infection of the lungs that can be caused by bacteria or viruses, fungi, exposure to certain chemicals, or inhaled substances. Symptoms include fever, chills, chest pain, difficulty breathing, headache, loss of appetite, muscle and joint pain, a cough usually accompanied by yellow or green sputum, and rales (the sound of movement of air and fluid in the bronchial tree). Diagnosis is made after reviewing client history and test results, most often a chest x-ray film showing an abnormal white area. Sputum is evaluated and blood tests often show an elevated white count. Primary treatment for bacterial pneumonia is an antibiotic, bed rest, and fluids. In serious cases the person must be hospitalized and given oxygen and antibiotics.

Pulmonary Embolism

In pulmonary embolism, a clot detaches from a deep vein in the leg or pelvis and travels to the right atrium, then to the right ventricles, and on to the pulmonary artery. Predisposing factors of clot formation are obesity, heart failure, surgery and immobilization, and a history of thrombophlebitis. If the clot lodges at the junction of the pulmonary trunk and the pulmonary arteries, it may cause death. If the clot moves into a pulmonary artery and impacts, destroying lung tissue, this is a pulmonary infarction. The person suddenly becomes short of breath. Other signs and symptoms are chest pain, fever, and wheezing. Diagnosis is made with the use of a lung scan and pulmonary angiogram. Treatment consists of intravenous anticoagulant (heparin) to prevent further clotting, and the use of a clot-dissolving medication. This is often followed by use of oral warfarin (Coumadin.)

Pulmonary Edema

Pulmonary edema is the accumulation of excess fluid in the lungs. The most common cause is heart failure, although it may be brought on by kidney disease, pneumonia, or other disorders. It is usually treated with diuretics and oxygen therapy.

Sinusitis

Sinusitis is inflammation of the sinuses that most commonly accompanies a nasal infection. Congestion, edema, and pain are present because of irritation of the sensory nerve endings in the periosteum. Pain takes the form of headache, particularly if the frontal sinus is involved. Drainage into the nasal cavity is blocked by congestion. The maxillary sinus lies over the upper teeth, and it is sometimes difficult for a person to tell whether the problem is a sinus attack or a toothache because of the similarity of the pain pattern. Treatment often consists of an antibiotic and a decongestant.

Sore Throat

Sore throat, or pharyngitis, is an inflammation of the pharynx. If tonsils are involved, the condition is tonsillitis. The cause is usually viral, but a throat culture may show *Streptococcus*, the organism that causes rheumatic fever, rheumatic heart disease, or glomerulonephritis as complications in certain individuals. Common signs and symptoms are a red, tender throat, enlarged cervical lymph nodes, and fever. Treatment consists of rest, an analgesic, saline gargles, and an antibiotic if the culture is positive for *Streptococcus*.

Tuberculosis

Tuberculosis is an infection that develops as chronic inflammatory lesions from the bacillus *Mycobacterium tuberculosis*. Once thought to be a rare occurrence, tuberculosis is on the rise again in adult populations who are immunosuppressed. Although any site of the body may be affected, pulmonary tuberculosis is by far the most common. In rare cases it may also affect the bones and kidneys. Early symptoms include listlessness and fatigue, chest pain, fever, and weight loss. The disease progresses to impair respiratory function severely and spreads to involve other body sites. This is a contagious disease spread by inhalation or ingestion of infected droplets dispersed by the infected person through coughing and nasal discharge. Treatment includes rest, nutritional support, and a medication regimen that must be continued for a long time, often more than a year. The disease is no longer infectious after the sputum tests free of bacteria, although it may lie dormant.

INDICATIONS CONTRAINDICATIONS

For Soft Tissue and Movement Therapies

Any of the listed disorders of the respiratory system of viral or bacterial cause are usually contraindicated for soft tissue or movement modalities until the disease runs its course. Whenever the body is under stress, as is found in dealing with respiratory infection, further stress in the system can worsen the condition. Simple palliative measures to provide comfort and encourage sleep are appropriate. All sanitary procedures and Universal Precautions are to be followed.

In chronic conditions such as asthma or emphysema, general stress management and maintenance of normal function of the muscles of respiration are beneficial, again gauging the appropriate added stress levels. In cystic fibrosis, percussion is used to help loosen the phlegm but should not be attempted without medical supervision and training.

Hyperventilation syndrome is often helped with both soft tissue approaches and moderate application of movement therapies.

Almost every meditation or relaxation system uses breathing patterns because they are a direct link to altering autonomic nervous system patterns, which in turn alters mood, feelings, and behavior. Other ways to modulate breathing are through singing and chanting.

The shoulders should not move during normal breathing. The accessory muscles of respiration located in the neck area should only be activated when increased oxygen is required for fight or flight. This is the pattern for sympathetic breathing. If the person does not use the additional oxygen through increased activity levels, he may hyperventilate. If the accessory muscles of respiration such as the scalenes, sternocleidomastoid, serratus posterior superior, levator scapulae, rhomboids, abdominals, and quadratus lumborum are constantly being activated for breathing when forced inhalation and expiration are not called for, dysfunctional muscle patterns will result. Soft tissue and movement therapies can bring balance into these areas to encourage a more effective breathing pattern. General stress management reduces anxiety and helps to normalize the breathing pattern.

Although detailed discussion of the many meditation, breathing modulation, or retraining measures is beyond the scope of this text, two basic types of systems exist: one leading to physiologic hyperarousal and one to hypoarousal. Both processes facilitate a reestablishment of homeostasis, just as a muscle can be encouraged to relax by either tensing it first and then releasing it or by using the antagonist pattern to initiate reciprocal inhibition to allow the muscle to relax. Hyperarousal systems increase sympathetic activity with a secondary parasympathetic balance. Aerobic exercise is an example. Hypoarousal systems will directly activate parasympathetic responses. Quiet reflection or meditative prayer combined with a chant are examples. Many resources use retraining programs to improve breathing patterns, and the recommendation is to find one that is comfortable and use it regularly.

Herbs such as eucalyptus are used as a vapor that is soothing to the respiratory system. Aromatherapy uses different scents that are taken into the body through the respiratory system. Some scents have a stimulating effect and others have a more calming effect. The efficacy of aromatherapy is valid when we understand the influence of the sense of smell on physiology. As with most forms of soft tissue and movement therapies, aromatherapy is nonspecific, supporting the body in balanced function (Activity 12-1).

ACTIVITY 12-1

It is important to be able to explain and justify the therapeutic value of the work we do. The following activity will assist you in developing the skills to explain the effectiveness of various modalities to clients and other health care professionals. Use the clinical reasoning model that follows to accomplish this task. The focus should be your primary modality or modalities applied to the respiratory system. An example is provided in the section opener on p. 450.

Modality/modalities

1. **What are the facts?**
   a. Which system is involved, and which structures of that system can be reached directly or indirectly?

   b. Which of these structures are most affected by this modality?

   c. Which physiologic functions are affected by this approach?

   d. When the treatment is applied, what changes in function will result in
      (1) This system

      (2) The whole body

   e. What is considered normal or balanced function?

   f. How are the functions of this system related to the body's homeostasis?

   g. What has worked or has not worked?

   h. Where could you find information that would support the use of this modality as a therapeutic intervention?

   i. What research is available to support the use of the therapeutic intervention?

ACTIVITY 12-1—cont'd

j. How does the intervention support a healthy state?

d. List at least three applications of this modality that would affect both the structure and function of this system.

k. Under which pathologic or dysfunctional conditions is the intervention most likely to be beneficial?

e. What are other ways to look at the situation?

f. What other methods could provide similar benefits?

2. What are the possibilities?

a. What do the data suggest?

3. What is the logical outcome of therapeutic intervention?
a. What would be the logical progression of the symptom pattern, contributing factors, and current behaviors?

b. What are the reasons for using the proposed methods?

b. What are the benefits and drawbacks of each intervention suggested?
Benefits:

c. What are the possible interventions?

Drawbacks:

b. Does the practitioner feel qualified to work with the situation and apply the identified modality to the particular situation?

c. What are the costs in terms of time, resources, and finances?

c. Does a feeling of cooperation and agreement exist among all those involved, and how would the practitioner recognize this feeling?

d. What is likely to happen if the modality is not used?

e. What is likely to happen if the modality is used?

Justification

Using the information developed in the clinical reasoning model, present a clear, concise statement of the ways in which the particular soft tissue or movement modality would be beneficial, either in supporting the particular body system in a healthy condition or as part of a treatment plan for a pathologic or dysfunctional condition. Based on the above information, give a brief summary of the effectiveness of the modality for this system.

4. For the intervention proposed, what would be the impact on the people involved, specifically the client, practitioner, and other professionals working with the client?

a. How does each of the people involved (including, besides those named above, the client's family and support system) feel about the possible interventions?

The Digestive System

Digestion is a physiologic process that involves the intake, assimilation, and egestion of nutrients. But the intake of food is much more than a means of gaining nutrients for growth, repair, and maintenance of the body. Eating is a pleasure activity and social event that involves many neurochemical interactions. Food choices can have an impact on our health risks. Biologic drives for food, especially foods high in fat and simple carbohydrates or sugars, played an important part in early human survival. These foods, which are rare in nature, supply quick and sustaining energy sources. No longer rare in our society, an overabundance of fats and sugars feeds the biologic cravings we still have even though the energy required to acquire these food sources has been decreased. The result is an epidemic of obesity.

Emotional eating is one type of substitution for lack of touch stimulation and loving relationships with others because the chemicals stimulated during all these processes are similar. Foods such as chocolate and other fat/carbohydrate combinations, along with some form of protein, generate serotonin and other feel-good neurochemicals just as effectively as a hug will. Food behaviors can become as addictive as any other pleasure activity. When we engage in exercise, it too results in a chemical pattern similar to eating or being touched.

Because biologic tendencies are for energy conservation, and our biologic patterns are for survival in a more primitive environment, the internal drive toward movement and activity was originally to provide for shelter, food, and protection. In today's society we find ourselves needing to move for the sake of movement without an immediate survival process attached to it. This is a physiologically confusing process and may be part of the reason that it is difficult for some people to find any motivation to exercise.

Both eating food and fasting as a cleansing or purification process are often at the heart of social and religious rituals. What would a holiday be without all the food? Healing practices usually involve the ingestion of a healing herb or brew. Mating behaviors, found as we pair into couples, often involve food and feeding behaviors. Who falls in love without sharing a meal—one milkshake with two straws—and, of course, there is the Western ritual of feeding each other the wedding cake.

One of the first acts of parental bonding is feeding the infant. Our lips and tongue remain forever sensitive to sensory stimulation connected with soothing and pleasure behaviors. The act of eating stimulates these areas and provides both comfort and sensory stimulation. So do childhood thumb-sucking and adult kissing.

Even the process of elimination and social constraints and rules around passage of intestinal gas becomes important. Is a belch rude behavior best kept in private or a compliment for a good meal? One cause of chronic constipation in Western society is the social stigma involved with the act of a bowel movement.

Food itself is interesting. Whether the food source is plant or animal, the life force is transferred from one being to another. It is the giving of one life for the continuation of another. "What greater gift is there than laying down your life for another?" is an inspiring quote. Human beings are at the top of the food chain. Regardless of what we eat, many lives—plant and animal—have been sacrificed so we may live. Ancient people and those who still attempt to live in the old ways remember this. The act of asking for a blessing on the food is the ritual of respect and honoring of the life force given so we may live.

As the parts and process of the digestive system are explored ever so briefly in this text, the student would do well to remember the bigger picture involved with the intake of food and water, and the process of receiving energy from one so that another may live.

ORGANS OF THE DIGESTIVE SYSTEM

The digestive system is one long tube with accessory organs that starts at the mouth and extends through the body to end at the anus (Figure 12-3). This tube is known as the *gastrointestinal tract,* or *GI tract,* also referred to as the *alimentary canal.* The GI tract is about 30 feet long and contains several special structures throughout its length. The entire lining is a mucous membrane made up of three layers of tissues: epithelium, connective tissue, and smooth muscle.

The digestive tract consists of the mouth, pharynx, esophagus, stomach, small intestine, large intestine, rectum, and anus. Accessory structures include the salivary glands, pancreas, liver, and gallbladder. The stomach and 24 to 30 feet of intestines lie in the abdominal cavity.

The abdomen, or abdominal cavity, contains the major organs of digestion. The cavity is lined with a mucous membrane that prevents friction called the *peritoneum.* The portion of the peritoneum lying against the body wall is the parietal peritoneum; the

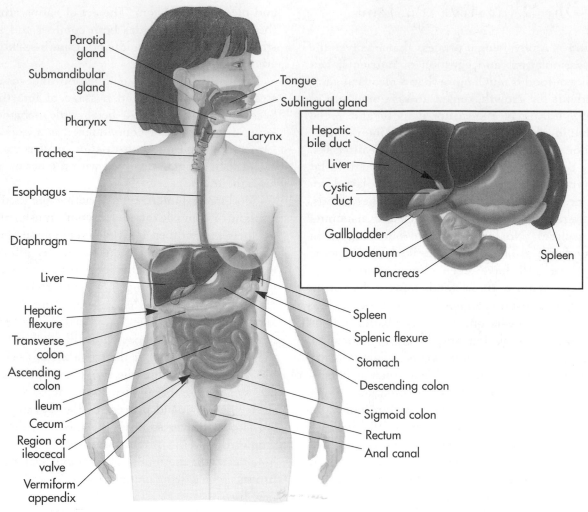

FIGURE 12-3   Location of digestive organs. (From Thibodeau GA, Patton KT: *The human body in health and disease*, ed 2, St Louis, 1997, Mosby.)

portion surrounding each organ is the visceral peritoneum. The intestines are suspended by a double layer of peritoneum: the mesentery (small intestine) and the mesocolon (transverse colon). Another double layer is the greater omentum (from the stomach to the transverse colon). Fat stored in the greater omentum accounts for much of the girth in obesity. The lesser omentum runs from the stomach and duodenum to the liver.

Mouth

The mouth is the oral cavity and makes up the first portion of the gastrointestinal tract. It includes the lips, cheeks, tongue, hard and soft palate, teeth, and salivary glands.

The tongue is a large strong muscle that mixes the food particles with saliva and helps us swallow. It also contains the taste buds.

The palate forms the roof of the mouth. The anterior hard part is the partition between the oral and nasal cavity and is made up of the palatine and maxillae bones. The posterior soft portion is the partition between the oropharynx and nasopharynx.

Teeth are accessory structures used to bite off and mechanically break up large pieces of food into smaller ones that can be swallowed. These bonelike structures are actually calcified connective tissue covered with enamel.

Salivary glands are located inside the mouth and provide secretions that keep the mucous membrane of the mouth moist and moisten and lubricate food to aid in swallowing. Saliva is mainly water mixed with a small amount of salts and organic substances. One of these is the enzyme amylase, which breaks down carbohydrates. Smell, sight, taste, and the thought of food stimulate parasympathetic fibers to increase the secretion of saliva. When the food is mechanically chewed, chemically broken down, and mixed with water, it is referred to as a *bolus*.

Pharynx

The pharynx is a cavity located behind the mouth that receives the bolus from the mouth.

Esophagus (Gullet)

A 10-inch, muscular, collapsible tube, directly behind the trachea, extending from the pharynx to the stomach. The opening into the stomach is the esophageal hiatus, and at the point of attachment is a thickened region called the *cardiac sphincter*, which keeps the entrance to the stomach closed and prevents gastric regurgitation.

Stomach

The stomach is a J-shaped, saclike organ that is actually an enlargement of the GI tract. Its widest part is located beneath the diaphragm. The narrow, distal end lies under the liver and empties into the duodenum. The bolus is received from the esophagus and the digestion process continues. As more liquids are added and the bolus breaks down, it becomes a semiliquid that is known as *chyme*. The stomach contains folds called *rugae* that enable the stomach to expand as food is ingested. The walls of the stomach contain gastric glands that secrete the hormone gastrin and gastric juices, including hydrochloric acid, enzymes, mucus, and water. The pylorus is the part of the stomach that narrows to connect with the duodenum. The stomach ends at the pyloric sphincter, a muscle that regulates the flow of chyme into the small intestine. Some gastric cells have histamine receptors. Irritation of the stomach appears to liberate histamine, a potent stimulator of gastric acid secretion. Cimetidine (Tagamet) competes with histamine for receptor sites, thus blocking the secretion of acid and making it an effective medication for treating ulcers.

Small Intestine

The small intestine is a coiled, muscular tube approximately 24 to 30 feet long. The small intestine receives the chyme from the stomach and continues the digestive process using intestinal juices from the small intestine and secretions from the pancreas, liver, and gallbladder to carry out digestion. The small intestine consists of three parts.

The **duodenum** is the shortest portion, making up the first 10 inches of the small intestine. It forms a C-shaped curve, circling the head of the pancreas where it turns into the jejunum. Ducts from the liver, gallbladder, and pancreas enter this structure.

The **jejunum** continues from the duodenum for the next 7 to 8 feet. It is supplied with blood vessels, lymph vessels, and nerves by a fold in the peritoneum called the *mesentery*. Numerous glands located in the walls of the jejunum provide secretions to the digestive process, the primary function of the jejunum. Most of the absorption of foodstuffs takes place in the jejunum, with some in the ileum.

The **ileum** makes up the final 12 feet of the small intestine. It connects the small intestine to the large intestine at the ileocecal valve, a sphincter. Mesenteries support the ileum and provide the means for blood vessels, lymph vessels, and nerves to supply the ileum. Absorption of food into the bloodstream and the lymphatic system is the major function of the ileum.

Pancreas

The pancreas is a long gland (about 5 inches by 1 inch). It lies behind the stomach and is connected to the duodenum by two pancreatic ducts. Most of the pancreas functions as an endocrine gland by producing digestive enzymes called *pancreatic juices*. About 1% of the cells of the pancreas, the islets of Langerhans, are scattered throughout the pancreas and secrete the hormones insulin, glucagon, and somatostatin.

Liver

The largest gland of the body, weighing about 3 pounds, the liver lies under the diaphragm. It has many important functions, including the following:

1. Active in protein metabolism
2. Breaks down fatty acids and stores the fat we need as fuel
3. Removes glucose from the blood and stores it as glycogen when blood sugar levels are high; converts it back to glucose when blood sugar levels are low
4. Secretes bile, which is important in the digestion of fats
5. Stores vitamins A, B_{12}, D, E, and K and iron and copper
6. Detoxifies the blood by removing drugs or hormones
7. Converts amino acids into glucose or fatty acids, depending on the body's needs
8. Destroys old red and white blood cells

Gallbladder

The gallbladder is a small 3- to 4-inch sac that lies on the undersurface of the liver; its function is to store and concentrate bile. The gallbladder releases bile into the small intestine by way of the cystic duct.

Large Intestine

The large intestine is a large muscular tube, about 4 to 5 feet long and 2½ inches in diameter. The large intestine has few digestive functions but does serve to reabsorb water and electrolytes, manufacture vitamins, and form and store the feces until defecation occurs. The large intestine, also called the *colon*, consists of eight parts.

The **cecum** begins as a blind pouch about 3 inches long and receives the digestive matter from the ileum of the small intestine.

The **appendix** is a narrow, twisted, close-ended tube that is attached to the cecum. It contains lymphatic tissue, but its function has not been clearly defined.

The **ascending colon** goes up on the right side of the abdomen to the underside of the liver, where it curves toward the left. This curve is known as the *hepatic flexure.*

The **transverse colon** goes across the abdomen from the hepatic flexure to the spleen, where it turns downward at the splenic flexure.

The **descending colon** extends down the left side of the body from the splenic flexure to about the top of the iliac crest.

The **sigmoid colon** forms an S-shaped curve beginning at the left iliac crest and continuing to the middle of the abdomen, where it connects the descending colon to the rectum.

The **rectum** is a straight, 5- to 6-inch continuation of the sigmoid colon, beginning at about the level of S3.

The **anal canal** is the last inch of the rectum, and it ends at the anus, a sphincter muscle of both smooth and skeletal muscle that controls the involuntary and voluntary elimination of feces.

The main function of the colon is the absorption of water and sodium.

Undigested matter passes as feces. The brown color of stool results from the breakdown products of bile pigments. Large numbers of bacteria are found in the colon. They may have a role in the production of vitamins.

Medicines are often given as rectal suppositories because the colon has great absorptive capacity.

A colostomy is an artificial opening between the colon and skin of the abdomen for the evacuation of feces. Usually done to relieve tumor obstruction, it is occasionally a temporary measure when inflammation or trauma is present.

Nerves

Parasympathetic stimulation from the vagus and pelvic nerves (from the sacral part of the spinal cord) increases peristalsis and secretion of mucus, which protects the intestinal wall. Sympathetic stimulation has the opposite effect.

DIGESTION

The function of the digestive system is to break down foods to be assimilated by the body. Digestion begins in the mouth and ends in the small intestine. It is accompanied by digestive enzymes (protein catalysts) that split large substances into small ones. The gastrointestinal tract contains glands that secrete mucus and digestive enzymes. Products of digestion are propelled along the tract from the esophagus to the anus by the rhythmic contraction of smooth muscle called **peristalsis.**

The four essential steps in the process of digestion are shown in Box 12-1.

NUTRITION

Nutrition is the use of food for growth and maintenance of the body. Poor nutrition has an effect on general health, stress response, and sleeping. In the elderly, decreased ability to digest and assimilate food accounts for much of their poor nutrition. Others may have diseases that can cause nutritional deficiencies. For most of us, our nutritional problems result from not following dietary recommendations. This is because nutrition involves food. Food involves eating. Eating affects the mood. Mood influ-

---

BOX 12-1

STEPS IN THE DIGESTION PROCESS

First step—**Ingestion:** Food entering the mouth (i.e., eating)

Second step—**Digestion:** The mechanical and chemical breakdown of food from its complex form into simple molecules

Third step—**Absorption:** The movement of the simple molecules from the digestive tract into the circulatory or lymphatic systems; vitamins and minerals are absorbed in the small intestine; amino acids, simple sugars, and small fatty acids pass through the intestinal villi into the bloodstream; larger fatty acids are reconstituted to fats in the intestinal wall and pass into the lymphatic system; capillaries of the intestinal villi become venules, then veins, and, finally, the large portal vein carries absorbed foodstuffs to the liver; the liver converts these substances into compounds required for body functions

Fourth step—**Elimination** (Egestion): Removal and release by defecation of solid waste products from food that cannot be digested or absorbed

ences feelings. Behavior supports feelings, and the whole issue of food is often an emotional topic.

The basics of good nutrition include eating a diet high in vegetables, grains, legumes, and fruit that is fresh, clean, and grown on nutrient-rich soil. Our protein requirement is moderate and may be met from animal or nonanimal sources. Fat and sugar requirements in the diet are small, but humans have a strong urge for sweets and fats. It is this instinctive craving for fat and sugar that causes many of our dietary problems. An ideal diet is low to moderate in fats and sugars, moderate in protein, with the bulk of the calories coming from complex carbohydrates. These recommendations can vary because differing genetic predisposition, age, and health can influence the ratio of fat, protein, and carbohydrate that best suits an individual.

The food we eat is only as good as the soil it is grown in or the food the animals were fed. Many suggest that much of the soil used in agriculture is worn out, depleted, and toxic from the continued use of artificial fertilizers and pesticides and overuse without rest time to replenish itself. If this is the condition of the soil, what is the nutritional value of the food grown on it? Food is most nutritious when freshly harvested and ripe. Food eaten a day after harvest will have lost a substantial amount of nutrients. Food, mostly fruit, picked green will not be as nutritious as fruit allowed to ripen on the vine. Food preservation methods all result in loss of nutritional value in the food. Under ideal conditions, we would harvest all of our food an hour before we eat, but this is not possible for most of us. We have to make a tradeoff between convenience and nutrition in many cases.

Many people take nutritional supplements, and many opinions exist on this topic. It is important to remember that these are supplements to our diet and should not be expected to replace proper food intake. The closer a supplement is to a "real food" the better it is able to be used by the body. Supplements are usually best taken with food to maximize absorption and use.

Drinking enough pure water is very important to optimal body function. Recommendations are for at least 64 ounces of water per day for efficient body function.

Main Food Groups
Proteins
Proteins are large high–molecular-weight substances containing carbon, hydrogen, oxygen, and nitrogen, as well as smaller amounts of other elements. Proteins break down into amino acids, which are then absorbed. The body uses 24 amino acids for its metabolic requirements. Most can be manufactured in the liver from other amino acids, but eight cannot. These are referred to as essential amino acids: phenylalanine, valine, threonine, leucine, isoleucine, methionine, tryptophan, and lysine. In addition, histidine and arginine are required for growth and development. Dietary proteins include animal products and bean and grain combinations.

Proteins are the chief structural components of the body. Enzymes, some hormones, muscle tissue, and a substantial portion of chromosomes are proteins. Proteins are essential components of the cell membrane. Important compounds such as epinephrine and acetylcholine are derived from amino acids.

Carbohydrates
Carbohydrates (CHO) have, as basic components, carbon, hydrogen, and oxygen in definite proportions. Complex carbohydrates are long chains of glucose molecules found in rice, vegetables, and so on. Animal starch or glycogen is the storage form of glucose in liver and muscle. Starch is digested in the mouth and small intestine and breaks down into monosaccharides and disaccharides, which are sugars or simple carbohydrates.

Glucose is the main fuel for the manufacture of adenosine triphosphate (ATP) in the cell. Sugars are converted to glucose in the liver. In some infants the enzyme that converts galactose to glucose is missing. Galactose from milk accumulates in tissues (galactosemia), a condition that may result in brain damage. Treatment is the use of a milk substitute.

Fats
The common fats or triglycerides break down into fatty acids and glycerol. A fatty acid is a molecule consisting of a chain of carbons, with no double-bonds (saturated) or several double-bonds (unsaturated). The unsaturated fats most closely resemble body fat and are more easily assimilated and used. Saturation (addition of hydrogen molecules) makes fat more solid and less desirable in the diet. Linoleic acid is an example of a fatty acid essential to human nutrition. In addition to serving as a reservoir of stored energy, fats are essential components of many hormones, the cell membrane, and the myelin sheath of the nerve fiber. Dietary fats are found in nuts, seeds, oils, and animal products.

Vitamins and minerals
Vitamins are growth factors needed in small amounts for daily body metabolism. They are classified as "fat

soluble" or "water soluble." Many vitamins act as enzyme activators (coenzymes). The fat-soluble vitamins are more toxic because the water-soluble ones are absorbed and excesses excreted more easily. Hypervitaminosis A (excessive intake of vitamin A) causes headache, as well as nausea, vomiting, vertigo, and bone pain. Hypervitaminosis D is sometimes seen in people who drink large quantities of milk. The increased vitamin D causes calcium to precipitate in the soft tissues of the body.

PATHOLOGY

Appendicitis

Appendicitis is an inflammation of the appendix usually from bacterial infection. Signs and symptoms begin with discomfort in the umbilical region that becomes pain localized in the lower right quadrant, fever, nausea, and vomiting. The appendix may be inflamed, abscessed, or it may burst. If it bursts, the pain initially decreases because of the pressure release, but the bacteria are spread to the abdominal cavity, resulting in peritonitis or infection of the peritoneal membrane that can be fatal.

Cirrhosis

Cirrhosis is the infiltration of connective tissue into the functioning cells of the liver that causes slow deterioration of the liver. The most common cause is alcoholism, although it is also seen in hepatitis. Many systemic functions are interrupted. If not too far advanced and causal factors can be eliminated, liver regeneration capacity is good.

Colon Cancer

Colon cancer is the most common cancer overall and usually affects the lowest part of the rectum. Males and females are equally susceptible. Tumors of the ascending colon (right-sided) usually cause rectal bleeding; those in the descending colon cause constipation and obstructive symptoms. Polyps and ulcerative colitis are important risk factors. Screening for blood in the stool, as well as sigmoidoscopy, detects most lesions; 70% are located in the sigmoid colon and rectum. Surgical removal of the bowel or removal of a section of the bowel with the ends reattached to maintain a passageway is often curative.

Constipation

Constipation is difficulty passing stools or an incomplete or infrequent passage of hard stool. Among the organic causes are intestinal obstruction, diverticulitis, and tumors. Functional impairment of the colon may occur in elderly or bedridden clients who fail to respond to the urge to defecate. Backache and headache may be present. Constipation or diarrhea are common side effects of many medications. Increase in fluid and dietary bulk and exercise are helpful, and stool softeners may be prescribed for the constipation. Education about regular bowel habits may be necessary.

Cystic Fibrosis

Cystic fibrosis is a genetic disease involving exocrine gland dysfunction. Secretions from the pancreas, mucus glands of the respiratory tract, and sweat glands are defective. When pancreatic enzymes are not produced, food cannot be broken down, so fats and nutrients will not be absorbed. Rarely does a child survive beyond his teens; most die from pulmonary infections. Treatment is a high-protein, high-caloric diet, accompanied by the replacement of pancreatic enzymes. Antibiotics, inhalation, and physical therapy are useful. Continuous home pulmonary care is often necessary.

Diverticular Disease

Diverticula are small, sac-like outpouchings of the intestinal wall found in weak areas of the colon near where vessels are located. Most occur in the sigmoid colon. When multiple diverticula are present, the condition is diverticulosis. If they become inflamed and infected, it is diverticulitis. Perforation of a diverticular sac may cause peritonitis, the inflammation of the peritoneum. Symptoms are similar to irritable bowel syndrome. Primary treatment consists of a high-fiber diet, increased intake of fluids, a bulk-forming laxative such as psyllium (Metamucil), and an antibiotic. In severe cases, hospitalization may be required.

Gallbladder Disease

Gallbladder disease is almost always the result of a gallstone composed of bile salts and/or cholesterol lodged in the cystic duct. A fatty meal often precedes an attack because the presence of fat stimulates contraction of the gallbladder. Signs and symptoms are as follows:

- Pain in the right upper quadrant of the abdomen, often radiating to the right scapula or upper back
- Nausea and vomiting
- Fever

Mild cases are treated with an analgesic. Fatty foods are eliminated from the diet. If infection is present, antibiotics are used. Surgical removal of the gallbladder may be necessary.

Gastroenteritis

Gastroenteritis is a general term for irritation, inflammation, and/or infection of the GI tract. If the stomach is involved, the condition is gastritis. Hemorrhagic gastritis is characterized by bleeding erosions. This condition is also called *acute erosive gastritis* or *multiple gastric erosions* and can occur without any apparent reason. It is associated, however, with aspirin ingestion, burns, traumatic injury, surgery, shock, liver disease, respiratory problems, and septicemia. It can cause vomiting and diarrhea and lead to dehydration. Gastroenteritis can become dangerous if infectious organisms or toxic substances enter the bloodstream.

If the intestine is affected, it is enteritis. Usually both the stomach and intestine are involved, so the term *gastroenteritis* is used. The most common cause is a virus. It can be passed from person to person. This "stomach flu" usually lasts 24 to 36 hours. If the cause is a bacterial toxin, the condition is food poisoning. Occasionally, it is caused by a bacterial infection, and rarely it is caused by a protozoal infection (dysentery). Diarrhea and generalized cramping abdominal pain are symptoms of the condition. Food poisoning from toxic foods, poisonous mushrooms, and so on is implicated in many cases. The inflammation may also be the result of illness or dietary changes, especially when eating foods or drinking water while traveling to foreign countries, or the result of extended use of antibiotics. Primary treatment is rehydration and relaxing the hyperactive bowel. Fluids only for 24 hours relax the intestine because food stimulates gastrointestinal hormone release and peristalsis. Several compounds slow the bowel: bismuth subsalicylate (Pepto-Bismol), diphenoxylate with atropine (Lomotil), and anticholinergic antispasmodics such as dicyclomine (Bentyl). If a stool culture shows a bacterial or protozoal infection, an antibiotic or antiprotozoal is given.

Hepatitis

Hepatitis is an infection of the liver. It is discussed in the immune section of Chapter 11.

Hemorrhoids

Hemorrhoids are dilated varicose veins of the anus. They often appear during pregnancy and delivery. External hemorrhoids lie distal to the anorectal margin; internal hemorrhoids lie proximal. Occasionally, a thrombus or clot forms, resulting in a painful, bluish mass. Hemorrhoids may cause pain, but the usual symptom is bleeding and/or itching caused by drying up of the protective mucus. Primary treatment is with sitz baths, suppositories, and stool soft-eners. The clot may be surgically removed under local anesthesia. Hemorrhoids may also be treated with a laser to seal the blood vessels, with cryosurgery, injection, or surgical removal.

Hernia

A hernia is the protrusion of soft tissues through a tear or weak spot in a muscle wall. They can occur anywhere but are most common in the abdomen. In a hiatal hernia the intestines bulge through an opening in the diaphragm. In an inguinal hernia there is a bulging of the abdominal organs or the inguinal canal. A reducible hernia means that the bulge can be pressed back through the opening. An irreducible hernia cannot be replaced and obstruction or strangulation may occur.

Inflammatory Bowel Disease

Two inflammatory diseases of the GI tract affect mainly young men and women, ages 20 to 40, causing ulcerative lesions and thickening of the intestinal wall. The cause for both is unknown, but an autoimmunity may be a factor. Ulcerative colitis primarily affects the sigmoid colon, with symptoms of lower abdominal pain and bloody diarrhea. Ulcers actually develop inside the large intestine. Regional enteritis is a chronic inflammation of the intestine, most commonly the ileum. It is known as *Crohn's disease*, and presents symptoms of cramping, right lower quadrant (RLQ) pain, and intermittent diarrhea. There may be one or two attacks, or they can occur regularly. Nutrients are not absorbed, and weight is lost. Primary treatment for both is an adequate diet, antibiotic therapy, and steroids. Occasionally surgical removal of the ileum is necessary.

Irritable Bowel Syndrome

Irritable bowel syndrome is also known as *spastic*, or *irritable, colon*. Symptoms include abdominal pain, alternating constipation and diarrhea, nausea, and gas. It can be brought on by poor diet, tension, and emotional problems. Peristaltic action is not well coordinated and results in changes in the pattern of bowel movements. Primary treatment includes a diet high in bran, restriction of alcohol and tobacco, a psyllium laxative such as Metamucil, and perhaps an anticholinergic tranquilizer such as Librax. A comprehensive stress management program is beneficial.

Malabsorption and Intolerance Syndromes

Malabsorption syndromes involve poor absorption of

nutrients. They can be caused by deficiency of digestive enzymes, inadequate transport of nutrients, or abnormalities in the structure of the intestine either through disease or surgery, and hypersensitivity reaction to a particular food. Wheat, corn, and dairy are the most common foods, and elimination diets may be beneficial. Malabsorption can be a result of cystic fibrosis, diabetes mellitus, or dietary intolerance such as celiac disease, a reaction to dietary gluten, or lactose intolerance as a result of lactose deficiency.

Obstructions

An obstruction is a partial or complete closure of the small or large intestine. As a result chyme backs up, the intestinal walls expand, local arteries may be compressed, and ischemic bowel disease can result. Obstructions are caused by any of the following:

- Adhesion—Bands of fibrous tissue from previous inflammation or surgical scars that grow between and around the loops of intestine and can cause strangulation
- Hernia—A protrusion of the intestine though a weakness in the abdominal wall; if the loop of intestine becomes trapped or strangulated, a medical emergency exists
- Tumors—Growths such as are seen in colon cancer can obstruct the intestine
- Volvulus—A knotting or twisting causing strangulation in the intestine

Pancreatitis

Most cases of acute pancreatitis involve alcoholism and gallstones. Lipase, amylase, and trypsin (digestive enzymes) back up in the pancreas and are released into the surrounding tissue. This causes autodigestion of the pancreas and necrosis of tissues, including the peritoneum. Hemorrhage and shock may develop. Massive destruction of tissue accompanied by fluid and blood loss may lead to shock and death. Signs and symptoms include the following:

- Intense pain in the center of the upper abdomen radiating to the back
- Nausea and vomiting
- Distended, tender, and bruised abdomen; the person feels better sitting than lying
- Elevated amylase and lipase levels in the bloodstream

Acute pancreatitis is a medical emergency. If suspected, immediate referral is necessary.

Chronic pancreatitis may occur after acute pancreatitis, gallstones, or alcohol abuse. Pancreatic function decreases and ultimately stops, so insulin and other pancreatic enzymes and hormones are not produced. There may be intense pain, and surgery may be needed to remove the pancreas or sever the nerves.

Peptic Ulcer Disease

A peptic ulcer is a gastric or duodenal ulcer that affects the lining of the esophagus, stomach, or duodenum. The sore can perforate the wall of the digestive tract. *Peptic ulcer disease (PUD)* is the name given to the process. The term *peptic* means that pepsin is involved. Risk factors include being male, smoking, heredity, alcohol, and stress. An increased secretion of hydrochloric acid (HCl) and pepsin, as well as decreased tissue resistance, contributes to the process. The normal protective mechanisms of the duodenal and gastric mucosa against HCl and pepsin are blocked. Excessive vagal stimulation is present. The ulcer causes pain and may erode into a vessel and cause bleeding. It may perforate through the intestinal or stomach wall, causing peritonitis and shock. Recent studies indicate a bacterial infection may cause many ulcers and treatment involves the use of antibiotics.

Common signs and symptoms include the following:

- Heartburn or burning pain ½ hour to 2 hours after a meal, relieved by antacids
- Vomiting of brownish-black–colored material (the color of coffee grounds) or the passage of dark stools, indicating the presence of blood
- Tenderness on palpation of the epigastric region of the abdomen
- Nausea, weight loss, and decreased appetite

Antacids such as magnesium–aluminum hydroxide mixtures (Maalox, Mylanta) are useful. Cimetidine (Tagamet) or ranitidine (Zantac) inhibit gastric acid secretion. Stopping smoking, decreasing or stopping alcohol consumption, and employing stress-management techniques are also indicated.

Reflux Esophagitis

Reflux esophagitis is the regurgitation of gastric acid up through an open esophageal sphincter, causing heartburn. It may be caused by a hiatal hernia. The discomfort is often aggravated when lying flat or bending over and relieved when sitting upright. It is frequently seen in obese people. Inflammation or ulceration of the esophagus is present. Primary treatment is weight loss to decrease the pressure on the abdominal structures and relieve the hiatal hernia, and an antacid.

Stomach Cancer

Stomach cancer is one of the more common causes of cancer death. Causal factors include exposure to environmental chemicals and chronic gastritis. Onset is slow and insidious with little advanced warning or detection mechanisms. Indigestion appears; other signs and symptoms are unexplained weight loss, epigastric pain, palpable upper abdominal mass, and iron-deficiency anemia from gastric bleeding.

INDICATIONS **CONTRAINDICATIONS**

For Soft Tissue and Movement Therapies

A client with abdominal pain or referred back pain may have one of several gastrointestinal disorders. In such cases referral is necessary for proper diagnosis. Many gastrointestinal diseases are bacterial or viral and contagious. Appropriate precautions need to be taken to maintain sanitary practice.

Most chronic gastrointestinal diseases have a strong correlation to stress. The intestinal tract is highly responsive to changes in autonomic function and endocrine patterns. Sympathetic arousal changes peristaltic action and can send the intestinal tract into all kinds of dysfunction. Comprehensive stress management programs, including soft tissue and movement methods, are often effective in the management of these conditions. Ginger is an herb that has been shown to be soothing to the digestive system.

A specific type of massage to the large intestine can assist in managing constipation. This method can be taught to the client for self-care. It is contraindicated in inflammatory bowel disease, and permission should be obtained from the physician for any other conditions. The massage consists of short scooping strokes firmly against the abdomen beginning on the left, always directed toward the rectum. Progress continues the length of the large intestine to the cecum in a fashion of two steps forward and one step back as the direction of the force is down and back toward the rectum. Beginning at the cecum on the right may push fecal material into a large mass especially at the flexure (Figure 12-4) (Activity 12-2).

Text continues on p. 540.

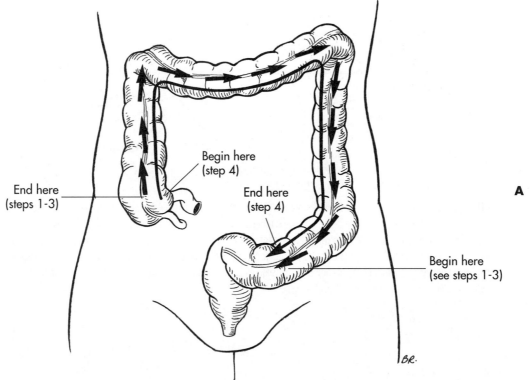

A

End here
(steps 1-3)

Begin here
(step 4)

End here
(step 4)

Begin here
(see steps 1-3)

FIGURE 12-4 A, Colon with flow pattern arrows. All massage manipulations are to be directed in a clockwise fashion. The manipulations begin in the lower right-hand quadrant (on the right side as you view the illustration) at the sigmoid colon. The methods progressively contact all of the large intestine as they eventually end up encompassing the entire colon area. (Modified from Fritz S: *Mosby's fundamentals of therapeutic massage,* St Louis, 1995, Mosby.)   *Continued*

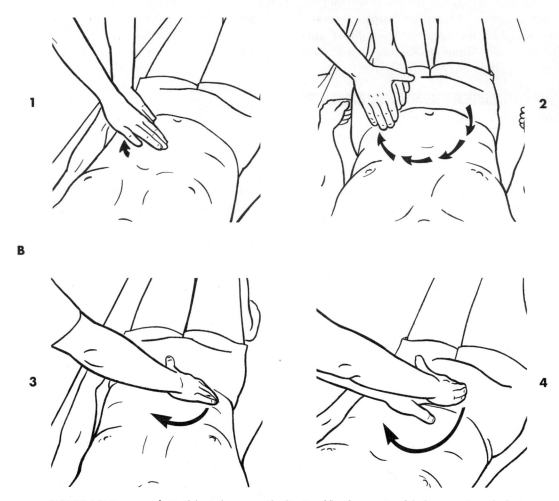

FIGURE 12-4—cont'd B, Abdominal sequence. The direction of flow for emptying of the large intestine and colon is: *1,* Massage down the left side of the descending colon using short strokes directed to the sigmoid colon. *2,* Massage across along the transverse colon to the left side using short strokes directed to the sigmoid colon. *3,* Massage up the ascending colon on the right side of the body using short strokes directed to the sigmoid colon. End at the right side ileocecal valve located in the lower right-hand quadrant of the abdomen. *4,* Massage entire flow pattern using long light strokes to moderate strokes from ileocecal valve to sigmoid colon. Repeat sequence.

ACTIVITY 12-2

It is important to be able to explain and justify the therapeutic value of the work we do. The following activity will assist you in developing the skills to explain the effectiveness of various modalities to clients and other health care professionals. Use the clinical reasoning model that follows to accomplish this task. The focus should be your primary modality or modalities applied to the digestive system. An example is provided in the section opener on p. 450.

Modality/modalities

1. What are the facts?

a. Which system is involved, and which structures of that system can be reached directly or indirectly?

b. Which of these structures are most affected by this modality?

c. Which physiologic functions are affected by this approach?

d. When the treatment is applied, what changes in function will result in
(1) This system

(2) The whole body

e. What is considered normal or balanced function?

f. How are the functions of this system related to the body's homeostasis?

g. What has worked or has not worked?

h. Where could you find information that would support the use of this modality as a therapeutic intervention?

i. What research is available to support the use of the therapeutic intervention?

Continued

ACTIVITY 12-2—cont'd

j. How does the intervention support a healthy state?

k. Under which pathologic or dysfunctional conditions is the intervention most likely to be beneficial?

2. What are the possibilities?

a. What do the data suggest?

b. What are the reasons for using the proposed methods?

c. What are the possible interventions?

d. List at least three applications of this modality that would affect both the structure and function of this system.

e. What are other ways to look at the situation?

f. What other methods could provide similar benefits?

3. What is the logical outcome of therapeutic intervention?

a. What would be the logical progression of the symptom pattern, contributing factors, and current behaviors?

b. What are the benefits and drawbacks of each intervention suggested?
   Benefits:

ACTIVITY 12-2—cont'd

Drawbacks:

b. Does the practitioner feel qualified to work with the situation and apply the identified modality to the particular situation?

c. What are the costs in terms of time, resources, and finances?

c. Does a feeling of cooperation and agreement exist among all those involved, and how would the practitioner recognize this feeling?

d. What is likely to happen if the modality is not used?

e. What is likely to happen if the modality is used?

Justification

Using the information developed in the clinical reasoning model, present a clear, concise statement of the ways in which the particular soft tissue or movement modality would be beneficial, either in supporting the particular body system in a healthy condition or as part of a treatment plan for a pathologic or dysfunctional condition. Based on the above information, give a brief summary of the effectiveness of the modality for this system.

4. **For the intervention proposed, what would be the impact on the people involved, specifically the client, practitioner, and other professionals working with the client?**
   a. How does each of the people involved (including, besides those named above, the client's family and support system) feel about the possible interventions?

The Urinary System

The urinary system consists of two kidneys, two ureters, one bladder, and one urethra (Figure 12-5). The kidneys maintain homeostasis by filtering waste products from the blood and keeping the proper amount of water and nutrients in the blood. Urine passes out of the kidneys and down through the ureters to the bladder, where it is stored. When a certain volume is reached, the urge to void is present. Urine is expelled from the bladder through the urethra.

FUNCTIONS OF THE URINARY SYSTEM

The important functions of the urinary system are as follows:

- The conservation of water
- The maintenance of the normal concentration of electrolytes
- The regulation of the acid-base balance
- The regulation of blood pressure
- Activation of vitamin D

Most waste is filtered and eliminated by the kidneys. In the average person about 100 liters of blood is filtered per day; 99 liters of filtrate are reabsorbed, leaving about 1 liter of urine. Substances secreted from the capillaries into the tubular filtrate include hydrogen, potassium, and ammonia.

Micturition (voiding, urination) is a parasympathetic action, modified by voluntary control. It is initiated when afferent impulses from stretch receptors in the bladder stimulate the sacral portion of the spinal cord. The detrusor muscle contracts and the sphincter relaxes.

ORGANS OF THE URINARY SYSTEM

Kidneys

The kidneys are two reddish-brown, bean-shaped organs located on the posterior wall of the abdomen against the back body wall musculature, just above the waist. The kidneys are imbedded in fat and located about the spinal level of T11 to L3 on each side of the vertebral column. The right kidney is lower than the left because of its displacement by the liver. An adrenal gland is found on top of each kidney.

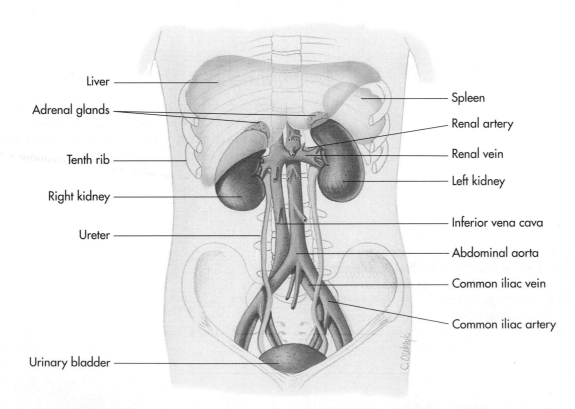

FIGURE 12-5 Urinary system. (From Thibodeau GA, Patton KT: *The human body in health and disease,* ed 2, St Louis, 1997, Mosby.)

The inside of a kidney is divided into a *cortex*, *medulla*, and *pelvis*. The cortex and medulla contain approximately one million *nephrons*, specialized tube-shaped filters that reabsorb or excrete substances to form urine. A nephron consists of a *glomerulus*, which is composed of a group of capillaries, and a renal tubule. Water and small solids from the blood pass across the membrane of the capillaries and enter the tubule. They enter the renal tubules, and travel through smaller loops and tubules to the collecting cups. Necessary substances such as water and electrolytes are returned to the blood while the urine drains through ducts and eventually reaches the ureters.

The renal artery, renal vein, and ureters enter or exit the kidney at the renal hilus. Although both sympathetic and parasympathetic nerve fibers are present in the kidney, the important component is sympathetic, causing vasoconstriction and the release of renin, a substance important in blood pressure control.

Several hormones affect the kidneys. The kidneys also function as endocrine glands, producing erythropoietin, a hormone released in response to lowered levels of oxygen in the blood. It stimulates the bone marrow to produce more red blood cells. The kidneys also contribute to the acid-base balance.

Ureters

The ureters are two narrow tubes extending from the kidney and connecting to the bladder. The two ureters lie in the psoas muscles. Each is a tube about 12 inches in length and $\frac{1}{8}$ to $\frac{1}{4}$ inch in diameter and abundantly supplied with nerves. Peristalsis moves urine down into the bladder. Ureter walls contain muscle cells that help move the urine into the bladder. As the bladder fills, it presses against the ureters, compressing them, and thus preventing a reverse flow of urine.

Bladder (Urinary Bladder)

The bladder is a muscular, baglike organ that lies in the pelvis and acts as a reservoir for urine. Urine flows continuously into the bladder from the ureters until a sufficient quantity of urine is collected for disposal through the urethra. When it is distended with about a cup of urine, the signal to empty the bladder occurs and a muscle called the *detrusor muscle* causes the bladder to contract.

Urethra

The urethra is the tube that carries urine from the bladder. The male urethra is about 8 inches long and serves to pass both urine and semen. The female urethra is about 1½ inches long, lies anterior to the vagina, and functions only to pass urine. The opening at the end of the urethra is called the *meatus*. The close proximity of the female urethra to the anus allows anal bacteria to migrate up the urethra to the bladder, ureters, and kidneys, predisposing females to ascending urinary tract infections.

PATHOLOGY

Bladder Infections

A bladder infection (cystitis) is a common infection that occurs most often in females. In women it is usually caused by bacteria in the bladder that spreads from the perineal region. Symptoms include pain in the lower abdomen, stinging or burning during urination, frequent urination (frequency) with only small amounts released, and a continuous sometimes uncontrollable urge to urinate (urgency). Antibiotics such as nitrofurantoin (Macrodantin), sulfa-containing agents such as trimethoprim/sulfamethoxazole (Bactrim, Septra), and synthetic penicillins (ampicillin or amoxicillin) are effective. Cranberry juice also seems to be beneficial in management of bladder infection.

Glomerulonephritis

Glomerulonephritis is a group of diseases involving antigen-antibody reactions affecting the glomeruli. The antigen may be an external one such as beta-hemolytic streptococci, or it may involve an autoimmune reaction. The most common type is poststreptococcal, in which antibodies are formed that react with streptococci. Immune complexes are deposited in the glomeruli. The condition may follow a "strep" infection such as pharyngitis, tonsillitis, or impetigo. For mild cases without bacterial infections, treatment is bed rest and salt restriction. Antibiotics are used if the cause is streptococcal, whereas immunosuppressant medications or steroids may be needed with autoimmune reactions.

Incontinence

Urinary incontinence is the inability to control urination and is most often caused by weak pelvic floor muscles or nerve damage. Causal factors include age, infection, obesity, brain or spinal cord lesion, damage to the nerve to the bladder, or injury to the sphincter usually occurring during childbirth. Stress incontinence is urine leakage during coughing, straining, sneezing, and so on when stress is placed on the muscles. This condition benefits from strengthening the pelvic floor muscles. Urge incontinence is a feeling of needing to void frequently. This condition may be caused by irritation or infection. It is also found in women during or after menopause because a decrease in the amount of estrogen in the body can weaken these muscles.

Kidney Failure

Kidney failure, also known as *renal failure*, is the inability to excrete waste products and retain electrolytes. In acute kidney failure, the kidneys suddenly stop working, frequently because of acute glomerulonephritis, allergic reactions to medications, shock, or obstruction. Waste products back up in the blood. This may cause hypertension, itching caused by the accumulation of waste products in the blood vessels of the skin, edema, and dehydration. When excess amounts of nitrogen wastes build up in the blood, that condition is known as *uremia*. Chronic kidney failure is caused by a gradual decrease in kidney function, often as a result of inflammation, glomerulonephritis, or diabetes mellitus. As in the acute stage, the kidneys are unable to excrete waste products or water, and these substances back up in the blood and tissues. In the chronic stage, scar tissue builds up in the kidneys, and they are unable to function. This leads to end-stage kidney failure in which the kidneys are unable to function at all, a life-threatening situation. The kidneys are damaged, and their functions must be replaced with dialysis, or the structures replaced with a kidney transplant.

Uremia (kidney failure) is the terminal stage of renal insufficiency from any cause, the most common being chronic pyelonephritis and chronic glomerulonephritis. The glomerular filtration rate, tubular absorption, and secretion are decreased. Signs and symptoms include the following:

- Weakness and fatigue from sodium, potassium, and calcium abnormalities such as anemia and acidosis
- Hypertension
- Itching from the accumulation of waste products in skin vessels
- Dehydration from the water loss
- Generalized edema

Treatment includes cautious administration of amino acids, adequate calories, sodium, and calcium, as well as antihypertensive medication. Blood trans-fusions may be necessary. Hemodialysis is the clearing of wastes from blood using an artificial kidney. Kidney transplants are among the most successful of organ transplants. Careful matching of similar blood and genetic types, as well as up-to-date immunosuppressive drug therapy, may result in long-term survival rates.

Kidney Stones

Kidney stones are small crystalline substances that develop in the kidney. Most kidney stones (calculi) consist of calcium, whereas others contain amino acids, uric acids, and other excretory products. The most frequent cause of stone formation is dehydration. Summer months are the time that most kidney stone problems occur. Other factors contributing to stone formation are urinary tract infection, impaired tubular reabsorption of calcium, gout, family history, medications such as diuretics, dietary imbalances, and immobilization. Although most kidney stones are composed of calcium, they usually result from the internal processing of calcium and not excessive intake. Kidney stones are usually undiscovered until one passes into a ureter, causing sudden, excruciating flank pain. Nausea and vomiting may also occur. Treatment includes increasing fluid intake to help pass the stone if it is small enough to pass through the ureters. If the stone is too large, surgical removal may be necessary. As a substitute for surgery, the person may have the stones crushed with an ultrasonic beam or shock-wave.

Obstruction

Obstruction of the urethra, causing retention of urine, is most common in older males who have prostate problems. (This is discussed further in the reproductive section of this chapter.)

Pyelonephritis

Pyelonephritis is an infection of the kidney that affects the nephrons, or filtering units. Bacteria may reach the kidney from the bladder or by spreading through the bloodstream from another infected site such as the tonsils, middle ear, sinuses, or prostate. Common symptoms are flank and back pain, usually on one side, abdominal pain that moves into the groin, and fever, sometimes with chills and nausea. Treatment includes the use of an appropriate antibiotic. If not treated, it may become chronic and lead to kidney failure.

INDICATIONS CONTRAINDICATIONS

For Soft Tissue and Movement Therapies

Soft tissue and movement therapy tends to increase blood volume through the kidneys, both a mechanical and reflexive process. In the healthy individual the filtration process is supported. For those with kidney disease the increased volume can strain the kidney function. General contraindications exist for anyone with kidney disease. Soft tissue and movement modalities may be useful for pain and stress manage-ment, but only with the careful supervision of the treating physician.

Acute infectious processes contraindicate body-work until the infection has run its course. Chronic infection treatment may be supported with these modalities as part of a supervised treatment plan. Stress is a contributing factor to incontinence. Any form of stress management will help somewhat with both stress and urge incontinence. Consideration needs to be given to incontinent clients for frequent and easy access to the restroom (Activity 12-3).

ACTIVITY 12-3

It is important to be able to explain and justify the therapeutic value of the work we do. The following activity will assist you in developing the skills to explain the effectiveness of various modalities to clients and other health care professionals. Use the clinical reasoning model that follows to accomplish this task. The focus should be your primary modality or modalities applied to the urinary system. An example is provided in the section opener on p. 450.

Modality/modalities

1. What are the facts?

a. Which system is involved, and which structures of that system can be reached directly or indirectly?

b. Which of these structures are most affected by this modality?

c. Which physiologic functions are affected by this approach?

d. When the treatment is applied, what changes in function will result in
(1) This system

(2) The whole body

e. What is considered normal or balanced function?

f. How are the functions of this system related to the body's homeostasis?

g. What has worked or has not worked?

Continued

h. Where could you find information that would support the use of this modality as a therapeutic intervention?

b. What are the reasons for using the proposed methods?

c. What are the possible interventions?

i. What research is available to support the use of the therapeutic intervention?

d. List at least three applications of this modality that would affect both the structure and function of this system.

j. How does the intervention support a healthy state?

e. What are other ways to look at the situation?

k. Under which pathologic or dysfunctional conditions is the intervention most likely to be beneficial?

f. What other methods could provide similar benefits?

2. What are the possibilities?

3. What is the logical outcome of therapeutic intervention?
   a. What would be the logical progression of the symptom pattern, contributing factors, and current behaviors?

a. What do the data suggest?

b. What are the benefits and drawbacks of each intervention suggested?
Benefits:

Drawbacks:

c. What are the costs in terms of time, resources, and finances?

d. What is likely to happen if the modality is not used?

e. What is likely to happen if the modality is used?

b. Does the practitioner feel qualified to work with the situation and apply the identified modality to the particular situation?

c. Does a feeling of cooperation and agreement exist among all those involved, and how would the practitioner recognize this feeling?

Justification

Using the information developed in the clinical reasoning model, present a clear, concise statement of the ways in which the particular soft tissue or movement modality would be beneficial, either in supporting the particular body system in a healthy condition or as part of a treatment plan for a pathologic or dysfunctional condition. Based on the above information, give a brief summary of the effectiveness of the modality for this system.

4. **For the intervention proposed, what would be the impact on the people involved, specifically the client, practitioner, and other professionals working with the client?**
   a. How does each of the people involved (including, besides those named above, the client's family and support system) feel about the possible interventions?

The Reproductive System

Continuation of the species is the biologic function of the reproductive system, yet our sexuality is more than reproduction and more than our genitals. This last section, the reproductive system, connects our study of the body back to the beginning, to the cell. The essence of reproduction is the duality of yin/yang and male/female, when at the moment of conception two cells create one whole.

This section focuses on the anatomy of the reproductive organs and the functions of procreation. A study of human sexuality, in its more holistic body/mind/spirit form, is beyond the scope of this text, yet it is important to raise the questions concerning the most intimate of physical acts in its expansive form as a communication of creation energy.

Along with the function of procreation, the sexual act can be identified as a pleasurable function, providing the same rewards as other pleasure functions. The act of sex and orgasm stimulates the same feel-good neurochemicals as other forms of touch, food, and exercise. Sexual arousal is a physiologic response generated primarily through parasympathetic activation—the very same pattern sought in most forms of stress management. Orgasm is a sympathetic autonomic nervous system tensing and relaxing of body-wide proportion.

Yet if the act of sex between human beings is only seen as biologic, what is the motivation in society to elevate the bonds between people who share sexual energy to a spiritual union? What makes sharing our bodies in a sexual union different than sharing a pizza? We do not have the answers, but we do know that the miracle and magic of the human experience is more than a sum of its parts. It is acknowledged that compassion cannot be totally explained by neurotransmitters, healing only by the repair mechanism of connective tissue and cellular division, growth purely by digestion and growth hormone, pain only in terms of neuropathways, anger as autonomic nervous system survival responses, and connectedness as entrainment. The experience of living is more than the biology that supports life, just as the clinical study of reproduction and birth cannot explain love, new life, and the sharing of creative energy. With all this said, it is necessary to understand the anatomy/form and physiology/function in the pure physical sense to be able to comprehend the beauty of the rest.

The human being is actually quite androgynous. Some generally recognized developmental behavioral differences exist between males and females in terms of brain development and function, social motivation, and communication styles, but these are insignificant in terms of general function. The gender differences do not limit what can be done. They are reflected more in the process than in the result. For example, the generic female is more interactive and will tend to problem solve in a group with much discussion of the feelings and satisfaction of those involved. The generic male will more likely problem solve independently, somewhat less concerned with the feelings of people and more concerned with the outcome of the process. Neither process is right or wrong, and women can certainly make decisions independently and men can work effectively in social groups.

The strongest and most obvious differences between males and females is the function and construction of the reproductive systems. It is in this anatomy and physiology that the gender differences are most evident. Even in the differentiation between male and female, a continuity of function exists. The same hormones from the hypothalamus stimulate both ovaries and testes. Musculature is similar, as is nervous system distribution. The main difference lies in development of the sex cells (ovum and sperm), the anatomy required to deliver the sperm to the ovum, and the organs to house the developing infant. The difference is not so prevalent in young children before puberty or in those in their mature years after 60 or so, but during the reproductive years the differences and in some ways the gender behavior are more evident.

THE MALE
REPRODUCTIVE SYSTEM

The male reproductive system is made up of the testicles, epididymis, vas deferens, ejaculatory duct, urethra, penis, and scrotum (Figure 12-6). The two testicles are enclosed in an external sac called the *scrotum*. Tiny seminiferous tubules in the testicles produce sperm.

Sperm travels from the testicles into the epididymis, where the sperm cells mature. Sperm then moves into the vas deferens, which extends upward into the body cavity, over the symphysis pubis and around the urinary bladder to connect with the two seminal vesicles.

The seminal vesicles produce and secrete a viscous fluid that makes up most of the semen and joins with the sperm to pass from the vas deferens into the ejaculatory duct. The ejaculatory duct passes through the prostate gland and joins with the urethra. The

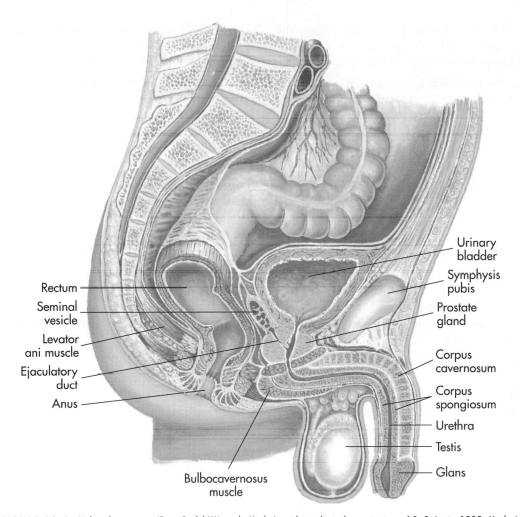

Rectum

Seminal
vesicle

Levator
ani muscle

Ejaculatory
duct

Anus

Urinary
bladder

Symphysis
pubis

Prostate
gland

Corpus
cavernosum

Corpus
spongiosum

Urethra

Testis

Glans

Bulbocavernosus
muscle

FIGURE 12-6   Male pelvic organs. (From Seidel HM et al: *Mosby's guide to physical examination,* ed 3, St Louis, 1995, Mosby.)

prostate gland is actually a group of small glands that surround the urethra as it exits the bladder and produce a milky alkaline fluid that becomes a component of semen.

The duct of the bulbourethral, or Cowper's, glands connects to the urethra below the prostate. These two small glands secrete a thick lubricating fluid, which is also a component of semen. On ejaculation, semen flows through the urethra to the outside of the body.

The penis is composed of a meshwork of erectile tissue (able to become firm by engorging with blood) and consists of a shaft whose end is covered with a loose flap of skin called the prepuce, or foreskin. This foreskin is often removed during a surgical process called *circumcision.* The end of the penis is called the *glans penis.* In the reproductive system the penis functions to deposit sperm cells into the vagina.

Hormonal Control

Testicular function is controlled by follicle-stimulating hormone (FSH) and luteinizing hormone (LH) from the pituitary gland. FSH stimulates sperm production, whereas LH stimulates the secretion of testosterone from interstitial cells. Gonadotropin-releasing hormone from the hypothalamus stimulates production of FSH and LH.

Before puberty, males produce little testosterone because no releasing hormone is secreted. During puberty or adolescence the hypothalamus matures and gonadotropin-releasing hormone stimulates the production of FSH and LH. LH increases the number of interstitial cells, and testosterone production is accelerated. Testosterone increases the synthesis of protein in cells, creating an anabolic effect. Male secondary sex characteristics appear. Body growth accelerates, muscle and bone mass increase, the penis and scrotum enlarge, the larynx develops and the voice deepens, and hair appears on the face, chest, axillae, abdomen, and pubis.

The sebaceous glands of the skin are stimulated, increasing the development of acne. Testosterone stimulates the male sexual drive or libido. Boys may begin to exhibit more aggressive social behavior. The production of sperm (spermatogenesis) is accelerated. Testosterone and sperm are produced throughout life, gradually diminishing after age 40. Spermatogenesis takes place at a temperature lower than body temperature, so the testes are located in the scrotal sac, where the temperature is cooler. During cold weather, the cremaster muscle contracts and elevates the testes closer to the body.

Erection is a parasympathetic response in which arteries of the penis dilate and veins constrict; blood flows into the erectile tissue, and venous outflow is blocked. A variety of stimuli cause erection. Emission involves the contraction of the epididymis, the vas deferens, the prostate, and the seminal vesicles. Semen moves into the urethra. Ejaculation consists of contraction of the muscles at the base of the penis (bulbocavernosus, ischiocavernosus). Approximately 3 milliliters of semen is propelled at high pressure through the penile urethra.

Male Contraceptive Methods

For men, there are several contraceptive methods available: abstinence, the condom, the condom with spermicidal jelly or foam, withdrawal, and vasectomy. The condom alone and the withdrawal method are not very reliable. The condom with a spermicide is a fairly reliable method. In addition, the condom protects against venereal disease. Vasectomy is a procedure done in the physician's office with the area under local anesthesia. It involves removal of a 2 cm piece of the vas, and tying the remaining ends This should be considered a permanent method of sterilization, even though it is possible to rejoin the cut ends. In most cases, after rejoining, fertility is less than 50%.

THE FEMALE REPRODUCTIVE SYSTEM

The female reproductive system is designed for child-bearing. The system consists of two ovaries, two fallopian tubes, a uterus, and a vagina. Also included in the system are the external genitalia and mammary glands (Figure 12-7).

Internal Organs

The ovaries are solid glands that produce the hormones estrogen and progesterone. The cortex of the ovaries contains numerous small masses of cells

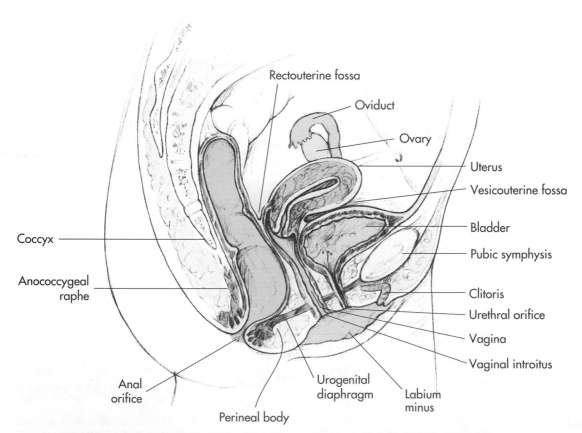

FIGURE 12-7 Female pelvic floor, midsagittal view. (From Mathers LH et al: *Clinical anatomy principles,* St Louis, 1996, Mosby.)

called *ovarian (graafian) follicles*. Each follicle contains an ovum. The two ovaries are held in position, one on each side of the uterus, by several ligaments. The largest of these ligaments is called the *broad ligament*. It holds the ovaries in close proximity to the fallopian tubes.

Each funnel-shaped fallopian tube is about 4 inches long and serves as a duct to transport the ovum to the uterus. The uterus, or womb, is a hollow, muscular organ in the shape of an inverted pear. The uterus lies between the urinary bladder and rectum. The upper part of the uterus is called the *fundus* and the middle part of the uterus is called the *corpus*. The lower, narrow portion of the uterus is the cervix, which opens into the vagina. The uterus receives the ovum and serves as the area in which the embryo grows and develops into a fetus. The inner lining is a soft, spongy layer, the endometrium, the surface of which is shed each month during menstruation. Uterine contractions at the end of the gestation period push the fetus into the vagina.

The vagina is a flexible, fibromuscular tube about 3½ inches long that receives the sperm from the male and serves as the birth canal. The region between the vagina and anus is the clinical perineum and may tear during the birth process because of overstretching.

The vagina has a dual function: sexual intercourse and delivery. Mucus in the vagina during nonsexual times comes from uterine glands. During sexual arousal, Bartholin's glands secrete mucus into the vagina. During orgasm, the muscular layer of the vagina contracts, moving semen into the cervix. Changes in the vaginal mucosa reflect cyclic endocrine changes that may be used to determine times of increased fertility.

External Organs

The external organs of the female reproductive system include the labia majora, labia minora, clitoris, mons pubis, vestibule, vaginal orifice, and Bartholin's (vestibular) glands. The aforementioned external genitalia are collectively known as the *vulva*. The mons pubis, located over the symphysis pubis, becomes covered with hair after puberty.

Each Bartholin's gland opens into the mucosal surface near the superior portion of the labia minora. A clear secretion is discharged during sexual arousal. Cysts and abscesses are common in these glands.

The mammary glands (breasts) are accessory organs that produce and secrete milk after pregnancy. The mammary glands are included in the integument and are discussed in that section of this book.

Beginning with puberty and for the next 35 to 40 years, the ovaries undergo cyclic changes in which a certain number of ovarian follicles develop. When one ovum completes the developmental process, it is released into one of the fallopian tubes. If fertilization does not occur, the developed ovum disintegrates and a new cycle begins.

A series of hormonal events takes place approximately every 28 days. Known as the *menstrual cycle*, day number 1 begins with the first day of uterine bleeding, called *menses* or *menstruation*. Cyclic hormonal changes occur in the pituitary, uterus, ovaries, and vagina. As in the male, FSH and LH from the pituitary gland affect the gonads. FSH stimulates growth of the follicle containing the egg and the secretion of female hormones collectively called *estrogen*. The main estrogen is estradiol, responsible for female secondary sex characteristics, growth of the maturing follicle, growth of the uterine lining (endometrium), and negative feedback control of FSH. LH has two main functions: ovulation and formation of the corpus luteum (from the old follicle). The corpus luteum secretes estrogen and another group of hormones, the progestins. The main progestin, progesterone, is responsible for the secretory phase of the uterine cycle, glandular growth in the breast, and negative feedback control of LH.

In the female, as in the male, almost no gonadal hormones are formed before age 9 or 10. As the hypothalamus matures, gonadotropin-releasing hormone stimulates production of FSH and LH. In response, the ovaries produce estradiol, then progesterone. Breast buds and pubic hair appear about age 11. The breasts grow, and axillary hair appears, with the adrenal cortex responsible for initial axillary and pubic hair growth in both sexes. The uterus and vagina enlarge. Uterine bleeding (the menarche) begins about 2 years after breast bud development and is often sporadic for several months. Ovulation takes place after the menarche.

As puberty progresses, the hips broaden, the forearms diverge more at the elbows, and scant body hair but much head hair is evident. The voice retains a high-pitched quality. Estradiol is not as anabolic as testosterone, and muscular development, bone size, and general body growth is not as great as in the male. Estrogens cause the skin to have a smooth texture. Prepubertal characteristics such as voice, head hairline, sparse body hair (compared with the male), and the distribution of body fat are retained and accentuated. Estradiol and testosterones are responsible for the female libido. In mammals, estrogens induce mating behavior, receptiveness of the female for the male, and nesting and maternal characteristics. As in the male, libido is influenced by cerebral control. Libido increases at ovulation and, sometimes, during menstruation.

After ages 40 to 50, a decrease in the responsiveness of the ovaries to FSH and LH, accompanied by irregular menstrual cycles, is the menopause. Although levels of estradiol and progesterone decrease, frequently little change in libido is noted.

Female Contraceptive Methods

In contrast to the male a multitude of contraceptive methods are available to the female. Removal of the uterus (hysterectomy) and tying or cauterizing the fallopian tubes (tubal ligation) should be considered permanent procedures. As with the vasectomy, even though the ends of the cut and tied fallopian tubes may later be rejoined, fertility is decreased. If the cauterization method was used, it is almost impossible to reverse the procedure. Currently used methods of birth control are the birth control pill, injections of hormones, implanted hormone-releasing devices, the intrauterine device, the diaphragm, spermicidal agents, postcoital douche, abstinence, and the rhythm method. The most reliable methods are the pill, injections, implants, the condom plus a spermicidal agent, the intrauterine device, and the diaphragm with a spermicidal agent, in decreasing order of effectiveness. In some women the pill contributes to venous thromboembolism. In others it may cause weight gain. The condom with a spermicidal agent has the added benefit of protection from venereal disease.

Pregnancy

Fertilization is the penetration of the egg by a sperm, restoring the diploid number (46) of chromosomes. This usually occurs as the egg moves down the fallopian tube. The ovum contains one X chromosome. A sperm contains either an X or a Y chromosome, so the male determines the sex of the baby. If a male sperm (Y) reaches the egg, a male baby results; if a female sperm (X) reaches the egg, a female baby is produced. After the head of the sperm enters the egg, the tail is lost and a barrier is set up, prohibiting the entrance of further sperm. The chromosomes of egg and sperm nuclei arrange themselves at the two poles of the fertilized egg, and it begins to divide.

Gestation takes approximately 10 lunar months (9 calendar months) and is divided into trimesters. The first trimester is the most important to the developing baby. During this phase, all of the body systems develop. The second trimester consists of rapid fetal growth and completion of systemic development. The third trimester is mostly a weight-gaining and maturing process, preparing the baby for life outside the womb.

Various physiologic changes occur for the mother during these markers as well. The first trimester is a time of radical hormonal changes. Mood, digestion, sleep, and energy levels are all influenced. In the second trimester, there is a settling into the pregnant state, development of maternal feelings, and often a general sense of well-being. Appetite increases, blood volume increases, and additional workload is placed on all physiologic functions. The last trimester finds the mother-to-be heavy with the baby, and posture changes are evident. Internal organs are crowded. Physiologic systems are strained with sustaining both mother and baby. The body's connective tissue structure alters by softening to allow for the expansion needed for the birth. This is a time of rest and waiting (Figure 12-8).

The main physiologic function of the mammary glands is to provide proper nutrition for the baby, as well as to protect the infant from infections during the first few months of life by transferring antibodies from mother to baby. The breasts enlarge substantially after the second month of pregnancy because of increased amounts of estrogens and progesterone. Prolactin causes the production and secretion of milk. The actual ejection (letdown) of milk from the nipple requires suckling and the release of oxytocin from the posterior pituitary gland. The cry of the infant, and in some cases emotional responses, may cause oxytocin release and lactation. Because milk production is based on a demand, if suckling continues, lactation will persist for months, even years. A yellow fluid, colostrum, is secreted during the last part of pregnancy and for the first day or two after delivery. It has a high protein content and contains antibodies. Milk is secreted 1 to 3 days after delivery.

Birth (Parturition)

The exact stimulus for birth is unknown, but increased fetal activity seems to play a role. Oxytocin stimulates contraction of the uterus. Oxytocin also causes delivery of the placenta after expulsion of the fetus.

There are three stages to labor. The first stage is dilatation, in which the cervix opens to allow passage of the baby into the birth canal. The second stage is expulsion and is the movement of the baby down the birth canal and the actual birth. The last stage is the placental stage when the placenta is expelled. Strong

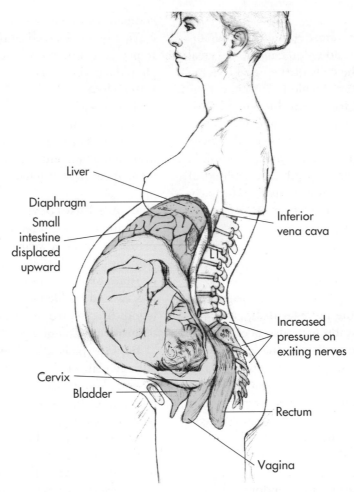

Liver

Diaphragm

Small intestine displaced upward

Inferior vena cava

Increased pressure on exiting nerves

Cervix

Bladder

Rectum

Vagina

FIGURE 12-8 Fetus in utero. This illustration shows the impressive degree to which the pregnant uterus displaces other abdominopelvic structures and puts pressure on important regions such as the pelvic diaphragm and the respiratory diaphragm. Venous return from pelvic and lower limb structures is made more difficult by pressure on the inferior vena cava, and women commonly develop hemorrhoids and varicose veins in the lower limbs. Breathing may be difficult because of pressure on the diaphragm and the inability to depress it fully to permit filling of the lungs. Back and lower limb pain is common because of pressure on exiting nerves of the lumbar and sacral plexuses. (From Mathers LH et al: *Clinical anatomy principles*, St Louis, 1996, Mosby.)

contractions of the uterus prevent hemorrhage. The stimulation at the breast by the baby further contracts the uterus.

Parental bonding with the infant immediately after birth seems to be important. The touch, sound, and smell of parents and infant in the first hours of birth establish biologic and emotional bonds. The hormone oxytocin seems to play a role in this bonding process for both mothers and fathers.

PATHOLOGY

Bartholin Cyst
Bartholin's glands are located on each side of the vaginal opening. Obstruction of a duct sometimes occurs from a bacterial infection. The area is painful and swollen. Treatment may require drainage.

Breast Lumps
Most breast lumps are not cancerous, although the incidence increases with age. See Chapter 11 on the integumentary system.

Cervicitis
Cervicitis is inflammation of the cervix. Acute cervicitis is usually caused by the same organisms that cause vaginitis (fungus, bacteria, or protozoa). Symptoms vary and can include redness, bleeding, pelvic pain, and discharge.

Chronic cervicitis is a recurrent inflammation of the cervix, frequently causing pelvic pain and often with a heavy discharge. Treatment of cervicitis includes medications if caused by organisms or cauterization if the condition becomes chronic.

Cervical Cancer

Cervical cancer is the third most common malignancy in women, after breast and colon cancer. Cervical dysplasia is a change in the cells of the cervix. Some of these abnormal cells can develop into cancerous cells. Early detection and treatment, by removing or destroying the cells, may prevent cancer. Factors contributing to the development of cervical cancer are becoming sexually active at an early age, multiple sexual partners, genital herpes, and a possible viral infection. If cervical cancer is not treated in the early stages, it can spread into other tissues, especially lymph nodes and the uterus.

Ectopic Pregnancy

An ectopic pregnancy is one in which the fertilized ovum is implanted and develops outside the uterus. Ninety percent occur in the fallopian tube; this is a tubal pregnancy. Implantation may also occur in the peritoneum. The embryo will eventually rupture, usually between the seventh and tenth week, and cause internal bleeding. Severe abdominal pain, which may be accompanied by hemorrhage and shock, is also present. This is a medical emergency. Surgical intervention is usually required.

Endometriosis

Endometriosis is a disease in which endometrial tissue is present in nonuterine locations, such as on the intestines, ovaries, or even in the fallopian tubes. It most often occurs in young women between the ages of 25 and 50, especially if they have no children. Although symptoms may be mild, common symptoms are heavy menstrual periods, intense back or pelvic pain, painful menstruation (dysmenorrhea), and painful intercourse (dyspareunia). Pregnancy often eliminates the problem. Birth control pills may help because they cause a change in the endometrial tissue. Sometimes surgical intervention is necessary.

Infertility

Infertility is a relative decrease in the ability to conceive, whereas sterility is a total loss of the ability. Infertility may be temporary and can result from structural or functional problems with the male, the female, or both. In males, common causes are impotency (the inability to have an erection), a decrease in sperm number, or abnormalities of sperm anatomy and motility. In females, common causes include a lack of ovulation, disorders of the fallopian tubes (often from a previous infection), and abnormal mucus secretion from the cervix, creating an environment hostile to sperm. A low sperm count may be caused by excessive use of alcohol, tobacco, and caffeine; poor nutrition; and fatigue. Tight underwear should not be worn by men because they pull the testes close to the body, increasing the temperature and decreasing the sperm count. In females, clomiphene citrate is sometimes effective in inducing ovulation. Surgery may be beneficial to correct tubal scarring. The administration of estrogen may restore normal cervical mucus.

Prostate Disorders

Prostatitis is an infection of the prostate, usually resulting from a urinary tract infection. Perineal pain, fever, chills, painful urination, and a tender prostate on rectal examination are common signs. If it is caused by bacteria, treatment with an antibiotic is indicated. Chronic prostatitis is commonly seen in older men with enlarged prostate glands.

Benign prostatic hypertrophy (BPH) is the enlargement of the prostate, a disorder of males age 45 and older, possibly caused by a relative decrease in the ratio of testosterone to estrogen. As testosterone declines, estrogen produced by the adrenal cortex seems to stimulate the central portion of the prostate, causing an overgrowth of prostate tissue. The amount of the enlargement is not as important as its ability to compress the urethra. This causes problems with urination such as straining, dribbling, and sometimes urinary retention. Medical treatment, including catheterization and surgery, is indicated in the most severe cases. The herb saw palmetto has been shown to be beneficial in decreasing hypertrophy.

Prostatic cancer is the most common malignancy in males (other than skin cancer). It is slow growing, often asymptomatic, and is most frequently found during a physical checkup. Early stage cancer is usually slow growing, whereas in later stages metastasis to bone commonly occurs, particularly in the thoracic and lumbar vertebrae and the sacrum. Symptoms include urinary retention if obstruction has taken place and lower back pain if metastasis has occurred. Primary treatment depends on the age of the person and stage of the cancer. It may focus on relieving symptoms or removing the cancer with such methods as prostatectomy, radiation therapy, and removal of the testes because cancer cells are stimulated by testosterone.

Sexually Transmitted Diseases

Sexually transmitted diseases include vaginal infections, hepatitis B infection, nongonococcal urethritis or chlamydia, genital warts, herpes genitalis, acquired immunodeficiency syndrome (AIDS), gonorrhea, syphilis, and body lice. Most of these diseases have been discussed elsewhere in the text.

Gonorrhea is an infectious disease caused by a bacterium. It is becoming more resistant to antibiotics because mutant strains have developed. The urethra of both sexes is infected, producing urethritis several days after exposure. The person may show no signs or mild symptoms, which are ignored while the bacteria spread.

In men, gonorrhea primarily affects the urethra, where it can cause scarring. If untreated, the bacteria can infect and inflame the prostate or the epididymis. Symptoms include difficult urination and a cloudy discharge.

In the female, gonorrhea usually infects the cervix, causing cervicitis. Untreated gonorrhea may infect the uterus or fallopian tubes, causing scarring that may result in infertility. Involvement of the tubes and surrounding pelvic area is pelvic inflammatory disease (PID). If it travels to the abdominal cavity, it can cause peritonitis. Signs and symptoms of gonorrhea in women include fever, abnormal bleeding, cloudy vaginal discharge, bilateral pelvic pain (usually during the menses), and tenderness on movement of the cervix (stretching the broad ligament).

Untreated gonorrhea in both sexes can infect the bloodstream, causing blood poisoning. It can also spread to the skin, bones, joints, and tendons.

Syphilis is a bacterial infection transmitted either sexually or from mother to fetus. Frequency declined with the discovery of penicillin, but as with gonorrhea, resistant strains are appearing. Syphilis appears in three stages:

Stage 1—Painless skin sores, treated primarily with antibiotics

Stage 2—Skin rash, which may be helped with antibiotics [both stages 1 and 2 are highly contagious]

Stage 3—Referred to as *late syphilis*, it is not as contagious unless there is blood exchanged between two people; if the person does not recognize the symptoms from Stages 1 or 2, this third stage can flare at any time and affect the brain, nervous system, aorta, and other organs of the body; syphilis cannot be reversed in the third stage

Herpes simplex is a deoxyribonucleic acid (DNA) virus that causes painful blisters and small ulcers in and around the mouth and on the genital area. Type 1 usually infects the upper body, and type 2 affects the genital area. Type 2 is a common sexually transmitted disease. The primary infection lasts about 1 to 4 weeks. Recurrent lesions are less painful and debilitating, often emerge every month or two, and last 7 to 10 days. The blisters form, then break open, and remain open for 2 to 3 weeks. This is very painful. Herpes is transmitted when it is active—that is, when the lesions are present and up to 7 days afterward. In some people, lesions recur. In others, recurrence takes place once or twice, and never again. They may be activated by fever, emotional stress, the menses, sunlight, infections, and trauma. Genital lesions in women consist of painful vesicles and erosions on the labia, vagina, or cervix. In males the lesions are often located on the penis. The antiviral drug acyclovir (Zovirax) is effective.

Uterine Disorders

A myoma, or fibroid, is a benign tumor in the uterus that grows inside the uterine muscle wall or attaches to the wall. They may be very small, grow slowly, and be asymptomatic. Those that grow large or rapidly cause heavy bleeding. If blood loss is extensive, anemia may occur. Fibroids are the most common disorder of the uterus. Seen in late reproductive years, the tumor is estrogen dependent. Prolonged or abnormal menstrual bleeding is usually the first sign. Treatment may be dietary for the anemia. In the rare cases that they grow large enough to cause severe bleeding, a hysterectomy is required.

Polyps are small growths of the endometrium extending into the body of the uterus. They are common in all age groups, especially in women with no children. The main symptom is increased menstrual bleeding between periods or postmenopausal bleeding. Removal of the polyps with a uterine curet (curettage) is indicated if symptoms are problematic. Cervical polyps occur when the lining of the cervix develops growths that hang outside the cervix.

Dysfunctional uterine bleeding is abnormal bleeding throughout much of the 28-day cycle. The main form of both diagnosis and treatment is dilatation and curettage.

Vaginitis

Vaginitis is inflammation of the vagina. Signs and symptoms are vaginal discharge, itching (pruritus), and irritation.

Yeast vaginitis (candidiasis, moniliasis) is a common fungal infection caused by the fungus *Candida albicans*. It responds to an antifungal ointment such as miconazole (Monistat) or nystatin.

Trichomonas vaginitis (trichomoniasis) is caused by a protozoal parasite that may infect the urinary tract of both sexes and is a sexually transmitted organism. Metronidazole (Flagyl) is effective. The sexual partner may also require treatment.

Gardnerella (Haemophilus) vaginitis is a bacterial infection of the vagina and responds to metronidazole.

INDICATIONS CONTRAINDICATIONS

For Soft Tissue and Movement Therapies

As with all acute infections, bodywork is contraindicated until any disease of the reproductive system runs it course. Bodywork in clients with malignancies is contraindicated unless approval and supervision is provided by the appropriate health care professional. Bodywork during a normal pregnancy is structured as part of a wellness program with accommodation for the changes in the pregnant woman. Permission should be obtained from the supervising health care professional. Certainly anyone working with pregnant women on a regular basis should learn more about pregnancy and fetal development than is provided in this text. Most reproductive system conditions present regional contraindications. As with most chronic illness and pain, soft tissue and movement modalities offer generalized support for homeostasis and can offer palliative or comfort care for the maintenance of these conditions (Activity 12-4).

ACTIVITY 12-4

It is important to be able to explain and justify the therapeutic value of the work we do. The following activity will assist you in developing the skills to explain the effectiveness of various modalities to clients and other health care professionals. Use the clinical reasoning model that follows to accomplish this task. The focus should be your primary modality or modalities applied to the reproductive system. An example is provided in the section opener on p. 450.

Modality/modalities

1. What are the facts?

a. Which system is involved, and which structures of that system can be reached directly or indirectly?

b. Which of these structures are most affected by this modality?

c. Which physiologic functions are affected by this approach?

d. When the treatment is applied, what changes in function will result in
(1) This system

(2) The whole body

e. What is considered normal or balanced function?

f. How are the functions of this system related to the body's homeostasis?

2. What are the possibilities?

a. What do the data suggest?

g. What has worked or has not worked?

b. What are the reasons for using the proposed methods?

h. Where could you find information that would support the use of this modality as a therapeutic intervention?

c. What are the possible interventions?

i. What research is available to support the use of the therapeutic intervention?

d. List at least three applications of this modality that would affect both the structure and function of this system.

j. How does the intervention support a healthy state?

e. What are other ways to look at the situation?

k. Under which pathologic or dysfunctional conditions is the intervention most likely to be beneficial?

f. What other methods could provide similar benefits?

Continued

ACTIVITY 12-4—cont'd

3. What is the logical outcome of therapeutic intervention?

a. What would be the logical progression of the symptom pattern, contributing factors, and current behaviors?

b. What are the benefits and drawbacks of each intervention suggested?
Benefits:

Drawbacks:

c. What are the costs in terms of time, resources, and finances?

d. What is likely to happen if the modality is not used?

e. What is likely to happen if the modality is used?

4. For the intervention proposed, what would be the impact on the people involved, specifically the client, practitioner, and other professionals working with the client?

a. How does each of the people involved (including, besides those named above, the client's family and support system) feel about the possible interventions?

b. Does the practitioner feel qualified to work with the situation and apply the identified modality to the particular situation?

c. Does a feeling of cooperation and agreement exist among all those involved, and how would the practitioner recognize this feeling?

Summary

On completion of this last set of justification exercises, a logical model of reasoning that honors intuition and the emotions and perceptions of the people involved should be familiar. As with all knowledge, question it, individualize the process, make it your own, and improve it. This model is only a framework; however, it helps us be more objective and address questions and issues we may not think of on our own.

This is good—to consider various perspectives and then make our own best decisions.

The respiratory, digestive, urinary, and reproductive systems all contribute to the complete function of the body as whole. These systems concern the movement of energy, water, and air and creation of new life in and out of the body. Again we see the interconnectedness of being alive and, with these systems, the need for interaction outside ourselves as we breathe in air, take in food and water, and connect with another to produce life.

ACTIVITY 12-4—cont'd

Justification

Using the information developed in the clinical reasoning model, present a clear, concise statement of the ways in which the particular soft tissue or movement modality would be beneficial, either in supporting the particular body system in a healthy condition or as part of a treatment plan for a pathologic or dysfunctional condition. Based on the above information, give a brief summary of the effectiveness of the modality for this system.

WORKBOOK SECTION

1. What are the parts of the upper and lower respiratory tract?

_____

_____

_____

2. How does the nose affect the breathing pattern when we sleep?

_____

_____

_____

_____

_____

_____

3. What happens in our bodies to prevent food from going into our lungs while we are eating?

_____

_____

_____

_____

_____

_____

4. How does the diaphragm work to help us breathe?

_____

_____

_____

_____

_____

_____

_____

5. Describe the mechanics of relaxed breathing.

_____

_____

_____

_____

_____

_____

6. What is a normal respiratory rate and how can it be affected?

_____

_____

_____

_____

_____

7. Where does digestion begin and end?

_____

_____

_____

_____

8. List the organs of digestion.

_____

_____

_____

9. What are the steps in digestion and what does each involve?

_____

_____

_____

_____

_____

_____

_____

10. What are the main food groups and why is each important? Give two examples of each.

_____

_____

_____

_____

_____

_____

_____

11. What are the organs of the urinary system and where are they located?

_____

_____

_____

_____

_____

_____

_____

_____

12. How much urine does the average person produce per day?

_____

_____

_____

13. What are the parts of the male reproductive system?

_____

_____

_____

14. What are the parts of the female reproductive system?

_____

_____

_____

15. What are the divisions of the gestational period in the human being, and what are the primary features of each period?

_____

_____

_____

_____

_____

_____

_____

16. What are the stages of labor?

_____

_____

_____

_____

_____

_____

FILL IN THE BLANK

_____ (1) is the movement of air in and out of the lungs, the exchange of oxygen and carbon dioxide between the lungs and blood, and the exchange between blood and body tissues.

_____ (2) is the exchange of oxygen and carbon dioxide between the lungs and the bloodstream.

The lower two thirds of the _____ (3) is composed mostly of cartilage. The upper third, or bridge of the nose, is formed from two small hard nasal bones. The tip of the nose is the apex, and the nostrils are the _____ (4).

The _____ (5) is the actual space inside both the external and internal nose structures. It is separated into left and right sides by the septum, a partition composed of cartilage and bone. At the upper portion of the nasal cavity, three thin, curled bones, the _____ (6), or conchae, project inward from the two outer walls.

Venous areas called _____ (7) are located on the turbinates.

The _____ (8) are four groups of air-filled spaces that open into the frontal, ethmoid, sphenoid, and maxillary bones of the skull. The _____ (9) is the continuation of the nasal cavity into the throat, or pharynx. The _____ (10), or voice box, connects the pharynx to the trachea. Its structure consists of cartilage, ligaments, connective tissue, muscles, and the vocal cords. The vocal cords and the spaces between the cords are located inside the _____ (11).

The _____ (12), or windpipe, is the main airway to the lungs. It is a 4- to 5-inch tube that begins at the glottis and ends at the junction of the two main bronchi near the level of the sternal angle.

The two _____ (13) are the primary organs of respiration. These soft, spongy, highly vascular structures are separated into the left and right lungs by the mediastinum. The _____ (14) is a dome-shaped sheet of muscle attached to the thoracic wall that separates the lungs and thoracic cavity from the abdominal cavity.

The _____ (15), or chest cavity, is the upper region of the torso enclosed by the sternum, ribs, and thoracic vertebrae. It contains the lungs, heart, and great vessels.

The _____ (16), or _____ (17), contains the major organs of digestion. The cavity is lined with a mucous membrane, the _____ (18), whose function is to prevent friction. Products of digestion are propelled along the tract from the esophagus to the anus by the rhythmic contraction of smooth muscle called _____ (19).

The testicles contain tiny seminiferous tubules that produce _____ (20).

The _____ (21) gland surrounds the urethra and produces a milky alkaline fluid.

The _____ (22) are solid glands that produce the hormones estrogen and progesterone. These external female genitalia are collectively known as the _____ (23).

Gestation takes approximately 10 lunar months (9 calendar months) and is divided into _____ (24). The hormone _____ (25) stimulates contraction of the uterus. There are three stages to labor. The first stage is _____ (26), where the cervix opens to allow passage of the baby into the birth canal. The second stage is _____ (27) and is the movement of the baby down the birth canal and the actual birth. The last stage is the _____ (28), when the placenta is expelled.

EXERCISE

In the illustration of the digestive system below, write the name of each part of the system next to its corresponding letter. Then color the illustration.

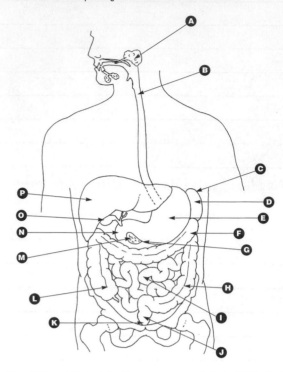

(From Williams RW: *Basic healthcare terminology,* St Louis, 1995, Mosby.)

PROFESSIONAL APPLICATION

What education and information should a soft tissue or movement therapist have to work with pregnant women?

_____

_____

_____

_____

_____

_____

_____

_____

_____

Answer Key

1. The upper respiratory tract consists of the nasal cavity and all its structures and the pharynx; the lower respiratory tract is made up of the larynx and trachea and the bronchi and alveoli in the lungs.

2. When a person lies with his head to one side, the swell bodies of the lower nostril become congested. The chamber narrows and the lumen is closed. When sleeping, we only breathe though one nostril at a time. The closure of the nostril then initiates movement of the head from one side to the other, which in turn causes a major movement and turning of the body. This head-body moving cycle initiated by the nose ensures maximal rest during sleep. A poorly functioning nose may allow the body and head to remain in one position and can cause symptoms such as backaches, numbness, cramps, and circulatory dysfunction.

3. The pharynx functions both as a passageway for food between the mouth and the esophagus and as a passageway for air between the nose, mouth, and trachea. At the entrance to the larynx is a small cartilaginous flap, the epiglottis. As we swallow food, the epiglottis closes over the glottis, preventing food or fluids from entering the lungs.

4. The diaphragm is a dome-shaped sheet of muscle attached to the thoracic wall that separates the lungs and thoracic cavity from the abdominal cavity. As the chest cavity enlarges, the diaphragm moves downward and creates a vacuum which allows air to flow into the lungs. As the chest contracts and the diaphragm relaxes, it arches upward, helping air to flow out of the lungs.

5. During the moments before we take a breath, the pressure both inside the lungs and outside the body are equal, whereas the pressure inside the pleural space is slightly lower. When we begin to inhale, the external intercostal muscles between the ribs contract, lifting the lower ribs up and out. This creates a vacuum that expands the lungs, causing the pressure inside the lungs to decrease. The diaphragm moves down, increasing the volume of the pleural cavities and decreasing their pressure even more. Elastic fibers in the alveolar walls stretch, permitting expansion of the air sacs. Air is drawn into the lungs until the pressure is equal again.

   As we exhale, the pressure inside the pleural cavity increases; the external intercostals, diaphragm, and alveolar walls relax; the volume inside the lungs decreases; and the pressure in the lungs raises until it again equalizes the air pressure.

6. The respiratory rate in adults is about 12 to 16 breaths per minute. In the newborn it is about 35 and gradually decreases to adult values at about age 20. Emotions are a powerful stimulus for respiratory changes. Fear, grief, and shock slow the rate; anger and sexual arousal increase the respiratory rate.

7. Digestion begins in the mouth and ends in the small intestine. It is accompanied by digestive enzymes (protein catalysts) that split large substances into small ones. The gastrointestinal tract contains glands that secrete mucus and digestive enzymes.

8. The digestive tract consists of the mouth, pharynx, esophagus, stomach, small intestine, large intestine, rectum, and anus. Accessory structures include the salivary glands, pancreas, liver, and gallbladder.

9. There are four essential steps in the process of digestion.
   Ingestion—Food entering the mouth
   Digestion—The mechanical and chemical breakdown of food from its complex form into simple molecules
   Absorption—The movement of these simple molecules from the digestive tract to the circulatory or lymphatic systems; vitamins and minerals are absorbed in the small intestine; amino acids, simple sugars, and small fatty acids pass through the intestinal villi into the bloodstream; the larger fatty acids are reconstituted to fats in the intestinal wall and pass into the lymphatic system; capillaries of the intestinal villi become venules, then veins, and, finally, the large portal vein carries absorbed foodstuffs to the liver; the liver converts these substances into compounds required for bodily functions
   Elimination (egestion)—Removal and release of solid waste products from food that cannot be digested or absorbed

10. Proteins—Proteins are large, high–molecular-weight substances containing carbon, hydrogen, oxygen, and nitrogen, as well as smaller amounts of other elements. Proteins break down into amino acids. The body uses 24 amino acids for its metabolic requirements. Dietary proteins include animal products and bean and grain combinations. Proteins are the chief structural components of the body.
   Carbohydrates—Complex carbohydrates are long chains of glucose molecules found in rice and vegetables. Glucose is the main fuel for the manufacture of adenosine triphosphate in the cell. Sugars are converted to glucose in the liver.
   Fats—In addition to serving as a reservoir of stored energy, fats are essential components of the cell membrane and myelin sheath of the nerve fiber. Dietary fats are found in nuts, seeds, oils, and animal products.

11. Kidneys—These are reddish brown, bean-shaped organs located on the posterior wall of the abdomen against the back body wall musculature, just above the waist. The kidneys are imbedded in fat and located about the spinal level of T11 to L3 on each side of the vertebral column. The right kidney is lower than the left because of its displacement by the liver. An adrenal gland is found on top of each kidney.
   Ureters—These are two narrow tubes extending from the kidney and connecting to the bladder. The two ureters lie in the psoas muscles.
   Bladder (urinary bladder)—The urinary bladder, a reservoir for urine, is a muscular, baglike organ that lies in the pelvis.
   Urethra—This is the tube that carries urine from the bladder. The opening at the end of the urethra is called the *meatus*.

12. In the average person, about 100 liters of blood are filtered per day; 99 liters of filtrate are reabsorbed, leaving about 1 liter of urine.

13. The male reproductive system consists of the testicles, epididymis, vas deferens, ejaculatory duct, urethra, penis, and scrotum.

14. The female reproductive system is designed for childbearing. The system consists of two ovaries, two fallopian tubes, a uterus, and a vagina. Also included in the system are the external genitalia and mammary glands.

15. Gestation takes approximately 10 lunar months (9 calendar months) and is divided into trimesters. The first trimester is the most important to the developing baby. It is during this phase that all the body systems develop. The second trimester consists of rapid fetal growth and completion of systemic development. The last trimester is mostly a weight-gaining and maturing process preparing the baby for life outside the womb. Various physiologic changes occur for the mother during these markers as well. The first trimester is a time of radical hormonal changes. Mood, digestion, sleep, and energy levels are all influenced. In the second trimester there is a settling into the pregnant state, development of maternal feelings, and often a general sense of well-being. Appetite increases, blood volume increases, and additional workload is placed on all physiologic functions. The last trimester finds the mother-to-be heavy with the baby, and posture changes are evident. Internal organs are crowded. Physiologic systems are strained with sustaining both mother and baby. The body's connective tissue structure alters by softening to allow for the expansion needed for the birth. This is a time of rest and waiting.

16. There are three stages to labor. The first stage is dilation, where the cervix opens to allow passage of the baby into the birth canal. The second stage is

expulsion and is the movement of the baby down the birth canal and the actual birth. The last stage is the placental stage, when the placenta is expelled. Strong contractions of the uterus prevent hemorrhage.

FILL IN THE BLANK

1. Respiration
2. External respiration
3. external nose
4. nares
5. nasal cavity
6. turbinates
7. swell bodies
8. sinuses
9. nasopharynx
10. larynx
11. glottis
12. trachea
13. lungs
14. diaphragm
15. thorax
16. abdomen
17. abdominal cavity
18. peritoneum
19. peristalsis
20. sperm
21. prostate
22. ovaries
23. vulva
24. trimesters
25. oxytocin
26. dilation
27. expulsion
28. placental stage

EXERCISE

A. Parotid gland
B. Esophagus
C. Diaphragm
D. Spleen
E. Stomach
F. Transverse colon
G. Duodenojejunal flexure
H. Descending colon
I. Ileum
J. Rectum
K. Anus
L. Cecum
M. Pancreas
N Duodenum
O. Gallbladder
P. Liver

Final Word

The learning journey continues. The student would be well served to obtain a comprehensive anatomy and physiology text to pursue further self-study and take additional courses on these topics.

This text has provided a map for an introductory journey through the body. The information has been presented with the bodywork and soft tissue and movement student and future professional in mind. The themes of dynamic balance, homeostasis, and clinical reasoning have been supported throughout the learning process. One goal has been to teach students to be their own teachers.

East/West philosophy and theory and ancient healing wisdom have been presented with a focus on science, but with a balance provided by acknowledging the body, mind, and spirit of being human. In the end, we can see that the concepts are similar, although the languages are different. The common ground is the body, and the anatomy and physiology are universal.

Another theme of this text can be recognized in retrospect: that the form and function of the human body can be wonderful examples and teachers for the form and function of life itself. The way in which the many systems of the body cooperate, and in so doing, support life, is similar to the way we as human beings can cooperate, respecting and supporting each other and other living creatures as we live and work together on this planet.

With just that vision, this text has been written.

Glossary

Abduction Lateral movement away from the midline of the trunk.

Absorption The movement of food molecules from the digestive tract to the circulatory or lymphatic systems.

Acetylcholine A neurotransmitter that stimulates the parasympathetic nervous system and the skeletal muscles. It is involved in memory.

Acne A chronic inflammation of the sebaceous glands and hair follicles caused by interactions between bacteria, sebum, and sex hormones.

Acupuncture The practice of Inserting needles in specific points on meridians, or channels, to stimulate or sedate energy flow to regulate or alter body function. A branch of Chinese medicine, it is the art and science of manipulating the flow of Qi, the basic life force, and Xue, the blood, body fluids, and nourishing essences. Western medicine uses it primarily to reduce pain. Acupressure, which uses digital pressure, follows the same Eastern principles.

Acute disease Disease that has a specific beginning, signs, and symptoms that develop quickly and last a short time, then disappear.

Acute pain Pain that is usually temporary, of sudden onset, and easily localized. It can be a symptom of a disease process or a temporary aspect of medical treatment. Acting as a warning signal, it activates the sympathetic nervous system.

Adduction A medial movement toward the midline of the body.

Adenosine triphosphate (ATP) A compound that stores energy in the muscles. When ATP is broken down during catabolic reactions, it releases energy.

Adrenergic Stimulation of the sympathetic nervous system, causing a release of epinephrine and similar neurotransmitters and hormones.

Afferent Toward a center or point of reference.

Afferent nerves (sensory nerves) Nerves that link sensory receptors with the central nervous system (CNS) and transmit the sensory information.

Agonist A muscle that causes or controls joint motion through a specified plane of motion; known as the primary or prime mover.

Alimentary canal The tube-shaped portion of the digestive system known as the gastrointestinal (GI) tract; it is about 30 feet long and contains several special structures throughout its length.

All or none response The property of muscle contraction by which, when the contraction is initiated, all the muscle fibers either contract to their full ability or do not contract at all.

Alopecia Hair loss or baldness on parts or all of the body.

Amphiarthrosis A slightly movable joint that connects bone to bone with fibrocartilage or hyaline growth cartilage. The two types in the human body are symphysis and synchondrosis.

Anabolism Chemical processes in the body that join simple compounds to form more complex compounds of carbohydrates, lipids, proteins, and nucleic acids. The processes require energy supplied from adenosine triphosphate (ATP).

Anaplasia Without shape; it describes abnormal or undifferentiated cells that fail to mature into specialized cell types. It is characteristic of malignant cells.

Anatomic range of motion (ROM) The amount of motion available to a joint based on the structure of the joint, and determined by the shape of the joint surfaces, the joint capsule, ligaments, muscle bulk, and surrounding musculotendinous and bony structures.

Anatomic position A standard position in which the person is standing upright with the feet slightly apart, arms hanging at the sides, palms facing forward, thumbs outward.

Anatomy The study of the body's structures and the relationship of its parts.

Androgens Male sex hormones.

Anemia A decrease in the normal number of red blood cells, or in the amount of hemoglobin or iron in the blood.

Aneurysm A permanent dilatation of part of a blood vessel caused by weakness or damage to its structure. The most common sites are the aorta and the arteries of the brain.

Antagonist A muscle usually located on the opposite side of a joint from the agonist and having the opposite action. The antagonist works with the agonist by relaxing and allowing movement.

Anterior pelvic rotation Anterior movement of the upper pelvis; the iliac crest tilts forward in a sagittal plane.

Antibody A specific protein that is produced to destroy or suppress antigens.

Antigen Any substance that causes the body to produce antibodies.

Aorta The large artery that carries oxygen and nutrients out of the heart.

Appendicular skeleton The part of the skeleton composed of the limbs and their attachments.

Appocrine A type of sweat gland that discharges a thicker and more odiferous form of sweat.

Arteriole The smallest of the arteries.

Arteriosclerosis A term meaning "hardening of the arteries"; it refers to arteries that have become brittle and have lost their elasticity.

Arterioles The smallest arteries.

Artery A blood vessel that transports either oxygenated blood from the heart to the body or deoxygenated blood from the heart to the lungs.

Arthritis The most common type of joint disorder, it literally means "inflammation of the joint."

Arthrokinematics Movements of the articulating surfaces of bones at joint surfaces.

Articulation Another word for joint, the structure created when bones connect to each other.

Atherosclerosis A condition in which fatty plaque is deposited in medium and large arteries.

Atom The smallest particle of an element that retains and exhibits the properties of that element. Atoms are made up of protons, neutrons, and electrons.

Atrium One of the two small, thin-walled, upper chambers of the heart; the right and left atria are separated by a thin interatrial septum.

Atrophy A decrease in the size of a body part or organ caused by a decrease in the size of the cells.

Attachments Connections of skeletal muscles to bones; often referred to as the origin and insertion.

Autonomic nervous system A division of the peripheral nervous system composed of nerves that connect the central nervous system to the glands, heart, and smooth muscles to maintain the internal body environment.

Avulsion The injury to a ligament or tendon when it is torn off its attachment.

Axial skeleton The axis of the body; the axial skeleton consists of the head, vertebral column (the spine), and the ribs and sternum. It provides the body with form and protection.

Axon A single elongated projection from the nerve cell body that transmits impulses away from the cell body.

Balance The ability to control equilibrium. There are two types of balance: static or still balance, and dynamic or moving balance.

Ball-and-socket joint Allows movement in many directions around a central point. Ball-and-socket joints are formed when a ball-shaped convex surface is fitted into a concave socket. This type of joint gives the greatest freedom of movement, but it is also the most easily dislocated.

Basement membrane A permeable membrane that attaches epithelial tissues to the underlying connective tissues.

Benign Usually describing a noncancerous tumor that is contained and does not spread.

Biological rhythms The internal periodic tuning component of an organism, also known as biorhythm. Circadian rhythms work on a 24-hour period to coordinate internal functions, such as sleep. Ultradian rhythms repeat themselves from every 90 minutes to every few hours, whereas seasonal rhythms function on a yearly basis.

Biomechanics The study of mechanical principles, movements, and actions applied to living bodies.

Blood A thick, red fluid that provides oxygen, nourishment, and protection to the cells and carries away waste products. Whole blood consists of two components, the formed cellular elements and the liquid plasma. Blood is a form of connective tissue.

Blood pressure The measurement of pressure exerted by the heart on the walls of the blood vessels. The highest pressure exerted is called *systolic pressure,* which results when the ventricles are contracted. Diastolic pressure, the lowest pressure, results when the ventricles are at rest. Blood forced into the aorta during systole sets up a pressure wave that travels down the arteries. The wave expands the arterial wall, and the expansion can be palpated by pressing the artery against tissue; the waves constitute the pulse rate.

Brain The largest and most complex unit of the nervous system; it is responsible for perception, sensation, emotion, intellect, and action.

Brainstem The primitive portion of the brain; it contains centers for vital functions and reflex actions, such as vomiting, coughing, sneezing, posture, and basic movement patterns.

Bursa A flat sac of synovial membrane in which the inner sides of the sac are separated by fluid film. Bursae are located where moving structures are apt to rub.

Bursitis Inflammation of a bursa.

Callus An area of thickened hardened skin that develops in an area of friction or region of recurrent pressure.

Cancer Malignant, non-encapsulated cells that invade surrounding tissue. They often break away, or metastasize, from the primary tumor and form secondary cancer masses.

Capillary One of the small blood vessels found between arteries and veins that allow the exchange of gases, nutrients, and waste products. The walls of capillaries are very thin, allowing molecules to diffuse easily.

Carbohydrate Sugars, starches, and cellulose composed of carbon, hydrogen, and oxygen.

Cardiac cycle A synchronized sequence of events that takes place during one full heartbeat.

Cardiac muscle Smaller, striated, involuntary muscle fibers (cells) in the heart that pump blood.

Cardiac output The amount of blood pumped by the left ventricle in one minute.

Carotene A yellow pigment found in the dermis, it provides a natural yellow tint to the skin of some individuals.

Cartilage A form of flexible connective tissue. Types of cartilage include hyaline, fibrocartilage, and elastic cartilage.

Catabolism Chemical processes in the body that release energy as complex compounds are broken down into simpler ones.

Catecholamines A group of neurotransmitters involved in sleep, mood, pleasure, and motor function.

Cell The basic structural unit of a living organism. A cell contains a nucleus and cytoplasm and is surrounded by a membrane.

Center of gravity An imaginary midpoint or center of the weight of a body or object. It is where the body or object could balance on a point.

Central nervous system The brain and spinal cord and their coverings.

Cerebellum The second largest part of the brain; it is involved with balance, posture, coordination, and movements.

Cerebrospinal fluid A clear, colorless fluid that flows throughout the brain and around the spinal cord, cushioning and protecting these structures and maintaining proper pH balance.

Cerebrum The largest of the brain divisions; it consists of two hemispheres that occupy the uppermost region of the cranium. The cerebrum receives, interprets, and associates incoming information with past memories, then transmits the appropriate motor response.

Cerumen A sticky substance released by glands in the ear. Also known as earwax, it protects the ear from the entry of foreign material and repels insects.

Ceruminous glands Modified apocrine glands found in the external ear canal that secrete cerumen.

Charting The process of keeping a written record of a client or patient. The most effective charting methods follow clinical reasoning, which emphasizes a problem-solving approach. Many systems are used, but these models all have similar components: POMR (problem-oriented medical record) and SOAP (subjective, objective, assessment/analysis, and plan—the four parts of the written record).

Chemical properties Those properties that demonstrate how a substance reacts with other substances or responds to a change in the environment.

Chronic disease Disease with a vague onset that develops slowly and lasts for a long time, sometimes for life.

Chronic pain Pain that continues or recurs over a prolonged time, usually for more than 6 months. The onset may be obscure, and the character and quality of the pain change over time. It is usually poorly localized and not as intense as acute pain, although for some it is exhausting and depressing. The sympathetic nervous system is not usually activated in chronic pain.

Circumduction Circular movement of a limb, combining the movement of flexion, extension, abduction, and adduction, to create a cone shape.

Close packed position The only position of a synovial joint where the surfaces fit precisely together and there is maximal contact between the opposing surfaces. Because the joint surfaces are compressed, it permits no movement, and the joint possesses its greatest stability.

Closed kinematic chain The positioning of joints in such a way that motion at one joint is accompanied by motion at an adjacent joint.

Collagen A protein substance composed of small fibrils that combine to create the connective tissue of fascia, tendons, and ligaments. When combined with water, it forms gelatin. Collagen constitutes one fourth of the protein in the body.

Collagenous fibers Strong fibers with little capacity for stretch. They have a high degree of tensile strength, which allows them to withstand longitudinal stress.

Combining vowel A vowel added between two roots or a root and a suffix to make pronunciation of the word easier.

Compact (dense) bone The hard portion of bone that protects spongy bone and provides the firm framework of the bone and the body. The osteocytes in this type of bone are located in concentric rings around a central haversian canal, through which nerves and blood vessels pass.

Concentric contraction The action of a prime mover or agonist where a muscle develops tension as it shortens in order to provide enough force to overcome resistance.

Condyle A rounded projection at the end of a bone.

Condyloid (condylar) joint Allows movement in two directions, but one motion predominates.

Connective tissue The most abundant type of tissue in the body, connective tissue supports and holds together the body and its parts, protects the body from foreign matter, and is organized to transport substances throughout the body.

Contractility The ability of a muscle to shorten forcibly with adequate stimulation. This property sets muscle apart from all other types of tissue.

Contracture The chronic shortening of a muscle, especially the connective tissue component.

Contusion A bruise.

Corn A painful conical thickening of skin over bony prominences of the feet caused by continued pressure and friction on normally thin skin. Soft corns are those located in moist areas, such as between the toes.

Coronary arteries The arteries that supply oxygenated blood to the heart muscle itself; they are located in grooves between the atria and ventricles and between the two ventricles.

Coronary veins Arteries that return the deoxygenated blood from the heart to the right atrium.

Cortisol A glucocorticoid, also known as hydrocortisone. Levels of stress are often measured by cortisol levels.

Cramps Painful muscle spasms or involuntary twitches that involve the whole muscle.

Cranial nerves Twelve pairs of nerves that originate from the olfactory bulbs, thalamus, visual cortex, and brainstem. They transmit information to and from the sense organs of the face, and the muscles of the face, neck, and upper shoulders.

Creep The slow movement of viscoelastic materials back to their original state and tissue structure after a deforming force is released.

Deep fascia A coarse sheet of fibrous connective tissue that binds muscles into functional groups and forms partitions, called *intermuscular septa,* between muscle groups.

Degenerative joint disease (DJD) Osteoarthritis.

Dendrites Branching projections from the nerve cell body that carry signals to the cell body.

Depression Downward or inferior movement.

Dermatitis A general term for acute or chronic skin inflammation characterized by redness, eruptions, edema, scaling, and itching. The three main types are atopic dermatitis, seborrheic dermatitis, and contact dermatitis. Eczema is a form of dermatitis.

Dermatome A cutaneous (skin) section supplied by a single spinal nerve.

Dermis The inner layer of skin; it contains collagen and elastin fibers, which provide much of the structure and strength of the skin, and is much thicker than the epidermis.

Diagnosis A labeling of signs and symptoms by a licensed medical professional.

Diagonal abduction Movement by a limb through a diagonal plane directly across and away from the midline of the body.

Diagonal adduction Movement by a limb through a diagonal plane toward and across the midline of the body.

Diaphragm A dome-shaped sheet of muscle attached to the thoracic wall that separates the lungs and thoracic cavity from the abdominal cavity. As the chest cavity enlarges, the diaphragm moves downward and creates a vacuum that allows air to flow into the lungs. As the chest contracts and the diaphragm relaxes, it arches upward, helping air to flow out of the lungs.

Diarthrosis A freely movable synovial joint.

Digestion The mechanical and chemical breakdown of food from its complex form into simple molecules.

Disease An abnormality in functions of the body especially when the abnormality threatens well-being.

Disharmony Distortions in health that result when the functions or systems are neither balanced nor working at their optimum. In Chinese medicine, disharmony can be created by the Six Pernicious Influences or the Seven Emotions.

Disk herniation A pathologic condition that occurs when there is a rupture of the fibrocartilage that surrounds the intervertebral disk, releasing the nucleus pulposus that cushions the vertebrae above and below. The resultant pressure on spinal nerve roots may cause pain and damage the surrounding nerves.

Dopamine A catecholamine found in the brain and autonomic system. Generally a stimulant, it is involved in emotions/moods and in regulating motor control and the executive functioning of the brain.

Dorsiflexion (dorsal flexion) Movement of the ankle that results in the top of the foot moving toward the anterior tibia.

Dynamic force Force applied to an object that produces movement in or of the object.

Eccentric contraction The action of an antagonist where a muscle lengthens while under tension and changes in tension to control the descent of the resistance. Eccentric contractions may be thought of as controlling movement against gravity or resistance and are described as negative contractions.

Eccrine A type of sweat gland that releases a watery fluid known as sweat, which cools the body and provides minor elimination of metabolic waste.

Edema The accumulation of abnormal amounts of fluid in tissue spaces.

Efferent Away from a center or point of reference.

Efferent nerves (motor nerves) Nerves that link the central nervous system to the effectors outside the CNS and transmit motor impulses.

Effort The force applied to overcome resistance.

Elastic fibers Connective tissue fibers that are extensible and elastic. They are made of a protein called *elastin,* which returns to its original length after being stretched.

Elasticity The ability of a muscle to recoil and resume its original resting length after being stretched.

Elastin A fibrous tissue that has elastic properties and allows flexibility of connective tissue structures.

Elevation Upward or superior movement.

Elimination (egestion) Removal and release of solid waste products from food that cannot be digested or absorbed.

Endocrine gland A ductless gland that secretes hormones directly into the bloodstream.

Endorphins Peptide hormones that mainly work like morphine to suppress pain. They influence mood, producing a mild euphoric feeling such as is seen in runner's high.

Endoskeleton The bony support structure found inside the human body; it accommodates growth.

Endosteum A thin membrane of connective tissue that lines the marrow cavity of a bone.

Energy The capacity to do work.

Entrainment A coordination or synchronization to a rhythm, especially when a person responds to certain patterns by moving in a coordinated manner to those patterns.

Epicondyle A bony projection above a condyle.

Epidermis The outer, or top, layer of skin, which is made up of sublayers, called *strata.* The epidermis contains no nerves or blood vessels.

Epinephrine A catecholamine released by the nervous system and involved in "fight-or-flight" responses such as dilatation of blood vessels to the skeletal muscles. It is classified as a hormone when secreted by the adrenal gland.

Epithelial tissues A specialized group of tissues that cover and protect the surface of the body and its parts, line body cavities, and form glands. Epithelial tissue usually is found in areas that move substances into and out of the body during secretion, absorption, and excretion.

Erythrocytes Red blood cells that contain hemoglobin and function to transport oxygen to the cells and carbon dioxide away from the cells.

Etiology The study of the factors involved in the development of disease, including the nature of the disease and the susceptibility of the person.

Eversion Movement of the sole of the foot outward away from the midline.

Excitability The ability of a muscle to receive and respond to a stimulus.

Exocrine gland A gland that secretes its hormones through ducts directly into specific areas. It is part of the endocrine system.

Extensibility The ability of a muscle to be stretched or extended.

Extension A movement that increases the angle between two bones, usually moving the body part back toward the anatomical position.

External respiration The exchange of oxygen and carbon dioxide between the lungs and the bloodstream.

External rotation Rotary movement around the longitudinal axis of a bone away from the midline of the body. Also known as rotation laterally, outward rotation, and lateral rotation.

Facet A smooth, flat surface on a bone.

Feedback loop A self-regulating control system in the body that receives information, integrates that information, and provides a response to maintian homeostasis. Negative feedback reverses the original stimulus, whereas positive feedback enhances and maintains the stimulus.

Fibrocartilage A connective tissue that permits little motion in joints and structures. It is found in such places as the intervertebral disks and forms our ears.

Fibromyalgia A syndrome with symptoms of widespread pain or aching, persistent fatigue, generalized morning stiffness, nonrestorative sleep, and multiple tender points. A disrupted sleep pattern, coupled with the dysfunction of myofascial repair mechanisms seems to be a factor.

Fibrous joint An articulation where fibrous tissue connects bone directly to bone.

Fixator One of the stabilizing muscles surrounding a joint or body part that contract to fixate, or stabilize, the area, enabling another limb or body segment to exert force and move.

Flaccid Term used to describe a muscle with decreased or absent tone.

Flexion A movement that decreases the angle between two bones as it moves the body part out of the anatomic position.

Fontanels Areas of the skull of an infant in which the bone formation is incomplete. The fontanels allow for compression of the skull as the infant travels through the birth canal and expansion as the brain grows.

Foramen An opening in a bone, such as the foramen magnum of the skull.

Force Any push or pull on an object in an attempt to affect motion or shape.

Fossa A depression in the surface or at the end of a bone.

Free nerve endings Sensory receptors that detect itch and tickle sensations.

Frontal (coronal) plane A vertical plane that divides the body into anterior and posterior (front and back) parts.

Gait The rhythmic and alternating motions of the legs, trunk, and arms resulting in the propulsion of the body.

Gait cycle Subdivided into the stance phase and swing phase, this cycle begins when the heel of one foot strikes the floor and continues until the same heel strikes the floor again.

Gallbladder A small 3- to 4-inch sac that stores and concentrates bile.

Ganglion Cystic, round, usually nontender swellings located along tendon sheaths or joint capsules.

General-adaptation syndrome (GAS) The method the body uses to mobilize different defense mechanisms when threatened by actual or perceived harmful stimuli.

Gestation The period of fetal growth from conception until birth.

Gibbus An angular deformity of a collapsed vertebra. Causes include metastatic cancer and tuberculosis of the spine.

Gliding joints Known also as synovial plane, the joints that allow only a gliding motion in various planes.

Grey matter Unmyelinated nervous tissue, particularly that found in the CNS.

Gross anatomy The study of body structures visible to the naked eye.

Half-life The amount of time required for half of a hormone to be eliminated from the bloodstream.

Health A condition of homeostasis resulting in a state of physical, emotional, social, and spiritual well-being.

Heart rate The number of cardiac cycles in one minute. In the average, healthy person, that works out to be 60 to 70 cycles or beats per minute.

Heart sounds The two main sounds resulting from the closure of the valves. Murmurs are extra sounds, such as those resulting from faulty valves.

Heart The pump of the cardiovascular system; it is hollow, cone-shaped, and about the size of a fist and is located in the mediastinum of the thoracic cavity. The myocardium is the heart muscle itself, the endocardium is the thin inner lining, and the epicardium is the outer membrane.

Heart valves Four sets of valves that keep the blood flowing in the correct direction through the heart.

Hemoglobin The oxygen-carrying, red-pigment molecule in the blood.

Hernia Weakness in a muscle or structure that allows for protrusion of a muscle, organ, or structure through the resulting opening.

Herpes simplex A DNA virus that causes painful blisters and small ulcers in and around the mouth, and on the genital area.

Hinge joint Allows flexion and extension movement in one direction, changing the angle of the bones at the joint, like a door hinge.

Histamine A neurotransmitter that is considered a stimulant. It is released by the mast cells as part of the inflammatory process and can cause itching.

Homeostasis The relatively constant state of the body's internal environment, which is maintained by adaptive responses. Specific control and feedback mechanisms are responsible for adjusting body systems to maintain this state.

Horizontal abduction Movement of the humerus in the horizontal plane away from the midline of the body. Also known as the horizontal extension or transverse abduction.

Horizontal adduction Movement of the humerus in the horizontal plane toward the midline of the body. Also known as horizontal flexion or transverse adduction.

Hyaline cartilage The thin covering of articular connective tissue on the ends of the bones in freely movable joints in the adult skeleton. It forms a smooth resilient, low-friction surface for the articulation of one bone with another, distributes force, and helps to absorb some of the pressure imposed on the joint surface.

Hyperalgesia An increased sensitivity to pain.

Hyperextension A movement that takes the area further in the direction of the extension, further out of anatomic position.

Hypermobility The range of motion of a joint is more than would normally be permitted by the structure. It results in instability.

Hyperplasia An uncontrolled increase in the number of cells of a body part.

Hypersecretion The excessive release of a hormone.

Hypertension An increase in both systolic and diastolic pressure.

Hypertrophy An increase in the size of a cell, which results in an increase in the size of a body part or organ.

Hyperventilation Abnormally deep or rapid breathing in excess of physical demands. It is a functional syndrome where all the parts are working effectively; therefore a pathologic condition does not exist. Instead, the breathing pattern is inappropriate for the situation, resulting in confused signals to the CNS, which sets up a whole chain of events.

Hyperventilation syndrome A complex set of behaviors that leads to overbreathing without a pathologic condition present. It results in restricted range of motion.

Hypomobility The range of motion of a joint is less than what would normally be permitted by the structure.

Hyposecretion The insufficient release of a hormone.

Hypotension A decrease in systolic and diastolic pressures. It is an important manifestation of shock, which causes inadequate blood supply to vital organs.

Immunity Resistance to disease, which is provided by the body through specific or nonspecific immunity. The immune system is a functional system, rather than an organ system in the anatomic sense. The most important immune cells are the lymphocytes and the macrophages. The key to immunity is the body's ability to distinguish self from nonself.

Incontinence The inability to control urination or defecation, most often due to weak pelvic floor muscles or nerve damage.

Inertia The reluctance of matter to change its state of motion.

Inflammation A protective response of the tissues to irritation or injury that may be chronic or acute. There are four primary signs: redness, heat, swelling, and pain.

Inflammatory response A sequence of events that involves chemical and cellular activation that destroys pathogens and aids in repairing tissues.

Ingestion Taking food into the mouth.

Insertion The distal attachment of a muscle; the part of a muscle that attaches farthest from the midline, or center, of the body.

Integument The skin and its appendages: hair, sebaceous and sweat glands, nails, and breasts.

Internal respiration The exchange of gases between the tissues and blood.

Internal rotation Medial rotary movement of a bone. Also known as rotation medially, inward rotation, and medial rotation.

Interphase The period during which a cell grows and carries on its activities.

Intractable pain The continuation of chronic pain without active disease present or when chronic pain persists even with treatment provided.

Inversion Movement of the sole of the foot inward toward the midline.

Ischemia A temporary deficiency or decreased supply of blood to a tissue.

Isometric contraction The action of the prime mover that occurs when tension develops within the muscle but no appreciable change occurs in the joint angle or the length of the muscle. Movement does not occur.

Isotonic contraction The action of the prime mover that occurs when tension is developed in the muscle while it either shortens or lengthens.

Joint capsule A connective tissue structure that indirectly connects the bony components of a joint.

Joint play The involuntary movement that occurs between articular surfaces that are separate from the range of motion of a joint produced by muscles. It is an essential component of joint motion and must occur for there to be normal functioning of the joint.

Keratin The fibrous protein produced in the epidermis that protects our skin and makes it waterproof.

Kyphosis A condition is which there is an exaggeration of the thoracic curve.

Lateral flexion (side bending) Movement of the head and/or trunk laterally away from the midline. Abduction of the spine.

Lateral recumbent (sidelying) Lying horizontally on either the right or left side.

Leukocytes White blood cells that protect the body from pathogens and remove dead cells and substances.

Lever A solid mass, such as a crowbar or a person's arm, that rotates around a fixed point called the *fulcrum*. The rotation is produced by a force applied to a lever at some distance from the fulcrum.

Ligaments Dense bundles of parallel connective tissue fibers, primarily collagen, that connect bones and strengthen and stabilize the joint.

Lipids Fats and oils.

List A lateral tilt of the spine.

Locomotion Moving from one place to another. Walking.

Loose packed position The position of a synovial joint where the joint capsule is most lax. Joints tend to assume this position when there is inflammation to accommodate the increased volume of synovial fluid.

Lordosis A condition in which there is an exaggeration of the normal lumbar curve.

Lower respiratory tract The larynx, trachea, bronchi, and alveoli.

Lungs The primary organs of respiration, they are soft, spongy, highly vascular structures separated into the left and right lungs by the mediastinum. Each lung is separated into lobes. The right lung has three lobes: an upper, middle, and lower; the left two lobes: an upper and lower.

Lymph A clear interstitial tissue fluid that bathes the cells. Lymph contains lymphocytes that provide immune response, it returns plasma proteins that have leaked out through capillary walls, and it transports fats from the gastrointestinal system to the bloodstream.

Lymph nodes Small, round structures distributed along the network of lymph vessels that provide a filtering system for removing waste products and transferring them to the bloodstream for removal to the spleen, intestines, and kidneys for detoxification. Lymph nodes are centers for lymphocyte production. Their main function is to prevent bacteria and viruses from gaining access to the bloodstream. Generally clustered at the joints for assistance in pumping when the joint moves, they are especially numerous in the axillae, groin, and neck and along certain blood vessels of the pelvic, abdominal, and thoracic cavities.

Matrix The basic substance between the cells of a tissue. Matrix is composed of amorphous ground substance consisting of molecules that expand when water molecules and electrolytes bind to them. Up to 90% of connective tissue is ground substance. Fibers make up the other component of matrix.

Maximal stimulus The point at which all motor units of a muscle have been recruited and the muscle is unable to increase in strength.

Mechanical receptors Sensory receptors that detect changes in pressure, movement, temperature, or other mechanical forces.

Meiosis A type of cell division in which a cell divides its chromosomes in half, forming two reproductive cells.

Melanin The pigment that colors our skin and works as a natural sunscreen to protect us from UV rays by darkening our skin.

Membrane A thin, sheetlike layer of tissue that covers a cell, an organ, or some other structure; that lines a tube or a cavity; or that divides or separates one part from another.

Metabolism Chemical processes in the body that convert food and oxygen into energy to support growth, distribution of nutrients, and elimination of waste.

Microorganisms Small life forms that may be damaging to the body or interfere with its function.

Micturition The clinical term for urination or voiding.

Mitosis The period of cell division in which the cell reproduces its DNA and divides into two identical daughter cells.

Mixed nerves Nerves that contain both sensory and motor axons.

Mole Also known as a nevus, it is a benign pigmented skin growth formed of melanocytes.

Molecule A combination of two or more atoms. A molecule is the smallest portion of a substance that can exist separately without losing the physical and chemical properties of that substance.

Motor point The location where the motor neuron enters the muscle and where a visible contraction can be elicited with a minimal amount of stimulation. Motor points are most often located in the belly of the muscle.

Motor unit All the muscle fibers innervated by a single motor neuron.

Muscle tissue A specialized form of tissue that contracts and shortens to provide movement, maintain posture, and produce heat.

Myelin A white, fatty, insulating substance formed by the Schwann cells that surrounds some axons. Also produced in the central nervous system by oligodendrocytes.

Myotome A skeletal muscle or group of skeletal muscles that receives motor axons from a particular spinal nerve.

Negative feedback system A control mechanism that provides a stimulus to decrease a function like a fire alarm that causes a series of reactions that work to reduce the fire.

Neoplasm The abnormal growth of new tissue. Also called a *tumor,* it may be benign or malignant.

Nerve A bundle of axons or dendrites, or both.

Nervous tissue A specialized tissue that coordinates and regulates body activity. It can develop more excitability and conductivity than other types of tissue.

Neurilemma The outer cell membrane of a Schwann cell that is essential in the regeneration of injured axons.

Neuroglia Specialized connective tissue cells that support, protect, and hold neurons together.

Neurons Nerve cells that conduct impulses.

Neurotransmitters Chemical compounds that generate action potentials when released in the synapses from presynaptic cells.

Nociceptors Sensory receptors that detect painful or intense stimuli.

Norepinephrine A catecholamine primarily involved in emotional responses. It is found in the CNS and the sympathetic division of the ANS and causes constriction of blood vessels in the skeletal muscles.

Nucleic acid The two types of nucleic acid are deoxyribonucleic acid (DNA) and ribonucleic acid (RNA).

Nutrition The use of food for growth and maintenance of the body.

Open kinematic chain A position in which the ends of the limbs or parts of the body are free to move without causing motion at another joint.

Opposition Movement of the thumb across the palmar aspect to make contact with the fingers.

Organelles The basic components of a cell that perform specific functions within the cell.

Origin The proximal attachment of a muscle; the part that attaches closest to the midline (center) of the body. The least movable part of a muscle.

Osteokinematics The movement of bones as opposed to the movement of articular surfaces; also known as range of motion.

Osteoporosis A disorder of the bone in which there is a lack of calcium and other minerals and a decrease in bone protein, leaving the bones soft, fragile, and more likely to break.

Oxygen debt The extra amount of oxygen that must be taken in to convert lactic acid to glucose or glycogen.

Pain An unpleasant sensation. It is a complex, private experience with physiologic, psychologic, and social aspects. Because it is subjective, it is often difficult to explain or describe.

Parasympathetic nervous system The energy conservation and restorative system associated with what is commonly called the *relaxation response*.

Pathogenesis The development of a disease.

Pathogens Microorganisms that are capable of producing disease.

Pathologic range of motion The amount of motion at a joint that either fails to reach the normal physiologic range or exceeds normal anatomic limits of motion of that joint.

Pathology The study of disease as it is observed in the structure and function of the body.

Pericardium A double membranous, serous sac surrounding the heart. The pericardium secretes a lubricating fluid to prevent friction from the movement of the heart.

Periosteum The thin membrane of connective tissue that covers bones except at articulations.

Peripheral nervous system (PNS) The system of somatic and autonomic neurons outside the central nervous system. The PNS comprises the afferent (sensory) division and the efferent (motor) division.

Peristalsis Rhythmic contraction of smooth muscles that propel products of digestion along the tract from the esophagus to the anus.

Peritoneum The mucous membrane that lines the abdominal cavity to prevent friction from the organs.

Phantom pain A form of pain or other sensation experienced in the missing extremity after a limb amputation.

Pharynx The throat.

Physiology The study of the processes and functions of the body involved in supporting life.

Physiologic range of motion The amount of motion available to a joint determined by the nervous system from information provided by joint sensory receptors. This information usually prevents a joint from being positioned where injury could occur.

Physiology The study of the processes and functions of the body involved in supporting life.

Piezoelectric The quality of bones that allows them to deform slightly and vibrate when electrical currents pass through them. Bone formation patterns follow lines of stress load directed by the piezoelectric currents.

Pivot joint Allows rotation around the length of the bone.

Plantar flexion Actually an extension movement of the ankle that results in the foot and/or toes moving away from the body.

Plasma A thick, straw-colored fluid that makes up about 55% of the blood.

Plastic range The range of movement of connective tissue when it is taken beyond the elastic limits. In this range, the tissue is permanently deformed and unable to return to its original state.

Plexus A network of intertwining nerves that innervates a particular region of the body.

Poliomyelitis Also known as polio, it is a viral infection that affects the nerves that control skeletal muscle movement.

Posterior pelvic rotation Posterior movement of the upper pelvis; the iliac crest tilts backward in a sagittal plane.

Prefix A word element added to the beginning of a root to change the meaning of the word.

Pressure The amount of force on a specific area.

Process Any prominent bony growth that projects out from the bone.

Pronation Internal rotary movement of the radius on the ulna that results in the hand moving from the palm-up to the palm-down position.

Prone Lying horizontal with the face down.

Proprioceptors Sensory receptors that provide the body with information about position, movement, muscle tension, joint activity, and equilibrium.

Protein A substance formed from amino acids.

Protraction Forward movement remaining in a horizontal plane.

Psoriasis A common, chronic, skin disease characterized by reddened skin that is covered by dry, silvery scales. It is most often found on the scalp, elbows, knees, back, or buttocks.

Pulmonary trunk The large artery that carries blood to lungs to release carbon dioxide and take in oxygen.

Pulmonary veins One of four veins from the lungs that bring oxygen-rich blood to the left atrium.

Qi Also known as *chi*; it refers to the life force.

Reciprocal inhibition Stimulation of an antagonist muscle to inhibit action in the prime mover.

Reciprocal innervation The circuitry of neurons that allows reciprocal inhibition to take place. It can be used therapeutically to assist in muscle relaxation.

Reduction Return of the spinal column to the anatomic position from lateral flexion. Adduction of the spine.

Referred pain Pain felt in a surface area far from the stimulated organ.

Reflex An automatic, involuntary reaction to a stimulus.

Reflex arc The pathway that a nerve impulse follows in a reflex action.

Regional anatomy The study of the structures of a particular area of the body.

Remission A reversal of signs and symptoms in chronic disease, it can be a temporary or permanent condition.

Respiration The movement of air in and out of the lungs, the exchange of oxygen and carbon dioxide between the lungs and blood, and the exchange between blood and body tissues.

Respiratory rate The number of breaths in one minute.

Reticular fibers Delicate, connective tissue fibers that occur in networks and support small structures, such as capillaries, nerve fibers, and the basement membrane. Reticular fibers are made of a specialized type of collagen called *reticulin*.

Retraction Backward movement in a horizontal plane.

Root A word element that contains the basic meaning of the word.

Rotation Partial turning or pivoting in an arc around a central axis.

Rupture The tearing and/or disruption of connective tissue fibers that takes place when they exceed the limits of the plastic range.

Saddle joint Both convex in one plane and concave in the other with the surface fit together like a rider on a saddle.

Schwann cell A specialized cell that forms myelin.

Scoliosis A lateral curvature of the spine.

Sebaceous glands The oil glands found in the skin.

Sebum The oily substance secreted by sebaceous glands that prevents dehydration, softens skin and hair, and slows the growth of bacteria.

Serotonin A neurotransmitter that works primarily as an inhibitor in the CNS. It is synthesized into melatonin and affects our sleep and moods.

Sesamoid bones Round bones that often are embedded in tendons and joint capsules.

The Seven Emotions The Oriental concept that joy, anger, fear, fright, sadness, worry, and grief are emotional responses that may trigger disharmony in the body, mind, or spirit under certain conditions.

Shock An inadequate blood supply to vital organs, causing reduced function in these organs.

Signs Objective changes that can be seen or measured by someone other than the client or patient.

Sinus Four groups of air-filled spaces that open into the internal nose. They are located in the frontal, ethmoid, sphenoid, and maxillary bones of the skull. Sinuses are lined with mucosa and function to lighten the weight of the skull, making it easier to hold the head up and help in the production of sound.

The Six Pernicious Influences The Oriental concept that heat, cold, wind, dampness, dryness, and summer heat, which are natural climate changes, may induce disease under certain conditions.

Skeletal muscle fibers Large, cross-striated cells that are connected to the skeleton and under voluntary control of the nervous system.

Smooth muscle fibers Muscle fibers that are neither striated nor voluntary. These muscle cells help regulate blood flow through the cardiovascular system, propel food through the gut, and squeeze secretions from glands.

SOAP notes Refers to *s*ubjective, *o*bjective, *a*nalysis assessment, and *p*lan, the four parts of the written account of the record keeping.

Somatic nervous system A system of nerves that keeps the body in balance with its external environment by transmitting impulses between the CNS, the skeletal muscles, and the skin.

Somatic pain Pain that arises from the body as opposed to the viscera. Superficial somatic pain comes from the stimulation of receptors in the skin, whereas deep somatic pain arises from stimulation of receptors in skeletal muscles, joints, tendons, and fascia.

Spastic Term used to describe a muscle with excessive tone.

Spinal cord Portion of the CNS that exits the skull into the vertebral column. The two major functions of the spinal cord are to conduct nerve impulses and to be a center for spinal reflexes.

Spinal nerves Thirty-one pairs of mixed nerves, originating in the spinal cord and emerging from the vertebral column, that make sensation and movement possible.

Spongy (cancellous) bone The lighter weight portion of bone made up of trabeculae.

Stabilizer A force or an object that helps maintain a position. Stabilization is essential to accurately assess movement patterns.

Static force Force applied to an object in such a way that it does not produce movement.

Stress Any external or internal stimulus that requires a change or response to prevent an imbalance in the internal environment of the body, mind, or emotions. It may be any activity that makes demands on mental and emotional resources. Some responses to stress may stimulate neurons of the hypothalamus to release corticotropin-releasing hormones, or CRH.

Subacute Diseases with characteristics between acute and chronic.

Suffix A word element added to the end of a root to change the meaning of the word.

Superficial fascia The subcutaneous tissue that composes the third layer of skin; it consists of loose connective tissue and contains fat or adipose tissue.

Supination External rotary movement of the radius on the ulna that results in the hand moving from the palm-down to the palm-up position.

Supine Lying horizontal with the face up.

Surface anatomy The study of internal organs and structures as they can be recognized and related to external features.

Suture A synarthrotic joint in which two bony components are united by a thin layer of dense fibrous tissue.

Sweat glands The sudoriferous glands in the skin; they are classified as either apocrine or eccrine on the basis of their location and structure.

Sympathetic nervous system The part of the autonomic nervous system that provides for most of our active function; when the body is under stress, the sympathetic nervous system predominates with fight-or-flight responses.

Symphysis A cartilaginous joint in which the two bony components are directly joined by fibrocartilage in the form of a disk or plate.

Symptoms The subjective changes noticed or felt only by the client or patient.

Synapse Spaces between neurons or between a neuron and an effector organ.

Synarthrosis A limited movement, nonsynovial joint.

Synchondrosis A joint in which the material used for connecting the two components is hyaline growth cartilage.

Syndesmosis A fibrous joint in which two bony components are joined directly by a ligament, cord, or aponeurotic membrane.

Syndrome A group of different signs and symptoms that identify a pathologic condition, especially when they have a common cause.

Synergist A muscle that aids or assists the action of the agonist but is not primarily responsible for the action; also known as a guiding muscle.

Synovial fluid A thick, colorless, lubricating fluid that is secreted by the membrane of the joint cavity.

Synovial joint A freely moving joint allowing motion in one or more planes of action.

Systemic anatomy The study of the structure of a particular body system.

Tao An ancient philosophic concept that represents the whole and its parts as one and the same.

Tendinitis Inflammation of a tendon.

Tenosynovitis Inflammation of a tendon sheath.

Thermal receptors Sensory receptors that detect changes in temperature.

Thorax Also known as the chest cavity, it is the upper region of the torso enclosed by the sternum, ribs, and thoracic vertebrae. It contains the lungs, heart, and great vessels.

Threshold stimulus The stimulus at which the first observable muscle contraction occurs.

Tissue A group of similar cells combined to perform a common function.

Tone A state of slight contraction in all skeletal muscles that enables the muscle to respond to stimulation.

Trabeculae An Irregular meshing of small, bony plates that makes up spongy bone; its spaces are filled with red marrow.

Tracts Collections of nerve fibers in the brain and spinal cord with a common function.

Trigger points "A myofascial trigger point is a hyperirritable locus within a taut band of skeletal muscle, located in the muscular tissue and/or its associated fascia. The spot is painful on compression and can evoke characteristic referred pain and autonomic phenomena." (Dr. Janet Travell)

Trochanter One of two large bony processes found only on the femur.

Tropic (or trophic) hormones Hormones produced by the endocrine glands that affect other endocrine glands.

Tubercle A small, rounded process on a bone.

Tuberosity A large rounded protuberance on a bone.

Tumor Also referred to as a *neoplasm*, a tumor is a growth of new tissues that may be benign (nonthreatening or noncancerous) or malignant (cancerous).

Ulcer A round open sore of the skin or mucous membrane.

Universal precautions Safety measures established in 1987 by the Centers for Disease Control and Prevention (CDC); they were instituted to prevent the spread of bacterial and viral infections by setting up specific methods of dealing with human fluids and waste products. Universal precautions protect both client and practitioner from pathogens.

Upper respiratory tract The nasal cavity and all its structures and the pharynx.

Upward rotation Scapular motion that turns the glenoid fossa upward and moves the inferior angle superiorly and laterally away from the spinal column.

Veins Blood vessels that collect blood from the capillaries and transport it back to the heart; 75% of the blood of the body is in the venous system. Larger veins often contain a set of valves, which ensures that blood flows in the correct direction to the heart and also prevents backflow.

Vena cava One of two large arteries that return poorly oxygenated blood to the right atrium of the heart.

Ventricles The two large, lower chambers of the heart; they are thick-walled and separated by a thick interventricular septum.

Venules The smallest veins.

Visceral pain Pain that is a result of the stimulation of receptors or an abnormal condition in the viscera (internal organs).

Viscoelasticity The combination of resistance offered by a fluid to a change of form and the ability of material to return to its original state after deformation. This term is used to describe connective tissue.

Whiplash An injury to the soft tissues of the neck caused by sudden hyperextension and/or flexion of the neck.

Word elements The parts of a word; the prefix, root, and suffix.

Yin/yang Yin and yang are terms used to describe polar relationships. Yin/yang refers to the dynamic balance between opposing forces and the continual process of creation and destruction. Yin/yang reflects the natural order and duality of the whole universe and everything in it, including the individual.

Works Consulted

Advice for the patient: drug information in lay language, vol 2, Rockfort, Maryland, 1990, United States Pharmaceutical Convention.

Agur AMR: *Grant's atlas of anatomy*, ed 9, Baltimore, 1991, Williams & Wilkins.

Basmajian JV, DeLuca CJ: *Muscles alive: their functions revealed by electromyography*, ed 5, Baltimore, 1985, Williams & Wilkins.

Basmajian JV, Nyberg R: *Rational manual therapies*, Baltimore, 1993, Williams & Wilkins.

Bates B: *A guide to physical examination and history taking*, ed 6, Philadelphia, 1995, Lippincott-Raven.

Best ML et al, editors: *The physician's assistant compendium of drug therapy*, New Jersey, 1994, Compendium.

Born BA: *An introduction to practical pathology for the myomassologist*, ed 7, Southfield, Mich, 1993.

Brennan R: *The Alexander technique workbook*, Rockport, Massachusetts, 1992, Element.

Bullock BL, Rosendahl PP: *Pathophysiology: adaptations and alterations in function*, ed 3, Philadelphia, 1992, JB Lippincott.

Burkitt GH, Young B, Heath J: *Wheater's functional histology*, ed 3, New York, 1993, Churchill Livingstone.

Butler DS: *Mobilization of the nervous system*, Melbourne, 1991, Churchill Livingstone.

Cailliet R: *Foot and ankle pain*, ed 3, Philadelphia, 1997, FA Davis.

Cailliet R: *Hand pain and impairment*, ed 4, Philadelphia, 1994, FA Davis.

Cailliet R: *Knee pain and disability*, ed 3, Philadelphia, 1992, FA Davis.

Cailliet R: *Low back pain syndrome*, ed 5, Philadelphia, 1995, FA Davis.

Cailliet R: *Neck and arm pain*, ed 3, Philadelphia, 1991, FA Davis.

Cailliet R: *Shoulder pain*, ed 3, Philadelphia, 1991, FA Davis.

Cailliet R: *Soft tissue pain and disability*, Philadelphia, 1996, FA Davis.

Castleman M: *Nature's cures*, Emmaus, Penn., 1996, Rodale Press.

Chaitow L: *Journal of bodywork and movement therapies*, New York, 1996, Churchill Livingstone.

Chaitow L: *Modern neuromuscular techniques*, New York, 1996, Churchill Livingstone.

Chaitow L: *Muscle energy techniques*, New York, 1996, Churchill Livingstone.

Chaitow L: *The book of natural pain relief*, New York, 1995, Harper Paperbacks.

Chaitow L: *The acupuncture treatment of pain*, Rochester, Vt, 1990, Healing Arts Press.

Chopra D: *Restful sleep*, New York, 1994, Crowne.

Clayton BD, Stock YN: *Basic pharmacology for nurses*, ed 11, St Louis, 1996, Mosby.

Colton H: *Touch therapy*, New York, 1983, Kensington.

Cooley C: *The book*, Scottsdale, Ariz, 1992, Big Guy Books!

Cowan P: *American Chronic Pain Association: staying well: advanced pain management for ACPA members*, 1994, California Dental Association.

Crawford AM: *The herbal menopause book*, Freedom, Calif, 1996, Crossing Press.

Daulby M, Mathison C: *Guide to spiritual healing*, London, 1996, Brockhampton Press.

Degenhardt B, Kuchera M: Update of osteopathic medical concepts and the lymphatic system, *J Am Osteopath Assoc* 96(2):97, 1996.

Di Lima SN, Painter SJ, Johns LT, editors: *Orthopaedic patient education resource manual*, Gaithersburg, Maryland, 1995, Aspen.

Doctor's little black bag of remedies and cures, vol 1, 1997, Boardroom.

Dossey L: *Space, time and medicine*, Boston, 1982, Random House.

Dvorak J, Vaclav D: *Medical checklists: manual medicine*, New York, 1991, Thieme Medical Publishers.

Editors of Consumers Guide: *Prescription drugs*, Lincolnwood, Ill, 1995, Publications International.

Falvo DR: *Medical and psychosocial aspects of chronic illness and disability*, Gaithersburg, Maryland, 1991, Aspen.

Garofano JS: *Therapeutic massage and bodywork*, Stamford, Conn, 1997, Appleton & Lange.

Golan R: *Optimal wellness*, New York, 1995, Ballantine Books.

Greenman PE: *Principles of manual medicine*, ed 2, Baltimore, 1996, Williams & Wilkins.

Gunn C: *Bones and joints*, ed 3, New York, 1996, Churchill Livingstone.

Gurevich D: *Russian medical massage*, Flint, Mich, 1992.

Heinerman J: *Healing powers of herbs*, Boca Raton, Florida, 1995, Globe Communications.

Hislop HJ, Montgomery J: *Daniel and Worthingham's muscle testing: techniques of manual examination*, ed 6, Philadelphia, 1995, WB Saunders.

Hoffman CJ: *HEV 370 nutrition*, ed 2, Michigan, 1996.

Hooper J, Teresi D: *The three pound universe*, New York, 1986, Dell.

Isselbacher KJ et al: *Harrison's principles of internal medicine*, ed 13, New York, 1994, McGraw-Hill.

Jacobs PH, Anhalt TS: *Handbook of skin clues of systemic diseases*, ed 2, Philadelphia, 1992, Lea & Febiger.

Kapit W, Rober I, Macey EM: *The physiology coloring book,* New York, 1987, HarperCollins.

Keen JH, Baird MS, Allen JH: *Mosby's critical care and emergency drug reference,* ed 2, St Louis, 1996, Mosby.

Keirsey D, Bates M: *Please understand me: temperament in leading,* Del Mar, Calif, 1996, Prometheus Nemesis.

Keirsey D, Bates M: *Please understand me: character and temperament types,* ed 2, Del Mar, Calif, 1984, Prometheus Nemesis.

Kendall F: *Florence Kendall's muscle testing video library,* vols 1-5, Baltimore, Williams & Wilkins (no date).

Kisner C, Colby LA: *Therapeutic exercise: foundations and techniques,* ed 3, Philadelphia, 1996, FA Davis.

Leadbeater CW: *The chakras,* Wheaton, Ill., 1927, Theosophical Publishing House.

Lee D: *Manual therapy for the thorax: a biomechanical approach,* 1994, British Columbia.

Leflet DH: *HEMME approach to modalities,* Bonifay, Fla, 1996, Hemme Approach Publications.

Leflet DH: *HEMME approach to soft tissue therapy,* Bonifay, Fla, 1992, HEMME Approach Publications.

Lillis CA: *A concise introduction to medical terminology,* ed 4, Stamford, Conn, 1997, Appleton & Lange.

Lindsay DT: *Functional human anatomy,* St Louis, 1996, Mosby.

Macnab I, McCulloch J: *Neck ache and shoulder pain,* Baltimore, 1994, Williams & Wilkins.

Lowe WW: *Functional assessment in massage therapy,* ed 2, Corvallis, Oregon, 1995, Pacific Orthopedic Massage.

Maciocia G *The foundations of Chinese medicine,* New York, 1994, Churchill Livingstone.

Macnab I, McCulloch J: *Neck ache and shoulder pain,* Baltimore, 1994, Williams & Wilkins

Marieb EN: *Human anatomy and physiology,* ed 4, Redwood City, Calif, 1997, Benjamin/Cummings.

McCraty R, Tiller WA, Atkinson M: *Head-heart entrainment: a preliminary survey,* Institute of HeartMath, PO Box 1463, 14700 West Park Ave, Boulder Creek CA 95006   Hrtmath@netcom.com   http://www.heartmath.org/researchpapers/Head/Hart/Headheart.html

McNaught AB, Callander R: *Illustrated physiology,* ed 4, New York, 1983, Churchill Livingstone.

Memmler RL, Cohen BH, Wood DL: *The human body in health and disease,* ed 7, Philadelphia, 1992, JB Lippincott.

Mennell JM: *The musculoskeletal system: differential diagnosis from symptoms and physical signs,* Gaithersburg, Maryland, 1992, Aspen.

Millenson JR: *Mind matters: psychological medicine in holistic practice,* Seattle, 1995, Eastland Press.

Netter FH: *The CIBA collection of medical illustrations,* ed 2, New Jersey, 1992, Hennegan.

Netter FH: *The CIBA collection of medical illustrations,* New Jersey, 1991, CIBA.

Newton D: *Pathology for massage therapists,* ed 2, Portland, 1995, Simran Publications.

Nikola RJ: *Creatures of water: hydrotherapy textbook,* Salt Lake City, 1995, Europa Therapeutic.

Norkin CC, Levangie PK: *Joint structure and function,* ed 2, Philadelphia, 1992, FA Davis.

Northrup C: *Heal your symptoms naturally,* Potomac, Maryland, 1996, Phillips.

Northrup C: *Women's bodies, women's wisdom,* New York, 1994, Bantam Books.

Ornstein R, Sobel D: *The healing brain,* New York, 1987, Simon & Schuster.

Osborne-Sheets C: *Deep tissue sculpting: a technical and artistic manual for therapeutic bodywork practitioners,* Poway, California, 1990, Body Therapy Associates.

Oschman JL: What is healing energy? Part 3: Silent pulses, *Journal of Bodywork and Movement Therapies,* 1(3):179, 1997.

Perry HM III, Morley JE, Coe RM: *Aging and musculoskeletal disorders,* New York, 1993, Springer.

The 1998 physician's GenRx, ed 8, St Louis, 1998, Mosby.

Premkumar K: *Pathology A to Z: a handbook for massage therapists,* Calgary, Canada, 1996, Vanpub Books, Banker's Hall, Box No 22325, Calgary AB T2P4J1.

Schlossberg L, Zuidema GD: *The Johns Hopkins atlas of human functional anatomy,* ed 2, Baltimore, 1981, Johns Hopkins University Press.

Schneider W, Tritschler T, Spring H: *Mobility: theory and practice,* New York, 1992, Thieme Medical Publishers.

Seeley RR, Stephens TD, Tate P: *Essentials of anatomy and physiology,* ed 2, St Louis, 1996, Mosby.

Selye H: *The stress of life,* New York, 1978, McGraw-Hill.

Sieg, adams: *Illustrated essentials of musculoskeletal anatomy,* ed 3, 1996, Megabooks.

Smith LK, Weiss E, Lehmkuhl L: *Brunnstrom's clinical kinesiology,* ed 5, Philadelphia, 1996, FA Davis.

Sorrentino SA: *Mosby's textbook for nursing assistants,* ed 4, St Louis, 1996, Mosby.

Stanway A: *The new natural family doctor,* Berkeley, 1987, North Atlantic Books.

Steefel L: Treating depression: helping the body heal the mind, *Alternative and complementary therapies* Jan/Feb 1996.

Stewart J: *Clinical anatomy and pathophysiology for the health professional,* Miami, 1994, MedMaster.

Sun C: *Chinese bodywork: a complete manual of Chinese therapeutic massage,* Berkeley, Calif, 1993, Pacific View Press.

Thibodeau GA, Patton KT: *Structure and function of the body,* ed 10, 1997, Mosby.

Thibodeau GA, Patton KT: *Anatomy and physiology,* ed 3, St Louis, 1996, Mosby.

Thibodeau GA, Patton KT: *The human body in health and disease,* ed 2, St Louis, 1997, Mosby.

Thomas CL: *Taber's cyclopedic medical dictionary,* ed 16, Philadelphia, 1985, FA Davis.

Thompson GW, Floyd RT: *Manual of structural kinesiology,* ed 12, St Louis, 1994, Mosby.

Timmons BH, Ley R: *Behavioral and psychological approaches to breathing disorders,* New York, 1994, Plenum Press.

Tortora GJ, Anagnostakos NP: *Anatomy and physiological laboratory manual,* ed 4, New York, 1993, Macmillan.

Tortora GJ, Grabowski SR: *Principles of anatomy and physiology,* ed 7, New York, 1993, HarperCollins.

Trew M, Everett T: *Human movement: an introductory text,* ed 3, New York, 1997, Churchill Livingstone.

Vardaxis NJ: *Pathology for the health sciences,* New York, 1995, Churchill Livingstone.

Warfield CA: *Principles and practice of pain management,* New York, 1993, McGraw-Hill.

Warfel JH: *The head, neck, and trunk*, ed 6, Philadelphia, 1993, Lea & Febiger.

Warfel JH: *The extremities: muscles and motor points*, ed 6, Philadelphia, 1992, Lea & Febiger.

Wheater P, Burkitt G, Stevens A, et al.: *Basic histopathology*, ed 2, New York, 1993, Churchill Livingstone.

Witters W, Venturelli P, Hanson G: *Drugs and society*, ed 3, Boston, 1986, Jones & Bartlett.

Williams RW: *Basic healthcare terminology*, St Louis, 1995, Mosby.

Whitney EN, Rolfes SR: *Understanding nutrition*, ed 7, Minneapolis, 1996, West Publishers.

Yates J: *A physician's guide to therapeutic massage: its physiological effects and their application to treatment*, Vancouver, British Columbia, 1990, Massage Therapist Association of British Columbia.

Zahourek J: *Myologik an atlas of human musculature in clay*, vols 1-5, Zoologik Systems Kinesthetic Anatomy Maniken, Zahourek Stytems, Loveland, CO, 1996.

Zi N: *The art of breathing*, Glendale, Calif, 1997, Vivi.

Zukav G: *The dancing wu li masters*, New York, 1980. Bantam Books.

Recommended Reading

Anderson KN, Anderson LE, Glanze WD, editors: *Mosby's medical, nursing, and allied health dictionary*, ed 5, St Louis, 1998, Mosby.

Calais-Germain B: *Anatomy of movement*, Seattle, 1993, Eastland Press.

Chaitow L: *Palpation skills: assessment and diagnosis through touch*, New York, 1997, Churchill Livingstone.

Cohen MR: *The Chinese way to healing: many paths to wholeness*, New York, 1996, Berkley Publishing Group.

Edwards D: *Mosby's anatomy flash cards: musculature, bones, and joints*, St Louis, 1998, Mosby.

Fritz S: *Mosby's fundamentals of therapeutic massage*, St Louis, 1995, Mosby.

Hinkle CZ: *Fundamentals of anatomy and movement: a workbook and guide*, St Louis, 1997, Mosby.

Kapit W, Lawrence ME: *The anatomy coloring book*, ed 2, New York, 1993, Harper Collins.

Li D: *Acupuncture meridian theory and acupuncture points*, Beijing, San Francisco, 1990, China Books & Periodicals.

Lowe WW: *Functional assessment in massage therapy*, ed 2, Corvallis, Oregon, 1995, Pacific Orthopedic Massage.

Maciocia G: *The foundations of Chinese medicine*, New York, 1994, Churchill Livingstone.

Olson TR: *ADAM student atlas of anatomy*, Pennsylvania, 1996, Williams & Wilkins.

The 1998 physician's GenRx, ed 8, St Louis, 1998, Mosby.

Sieg, Adams: *Illustrated essentials of musculoskeletal anatomy*, ed 2, 1994, Megabooks.

Thompson DL: *Hands heal: documentation for massage therapy*, Seattle, 1993, Thompson.

Travell JG, Simons DG: *Myofascial pain and dysfunction: the trigger point manual (the lower extremities)*, Baltimore, 1992, Williams & Wilkins.

Travell JG, Simons DG: *Myofascial pain and dysfunction: the trigger point manual (upper half)*, vol 1, Baltimore, 1983, Williams & Wilkins.

Zahourek J: *Myologik an Atlas of Human Musculature in Clay*, vols 1-5, Zoologik Systems Kinesthetic Anatomy Maniken, Zahourek Stytems, Loveland, CO, 1996.

Index

Psychophysiology, 49
Pterygoid hamulus, 218
Pterygomandibular septa, 273
-ptosis, suffix, 62
Puberty
  female, 549
  male, 547
  sex hormones, 198
Pubic symphysis, 279, 548
Pubic tubercle, 279
Pubis, 232
Pubofemoral ligament, 278, 279
Pudendal nerve, 143
pulmo-, root word, 61
Pulmonary artery, 469, 517, 518
Pulmonary edema, 522
Pulmonary embolism, 522
Pulmonary infarction, 522
Pulmonary trunk, 469
Pulmonary valve, 469
Pulmonary vein, 470, 517, 518
Pulse, 474-476
Pupil, 164
Purkinje's fibers, 469
Pyelonephritis, 542
Pyloric sphincter, 529
Pylorus, 529
py(o)-, root word, 61
Pyramidal fiber, 119
Pyramidal tract, 121
Pyramidalis, 338

Q

Q angle, 436, 437
Qi, 17, 59, 84, 86
Qi Gong, 86
quadr(a,i)-, prefix, 60
Quadrants of abdomen, 72
Quadratus femoris, 364, 433
Quadratus lumborum, 335-336
Quadratus plantae, 376, 443
Quadriceps, 436, 438
Quadriceps femoris, 368-369
Quadriplegia, 122
Quantum mechanics, 93, 94
Quartz, 211
Quiet expiration, 333

R

Radial artery, 477
Radial artery pulse, 475
Radial collateral ligament, 277
Radial flexion, 267
Radial fossa, 229
Radial groove, 229

Radial head, 228
Radial nerve, 142, 143
Radial tuberosity, 277
Radiation therapy, 238
Radical mastectomy, 464
Radiocarpal wrist joint, 276
Radiohumeral joint, 275
Radioulnar joint, 275
  biomechanics, 423
  muscles, 349-353
  syndesmoses, 262
Radius, 217, 230
  elbow, 275
  syndesmoses, 262
Ramus of mandible, 218
Range of motion, 266
  anatomic, 253, 266
  biomechanical assessment, 407, 408
  combinations of rolling, sliding and spinning, 265
  joint positions and stability, 265
  knee, 436
  pathologic, 254, 266
  physiologic, 254, 266
Rapid eye movement sleep, 115
RAS; *see* Reticular activating system
Raynaud's disease, 483
Raynaud's phenomenon, 483
Raynaud's syndrome, 463
re-, prefix, 60
Reactive anxiety, 170
Reasoning, 65-67
Receptor
  baroreceptor, 30, 476
  body rhythms, 30
  chemoreceptor, 519
  histamine, 529
  homeostasis, 29
  hormone, 183
  involuntary reflexes, 145
  joint, 263, 312
  ligament, 148
  locomotion, 400-401
  mechanoreceptor, 137, 147, 312
  neuropeptides, 497
  pain, 39
  pressure, 147
  sensory
    hand, 457
    lung, 152
    peripheral nervous system, 145-149
    smooth muscle, 152
  smell, 166-167
  stretch, 476
  thermal, 137, 147
  touch, 147
  vibrations and motion, 163